The Healthy Diets Collection

The Newest Guides on The Ketogenic Diet, The Frugal Renal Diet, Plant-Based Diet, Meal Prep for Weight Loss and The Wholesome Optavia Diet.
Discover How to Exploit These Incredible Diets for a Prograssive Weight Loss

THE KETO DIET
[3 IN 1]

The Complete Guide to Understand the Basic Principles to Get Into Ketosis. 315+Ketogenic Recipes to Induce Your Body Into a Progressive Loss of Weight

Amanda Davis

Introduction

Congratulations on purchasing *Keto Diet for Beginners: An Ultimate Keto Diet Guide for Beginners Code to Use Keto Aliments, Alkaline Plant and Vegetable to Eliminate Obesity and Weight Loss Fast Improve Your Health Eating Healthy Food* and thank you for doing so.

The following chapters will discuss everything a beginner would need to know concerning the Keto Diet, and the impact such a diet would have on an individual's desire to lose weight and live a healthy life.

The first chapter is an introduction to the Keto diet. This chapter begins with a definition and an explanation of the keto diet. The chapter goes into detail to explain the science behind the diet, the advantages an individual committing to the diet will enjoy, and the overall health benefits of the diet.

Furthermore, the chapter explores the mechanism behind the diet, the common mistakes people make when trying to follow the diet, and the different types of keto diets out there. The chapter ends with an overview of the skills an individual would need to cultivate to gain success in this diet.

The second chapter is an in-depth explanation of the ketosis process. The chapter begins with tips on how an individual can start and get to a ketosis process. The chapter continues to explain the reasons keto is convenient, the process of testing for the ketosis process and the different ways people can use to eliminate the wrong type of fat.

The chapter concludes with the process that an individual can control his or her calories with low carb, an explanation of keto health, and the secret behind weight loss using keto.

The third chapter is a guide for someone who would want to start living the keto lifestyle. The chapter begins with encouraging an individual to consider the diet he or she is on, and then continues to point out the eating habits that such an individual would need to give up. The chapter continues to explain the food combinations people follow that are wrong in so many ways, and then concludes with a description of a healthy keto food combination.

The fourth chapter is about the keto shopping list. The chapter begins with an explanation of the different keto supplements an individual should look for in the market and the hormones balance in keto. The chapter continues to explain how keto in its totality can help with the fight against cancer, the benefits it has on the body, the brain, and the heart.

The fifth chapter is a breakdown of the different types of keto diet plans. The chapter begins with a description of the type of diet a beginner should subscribe to as he or she starts to get used to keto. The chapter continues to explain the basic plan, it explains the snacks an individual can take, and even the plan one would need to follow if he or she were fasting. The chapter concludes with the keto plans for vegetarians and vegans.

The sixth chapter is the place to get to for anyone who is interested to find out as much as he or she can concern keto cycling. The chapter begins with a definition of keto cycling, it explains the specific aspects of the cycle program and explains the benefits of keto cycling. The chapter concludes with distinguishing between keto cycling and carb cycling and then takes you on a journey to discover whether keto cycling is good for you.

There are plenty of books on this subject on the market, thanks again for choosing this one! Every effort was made to ensure it is full of as much useful information as possible, please enjoy it!

Chapter 1: Introduction to Keto Diet

At the beginning of every year, and every day in between, people hear about a new diet, detox plan, or gym membership that promises to be the secret to a successful year or a healthy life. Sometimes, it seems like the whole world is trying to get rid of a few extra pounds as fast as possible. Often people are willing to try anything that sounds remotely promising.

Enter the keto diet. This diet plan is one of the hottest trends currently. Interestingly, its origins date back to the 1920s as a treatment plan for childhood epilepsy. Due to its overwhelming popularity and success rate, many people still use it to deal with this condition today.

According to some studies, people who follow this diet experience up to 40% fewer epileptic seizures. Its use, however, is more common in the generally healthy population seeking to get more out of life or drop a few pounds. This diet plan promises a wide range of benefits from increased mental focus to faster weight loss.

The keto diet aims to decrease insulin and blood sugar levels by shifting the body's metabolism to burn fat more effectively to generate energy, which leads to the production of ketones. In addition, proponents of this diet plan insist that it can help people lose weight quite fast, which is one of the reasons why it is so popular.

However, to determine whether this diet plan is good for them, people need to learn as much as possible about the keto diet. They need to determine whether science backs it before joining the cause and adopting it into their lifestyle.

What Is the Keto Diet Plan?

The word keto comes from the fact that this diet plan drives the body to produce ketones, which are tiny energy/fuel molecules. The body turns to this fuel source when the level of blood sugar is low. The human brain is a constantly hungry organ that needs a lot of energy, which is understandable given the work it does every second. However, it cannot run on fat; rather, it needs glucose or ketones.

This diet plan consists of consuming food that is low in carbohydrates, moderate in protein, and significantly high in fat. Actually, according to some keto diet variations, the fat content should make up to 80% of a person's daily calories. The carbohydrates, on the other hand, should be less than 5% of the calories. Protein should contribute between 15% and 20% of the calories.

It is easy to see why many people are apprehensive about this diet plan. The keto diet drastically departs from the generally accepted macronutrient distribution of 10% to 35% fat, 45% to 65% carbs, and 20% to 35% protein. However, the most important aspect of this diet is the normal and natural process known as ketosis.

The healthy human body runs quite well on the glucose produced when the body burns or breaks down carbohydrates. Actually, the human body prefers to generate energy through the breakdown of carbohydrates. However, when a person is hungry or cutting back on carbohydrates, his/her body will seek other sources of energy.

Fat is an alternative source of energy for the body. When a person's blood sugar is low because he/she is not feeding his/her body with carbohydrates, his/her cells will release fat and flood the liver.

Consequently, the liver will turn the fat into ketone bodies, which the body will use as its secondary energy source.

In other words, the ketogenic diet aims to substitute the body's primary sources of energy with fats. Actually, this process is surprisingly efficient, which is why it leads to weight loss and other health benefits. Another subtle benefit of this diet plan is that one will have a constant supply of energy and feel hungry less often.

Consequently, one will feel focused and sharp all day. As stated earlier, the keto diet helps decrease insulin and blood sugar levels. Sugar, however, is the brain's main fuel or food. Fortunately, ketones produced by the liver from fat will feed the brain. Most people who follow this diet plan insist it is quite safe.

Nevertheless, the ketogenic diet is still controversial. Actually, three groups of people should keep away from this diet. These are breastfeeding women, people with high blood pressure taking antihypertensive medication, and people with diabetes who take insulin. Before adopting this diet, people in these situations should seek their doctors' advice.

People on a keto diet force their bodies to run on fat, essentially, their bodies burn fat 24 hours a day, seven days a week, as long as they are following this diet plan religiously. The fastest way to get the body into a state of ketosis is through fasting. However, it is extremely difficult to fast for several days.

This is where the keto diet comes in handy. This diet plan helps the body reach this state surprisingly fast, and people can adopt and follow it indefinitely. A typical ketogenic diet consists of foods such as butter, meat, cheese, fish, eggs, heavy cream, avocado, oils, seeds, nuts, and low-carb green veggies.

Looking at this list, one will notice that it does not include people's favorite carbohydrate-rich foods such as fruits, grains, cereals, rice, milk, beans, sweets, potatoes, and even some veggies.

The Science of Keto

Every year, new diet fads rise and fall with little to commend them. Nothing new there; however, the keto diet has been around for a remarkably long time and continues to gain popularity because of the science behind it. Many prominent medical professionals believe in the benefits of ketosis, which is reason enough for one to take a closer look at this diet.

After years of trying any weight loss diets, most overweight individuals come to believe that nothing makes a difference. They only lose some weight if they consume fewer calories than they used to, but when they do this, then they feel hungry all the time, which causes them to binge eat on certain occasions. When such individuals learn about the ketogenic diet, few can resist its attraction.

The concept behind this diet plan makes a lot of sense. The weirdly named ketone bodies are tiny molecules that serve as the natural back-up fuel supply for the body when glucose is in short supply. As stated earlier, people normally enter ketosis when they starve themselves for several days at a time.

Ketosis is the state where ketone bodies build up in the bloodstream. When the body reaches ketosis, metabolism switches to fat-burning to convert accumulated fat molecules into ketone bodies, which help power the brain and muscles. Being in a state of ketosis, therefore, sounds like an awesome way to get rid of excess fat.

Not eating for days, on the other hand, is not something most people would be willing to do. Fortunately, the keto diet seems to be the answer to this dilemma. People do not need to starve themselves to reach ketosis. Instead, all they need to do is drastically reduce the carbohydrates in their diet, and this includes refined carbs, complex carbs, as well as starches.

When the body lacks a source of glucose, it has to go into a state of ketosis since the brain needs fuel in the form of either glucose or ketone bodies to function and survive. Therefore, no matter how much fat or protein one eats, the body will still need to break down fat to ketone bodies to produce the fuel it needs.

As earlier stated, there are many variations of the keto diet. All of them, however, aim to switch the body's metabolism to ketosis. Actually, the keto diets doing the rounds out there are not the only ones or the first to do that. The Atkins diet, for example, rose to prominence a few decades ago and helped many people lose weight.

The Atkins diet, in reality, is another variation of the keto diet since it removes carbohydrates from the diet and substitutes them with protein. Interestingly, followers of this diet discovered that they felt less hungry than they feared, which means that the calories from increased protein intake made the feel satisfied for longer.

When one is feeling full, one will eat less, which will translate to significant weight loss. The Atkins diet, however, has certain side effects for people who follow it for an extended period. The most troubling of these side effects is its impact on the balance of nitrogen from the consumption of too much protein.

For example, there is an increased risk of dehydration for those who adhere to the Atkins diet. In serious cases, the need to get rid of excess

nitrogen as urine leads to the formation of kidney stones. In a certain sense, the keto diet is the 21st-century version of the Atkins diet. Instead of replacing carbohydrates with protein, the keto diet replaces them with fats.

The regimen of a typical Atkins diet consisted of less than 5% of calories from carbohydrates, 25% from fats, and about 75% from protein. The modern keto diet regimen, in contrast, suggests 25% of calories from protein, less than 5% from carbohydrates, and about 75% from fats.

Since the intake of protein in the keto diet is the same as the recommended protein intake in a typical balanced diet, it neatly sidesteps the side effects resulting from nitrogen imbalance. However, the recommended fat intake in the keto diet is a huge concern for many people.

It seems more than a bit ironic that it advocates for people who want to get rid of excess fat to include more fats in their diet. To many people, it seems quite unhealthy. To help understand this conundrum, consider the case if the lipid profiles of the brave individuals who explore and cross the Antarctic on foot while dragging sleds packed with food and supplies.

To achieve this feat, they need to take food with a very high calorie to weight ratio. Essentially, this means eating a lot of butter. It takes several months to cross the continent on foot, which means living on an all-butter diet for months. Interestingly, after months on this diet, the level of bad cholesterol in their bodies, known as LDL-cholesterol, actually decreases significantly.

This may surprise many people, but it is not as surprising as it sounds. When the body goes into ketosis, it moves fats towards the liver, where the transformation of fats into ketone bodies happens, which is the work of

HDL-cholesterol. Usually, LDL-cholesterol transports excess fat from the liver to deposits in different parts of the body.

Essentially, this type of cholesterol moves fat in the opposite direction. In ketosis, therefore, no matter how much fat one is consuming, one will have a lipid profile usually considered healthier. In other words, one will have lower LDL and higher HDL, which is quite remarkable.

However, as discussed earlier, one of the benefits of following the Atkins diet was reduced feelings of hunger due to the sustaining power of protein. People often wonder how the keto diet can achieve this without increasing the protein content of their diet. As it turns out, reduced hunger stems from the state of ketosis itself.

In a certain sense, it might not matter how one achieves this state. Therefore, theoretically, science seems to back up the modern keto diet. However, it would be somewhat interesting to imagine how it would feel to follow the keto diet in place of the commonly touted, calorie-deficient, low-everything diet.

Consider a man weighing 195 pounds on a 5-foot, 9-inch frame at the beginning of the year. This would put his body mass index at about 30, which is quite close to being obese. Anyway, on the first day of the year, he reads about the keto diet, does some research, and decides to try it.

He purchases one of the deliciously sounding cookbooks from Amazon and begins the keto journey. His intake of carbohydrates immediately falls below 5%, which means, among other things, eating a rib-eye steak topped with chili-butter, followed with cheese and scrambled eggs in the morning. This sounds somewhat awesome.

Anyway, people who believe that fats are an important ingredient in great tasting food should find the keto diet quite appealing and easy to follow.

This man usually works out for 30 minutes each day on a rowing machine. To improve the effectiveness of his new diet, he decides to increase his workout time to 45 minutes.

This workout will help get rid of excess carbohydrates in his body stored as glycogen in the liver, which will release quickly to power his muscles. Within 2 days, he reaches ketosis. Using urine dipsticks, he determines that his ketone body level indicates a state of deep ketosis.

The level of ketone bodies stayed constant for more than a month while he enjoyed the culinary delights of meals such as cream pork stroganoff accompanied by zucchini ribbons sour cream and avocado dressings, and burgers. Essentially, he was eating three fat-rich meals each day.

In this example, it is important to look at the benefits he enjoyed before looking at any disadvantages. Once he went into a state of ketosis a few days on, he founds that he was never hungry. Essentially, he stopped snacking between meals as he usually did. Actually, he found himself thinking less about eating.

Soon, missing lunch altogether by accident became something quite normal. There was a significant improvement in his focus and concentration as well, in addition to having more energy, which also increased his productivity. In other words, using his back-up batteries, which are the tiny ketone bodies, seemed to be better than using carbohydrates for fuel.

There is a good reason why this might happen, especially for a chubby individual like the person in this example. Essentially, the ketone levels never decline. By contrast, when people eat carbohydrate-rich foods, the metabolism system immediately turns the excess carbohydrates into fat. In a sense, it stores it for a rainy day.

Therefore, after eating a carbohydrate-rich meal, a person's blood glucose level starts to decrease a few hours after, which triggers feelings of hunger and the urge to eat again. In addition, it also triggers a sense of declining concentration and energy, which 'carbavores' and late afternoon dippers know so well.

Going back to the hypothetical man in the example above, eating less actually led to a significant loss of weight. For this example, based on a testimonial from the real individual, he lost 10 pounds in less than a month, mostly from unhealthy-looking and unattractive fat deposits on his body.

According to his testimonial, his waistline decreased by two notches, which is twice as much as his previous diet achieved by keeping hi constantly hungry. In addition, the keto diet brought other unexpected benefits as well. The amount of plaque on his teeth, for example, reduced quite significantly, maybe because carbohydrates need to feed off dietary carbohydrates.

When it comes to the downside of the keto diet, at least according to him, there were just a few. The first is about staying away from carbohydrates, keeping them below 5% proved to be quite challenging after a couple of weeks. He had to check the content of carbohydrates in everything he ate, which was difficult because he found them in almost everything he chose to eat.

Eating out was also a challenge, not to mention having to attend dinner parties at a family member or friend's house unless they were unusually accommodating. As a result, planning and preparing food took on a new level of significance and demand for his resources and time than previously.

Secondly is the issue of accurate portion control. Since the keto diet includes high-fat meals with high-calorie content, he often feared he would unintentionally consume too many calories. To lose weight people need to eat fewer calories than they need. Even the ketogenic diet cannot break this law.

The last downside was a bit easier to avoid. While following the keto diet, it is difficult to get enough fiber mainly because most of the fiber sources commonly available also contain carbohydrates. Essentially, since fiber is an indigestible or insoluble carbohydrate polymer, it naturally contains digestible carbohydrates. His solution was to take a fiber supplement.

If this man were to conduct an experiment to determine the impact of eating some carbs after following a carbohydrate-free diet for a month, just a small portion of carbohydrates would immediately kill ketosis. He would then need to re-establish ketosis after one moment of weakness. Following the keto diet, therefore, requires Zen-like discipline.

This experiment shows that ketosis is difficult and slow to establish, but very easy to turn off. Scientists call this phenomenon hysteresis. There are good reasons for this. Although carbohydrates and glucose good sources of fuel, they can damage the proteins that make up the body's tissues and cells.

When the levels of glucose go up too much, this tissue and cell damage may be irreversible, which can happen in diabetes. To prevent this from happening, the body produces insulin as soon as the levels of blood glucose start to go up. Insulin limits glucose levels in the blood by instructing the liver to turn excess glucose into fat.

In the process, however, insulin kills ketosis, which is why ketosis ends so quickly when people following the keto diet slip up. Nowadays, there is unlimited availability of calories.

The body stores every ounce of excess carbohydrates as fat. Without establishing ketosis, the body will not re-assess these fat deposits when glucose runs out; instead, one will simply feel hungry. With fast-food joints around every corner, it is extremely tempting to refuel with carbohydrates again.

As stated earlier, one reason why people lose weight while on a keto diet is that feelings of hunger go way down, which forces more fat out of fat deposits for energy than the fat that goes in. Without spikes in insulin, the body takes advantage of leptin-induced satiety ore easily.

The keto diet also helps people wean off dopamine addiction caused by spiking blood sugar, which raises HDL and reduces LDL and triglycerides in obese people. However, people who want to try the keto diet should first discuss it with their doctor to determine whether it is good for them.

Benefits of Keto Diet

The keto diet is one of the most popular diets today, which is why there are more than a million Google searches every month for this diet. Some of the reasons for its popularity include:

1. It Helps People Lose Weight

Initially, weight loss results from loss of water because of the drastic reduction in carbohydrate intake. The keto diet also encourages people to consume foods rich in fat and cut back on carbohydrates, sugar, and

refined carbohydrates. This will lead to a constant supply of energy and fewer sugar highs and crashes.

Actually, the first thing people on this diet report is having steady energy and not needing to snack all the time due to waning energy. Essentially, the keto diet often lowers the desire to eat and leads to fewer

hunger pangs. If one is not hungry all the time, one will eat less, which will lead to weight loss.

Interestingly, although the keto diet is high in fat content, it is often more effective when it comes to helping people lose weight than a low-fat diet. However, it is not right for everyone. While it may lead to short-term weight loss, it is extremely difficult to follow.

2. Treating Epilepsy in Kids

The only clear and proven health benefit of the keto diet is its ability to reduce epileptic seizures in kids. In fact, since 1920, doctors have been using it therapeutically for this very purpose. Experts recommend the keto diet for children suffering from certain conditions, such as Rett syndrome or Lennox-Gastaut syndrome, and do not respond to medication for seizure.

The Epilepsy Foundation suggests that the ketogenic diet can decrease the number of seizures kids have by up to 50%, with about 10% to 15% of children becoming seizure-free. The foundation also notes that this diet can also be beneficial for adults who suffer from epilepsy, although it is quite difficult and restrictive to stick with.

3. May Improve Heart Health

When a person follows the keto diet in a healthy manner, it can improve the health of his/her heart by reducing bad cholesterol. In addition, this diet also increases the levels of HDL-cholesterol, which is good cholesterol.

4. Reduces Acne

There are many different forms of acne, and some may have a connection to blood sugar and diet. A diet rich in refined and processed carbohydrates, for example, can alter the bacteria in the gut and dramatic fluctuations in the levels of blood sugar, which can have a negative effect on skin health. Limiting carbohydrates intake; therefore, can help reduce some forms of acne.

5. Metabolic Syndrome

Limited research suggests that adults suffering from the metabolic disease can benefit from the keto diet because it can help them get rid of more body fat and weight, compared to people who eat a diet heavy in added sugars and processed foods.

6. Type 2 Diabetes

In September 2016, the Journal of Obesity and Eating Disorders published research suggesting that the keto diet could be helpful to people with type 2 diabetes and lead to improvements in the levels of HbA1c. However, it is important to understand that it can also lead to low blood sugar levels, also called hypoglycemia, if the patient also takes medication to lower his/her blood sugar.

7. Bipolar Disorder

The keto diet may be a mood stabilizer for individuals with type 2 bipolar disorder. According to a study published in the journal Neurocase in October 2012, in certain cases, it may be more effective than medication.

8. Obesity

According to one study published in the journal Endocrine in December 2016, obese people on a low-calorie keto diet lose ore inflammatory belly fat as compared to those on a normal low-calorie diet. In addition, according to a February 2018 article published in the journal Nutrition and Metabolism, this diet may also help maintain a lean body mass during weight loss.

9. Alzheimer's Disease and Dementia

An article in the journal Neurobiology of Aging published in February 2013 suggested that higher-risk older adults on a ketogenic diet experienced significantly better memory functioning after one and a half months.

Certain experts in the field of Alzheimer's, such as the director of the Alzheimer's Prevention Clinic at Weill Cornell Medicine and New York Presbyterian, Richard Issacson, MD, suggest low-carbohydrate diets as one of the ways to delay brain aging, and maybe even Alzheimer's, which is a form of dementia.

10. Parkinson's Disease

Since people with this condition tend to have a higher risk of developing dementia, experts like Robert Krikorian, Ph.D., a professor of clinical psychiatry, are conducting studies looking at whether inducing dietary ketosis can preserve cognitive functioning. Only time and more research will tell.

11. Certain Forms of Cancer

Some studies, such as one published in the journal Oncology in November 2018; suggest that doctors should use the ketogenic diet in conjunction with radiation and chemotherapy to treat certain forms of cancer.

However, to determine whether this diet can play a helpful role in cancer therapy, scientists need to conduct more studies. More importantly, without a doctor's consent, patients should not use the keto diet as a stand-alone treatment for any disease.

12. Polycystic Ovary Syndrome

Women with this infertility condition have a higher risk of developing obesity and diabetes. This is why some medical professionals recommend the ketogenic diet. However, researchers need to conduct long-term research on the safety of using the keto diet to deal with this condition.

• Other Unexpected Benefits

Some researchers suggest the possibility of gaining several other unexpected benefits from the keto diet. These findings, however, are preliminary and require more research. These include:

1. The diminishment of anxiety and depression
2. A healthier liver
3. A fall in inflammation markers
4. Sound sleep

Advantages of The Keto Diet

In the beginning, the ketogenic diet can be quite overwhelming. Before people give it a go, they need to understand what it involves, how the diet works, and, most importantly, what doctors and nutritionists think about

the ketogenic diet. According to many people who follow the keto diet plan, it provides impressive results within a very short time.

Research also suggests that the keto diet may even improve workout performance in athletes and help them lose body fat while maintaining muscle mass. However, it is important to note that conflicting evidence exists to support these claims. Some experts, for example, express concerns about the sustainability of this diet plan, as well as its long-term effects on the body.

Some of the common advantages of the keto diet include:

1. Quick weight loss
2. Tons of online recipes and resources
3. Ability to boost satiety
4. Improved athletic performance in certain people
5. Reduced abdominal fat
6. Ay improve health markers like cholesterol levels, triglyceride, and blood pressure

Mechanism of Keto Diet

The keto diet restricts the intake of proteins and especially carbohydrates while encouraging the consumption of fat. For several decades, doctors have been using this diet plan in the management and treatment of drug- resistant epilepsy. This is because its action mechanism leads to changes in ketone levels and other substances, thereby reducing the frequency of seizures.

• Seizure Pathophysiology

The brain has a complex network of neurons that transmit signals and nerve impulses. These transmitters play a critical role in the dissemination of these nerve impulses, which carry messages across the neuron synapse. Neurotransmitters are inhibitory or excitatory based on their effect on the triggering of impulses.

A common excitatory neurotransmitter is a glutamate, which aids the distribution of impulses. On the other hand, GABA serves to inhibit nerve impulses. Any imbalance between the brain's neurotransmitters causes a seizure, especially due to the firing of too many nervous messages and over-excitement of the nerves.

Therefore, GABA helps to control the frequency of epileptic seizures, while anticonvulsant medication helps to boost inhibitory neurotransmitters. Scientists do not know the keto diet's precise mechanism; however, they propose several possible explanations.

Many changes take place in the brain and body because of the keto diet. However, science is yet to identify the change that leads to the anticonvulsant effect. That said, the action mechanism of most pharmacological anticonvulsant medication is similarly mysterious.

The most important aspect of the keto diet is the drastic restriction of carbohydrates from the diet. To compensate for this reduction, the conversion of fatty acids into sources of fuel takes place through oxidation in the mitochondria. The lack of carbohydrates in the diet leads to the absence of glucose.

Acetone, acetoacetate, and hydroxybutyrate, which are ketone bodies, synthesize and pass through the blood-brain barrier to provide an alternative energy source for the brain. Scientists think they possess anticonvulsant properties needed to prevent seizures in test animals.

The propagation of nerve messages and stabilization of neurons may happen because of the ketone bodies' efficiency as a source of fuel. As the body adapts to the conversion of fat to produce ketone bodies for energy, the increase in the number of mitochondria takes place.

Both the keto diet and pharmacological anticonvulsants work because of their ability to suppress seizures. Unlike anticonvulsant medication, however, the keto diet seems to have anti-epileptogenic properties and the ability to hinder the progress of epilepsy, at least according to a study of rats.

There are several other theories about the keto diet's action mechanism, such as hypoglycemia, electrolyte changes, and systemic acidosis, which is increased blood acidity. However, science is yet to prove the accuracy of most of these theories. In addition, some evidence suggests that these hypotheses may not have anything to do with the diet's mechanism.

Within the past twenty years or so, interest in determining the therapeutic mechanism of the keto diet has been growing steadily. Fortunately, modern advances in the scientific and medical fields are yielding critical insight into the biochemical basis of many brain functions, both pathologic and normal.

Some of the metabolic changes likely connected to the keto diet's anticonvulsant properties include increased bioenergetics reserves, increased fatty acid levels, reduced glucose levels, and ketosis.

According to some experts in the field of neuroscience, some of the effects induced by the keto diet may include GABA neurotransmission and enhanced purinergic, sensitive potassium channel modulation, and boosted brain-derived neurotrophic factor expression because of glycolytic limitation.

More importantly, in addition to its use as an anticonvulsant, the keto diet may also promote neuroprotective properties, which can help boost the clinical potential of the diet as an illness-prevention approach or intervention.

Since scientific evidence proves that changes in diet can trigger a wide range of complex metabolic alterations, future scientific research should reveal a more detailed framework for the keto diet mechanism in action, which will allow for the formulation of an improved offering with fewer side effects for a wide range of physical disorders.

Some scientists proposed the modulation of the levels of biogenetic monoamine as a plausible action mechanism for the anticonvulsant properties of the keto diet. The specific workings underlying such properties, however, remain unclear. Norepinephrine levels in test animals seem to show an increase in rats consuming this diet.

When researchers inhibited the transport of norepinephrine, there was no observable benefit from the keto diet. This seems to suggest the need for a noradrenergic system for the neuroprotective properties of the ketogenic diet to take place. From this brief discussion, it is clear to see the complexity of the keto diet's mechanism of action.

Common Mistakes of Keto

The hottest diet last year, which is the ketogenic diet, is only gaining momentum this year. It attracts more than one million searches on Google each month, which is a testament to its popularity. However, this popularity tends to make people who want to try it out make various mistakes.

Unfortunately, people tend to jump headlong into any weight loss and wellness diet that promises amazing results without doing adequate research to determine whether the diet is right for them. This is also true when it comes to the keto diet. It is difficult to know what to expect when one decides to follow the keto diet without proper research.

The most important thing to understand about this low-carb, high-fat diet is that it is extremely restrictive; therefore, getting it right can be quite difficult. For example, in addition to the obvious carbohydrates, people who want to adopt this diet need to avoid starchy vegetables and limit grains, fruits, sweets, and juices.

In addition, they will need to bulk up on fats, according to the recommended keto food list. By doing this, they will go into ketosis within a very short time, which, as discussed earlier, is the metabolic state that forces their bodies to burn fat to generate fuel, instead of burning carbohydrates. In most cases, this will speed up their weight-loss goals.

Since carbohydrates are in just about everything people eat today and fats come in several different forms, it is easy to make mistakes, especially if one does not know much about the ketogenic lifestyle. At this point, it is important to understand that not all fats are healthy.

To live the keto lifestyle safely, one needs to understand the common mistakes people make, including:

1. Increasing Fat Intake and reducing Carbohydrate Intake too Quickly and too Much

One day, one is eating cereal in the morning, sandwiches at lunch, and pasta for dinner. Suddenly, having decided to adopt the keto diet, one will need to consume less than 20 grams of carbohydrates every day, based on

the starting amount recommended by the keto diet. This is harder to achieve than it sounds.

A medium apple, for example, contains approximately 25 grams of carbohydrates.

This is a good point of reference for people who decide to follow the keto diet. Essentially, this diet requires drastic dietary and lifestyle changes. Therefore, it is important to ease into the diet. Before adopting this diet fully, people should begin by decreasing their carbohydrates intake gradually, instead of doing it cold turkey.

2. Failing to Drink Adequate Water

When most people start weight loss or wellness diets, including the keto diet, they tend to focus on what they are eating and forget about what they are drinking. People on the ketogenic diet have an increased risk of dehydration due to the extreme decrease in their carbohydrate intake.

This can easily lead to a shift in electrolyte and fluid balance. The body stores carbohydrates along with water; therefore, as the deposits of carbohydrates in the body run dry, excess water in the body also depletes. In addition, the body gets rid of excess ketones through urine, which depletes sodium and water from the body.

Therefore, it is important to drink a lot of water to prevent dehydration. When one wakes up, for example, one should drink a glass of water and sip water regularly throughout the day, which will help one reach the goal of drinking half of one's body weight in ounces of water every day.

3. Failing to Prepare for the Keto Flu

As one's body transitions from a carb engine to a fat engine, one might experience the keto flu, which comes with flu-like symptoms such as fatigue, body aches, nausea, and cramps. This often happens during the

first couple of weeks; however, these symptoms do not affect everyone who adopts this diet.

People who lack knowledge about the keto diet and fail to prepare themselves for these symptoms often think there is something very wrong, which makes them give up on the diet altogether.

However, such people can overcome these symptoms by planning their prepping and meal preparation in advance. It is also wise to eat foods rich in sodium, magnesium, and potassium, in addition to drinking water to help deal with any negative symptoms of this diet.

Other common mistakes people make when they decide to adopt the keto diet include:

- Failing to eat foods rich in omega-3 fatty acids
- Failing to salt their food adequately
- Failing to consult their doctor about the diet and trying to do it alone
- Failing to pay attention to their vegetable intake

- Focusing on the carbohydrate intake and forgetting about the quality of food
- Drinking too much dairy
- Snacking too much
- Being obsessive about the scale
- Not sleeping enough

How to Recognize Good Fats from Bad Fats The word 'fat' is something people do not want to be associated with; however, fat plays an integral role in the functioning of the human body. When people hear the word "fat," nothing good comes to their minds, but it is scientifically proven that meals that contain high amounts of fat and low amounts of carbs actually help to reduce weight more effectively than meals that contain low fat.

Fat is an essential element in the human body, and it is impossible to survive without it. However, the problem is that people do not understand the difference between good fats and bad fats. Thus, it is important to understand, and be able to distinguish between good and bad fats, so that people can make the best choices with regards to diets.

What exactly are good fats?

Good fats are mainly saturated fats, unsaturated fats, and trans fats that exist naturally. In the unsaturated fats category, there are polyunsaturated fats and monounsaturated fats. Good fats contain elements that support heart health and generally lower cholesterol levels in the body, and that is one of the reasons why they should replace all forms of unhealthy saturated fats present in a plethora of diets these days.

It might sound a little bit off-key, but there are zero links between saturated fats and the increase in heart diseases. New studies are starting to change our views on the so-called traditional "bad" fats in our diet.

Polyunsaturated Fats

Polyunsaturated fats are predominantly found in vegetable oils. They contain elements that help reduce triglyceride and cholesterol levels and

are the perfect substitutes for saturated fats. Just like every other thing in life, the keto diet seeks balance, and that's why it is important to maintain a good balance of these fats.

Omega-3 fatty acids are essential to the human body because they contain elements that support heart health, which generally improves human health and sustainability. They are predominantly found in fishes like catfish, mackerel, trout, and salmon, etc. Some plant-based foods that contain these good fats are walnuts and flaxseed.

If you have a deficiency, you can use supplements, but there is nothing better than obtaining your Omega-3 fatty acids from food.

Monounsaturated Fats

Monounsaturated fats are renowned for their unique ability to mitigate and reduce the risk and impact of heart disease. Mediterranean foods contain a lot of it, and that's because they use a lot of olive oil in the preparation of their dishes. Monounsaturated fats have been credited with the extremely low occurrence of heart diseases in and around the Mediterranean countries. The thing about theses fats is that they become solid when refrigerated, but when stored at room temperature, they maintain their liquid form. When olive oil starts to solidify below 75 degrees Fahrenheit, it points to the fact that you have monounsaturated oil. Vitamin E is another healthy nutrient present in these fats, and it is always better to eat foods that contain these nutrients, as opposed to taking supplements (this is to ensure the best possible effect). Some of the foods that contain these fats include; sesame seeds, nuts, cashew,

pumpkin seeds, and olives. Other good sources include peanut oil, canola oil, and olive oil.

Keto and Unsaturated Fats

There are people on the keto diet that make the blunder of consuming huge amounts of fat without much emphasis on the quality, and this is somewhat counterproductive. Thus, it is important to choose your fats correctly because not all fats are the same, and some are far better than others, e.g., fats that emanate from coconut oil and olive oil are good. Also, fats from nuts are good too. While on Keto, it is important always to read nutritional labels to ascertain the type of fats present in your diets; because it will help you stay on course. Finally, it is important to note that most fried foods do not come with enough healthy fats.

Saturated Fat

Over time, it has been said that no matter what happens, people should avoid consuming saturated fats at all costs. However, recent studies have shown that the consumption of saturated fats is in no way associated with greater risks for stroke, heart diseases, and other earlier associated health conditions (and it has nothing to do with gender or age).

Slowly but surely, the perception towards saturated fats is changing, and even the medical community is now getting used to the fact that saturated fats are not as bad as previously thought.

Saturated fats have always been part of human history; for example, coconut oil contains a unique type of saturated fat referred to as medium-

chain triglycerides. These fats are extremely easy to digest and transformed into

energy. Since modern research findings have proven that saturated fats are beneficial in healthy dieting, it is now clear that saturated fats are necessary components of a healthy diet.

Saturated Fats and its Health Benefits

Before, the consensus was that saturated fats are completely bad for human health. However, new studies have shown that the position to be wrong and even gone on to show the numerous benefits of saturated fats. In Keto, some of the best sources of saturated fats are cocoa butter, eggs, cream, coconut oil, lard, red meat, and butter, etc. Some of the health benefits include;

Saturated fats help to raise the good blood cholesterol in other to stop the buildup LDL in the arteries. Saturated fats help in the production of hormones like testosterone and Cortisol. They also help in boosting the immune system to combat infections and diseases.

Saturated fats support bone density, and are also responsible for improved HDL and LDL cholesterol levels.

Natural Trans Fats

Trans fats are mostly bad fats, and it is strange to see them listed in this section. However, the reason they are listed in this section is that there are foods that contain a particular type of "natural" trans fat. These foods contain trans fat referred to as Vaccenic acid, and they help maintain heart health, as well as reduce the risk of obesity and diabetes. Healthy trans fats are mostly found in dairy products and grass-fed meat and are even known to suppress intestinal inflammation and protect against cancer.

What are the bad fats?

For people that intend to lose weight, it is possible to lose weight on the keto diet while consuming bad fats, but there are multiples risks involved. The truth is that you might achieve your primary aim but end up jeopardizing your overall wellbeing, for example, bad fats are known to increase inflammation and are also associated with an increased risk of certain cancer types, including prostate and colon cancer.

The Keto diet is not just about weight loss, and the idea is to live healthy and happy. Thus it is necessary to remove bad fats from your diet completely.

Processed Trans Fats

Not all Trans fats are bad, but the processed ones are as bad as they come. These synthetic fats are bad for human health. Thus it is important to always go for natural Trans fats, as opposed to the processed ones. Most of these processed trans fats are produced from oils made from genetically altered seeds when you consume them, and you are exposed to radical elements that can easily wreak havoc on your body.

Keep away from processed Trans fats.

Dangers of Consuming Trans Fats

There are huge amounts of risks associated with the consumption of processed and adulterated trans fats, and the likelihood of heart disease is

just one of them. People that consume processed foods that contain Trans fats are at a greater risk of developing different forms of cancer. Thus, it is extremely important to consume meats that haven't been processed with chemicals and hormones.

When people consume bad fats, they risk upsetting the equilibrium between good and bad cholesterol levels, which can easily cause inflammation in the body. Furthermore, your gut flora can be destroyed by Trans fats, which also increases the risk of being exposed to all sorts of diseases.

Like I mentioned earlier, there are good and bad trans fats; you only have to pay close attention in other to figure out which is which. If you come in contact with any type of hydrogenated oil or partially hydrogenated oil, it is important to boycott them. Most times, you'll find them in foods like cookies, margarine, crackers, and some fast food. Some other forms of processed oils you should be on the lookout for include safflower oil, cottonseed oil, canola oil, and sunflower oil. It is important to completely remove these oils from your diet in other to maintain a healthier mind and body.

The Low-Fat Misconception

Most labels on food products come with so much misinformation that it is now difficult to truly ascertain what you're purchasing. It is normal for these companies to withhold names of ingredients and chemicals that were used during production because they believe the quantities are under a

certain threshold. Sometimes you'll see labels that read natural and fat- free, but the truth is that they are not always as stated, and some of the added ingredients might even be harmful to human health.

In today's world, there is so much misinformation concerning the types of fat that are safe to consume. However, for people that are on a keto diet, it is important to boycott everything and anything hydrogenated or processed because that is when you'll truly see the effects of a low-carb diet. Don't just buy anything from the mall. Before you do, carefully check the labels and if you find any ingredient you're not familiar with, use the internet to check if its something you can safely consume.

Finally, one of the things you should lookout for a while checking labels is the length of the ingredients. If you come across an item that has too many ingredients, it is safe to say that you should boycott it, and move on

to something with a more streamlined ingredients list.

Types of Keto Diet

Since the end goal of different variations of the keto diet is the same, these variations share certain similarities, the most notable of which is high dietary fats and low carbohydrates. To put together the right diet, it is important to speak to a doctor or dietician who will give one personalized guidance and advice based on one's individual needs.

Some of the most common types of keto diets include:

1. The common keto diet composed of 20% protein, 70% to 75% fat, and 5% to 10% protein
2. The extremely low carbohydrate keto diet with less than 5% carbohydrate content
3. The well-formulated keto diet with macronutrients of carbohydrates, protein, and fat that meet the requirements or standards of the keto diet
4. The medium-chain triglycerides keto diet
5. Calorie-restricted keto diet
6. Cyclical keto diet
7. Targeted keto diet
8. The high protein keto diet

Skills for Success in Keto Diet

The keto diet can be extremely difficult to start and maintain since it radically departs from the way people eat these days. The typical American diet, for instance, is high in both processed foods and carbohydrates. The keto diet, however, involves putting the body into a state of ketosis to force it into burning fat for energy.

Some of the skills needed to follow and maintain the keto diet include:

1. Knowing the foods to avoid and eat
2. Understanding one's relationship with fat
3. Improving one's cooking skills
4. Drinking bulletproof coffee, which is one of the best ketogenic- friendly drinks
5. Seeking support from family members and friends

The ketogenic diet or keto, in short, went viral last year. Actually, 2018 was the year of the ketogenic diet. Even today, it shows no signs of slowing down. The internet has tons of guides about this diet because it is somewhat difficult to follow and maintain. There are many different variations of the keto diet plan on the internet. Therefore, it is important to talk to a doctor or dietician before embarking on the ketogenic journey.

Chapter 2: What Is the Ketosis Process?

If you have searched for ways to lose weight, you might have come across this word Ketosis. Ketosis refers to a natural metabolic process whereby the body burns stored fats to get energy when there is not enough supply of glucose or carbohydrates in the body. You can achieve this by observing a low-carb diet, Ketogenic diet or intermittent fasting. These types of diets will enable your body to burn the unwanted fats in your body for energy because the supply of carbohydrates is not enough.

When the fats are broken down to produce the energy needed by the body, it releases a type of acid known as ketones that the body can excrete through urine. However, the amount of these ketones should not be too much because it will raise the acidity level in blood. This will cause a condition known as ketoacidosis that is dangerous.

How to Get a Ketosis Process?

Reaching a ketosis state is not something that you can achieve instantly, but it can take you several hours or even days to get to that high fat-

burning state. The following are tips that can stimulate your ketosis process.

1. Reduce Your Carb Intake and Concentrate on Keto Friendly Foods

Eating a low-carb diet will accelerate your Ketosis. Naturally, your body cells will use glucose and sugars to get energy. However, the body can also get energy from Ketones also known as the fatty acids that the liver converts into energy. Keto-friendly foods are low in carbs and high in healthy fats. You should also include high-quality protein like meat, fish, eggs, and chicken in moderation. Therefore, you should strive at eating 70% fat, 25% protein, and 5% carbs. This kind of meals will help you to stay full for longer.

You should not unless you are feeling hungry. This will ensure that the body keeps very little glucose hence you reach Ketosis faster. You will be feeling so much hunger pangs when starting, but this will reduce once you are on Ketosis. However, if you feel that hunger is too much for you, then eat Keto-friendly foods that are high in fat and have moderate protein. Remember that the portion of your meals should not increase just because you have reduced the carb intake.

You should avoid the following foods that are rich in carbs if you want to get into ketosis:

- Sweetened beverages like sodas, juice, alcoholic beverages.
- Sugary foods like ice cream.
- Starchy vegetables like potatoes, peas, beans, corn.
- Wheat products like bread, pasta, cookies, and doughnuts.
- Cereals like rice, wheat, corn, and their products.

- Unhealthy fats like margarine and corn oil
- Processed foods like canned foods or packaged fast foods.
- Avoid foods that contain preservatives, artificial coloring, and sweeteners. Here is an example of a Keto meal plan: Breakfast
- You can have Spinach, eggs, bacon and unsweetened coffee or tea. Lunch
- You can have vegetable salads, meat, avocado, and broccoli and dress it with olive oil. Dinner
- You can prepare grilled chicken, zucchini, cauliflower gratin, and some salad dressing.

2. Increase your physical activity

Doing physical exercises can help you get rid of stored glycogen in your body. When our bodies get busy in any physical activity, it uses muscle glycogen as a source of energy. Therefore, when the glycogen reserve decreases, the body will resort to burning fat to get the needed energy. Therefore, increasing your physical activities will accelerate your ketosis process.

3. Try intermittent fasting

Intermittent fasting is the trending thing for those people who are trying to lose weight. It refers to going for some hours or even days without food. When you do not supply food to your body, it will resort to stored fats to convert it into energy. This will help you in getting rid of unwanted fats in

your body hence you will shed some weight in the process. There are several types of intermittent fasting. You can do the 16:8 plan, which means that you will eat within eight hours and then you fast in the remaining 16 hours. You can also go for 24 hours or more without food.

These short and long fasts will put you in a ketosis state. Although most people do intermittent fasting for weight loss, research has shown that it has other health benefits. People suffering from diabetes have found that intermittent fasting decreases blood sugar levels. It also helps in reducing cholesterol and slows down the aging symptoms. As you do the fasting, it is important to listen to your body! If you feel sick or nauseated during the fast, then you should break the fast with some healthy food.

4. Drink enough water

We all know that water is life! Water helps in digestion and the removal of toxins from the body system. It is also responsible for transporting important nutrients in the blood cells and other body cells. It also aids the liver in the metabolism process as well as the operations of the kidneys. Therefore, we should always keep our bodies hydrated to enable the proper functioning of the various body organs. Drinking water can also help you in your keto process by preventing the keto side effects like bad breath and dry mouth.

5. **Eat enough protein**

Although we are supposed to eat protein to achieve ketosis, we should not eat an excess of it because the body will convert the excess proteins into fats. Protein should be taken in moderation so that it can help the liver with a supply of amino acids that can be converted into glucose to be used by red blood cells and the brain cells. Proteins will also help you in

building muscle mass but excessive of it will alter the production of Ketones in your body.

6. **Watch your electrolyte intake**

When you switch to a low-carb keto diet, the kidneys will get rid of some minerals and water from your system. These minerals are electrolytes and they are magnesium, salts, potassium, and calcium. These minerals are very important in our body system because without them, you will be feeling some fatigue, dizziness, cramps, and mood swings. You can find most of these minerals in the bone broth and some keto-friendly foods. You should use the lite-salt because it has both sodium and potassium in it.

7. **Increase the healthy fat intake**

Eating healthy fats will help you to stay full for longer hence it will prevent unnecessary eating. These fats or oils will help you to reach a ketosis state easily. Some of the healthy fats include:

- Avocado
- Coconut oil
- Olive oil
- Flaxseed

How to Start a Ketosis Process?
1. **Make a plan• Plan keto-friendly meals**

You can make a meal plan for a few days, to begin with. Look for keto meal plans and their recipes online. Some of the most popular keto-friendly

foods are eggs, beef, vegetable salads, cucumbers, zucchini, chicken, fish, broccoli, cheese, plain yogurt, mushroom, and cauliflower among others. When preparing these foods, ensure that you use healthy oils like olive oils, coconut oils, and avocado oils.

- **Visit the grocery with the keto-food list**

When going shopping, ensure that you have prepared a keto-friendly shopping list. You can also search online for a keto shopping list to guide you on what to buy. Ensure that you check their labels for information about calories, fat, carb, and protein levels that they contain.

- **Purchase a home testing Ketone kit**

It is good to measure your blood ketone level so that you can know your progress and adjust where appropriate. You can do it with the help of indicator strips or ketone meters. You should do the test at least once daily. If you are on ketosis state, the readings in your ketone testing kit should be between 0.5 mmol/l – 3 mmol/l. You can also check the ketone levels in your blood by testing the blood samples and you can request your doctor to do it.

• Maintain a ketogenic diet for a week

After a few days of switching to a keto diet, you may get into a ketosis state. You can then decide on how many days you want to stay on ketosis. However, you should consult your nutritionist or doctor about how long you can safely maintain a ketogenic diet.

2. Shift to a ketogenic diet• Aim at consuming fewer carbs every day

You need to reduce your carb intake to less than 50 grams per day. You can achieve this by avoiding high carb foods like pasta, rice, potatoes,

wheat products, corn, legumes, and beans. You can replace these foods with low-carb foods.

• Eat healthy fats

We mentioned earlier that eating enough healthy fats will keep you feeling full and satisfied for a longer period. Examples of these healthy fat foods include avocados, olive oil, cheese, butter, and coconut oils. You can add these healthy fats into your keto diet to keep you satisfied for longer hours. You can also add whipping cream to your sugarless coffee or tea. Feeling more hunger pangs after switching to a keto diet is an indication that you are not eating enough healthy fats.

• Avoid starchy vegetables

The vegetable is very important in our bodies because they carry very essential nutrients however, you should reduce the intake of starchy vegetables so that you can reach ketosis. You should instead eat those vegetables that are very low in carbohydrates like cruciferous vegetables (cabbage, broccoli, cauliflower, and Brussels sprouts), zucchini, cucumbers, spinach, green leaves vegetables, mushroom, and tomatoes.

• Eat proteins in moderation

Proteins are very important in a ketogenic diet. However, eating proteins in excess will alter the production of ketones in your body because the body will convert it into glucose. The excess glucose will then be converted and stored as fats. A good source of protein is beef, fish, eggs among others.

• Include high fiber foods in your diet

Adding high fiber foods to your diet is important because it aids in digestion.

Although most high fiber foods are carbs, you can still find carb-

free foods that are high in fiber like flaxseeds, chia seeds, and almonds. Eating high fiber food will help you prevent constipation.

- **Take more coconut oil**

Using extra virgin coconut oil will help you reach your ketosis easily and it comes with other health benefits.

3. **Make lifestyle adjustments • Avoid snacking**

For optimum ketosis state, you should minimize the number of times that you eat in a day. Eating several snacks will hinder you from achieving your ketosis state. You should minimize the snack time you have per day and when you take snacks, ensure that they are keto-friendly. Avoid packaged snacks because most of them contain carbs. You can take low carb snacks like plain yogurt, macadamia nuts or a boiled egg.

- **Drink enough water to stay hydrated**

You need to take enough water every day so that your body organs can function well. You should not drink more than enough water because it will strain the kidneys. Bone broth is also very helpful because it hydrates you as well as provides you with some minerals.

- **Exercise**

When you engage in any physical activity, your body burns carbs into energy and if there is not enough supply of carbs, the body will resort to stored fats for energy. Therefore, exercising can hasten your ketosis process. Exercising for at least 30 minutes daily can give the best results. You can vary your type of exercise to prevent monotony. You can talk a walk, jog around or even run.

- **Get enough sleep**

Getting enough sleep can lower your stress levels. High-stress levels can increase the level of sugar in your blood and this can hinder you from achieving ketosis faster. You should aim at sleeping a minimum of 8 hours daily. This will ensure that your body gets enough rest and re-energizes.

Why Keto Is Convenient

Keto diet is gaining popularity because of its ability to aid in weight loss as well as enhancing the wellbeing of your physical and mental health. The following are some of the reasons why we think keto is convenient.

1. **It helps in weight loss program**

Keto diet is a low carb high-fat diet. Research shows that people who are on a keto diet lose weight faster than those other people who are on a low- fat diet. Since you will be taking high fat and low carb, you will reduce the number of times you eat per day because the high fat and protein will keep you full for longer. The reduction of carbs supply in your body will enable the body to burn stored fats for energy. This will get rid of unwanted fats in your body hence you will shed some weight because of the burned fats.

2. Reduced blood sugar and insulin levels

Keto has become very popular among individuals living with diabetes. This is because reducing carbs intake lowers blood sugar and insulin levels and most diabetic people confess that keto has reduced their insulin dosage by a great percentage. Research shows that the keto diet helps in controlling blood sugar and most diabetic patients who are on keto no longer use glucose-lowering medicines. Therefore, reducing carbs intake will give you good blood sugar levels and it can reverse type 2 diabetes. Keto diet has

also proven to help in controlling insulin levels in patients with type 1 diabetes.

3. Helps in treating Epilepsy in children

A research done in 1998 on 150 children who took carbs restricted diet shows that it was effective in decreasing their seizures by 90%. The keto diet proved to be more helpful on the epilepsy patients more than the anticonvulsant drugs.

4. Improves blood pressure

A research done in 2007 showed that a low carb diet was effective in controlling blood pressure. This is because keto diet helps in reducing body mass, LDL cholesterol, and triglycerides. An increase in blood pressure can put you at risk of getting heart diseases and kidney failure. Triglyceride, which is the fat molecules, that circulates in the bloodstream is dangerous because it can cause heart disease.

Reducing carb intake will lower these fat molecules from your bloodstream drastically. On the other hand, LDL is bad cholesterol that circulates in the bloodstream and it can cause heart diseases. Eating a low carb diet will help you to prevent these unpleasant health conditions.

5. Improves the mental Health

Taking too much sugar is not good for your brain and high carbs intake has proved to worsen the condition of Alzheimer patients. Research shows that a keto diet helps to reverse Alzheimer's because the ketone bodies help in improving the memory operations of Alzheimer patients.

Ketone bodies have numerous health benefits to the brain like protecting the brain cells, preserving the neuron, and preventing its loss. Therefore, a

low carb diet will significantly improve the health and functions of the brain cells.

6. Helps in the treatment of polycystic ovary syndrome and infertility

Polycystic ovary syndrome (PCOS) is a condition that causes infertility in most women because of the enlarged ovaries that contain cysts. High levels of insulin trigger this condition and it makes the ovaries to release androgens as well as lowering the production of sex hormone. The sex hormone glycoprotein blocks testosterone from getting into the cells. Although there is no such study that shows the relationship between PCOS and diet, keto diet help reduce insulin levels that cause PCOS. Therefore, keto can improve fertility in women.

Testing for Ketosis Process

If you are on a keto diet or fasting, chances are your body is producing ketones. However, you should be in nutritional ketosis where you will reap the most benefits. Therefore, you need to test so that you can know your level of ketosis. Keto diet alone does not determine your level of ketosis. We have other factors like your reaction to food and the activities that you engage in can determine the success of your ketosis.

Testing your ketone levels will help you to understand your progress and adjust your food where necessary. You can adjust your diet and do the testing so that you can know which kinds of food are the most effective in producing more ketones. There are three types of ketone testing:

- The blood tests
- Urine test
- Breath analyzer

The blood test will give the best and most reliable result of the three methods. Our bodies can release three types of ketone bodies namely:

- Acetoacetate: this is the first ketone body that the body produces when there is no longer a supply of glucose for energy. The liver will convert fats into fatty acids, then further converts the fatty acids into ketones. These types of ketones are present in the initial stages of ketosis and it can be detected in urine.

- Acetate (acetone): we get this ketone when acetoacetate is broken down and we exhale it through the lungs as a waste product.

- Beta-hydroxybutyrate (BHB): this is the most common ketone body that is present in blood and goes to cells in the form of energy. It provides the brain cells, muscles, and other body organs with the needed energy. After reviewing the different types of ketones, we can now look at the various methods that we can use to test ketones in our bodies.

1. Urine strips

Urine strips are popular among diabetes patients because they use them to check the diabetes ketones. You can buy urine strips over the counter on any drug store or supermarket pharmacies. You will use it by dipping the strip in the urine collected and wait for a few minutes then read the color of the strip and compare it with the illustrated colors in the package. The color starts from faint to darker and the darker the strip the more ketones you have in your body.

However, urine strips do not give accurate results. This is because when entering into ketosis, acetoacetate ketones spill into the urine and this

might give you a wrong impression on your level of ketosis. The level of hydration in your body will also affect the results of the strip because if you test the urine when you are highly hydrated, the results will not be the same as during dehydration. Therefore, urine strips can only give accurate results for diabetes ketones but not nutritional ketones.

2. **Breath test: Acetone indicator**

The breath test is for testing acetone, which is a byproduct of breaking down acetoacetate. However, you cannot use it to measure the number of ketones in your body that is working as fuel. You will need a breath meter that you plug into a battery source. You use the breath meter by blowing into it until the flashing light starts reading your breath acetones then you can check the color blinking and the number of times it is blinking then compare with the one illustrated in the package.

There are external factors that can alter the results of the test like chewing gums, cigarettes, toothpaste, garlic, alcohol, and other food substances that can make the sensor malfunction. Your breathing pace can also affect the acetone level. Therefore, when doing the breath test you need to consider factors like the environment condition, the breathing pace as well as the sensor validity.

You will need to practice breathing techniques severally to get reliable results. You should also purchase a breath meter that allows you to change the sensor and one that you can adjust to a known control.

3. **The blood ketone meter**

This is the most reliable method of the three. We use the blood ketone meter to measure BHB (beta-hydroxybutyrate) which is the most active ketone body, it circulates in the blood to the cells, and it converts into useful energy. You can do this by taking your blood sample through

pricking your finger then squeeze the blood out onto a little strip from the machine and wait for a few seconds to read the machine. Remember to use alcohol to disinfect the area you are pricking to prevent any infection.

There you go; you can now know the BHB level in your blood! You will be able to know the number of ketone bodies that are fueling your body. The advantage of blood ketone meter is that factors like hydration or temperature do not interfere with the outcome unlike in breath tests. Although this method is expensive, it is the best way that you can know your actual ketone levels.

Eliminate the Wrong Convictions of Fat

I grew up with a mentality that fats are not healthy and that I should take a low-fat diet so that I can live a healthy life but I was wrong and I know that I am not alone in this wrong myth. The truth is that there are fats that are good for you and others are bad for your health. Therefore, the belief that a low-fat diet is healthier than a high-fat diet is not justified because it all depends on what kinds of fats you are eating.

There are different types of fats: bad ones and good ones. Monounsaturated fats and polyunsaturated are healthy fats. These fats come from vegetables, nuts, fish, and seeds. The bad fats include the industrial made Trans fats that come in solid kinds of margarine and vegetable shortening while the saturated fats are neither good nor bad and they mostly come from animal products like meat and whole milk.

Our bodies require fats because it helps in absorbing minerals and vitamins. They are also vital in building the cell membranes as well as the sheaths encircling the nerves. The belief that you should eat a low-fat diet

to lower your cholesterol is also not true. The following are some of the myths about fats that nutritionist have proven to be wrong.

1. Eating fat will make you fat

Eating healthy fats like avocados, olive oil, coconut oil, and butter will help you stay full longer hence; it suppresses your craving for food and the urge to overeat. This can be a useful trick in weight loss management.

2. Fats are not important in our bodies

This is not true because healthy fats help us in absorbing important nutrients and vitamins as well as antioxidants and it supplies our bodies with energy. Fats extracted from fish, nuts, and seeds are good for the heart and the brain cells. They also help in weight loss and maintenance. Fats are also responsible for regulating body temperature and hormones.

3. A low-fat diet is good for weight loss

This is false. Our bodies require enough fats for energy purposes and the growth of cells. You need to know which good fats are and which ones are not good. Healthy fats like monounsaturated and polyunsaturated fats can be useful in weight loss if you include them in your diets. Most of the packaged foods that write low fat in their label contain sugars. We all know that sugar will hinder weight loss. Other factors can lead to weight gains like excess intake of carbs and calories.

4. Fats increase cholesterol levels in the bloodstream

Healthy fats like monounsaturated fats and polyunsaturated fats do not raise the bad cholesterol in your bloodstream but Trans-fats do and you should avoid them. You should also limit the consumption of saturated fats.

5. Saturated fats clog the arteries

A research done by a team of cardiologists shows that there is no evidence for this claim because they did not find any relationship between the consumption of saturated fats and the risk of heart diseases. They instead said that people should eat healthy food and exercise to prevent coronary diseases instead of blaming it on the dietary saturated fats. They also noted that patients living with chronic inflammatory disease responded well with eating healthy fats like olive oil, and the oils from nuts and fish. The omega 3 fatty acids found in these oils helps in preventing heart diseases.

Take away

It is important to know what kind of fat you are consuming because healthy fats are very crucial for healthy living while Trans fats can cause problems for your health.

Control Calories with Low Carb

Calories refer to the amount of energy that you get from food and the energy you use on physical activities. For weight gain, you subtract the calorie going out from the calorie coming in. If you want to lose weight then you should control your calorie intake even if you are on a keto diet or you can increase your physical activities so that you can burn the excess calories. The number of calories that you can consume will depend on what you want to achieve, how physically active you are and your basal metabolic rate (BMR).

Eating a low carb diet can generally reduce the number of calories that you consume because the macronutrients from high fat, protein, and low carb suppress the cravings for food. However, if you take the high-fat diet in excess, it can add up to more calorie intake. Most of the Keto-friendly

foods like avocados, olive oil, and full-fat dairy contain a high amount of calories so you should eat them in moderation if you plan to lose weight.

To control the calories in a keto diet, you need to be very meticulous when it comes to your food portion. You also need to consider engaging in physical exercises to ensure that you burn more calories than the amount you take. If your plan is just to reach ketosis and improve your well-being, then your attention should be on the quality of the food you eat and not calories. However, if your main aim is to cut some weight, then you will need to watch your calorie intake and adjust appropriately.

You may not alter the amount of protein and carbs you take while on keto but you can adjust the amounts of fat so that you can monitor the caloric intake. The carb levels should be low and you can focus on the green leafy vegetables while you eat proteins in moderation to help you in building your mass muscles.

Therefore, it is important to track the number of calories that you take as well as the macronutrient's quality. This will ensure that you do not experience some nutrient deficiencies as well as gain weight from consuming too many calories. On the other hand, you should engage in physical exercises to keep you fit.

Keto Health

Keto diet is among the trending diet plans available. It is popular among diabetic patients and those people who wish to lose weight. It involves taking 75% high-fat food, 20% protein, and only 5% carbs. After a few days of observing this percentage of foods in your diet, your body will get into a state called ketosis whereby the body burns stored fat in the body.

Therefore, this diet plan restricts carb intake and focuses on taking a high- fat diet.

The following are some health benefits of keto:

1. Helps in weight loss

Perhaps this is the #1 reason why keto gained popularity. Keto helps in burning stored fats and suppressing the cravings for food so this will prevent frequent snacking. Eating fewer carbs also will help in reducing the amount of calorie intake and the protein and fat in the diet will provide a satiating effect.

When carbs intake reduces, the body's metabolism changes and accelerates the burning of fat to get energy. Therefore, the body uses most of the fat sources and converts it into energy. This process of burning fat will enable the body to burn calories too. However, to get rid of more calories you need to ensure that you limit the calorie intake and do more activities that are physical.

2. Blood sugar control

Keto helps in stabilizing blood sugar and the mood swings that come with the fluctuation of blood sugar levels. Keto diet is helpful to diabetes patients because the low carb intake prevents the huge spikes in blood sugar hence lowering the need for insulin. However, you should be careful not to combine a keto diet with insulin because it can lead to hypoglycemia a condition for low blood sugar. Ensure that you talk with your doctor concerning your switch of diet while on medication.

3. Keto improves brain function and mental health

Ketosis helps in protecting the brain from damage by shifting the energy source and regulating the energy metabolism genes. It also protects it from

oxidative stress that can damage it. Oxidative stress promotes brain aging, depression, and anxiety. Ketones provide the brain with energy when it cannot get it from glucose and this helps to improve memory performance by balancing the brain chemicals.

People doing keto confess that it provides them with mental sharpness and creativity that helps them to handle multitasking while they maintain a motivated attitude. It increases blood flow to the brain hence reinforcing the various memory and sensory operations. Keto can treat epilepsy in children because of its ability to reconnect brain energy metabolism. Epileptic kids who shift to keto decrease their seizure by a greater percentage.

4. Eliminates food cravings

Eating a high fat, moderate protein, and low carb diet will give you a satiating effect. It will make you feel full for longer hence your appetite for frequent snacking will no longer be there. This will help you to focus on eating healthy low carb diets during the main meals. You will no longer have to worry about your addiction to overeating because keto will put your appetite under control.

5. Reduces anxiety and depression

Keto helps protect the brain from the damage of oxidative stress that can cause depression and anxiety. Keto diet stabilizes blood sugar that can cause fluctuation in mood swings. Therefore, being on keto can keep your moods on track!

6. Good for your heart

Keto can help you to lose weight that can lead to cardiovascular diseases such as high blood pressure, high blood sugar that can cause the

inflammation of the arteries and increase in bad cholesterol. These conditions are not good for the heart. Therefore, keto helps in preventing the conditions that can be harmful to the heart.

The Downside of Keto

Although you can reap many benefits from a keto diet, there is an unpleasant downside of this diet plan and you should study it carefully if you plan to do it on a long-term basis. Some of the side effects occur naturally while you are on keto while others can occur if you do it the wrong way. The medical community, however, points out that keto might not be a safe long-term diet plan. Here are some of the unpleasant downsides that you will experience while on keto.

1. Keto flu

During the first weeks of being on keto, your body will be struggling to adapt to the new diet and the carb reduction. As a result, you will lose some water and electrolytes and this might make you feel sick. The keto flu symptoms are:

- Frequent headaches
- Fatigue
- Nausea
- Dizziness
- Brain fog
- Irritability

These symptoms can subsidize when your body enters ketosis state. You will need to press on until your body gets used to a low supply of carbohydrates.

2. Nutritional deficiencies

Keto diet is a restricted diet. That means there are some foods that you are not supposed to eat while on keto. The foods that you restrict or ban from your diet contain some essential nutrients to your well-being. Beans, legumes, fruits, and some vegetables provide us with vitamin C and fiber yet keto restricts its intake. Therefore, keto will deprive you of getting very important nutrients by eliminating certain food from your diet.

3. Limited food choice

Keto involves restriction of carbs yet most of the foods available contain carbs. If you are restricting carb intake, then it means that you will have a list of foods to choose from in your diet. You will need to cut off all the grains and their products as well as all the starchy vegetables and all the sugars. This diet plan may not be sustainable in the end because you will be craving for foods that you eliminated.

4. Expensive

Most of the keto meal plans are expensive compared to non-keto meals. The oils used in the keto diet like olive oils, coconut oils, and fish oils are also quite expensive when you compare to the ordinary cooking oils. You can find avocados when they are in season but the avocado oil can be hard to find not to mention its high cost.

5. Loss of electrolytes

When your body reaches a ketosis state, it will start eliminating glycogen from the muscles and the liver and this can lead to frequent urination.

When you lose more water in your body, you also lose electrolytes like sodium, potassium, and magnesium that are very crucial for heart operations. Therefore, you will have to look for electrolyte supplements to replace the lost ones.

6. Health concerns

There is no existing study on the long-term safety of keto use but the medical community suggests that long-term use may not be healthy. People who have used keto for long reported digestion problems like constipation, diarrhea, and bloating. Lack of enough fiber in the diet is the main reason for such stomach problems.

Kidney stones are another common problem for someone who uses a keto diet for several months or even years. People reported to having abdominal pains that later turned to be kidney stones. This could be the effects of consuming too much animal proteins.

Ketoacidosis is also a problem that can occur while you are on a keto diet. This occurs when the body produces too much ketone bodies and the blood become too acidic. This condition is dangerous because it can damage the kidneys, liver and even the brain. Ketoacidosis can affect most people with diabetes and are on a keto diet. Therefore, diabetic individuals need to be extra watchful of their glucose levels while on keto.

Patients suffering from liver failure, pancreatitis, a disorder of fat metabolism, should consult their doctors before getting into keto. Although keto helps improve fertility in women, research shows that it can harm the growing fetus because it will lack some important nutrients that are crucial for its growth and development. You also need to check your body regularly if you have a history of anemia in your family. This is because a nutritional deficiency can put you at risk of contracting it.

7. Weakened immune system

Eating high fat and less fiber can mess with the balance of good and bad bacteria in your gastrointestinal tract. Since the GI protects your immune system, the imbalance of bacteria in it can have an impact on the gut-brain connection as well as the immune connection and this can cause diseases.

Fruits and vegetables are good for protecting the immune system. However, keto restricts the intake of vegetables and fruits that contains carbs this can make you susceptible to chronic illness or long-term diseases.

Keto for Weight Loss

Keto diet is high in healthy fat with moderate protein and low carbs. Since your body will cut down the supply of carbs that is supposed to provide glucose for energy, the body will source for glucose elsewhere within the body. The liver can rescue your body with energy by converting the stored fats into ketone bodies. This process is ketosis.

To reach ketosis, you will need to restrict your daily carb intake to less than 50 grams. If you aim to lose weight, then you have to watch the calories you consume through fats. You also have to ensure that the fats that you consume are healthy ones like olive oil, avocado oils, and nuts. Remember that it is important to engage in physical exercises so that your body can burn excess calories.

Keto is a great tool for weight loss because the high fat and the protein in the diet will keep you feeling full for longer hence you will reduce the number of snack times as well as the calorie intake. Keto will help you to suppress your appetite for food giving you more self-control on what you

can eat. It will also supply you with the needed energy for physical activities. Therefore, the keto diet is good enough for those people who wish to cut some weight.

Chapter 3: Ketogenic Diet for Women after 50

Ketogenic Diet and Diabetes

The Ketogenic diet is something that makes headlines these days, and that's because approvals by celebrities and supermodels have pushed it into popular culture. However, one of the questions being asked is,"Is the ketogenic diet plan effective for people with diabetes?"

Medically, the Ketogenic diet is not highly recommended for people with type 1 diabetes' however, in terms of the management of type 2 diabetes, there is no straightforward answer.

Some data shows that the ketogenic diet might be helpful, while others like a study on Nutrients published in September 2016, highlights the significance of whole grains as a dietary requirement for people living with diabetes – an unacceptable category of food in the keto diet.Though the Ketogenic diet comes with a lot of potential benefits for the management of diabetes, a lot of discipline and commitment is required in other to reap the rewards.

Thus, if you're someone suffering from diabetes, it is important to explore the following questions in other to ascertain whether it's right for you.

What exactly are the health benefits of a Keto Diet for Diabetes?

According to Lori Zanini, RD, CDE, the author of Eat What You Love Diabetes Cookbook, if you are trying to manage type 2 diabetes, this is how the ketogenic diet may help, "With a higher protein and fat intake, individuals may feel less hungry and are often able to lose weight, since protein and fat take longer to digest than carbohydrates." It also helps to boost and maintain energy levels.

The ketogenic diet also contains other possible benefits. For example, a September 2016 review posits that a Keto diet may improve A1C test results for people with diabetes (A result that shows average blood sugar levels within 3 months) better than low-calorie diets. The diet can also help reduce triglycerides better than a low-fat diet, which is beneficial for diabetes patients that are exposed to a higher risk for heart disease.

In addition, a keto diet is likely to be three times more efficient for weight loss than a low-fat diet – impressive because the loss of even five to ten percent of total body weight can come with health benefits such as improved blood pressure, cholesterol, and blood sugar mitigation (as stated by the Center for Disease Control and Prevention). Furthermore,

_____ _____

the European Journal of Clinical Nutrition in August 2013 published a review that posited that a Keto diet might be capable of controlling blood sugar levels and improving cholesterol levels.

Is the Keto diet the most effecting eating approach for Type 2 Diabetes?

Several modern research studies support the use of the ketogenic diet in the management of diabetes, and some hospitals have gone as far as implementing therapeutic keto programs. Virta Health, which offers a telemedicine lifestyle and diet program, has projected research that shows that embracing online support may help diabetic patients lower their A1C, lose weight and get off diabetes medication more successfully than the American Diabetes Association recommended the diet. Diabetes Therapy published the study in February 2018.

However, it is important to understand that the Keto diet isn't the best possible path for every diabetic patient. Some studies project other plans like the Mediterranean diet – which is rich in vegetables, lean meats, fruits, nuts, whole grains, olive oil, and fish- to be more suited for diabetic patients. In the April 2014 issue of the Nutrients, a published review posited that the Mediterranean diet helps to lower the risk of developing type 2 Diabetes.

In the January issue of Diabetes Care, a randomized controlled trial posited that adherence to a Mediterranean diet without any calorie ceiling might help prevent diabetes. The diet plan may also help people already inflicted with the sickness. The review also quoted some studies that linked the Mediterranean diet with better blood sugar control.

There are risks associated with the Keto diet. In 2016, the Journal of Obesity and Eating Disorders published a study that posits that type 2 diabetic patients who take oral medication to reduce their blood sugar may be prone to low blood sugar or hypoglycemia when following a keto diet. Also, a keto diet can lead to side effects like chills, fever, fast heartbeat, excessive hunger and thirst, confusion, fatigue, headache, nausea, dizziness, and bad breath, etc.

If you are suffering from Type 2 Diabetes, what is the best way to start a Keto Diet?

If you're living with type 2 diabetes, it is advisable to check in with your medical support team before you explore the Keto diet plan. Also, it is important to slowly implement the diet, gradually reducing carbs, because radical reductions may cause low blood sugar or hypoglycemia, especially for people on insulin or oral diabetes medications. Sylvia White, RD, CDE, a nurse In Memphis, Tennessee, says, "if your blood sugar level dips, glucagon, the emergency medication, might not even be able to boost it."

She went on to stress the need for regular checks on ketone and blood sugar levels to ward off serious side effects. "It is important to do so to avoid diabetic ketoacidosis. Some early symptoms of diabetic ketoacidosis include consistent high ketone levels, high blood sugar, frequent urination, dry mouth, vomiting, and nausea. These complications can result in a diabetic coma.

It is also important to consume a balance of nutrients, especially fiber, minerals, vitamins, and others – as well as the right amount of healthy

keto-friendly fats and calories. Generally, healthy fats include omega-3s and monounsaturated fats, which are known to improve cholesterol levels and reduce inflammation. Consume sunflower seeds, peanut butter, almonds, and avocados for monounsaturated fats, and a fatty fish like salmon for omega-3s.

If you're confused, reach out to your dietician, because most times people only focus on what not to eat, without paying attention to foods that should be included in their diets, including lean proteins, healthy monounsaturated fats, vegetables, and many more.

How do you stick to the low carb count on the Keto Diet?

No matter how you look at it, it's not an easy task to eat just twenty to sixty grams of carbs per day (the permitted amount of carbs on the keto diet). Thus, for people to observe

this rigid guideline, they need to change the food they eat and their entire lifestyle.

Typical foods that constitute the American diet like milkshakes, Big Macs, and for-long subs, don't fit into the ketogenic diet plan – also, foods known as staples of a balanced diet such as whole-grain bread and sweet potatoes may need to be controlled. These modifications can be hard to execute, even for people already eating healthy diets. A practice that comes in handy is tracking the food you eat. You can either use apps on your smartphone or with a paper food diary.

The plan doesn't allow you to take days off. You have to be disciplined if you intend to achieve results – or else you'll just be eating a high-protein, high-fat diet.

Is the Keto diet safe for everyone who has Type 2 Diabetes?

The ketogenic diet is not safe for everyone with Type 2 diabetes; it is particularly bad for people that have already developed kidney issues because then, protein intake has to be limited.

People with type 1 diabetes also need to be wary of the keto diet. The American Diabetes Association warns that Ketones (synthesized during ketosis) are mainly a risk factor for DKA, which is prominent in people with type 1 diabetic patients than type 2 diabetic patients.

It is also important to diligently look out for other possible symptoms of DKA.

Furthermore, another set of people that should be wary of the Keto diet are those with a history of heart disease. During the initial stages of the Keto diet, cholesterol levels tend to increase, and this can increase the risk of heart disease. Also, yo-yo dieting, which can easily occur on a keto diet plan, is capable of straining the heart, possibly causing a heart attack or stroke.

It is important to work with a dietician or doctor to work out the right diet plan for you, especially if you have a history of struggling with an eating disorder. Irrespective of what you've heard or read on the internet, you have to understand that a history of binge eating disorder and the Keto diet do no match at all. The restrictions imposed by the ketogenic diet on carbs increases the risks of compulsive overeating, bingeing, and other eating disorders.

Chapter 4: Ways to Start the Keto Lifestyle

Past Perspective on Your Diet

Food is generally supposed to be eaten to provide nourishment to the body. It is the source of energy as well as the fuel for growth. Human beings eat food for a number of reasons. They can eat to celebrate a certain occasion while they make merry with friends and family. They also eat for pleasure especially when they are socializing. Sometimes, people eat because they have nothing else to do, they can do so out of boredom or loneliness. Food can also be consumed out of habit or because a person is accustomed to certain traditions.

A good number of people turn to food when they are stressed or anxious about something. Food in such cases becomes a drug for comfort. Rather than turn to habits such as drinking or smoking these kinds of people get their high from food. Notably, just as with the case of drunks and smokers, emotional eaters also regret their choices soon after they indulge in an unhealthy meal. Eventually, they also suffer the consequences of their 'substance abuse'.

People's intake of food also depends on an individual's lifestyle. For example, there are those people who like staying fit so they are very cautious about what they put in their mouths. They also exercise on a regular basis to keep their weight on check. Although they may appear to be healthy, some of them struggle to maintain their lifestyle. They agonize over what they are missing out, how to avoid social gatherings or people who may mislead them from their diet plans. Spending too much time planning for the next meal in addition to the agony of wanting to burn off excess calories after indulging in a treat eventually begins to stress them out.

For another set of people, their lives are too chaotic for them to sit and have a decent meal. A working mom, for example, who juggles a hectic work schedule, family time and volunteer work, might not find time to eat healthily. She may result in eating while on the move or multitask while eating. This means that she eats while driving or walking to a meeting or when answering phone calls and emails. This mom will only eat a proper meal when she gets back to the house. If she is too tired to eat, she will have another snack and retire to bed. She may also want to eat healthily and is clearly aware that she should eat more nutritional food but is unable to do so because of her crazy work schedule.

There is also another group of people who seem to be unaffected by what they eat. They are not bothered by what they eat nor do they care to follow diets or engage in exercise. Those who manage to remain slender after all the eating is the envy of many. A majority of natural eaters, however, appear soft and round. Some may appear strong and built because of either their genes or engaging in some form of physical activity that builds muscle.

Wherever you fall in the above categories, you should always ensure that your diet has the right amount of calories. A proper diet should not too little calories or too many calories. The exercise junky might be getting too few calories while the natural eater might be consuming too many calories. People who do not get enough calories end up losing muscle mass and succumb to health problems. Eating too many calories leads to high blood pressure, heart disease, diabetes or even death.

A healthy diet should also have the right amounts of fat and the right type of fat. Generally, it is advisable to avoid unhealthy fats such as saturated fats found in fatty meat and dairy products such as butter and cream. Trans-fats found in commercial foods such as cakes and fried junk food should be kept to a minimal. Fats increase cholesterol levels in the blood and can block arteries or cause heart attacks and stroke.

High amounts of sugar in a diet also put you at risk of gaining weight and developing health problems similar to the ones listed above. Sugar comes in many forms and therefore has different names. Added sugar is a very common ingredient in modern diets and people should avoid anything that has added sugar. High consumption of sugar leads to weight gain and is associated with diseases such as type 2 diabetes and heart disease.

Fruits and vegetables should be consumed in large amounts but they seem to make the least appearance in most people's diets. People are also choosing to substitute water with other unhealthy drinks that are harmful to the body. Salt is also consumed but sometimes at extreme levels while nuts and seeds are not incorporated on a regular basis.

In an attempt to overcome unhealthy eating habits people also get into all sorts of diets. Fad diets are unrealistic and as much as they may help a person lose weight on the onset, most are not sustainable. They also deprive people of healthy foods that are important to the body. Any person who wants to start a diet allows them to consume foods from most if not all food groups but of course, everything should be consumed in moderation. Exercise is also important in maintaining a healthy weight and general health of the body.

It is important to review your diet and reason out whether the diet you are following offers the right amounts of nutrients that are able to feed and

nourish your cells as well as give you a general feeling of happiness. A good diet should also enable you to eliminate waste on a regular basis and give you energy.

Wrong Eating Habits

Most people have an idea of what they should and should not eat. Some have even gone a step further to carefully plan their meals and sign up for fitness classes. However, for some reason, they are still not able to achieve healthy weight levels. Healthy eating does not just involve eating the right types of foods; how people eat and the habits they form around food contribute a great deal, to whether or not they live happy and healthy lifestyles.

The number one cause of unhealthy diets is, of course, unhealthy food. Foods that contain high amounts of fat, calories, and sugar are considered unhealthy. The quality of food that you put in your mouth matters and affects your health. The best diets include foods from every group. They also include both animal and plant sources. Eating unhealthy fats raises your cholesterol levels so does eating excess carbohydrates and proteins. Occasionally, you can indulge in your favorite snack but you should remember to do it in moderation. Other healthy foods such as vegetables, fruits, and nuts are eaten in minimal quantities when they should occupy the most amount of space on your plate.

Some wrong eating habits that people have gotten accustomed to include:

1. Stocking up on tempting snacks

It is very hard to keep away from the food that you can see and is within your reach. Sometimes even storing unhealthy snacks inside the cupboard

or just in the house can tempt you to eat them. It is best to avoid stacking snacks in the house. If you have to snack keep fresh pre-chopped vegetables and fruits on the countertop.

2. Skipping breakfast

Breakfast is the most important meal of the day. When you load on a healthy breakfast, you get enough energy to take on the day. When you skip it, your metabolism slows down and you increase your chances of binging on an unhealthy snack or meal later on in the day because you are too hungry. Skipping breakfast eventually leads to weight gain in the end. Rushing through breakfast is also not advised.

3. Mindless eating

Mindless eating or snacking leads to unhealthy weight gain and it occurs when a TV, video game, or working on a computer, distracts people. Binging in front of the TV makes you gain weight in two ways. Eating while distracted by something else makes you eat more. You unknowingly consume larger portions of food especially if you are eating from a large bowl or out of a box. Most of the time when you eat out of a bag, you normally eat more than one serving, even several without knowing. This contributes to weight gain. If you have a habit of sitting or lying down for long hours, physical inactivity can make you retain a lot of weight.

4. Midnight and endless snacking

Eating at night is never a good idea. When people eat dinner and then go to bed immediately, their food does not get digested properly. When you also snack in the middle of the night, you also do not give the food time to digest well. Sleeping also puts the body in a state of inactivity meaning that the food consumed does not burn to energy so it has to be stored in the body and this contributes to weight gain. The other problem with midnight

snacking is the fact that people rarely snack on healthy foods. Most commercial snacks are unhealthy, they are either high in unhealthy fats, calories or contain added sugar and high amounts of salt. Unhealthy snacking during the day is also not advisable.

5. Eating on the move

When you eat while driving or walking in most cases, you are not conscious of how much you are putting in your mouth, so you end up eating a lot of food. The other activity you are engaged in also acts as a distraction so you end up consuming more food unknowingly. The other challenge with eating while distracted with another activity and eating quickly for that matter is that you

do not give your body enough time to register that you are full. Your brain takes time to receive the message that you are full and needs time to signal to you that you should stop eating. When you eat slowly and chew your food the right away, you give your body organs time to communicate with one another. Even the simple act of putting the spoon down or taking a sip of water slows you down to think whether you are full or not.

6. Eat out or order in too much

Most foods prepared in restaurants and fast foods are not prepared with healthy eating in mind. These foods are prepared to fulfill taste and flavor rather than nutrition. Restaurant meals are also normally served with extra sauces drizzled with excess oil and the quantities are usually more. It is very easy to gain weight when you constantly eat out or order in food. Most takeout meals or foods that are delivered are normally junk food, such as burgers, fries, or pizzas. Unlike when food is prepared at home, you also do not have much control over what unhealthy food items or spices are put in your food.

7. Take unhealthy drinks

Your favorite latte in the morning or cappuccino could just be as unhealthy as eating junk food and so is downing a flavored drink. It is very possible to consume more calories from a drink than a meal. In addition to the calories, some drinks contain high levels of sugar and the frothy drinks contain unhealthy fats. These drinks also replace water intake, which is very crucial in maintaining good health. Alcoholic drinks, on the other hand, add to the calories you consume.

Keto Friendly Foods Dairy & Eggs

Make sure you always get full-fat cheese and boycott low fat labeled products. Make it a tradition always to read labels because different brands count their carbs differently. All in all, just stay away from foods that come with an ingredient list

- Sour cream
- Eggs
- Ghee
- Heavy whipping cream
- Full fat cheese: cream cheese, parmesan cheese, cheddar cheese
- Butter
- Full fat yogurt

Fish and Meat

It is a well-known fact that meats contain zero (0) carbs, and the higher fat cuts are better for the keto diet. However, processed meats such as sausage, deli, or bacon sometimes contain carbs and hidden sugar contents.

- Duck
- Lamb

- Chicken meat
- Pork ribs
- Ground beef
- Organ meats
- Pork chops
- Salmon
- Sausage
- Pork Roast
- Shrimp
- Bacon
- Cold cuts
- Pork Chops

Keto Fats and Oils

In the keto diet, fat is extremely important, but as mentioned earlier, some fats are bad. Thus, you must boycott margarine and canola oil because they contain high amounts of polyunsaturated fats that escalate inflammation.

- Cocoa Butter
- Sesame oil
- Lard
- Avocado oil
- MCT oil
- Coconut oil
- Olive oil

Keto Vegetables & Fruits Shopping List

Don't ever make the mistake of skipping vegetables from your shopping list. It is important to make use of different vegetables and greens in your keto meals because they are rich in nutrients, fiber, and will help you remain in ketosis. Remember, some vegetables contain higher carbs than others. Thus it is important to work with the keto vegetable list. Below are some of the vegetables with low carbs fruits for making enjoyable keto dishes/

- Low Carb Vegetables
- Asparagus
- Broccoli
- Garlic
- Cauliflower
- Onions
- Cabbage
- Zucchini
- Cucumber
- Spaghetti squash
- Eggplant
- Salad mix
- Bell Pepper
- Lettuce

Low Carb Fruits

Generally, fruits possess some amounts of carb, and that is why you have to consume them moderately, especially in keto desserts or as a treat.

- Limes
- Avocados
- Lemon
- Blueberries
- Strawberries
- Raspberries
- Blackberries

Keto Seeds and Nuts for the Grocery List

- Nut butter
- Macadamia nuts
- Chia seeds
- Pistachios
- Almonds
- Pecans
- Sunflower seeds
- Peanuts
- Hazelnuts

Keto Pantry Items for a Grocery list

When you embrace the keto lifestyle, these are items you can use to make your meals taste good while you chase your primary motives. They are the following; • Basil

- Pickle juice
- Black pepper
- Hot sauce
- Mustard
- Beef jerky
- Curry powder
- Pork rinds
- Cayenne powder
- Coconut milk
- Chili powder

- Almond milk
- Italian seasoning
- Cashew milk
- Basil
- Coffee
- Black pepper
- Himalayan pink salt

Foods to Avoid

In the keto diet, it is not so difficult to identify foods that are not so good. All you have to do is to identify foods that contain high amounts of carbs and boycott them because they stand as an albatross on your quest to attain ketosis. Thus, the following are foods that you must not add to your ketogenic diet shopping list;

- Legumes, soybeans, beans, green peas, lentils, chickpeas;
- Grains – rye, oats, rice corn, wheat
- Starchy vegetables – corn, beets, yams, sweet potatoes, white potatoes;
- Sugar – coconut sugar, maple syrup, agave syrup, honey
- Pseudocereal grains – buckwheat, quinoa, amaranth
- Fruits – watermelon, oranges, plantains, pineapple, pears, bananas, apples

Wrong Food Combinations

All health experts condone overindulging in unhealthy meals. Most people are aware of the health risks and dangers associated with consuming unhealthy meals. Healthy meals that are combined in the wrong way are at times just as harmful as eating unhealthy meals.

1. Carbs and animal protein

A combination of steak and fries is bad. The starch in potatoes normally requires alkaline juices to digest while proteins require an acidic environment to be broken down. When the two are eaten together, they remain in the stomach and bring discomforts such as gas, flatulence, and heartburn. The same goes for a combination such as pasta and minced meat. The starch in pasta is converted to sugar and when combined with the meat, a person can develop diabetes. With time, a person who eats such combinations develops immunity but the excess intake, especially with a combination of fatty oils from both foods, leads to elevated cholesterol levels and unhealthy weight gain. It is okay to combine carbs with healthy plant protein such as beans that is why a combination such as rice and beans is not only delicious but also yummy.

2. Two high proteins

People are notorious for eating more than one protein and heavy ones for that matter during breakfast. One of the most popular combinations is bacon and eggs. As much as a person remains full for longer, the combination overworks the digestive system. This combination also gives a high-energy boost immediately after the meal but it also disappears after a short denying you proper energy to begin the day. Two proteins also take longer to digest. When you eat two proteins at the same time, it is advisable that you combine a light protein and heavy one but not two heavy proteins. The lighter one should be eaten first followed by the heavy one and the two should not be spaced out too much. They should also be eaten within 10 minutes of each other. A combination such as beans and cheese also fall in this category of two high proteins. They are both heavy to digest. Cheese and meat are also two high proteins that are difficult to digest.

3. Food with drinks

Food should never be taken with any beverage, even water. Water normally dilutes stomach acids, which digest food. It reduces the ability of the acid to breakdown the food in the stomach. Water or juices took immediately after meals also have the same effects on the digestive system.

4. Fruits after meals

We all love to fish with a juicy mango salad but experts advise that this is another disastrous food combination that people should avoid. Essentially fruits should be eaten before meals as they pass through the digestive system faster. When they are combined with a meal and especially a heavy protein, they have to stay in the digestive tract for long and the sugar in them

begins to ferment. You may think that you are making a healthy food

choice when you eat fruit instead of a slice of cake after a meal but you are also not doing the right thing for your body. If you have to eat fruit with a meal, it is always good to eat it before the meal.

5. Yogurt with fruit

Most of us have eaten this combination without giving it a second thought; both items are healthy with the yogurt providing a good dose of protein and calcium as well as good bacteria and the fruits bursting with vitamins. However, the two together are a bad idea. Milk and acid generally do not mix well. Since fruits are acidic, they are never a good fit for yogurt. The bacterium in yogurt also likes the sugar in fruit and does not hesitate to act on it. Dairy is also known for causing sinuses and cold allergies when it is combined with fruit, its effects worsen.

6. Cereal with juice

Cereal is a popular food item during breakfast and it normally goes well with milk. There are people who add juice to this combination, however, as earlier deduced the acid in juice is never a good combination with dairy products. The casein in milk and the acid together, normally curdle milk. The combination also destroys enzymes found in the starch of the cereal. The carbohydrate in cereal is therefore not broken down well.

The discomfort after eating this combination is characterized by a feeling of heaviness.

7. Tomatoes with pasta

Although this is a favorite among many people, the combination causes havoc in the stomach. Worse still is when the meal is combined with cheese. The acid in tomatoes curdles the dairy in cheese and interferes with the enzymes that digest starch in the pasta. Meats and carbs as earlier stated are also not one of the best combinations of foods.

8. Milk with banana

This is another popular combination probably because it is very easy to prepare. The sugar in the banana also adds a sweet taste to the milk. Banana is a fruit and like many fruits, it should not be consumed with dairy products. When fruits and especially sweet ones are combined with other foods, milk included, they stay in the digestive system for longer. Rather than add fruits to milk, a pinch of nutmeg or cinnamon stimulates the digestive system and does not slow it down.

Healthy Keto Food Combinations

The keto diet is becoming popular. However, a number of people are still not been able to achieve any substantial results with it. If people are not keen on both how and what they eat and the combinations of food that they eat, then they can hardly sustain the diets that they are following.

A proper keto diet should be high in healthy fats, it should have moderate amounts of protein and carbohydrates should be low. The fact that a keto diet helps you get rid of carbohydrates and bulks you on protein and starch should not be a reason for you to stock up on bacon and burgers. Although there is nothing wrong with a little bacon and butter, most of the food in the keto diet should be plant-based and then the protein and fat can be added on top of greens.

Vegetables provide healthy carbohydrates as well as fiber. Insoluble fiber cannot be broken down by bacteria neither does it dissolve in water. This means that it stays in the gut and cleans it up. It also helps the gut retain a lot of water, which makes waste softer and enables it to pass through easily.

Keto diets should also have resistant starches, which keep you fuller for longer. Some foods that have resistant starch in abundance include legumes, bananas, peas, and oats. Eating these types of foods prevent you from overeating proteins and carbohydrates. Aside from suppressing hunger, they also do not elevate blood glucose levels, unlike excess protein and carbs. Excess protein raises insulin levels the same way carbohydrates do. It is normally converted to glucose and stored as fat in the body.

Therefore, as you think of starting or resuming a keto diet, you should keep in mind that plants should take up more space followed by fats and then protein. Here are some good keto combinations

1. Vegetables drizzled with oil

Low carb vegetables such as broccoli, mushroom, celery, kale, or peppers are good choices in a keto diet. Pouring a generous amount of healthy oil such as olive oil on top of the vegetable makes a good keto meal. Ghee can also be used in place of the olive oil. Coconut oil can also make a great substitute. Since ketogenic diets also allow for moderate amounts of protein, cheese sprinkles can be added to the vegetables to provide nutrition and flavor. Unhealthy oils such as margarine should be avoided. Shortening oils and vegetable oils are also not healthy compared to super oils such as coconut and olive oils. You can prepare a combination of vegetables as long as you keep carbs on the check.

2. Chicken and avocado

Chicken is a very good source of protein while avocado is a good source of healthy fat, which makes this combination perfect for a person following the keto diet. Chicken can also be prepared in very many ways and according to a person's taste. Its diversity also ensures that a person is able to eat this meal in different ways, which means that they do not easily get

bored with it. The chicken can be boiled, grilled, or roasted and can be substituted with fish to make a healthy complete keto meal. Turkey can also be used in place of the chicken.

3. Fish and sour cream

If the taste of fish with avocado does not tingle your taste buds, you can try fish with some sour cream. A number of people like their fish with a slice of lemon but this would not make a complete keto meal. It lacks a vegetable and healthy fat. Fish is rich in protein and in addition to being a good source of protein, fish also has omega 3 which are healthy for the brain. The sour cream, on the other hand, brings in fat, which is essential in a keto diet. It also enhances the flavor of the fish. You can also ditch the sour cream altogether and have a grilled salmon combined with sautéed vegetables. Coconut oil can be used to sauté a good serving of spinach.

4. Pork chops with green beans

This combination can be eaten for dinner and is very filling. The pork, of course, provides the protein while the green beans sautéed in healthy oil such as coconut oil bring in the element of fat and vegetable nutrition.

5. Eggsandcheese

If you are looking for something healthy to have for breakfast while on a keto diet, eggs and cheese are a healthy combination. Rather than have eggs and bacon which are two high proteins, eggs and cheese is a much healthier combination. The egg provides the protein while the cheese provides an excellent source of fat. Cheese also contains protein but when combined with eggs, the protein intake is not too high as with other combinations such as meat and cheese. Eggs and cheese can also be used together in a Cobb salad. In addition to these two ingredients, a Cobb salad can have slices of turkey and a green vegetable especially one that is low on

carbs. You can also substitute the cheese and use a plant protein such as a mushroom; these two food items together with a bit of oil can make a tasty mushroom omelet. Eggs served with sautéed greens can also provide a healthy keto breakfast.

6. Healthy keto smoothies

Yogurt and fruits are not a good combination as earlier stated but yogurt and nuts go very well together. Greek yogurt enriched with nuts such as almonds, cashews or walnuts is a very healthy snack perfect for anyone on a keto diet. Yogurt is dairy and therefore provides a good dose of protein. It also has friendly bacteria that are good for your gut. Since regular dairy milk is not healthy if combined with fruits, an avocado can be combined with coconut milk to produce healthy coconut milk and avocado smoothie.

Water is very important in any diet and more so in a keto diet that is low in carbs. Carbs not only provide energy for the body but they also help the body to retain water. Any extra carbs are normally stored as glycogen in the liver. For the glycogen to stay together it needs water. Since ketogenic diets are low on carbs, there are normally no extra carbs to store in the liver, which means that the water molecules are also not needed. Therefore, a person on any low carb diet should ensure that they drink a lot of water, even more than the recommended eight glasses of water. Most alcoholic drinks and sweet drinks should be avoided mainly because they add carbs to the die. To have a variety of beverages, you can flavor your water or take sparkling water in place of soda. If you enjoy coffee and tea, you should keep it as plain as possible and avoid adding sugar.

Of course, electrolytes which include sodium, potassium, and magnesium should also be present in any diet include a keto diet. It is very easy to lose these minerals because of the way the diet flashes out water from the body.

To avoid this, a person on a low carb diet can consciously add salt or take supplements, otherwise, they risk contracting what is commonly known as the keto flu.

Chapter 5: Keto Shopping List

What healthy options should you consider having in your grocery- shopping list? Spinach and arugula, avocados, cucumbers, berries, olive oil, almond butter, parmesan and gouda cheese, natural yogurt, lamb chops, chicken, turkey, tuna, salmon, sardines, cod, bacon, walnuts, chia seeds, and flax seeds.

Keto is a high fat, high-protein, and low-carb eating plan that enables a person's body to burn fat instead of carbs for fuel, and ultimately leading to substantial weight loss.

The human body breaks down, carbohydrates into glucose, which the body uses for energy. When the body does not have enough energy, it goes into a state called Ketosis. During ketosis, the body burns fat and uses it for energy, in place of the glucose.

Ketosis, therefore, makes the ketogenic diet a popular option for people who want to lose weight. However, a person's body needs to go into ketosis before a person can begin to lose weight on the keto diet. That means reducing the intake of carbohydrates to the minimum. A diet that provides fewer than 50 grams of carbs per day can cause ketosis.

Keto Supplements

Certain supplements help to support a person's immune system and prevent nutrient deficiencies.

Here are the best supplements to consider having in your keto diet.

1. **Plant-based MCT oil**: Medium-Chain-Triglycerides (MCT) comes from coconut or palm oil. A person can put a tablespoon or two to a coffee or a smoothie to reach ketosis and improve mental energy. MCT oil gives high levels of circulating ketones in the blood, which fuels the brain cells and curb a person's appetite. A person should start with small doses to avoid stomach pain.

2. **Omega-3 fatty acids**: Fish oils are a valuable source of heart- healthy omega 3- fatty acids. The fats are essential for reducing cholesterol numbers connected to cardiovascular disease. Exposure to plant oils and clean sources of fish oils increases the chances of lowering cholesterol levels in a person's body.

3. **Magnesium supplements**: Magnesium is an essential nutrient for muscle and bone health and regulation of blood pressure. However, magnesium-rich foods like fruits and beans are high in carbs and can kick a person out of ketosis. Therefore, a person can substitute such foods for foods such as avocados and spinach that are low on magnesium.

4. **BHB Salts**: Beta-hydroxybutyrate (BHB) is an energy particle that a person's body produces when breaking down and burning fat. When a person is in ketosis, he or she has higher levels of BHB.

BHB salts facilitate a person's brain to lower the production of glucose and turn to burn fat instead.

5. **Collagen supplements**: Collagen is an animal protein that comes from the bones, bone marrows and the connective tissues of the animal. Collagen is a high source of energy that helps to strengthen muscles because ketosis can feed on the muscle if a person does not have enough fat for fuel. Collagen supplements have to contain MCT oil powder to make it keto-friendly.

6. **Calcium supplements**: Cheese, yogurt, and milk are rich in calcium but also high in carbs. Therefore, a person has to reduce the intake of such calcium-rich foods to minimize carbs. Alternatively, a person can obtain calcium from sardines, salmon, and mackerel with edible bones. In addition, the person can get calcium from calcium citrate or calcium carbonate supplements, which he or she should eat, with food to ensure maximum absorption.

7. **Digestive enzymes**: Digestive enzymes break down fats and proteins to facilitate a person's digestion and to prevent constipation. Fatty foods can increase chances of constipation, but digestive enzymes have lipase and protease that help to improve a person's digestion, in the absence of fiber-rich carbohydrates.

8. **Fiber supplements**: Fiber supplements such as psyllium increase fiber in ketogenic diets. A person should allow time for his or her gastrointestinal (GI) tract to adapt to the high fiber intake, to avoid cramping and gas.

Other keto-friendly fiber sources include cauliflower and brussels sprouts.

9. **Multivitamins Supplements**: Multivitamin keto supplements help to keep a person's body functioning normally by supplying the specific nutrients level that the body needs.

A person can take multivitamins that provide the B vitamins, to make up for his or her reduced intake of whole grains and legumes.

10. **Vitamin B complex supplements**: Vitamin B supplements help to reduce exhaustion, cramping, and brain fog. These are the symptoms a person experiences when switching to a low-carb eating plan.

Vitamin B increases blood sugar and brain energy levels as fats replace carbs as the body's primary source of energy.

11. **Electrolyte supplements**: Electrolyte supplements help to replace the levels of sodium, magnesium, and potassium that a person loses when taking the keto diet.

A person can begin to cut off water weight when the level of electrolytes goes down. A person loses great amounts of fluid through the keto diet, but the electrolyte supplements help to prevent such loss of electrolytes.

12. **Vitamin D3 supplements**: Vitamin D3 is essential for helping a person's body to absorb calcium. In that way, Vitamin D3 boosts the growth of body cells, reduces inflammation, and maintains the health of a person's bones.

Alternatively, a person can get this sunshine vitamin by exposing himself or herself to the sunrays. However, that exposure may not be enough to help a person's body to produce Vitamin D naturally.

Hormones Balance in Keto

A ketogenic diet helps to regulate specific hormone imbalances naturally. Here are ways in which going keto helps to put a person's body back in order.

1. Keto diet cools hot flashes

High estrogen levels cause the part of the brain that controls stress to become unstable when prompted abruptly. As a result, the body's temperature increases and then decreases within minutes.

Keto diet supplies the body with a continuous source of fuel, ketones, for the brain. In so doing, the hot flashes cool down. Hot flashes make menopausal women and those with Polycystic ovary syndrome (PCOS) to have distressing periods of a sudden rise in their body temperature.

2. Keto diet decreases inflammations

Inflammation can be good when it is an immune response to protect the body from disease and infection, and harmful when it causes inflammatory disorders.

Studies show that low-carb diets reduce the chances of inflammation by a more considerable margin than consuming low-fat diets. Ketogenic diets prevent factors responsible for chronic inflammation by activating a complex biochemical process that fights inflammation directly.

In addition, biochemical activity helps to reduce chronic inflammations related to health problems.

3. Keto diet facilitates weight loss

Since keto can regulate ghrelin and leptin, the hormones that bring an appetite, therefore a person following a keto diet can feel less hungry.

When ghrelin and leptin are not balanced, a person usually feels always hungry even when he or she eats something. The irregular increase in levels of hunger and decrease in fullness after eating prompts a person's craving to ingest more glucose.

Because the keto diet helps to balance these hormones, a person on a keto diet will, therefore, eat less and lose weight more naturally.

4. Keto diet increases energy levels

High energy levels during the day help people to sleep better at night. That is because keto helps to control levels of cortisol in the body, thus reducing stress levels and increasing energy production.

Keto diets provide slower-burning forms of energy that regulate blood sugar levels and produce enough energy for the day. Hormonal imbalance can increase the levels of cortisol production in the body. The stress hormone can suck up a person's energy and bring about restless sleep.

5. Ketodietlowersbloodpressure

A ketogenic diet lowers blood pressure by helping in weight loss. Being overweight is one of the top causes of high blood pressure.

A keto diet that takes processed foods off the shopping list, promotes foods that lower high levels of blood sugar in a person's body and reduces cholesterol levels and blood pressure.

High blood pressure is a risk feature for cardiovascular disease and can harm the well-being of a person's heart.

6. Promotes mental health

Hormonal imbalance can affect brain activity negatively. That is because the imbalance can reduce brain function.

Such cognitive glitches come about because of the brain's need for fuel. The brain struggles to get fuel when there is low production of hormones. However, the keto diet provides alternative sources of fuel that regulate energy stability in the body.

When a person has stable energy levels, hormones regain balance and thus improve the cognitive function.

Keto Aliments Can Kill Cancer

Although no single food can cure disease, research shows that the keto diet shows some degree of potential in reducing the growth of certain tumors. That includes slowing the growth of tumors, prolonging the survival rate of cancer patients, and delaying the initial growth stages of tumors.

Keto aliments improve the effectiveness of standard chemotherapy because the diet helps to keep the blood sugar in check. Cancer patients can benefit from the ketogenic diet by following the diet, along with their chemotherapy or cancer treatments.

Chemotherapy and cancer treatments are much more effective when a cancer patient takes in low-carb meals. Health practitioners recommend patients to eat 70 to 80 percent fat, and 10 to 25 percent protein to help with cancer treatment. However, health experts do not guarantee that the keto diet can help to prevent cancer.

Keto diet strengthens regular cancer treatment by inducing metabolic oxidative stress in cancer cells, but not in the healthy cells. In addition, some cancer cells rely heavily on glucose for energy. Therefore, limiting

the access of cancer cells to glucose may cause the cancer cells to respond positively to chemotherapy.

According to research, the keto diet, along with the medical restriction of blood glucose prevents the growth of squamous cell carcinoma (SCC) in mice with lung cancer. Even though such interventions did not reduce the size of the tumors in the mice, they prevented the tumors from developing. That only applied to the SCC cancers and not to the lung adenocarcinoma cancers.

However, it is still too early to tell whether the outcomes of the research can apply to humans. For now, the keto diet may only act as a complementary therapy for some patients going through cancer treatment.

That is to say that when cancer patients follow a ketogenic diet, they help to strengthen their metabolic network systems throughout the body. As long as a person's mitochondria stay healthy and useful, it is very unlikely that the person will develop cancer.

In the meantime, health specialists will continue to carry out more comprehensive and detailed clinical studies on the subject.

Keto Aliments for Brain Health

Keto diets provide energy to the brain through a process called ketogenesis. Glucose is the primary source of energy for the brain, and the brain cannot use fat as a source of energy.

However, the brain can use ketones that the liver produces when the level of glucose and insulin in a person's body is low. When a person eliminates carbs from his or her diet, ketones can give up to 70 percent of the brain's

energy. However, that means that the body is still getting 20 to 25 percent of its energy from glucose.

Therefore, even when a person is in ketosis, his or her body is still finding a way to generate blood sugar and have glucose in the system. The brain will always have glucose demands. Similarly, a person will eliminate glucose from his or her body.

A ketogenic diet helps to multiply the number of mitochondria in the brain cells, which helps to improve mild cognitive impairment and memory scores. Ketones elicit more response than glucose does inside the mitochondria. That is because there is more energy per unit of oxygen combined with the ketone than there is energy created when oxygen combines with glucose.

Given that most of the human brain, the tissue comprises fatty acid, taking omega-3 and omega-6 boosts learning and sensory execution.

In addition, ketones in a ketogenic diet help the brain to generate adenosine triphosphate (ATP), the brain particle that transmits energy for metabolism within the cells. Ketones also decrease the number of destructive cells that the body produces.

Whenever a person talks, thinks, or processes information, glutamate receptors are involved. Glutamate is a neurotransmitter that boosts stimulation in the body and is crucial in cognitive function and learning.

Glutamate should convert into GABA, but sometimes the change does not take place as successfully as it should. Therefore, ketones give an alternative source of energy that allows the brain to convert the extra glutamate into GABA efficiently.

Subsequently, the keto diet helps to increase the production of gamma- aminobutyric acid (GABA) and to reduce the number of excess neurons that fire in the brain. That helps to boost mental focus and helps to decrease the presence of stress and anxiety.

Additionally, the ketogenic diet helps to treat congenital hyperinsulinism, relieves migraine headaches, reducing the effects of Parkinson's disease, and speeds up the recovery of traumatic brain injuries.

Keto Aliments for Body Health

The ketogenic diet is an excellent means for enhancing a person's body functions by burning excess fat, balancing hormones, and reducing cravings.

Keto promotes body health by turning fat into energy and speeding up weight loss. The diet achieves this by reducing the hunger levels in a person while maintaining a healthy nutritional balance in that person's body.

Additionally, the keto diet reduces acne. When a person eats foods that are high in processed and refined carbohydrates, he or she can change gut bacteria and bring about sudden fluctuations in blood sugar, which can have an impact on skin health. Reduced carb intake can prevent the development of acne.

Fats, protein, and carbohydrates change the way the body utilizes energy, bringing about ketosis. Studies show that ketosis reduces seizures in children who experience focal seizures. Doctors advise children who have not responded to various seizure medicines to adopt a ketogenic diet.

Some of the ketogenic foods with health benefits include:

- Seafood - Fish and shellfish are healthy sources vitamins, minerals, and omega-3 fatty acids
- Low-carb vegetables - non-starchy vegetables are versatile, and they help to reduce the risk of illnesses
- Cheese is rich in calcium, protein, and healthy fatty acids with a minimal amount of carbs
- Plain yogurt and cottage cheese help to reduce appetite and promote fullness
- Avocados are rich in potassium and fiber, which improve heart function.
- Grass-fed meat and poultry are high-protein foods rich in omega-3 fatty acids, conjugated linoleic acids, and antioxidants, and are low in carbs
- Egg yolks contain lutein and zeaxanthin which help to keep the eye healthy
- Coconut oil is rich in MCTs which increase ketone production and promote loss of weight and belly fat
- Extra virgin oil is high in fats and antioxidants keeps the heart- healthy
- Nuts and seeds are high in fiber and facilitate healthier
- Berries provide nutrients that reduce the risk of disease

- Olives are rich in antioxidants that promote healthy bones
- Unsweetened tea and coffee boost the body's metabolic rate, physical and mental health

Keto Aliments for Heart Health

Keto diet helps to reduce inflammations, lower blood pressure and to increase insulin function. The diet accomplishes that by reducing the amount of fat in the body. There are two types of fats in the human body; triglycerides and cholesterol.

Triglycerides are fatty-acid molecules that reserve energy for later use. Too many triglycerides in the blood can increase the risk of getting diabetes, cardiovascular illnesses, and other life-threatening diseases.

Cholesterol is a waxy lipid produced in the liver that supports functions in the body. Such functions include building hormones, maintaining the proper functioning of cell membranes, and facilitating the absorption of vitamins. A person's body produces about 75 percent of cholesterol. The remaining 25 percent comes from animal protein.

Lipoproteins help to transport cholesterol around a person's body. The lipoproteins include the high-density lipoprotein (HDL) or the good cholesterol, and the low-density lipoprotein (LDL) or the bad cholesterol.

HDL transports cholesterol around the body, collects, and returns good cholesterol to the liver for recycling or discarding. In that way,

HDL prevents cholesterol from accumulating and clogging arteries.

Unlike HDL, LDL moves slowly through the bloodstream and is vulnerable to free radicals, which are oxidizing agents. Once oxidized, LDL can quickly burrow itself into the walls of a person's artery and impede cardiovascular function. That triggers an inflammatory response in which white blood cells rush to eat up the LDL, which can cause further build-up.

Healthcare associates HDL with a lower risk of cardiovascular disease. The HDL - increasing lifestyle makes a person's heart healthier and not necessarily the drugs that raise HDL. A person can naturally raise HDL by following a ketogenic diet, which decreases LDL while increasing HDL.

Recent research shows that although higher levels of LDL can be harmful to heart health, the size, and the density of the LDL particles matter. It is essential for a person to know both the size and density of LDL particles. That is because larger LDL particles are healthier for the body.

However, while a person's diet is vital in preventing heart diseases, blood pressure, cholesterol, blood sugar, stress, smoking, and family history are factors that can contribute to the possibility of a person developing heart disease.

Therefore, if a person is at risk of developing heart disease, he or she should seek advice from a cardiologist, before he or she goes on a keto diet especially when the person has a family history of the disease.

In conclusion, the ketogenic diet helps a person to lose weight. However, it may be a short-term solution and not really a sustainable diet plan in real- life experiences. While a keto diet can help to reduce excess body fat, the goal should be to keep away the lost weight.

It is therefore advisable for a person who wishes to follow a keto diet to consult a knowledgeable health practitioner or dietician with experience in prescribing the diet plan, and in ensuring that the diet will have no adverse effects on a person.

Therefore, a person following the ketogenic diet should utilize fat wisely rather than excessively and seek nutritional ketosis rather than higher ketone levels.

Chapter 6: Keto Diet 31 days Plan

In the ketogenic diet plan, one of the best things to do is to remain steadfast and disciplined because that is the only way to achieve positive results. For people that deviate from time to time and eat unhealthy meals, the truth is that it is almost impossible to achieve results; most undisciplined people end up eating foods with low carbs and high fats without truly unlocking the benefits of the ketogenic diet because their indiscipline prevents them from attaining Ketosis.

With that said, this well thought out keto diet plan is aimed at assisting people in preparing and eating keto diets 7 days a week. If strictly adhered to, the attainment of ketosis becomes a possibility. The recipes listed all have one thing in common; they all have huge amounts of healthy fats, moderate amounts of protein, and low carbs.

Week 1:MondayBreakfast: Pancakes with almond flour and coconut flour-paleo

Coconuts are not only versatile; they are also nutritious and tasty. In terms of health benefits, they are rich in antioxidants, boost the immune system, and also protect against kidney and gall bladder diseases. Likewise, almonds are known to have several health benefits, including; blood sugar control, blood pressure control, and mitigation of cholesterol levels, etc.

Lunch: Keto Brunch Spread

One of the ingredients used in the making of this recipe is eggs, and they are generally known to be nutritious. Eggs promote the level of good cholesterol in the body. They also contain elements that aid heart health. Asparagus, another ingredient in this recipe, aids weight loss and supplies the body with much-needed Vitamins E.

Dinner: Keto Lasagna

Keto Lasagna contains several healthy food ingredients, but one that stands out is garlic. Garlic is a potent food that contains several health benefits, ranging from the reduction of blood pressure to the prevention of dementia, and detoxification of heavy metals in the body. Basil, another ingredient in this recipe, contains elements that fight arthritis, brain diseases, epilepsy, eye diseases, and many others.

TuesdayBreakfast: Paleo Egg Muffins The Paleo Egg Muffins are made with eggs and other healthy food ingredients. Eggs can promote eye health, reduce the risk of stroke, and aid weight loss, etc. Avocado oil, another ingredient in this recipe, doesn't only boost the taste of the meal; it also contains healthy fat and other medical properties, including the reduction of cholesterol and symptoms of arthritis.

Lunch: Turkey Sausage Frittata

This nutrient-packed keto lunch recipe is made with bell peppers and eggs, among other ingredients. Eggs are a miracle food that contains many health benefits like; reduction of heart disease risk, as well as the supply of essential amino acids. Bell peppers do not only improve the taste of this

dish, but they also contain medical properties that aid weight loss, nourish the fetus (for pregnant women), and aid respiratory health.

Dinner: Cauliflower Bake

Cauliflower is a highly nutritious vegetable that contains sulforaphane, choline, fiber, and many other trace elements. It is a good source of antioxidants and greatly aids weight loss. The Cauliflower bake is a perfect meal for dinner because it is easily digestible and hearty. Also, due to its awesomeness, don't be surprised when non-keto eaters in your family decide to request for more.

WednesdayBreakfast: Ham Egg & Cheese Roll-UpsHam, a prominent food ingredient in this recipe is a good source of vitamins B, protein, amino acids, zinc, and magnesium. Eggs contain omega-3 fatty acids, phosphorus, and selenium, etc. This is the perfect keto breakfast meal to keep the liver busy with healthy fats all morning.

Lunch: Keto Cloud Bread

Keto Cloud Bread is a healthy keto recipe that contains several healthy elements that aid heart health, reduce cholesterol level, and boost skin health. The Cloud bread recipe is tasty and will surely play its small part in pushing your body towards ketosis.

Dinner: Keto Mayo

This easy to make recipe is tasty and nutrient-rich. It is light and can be eaten alone or alongside something else. The Keto Mayo is simple but highly rewarding, and that is why it is boldly on this list.

ThursdayBreakfast: Keto French OmeletThis is another keto breakfast recipe that contains reasonable amounts of healthy fats. It is perfect for beginners and veterans in the world of the keto diet. Apart from its impact on sustainable weight loss, there are other health benefits tied to this content-rich diet.

Lunch: Ketofied Chick-Fil-A-style Chicken

This lunch recipe is rich in protein, healthy fats, and many other nutrients. It is also delicious and filling. The food ingredients in this meal contain properties that combat common cold, skin diseases, diabetes, and heart diseases.

Dinner: Portobello Bun Cheeseburgers

Avocado oil and bell peppers are two prominent food ingredients in this tasty and delicious recipe. These healthy foods are known to contain Oleic acid, Lutein, Vitamin B12, Selenium, Fiber, Folate, Copper, Phosphorus, and magnesium, etc. These elements and others help to maintain eye health, boost the immune system, support digestive health, and enhance healing of wounds, etc.

FridayBreakfast: Keto Sage Sausage Patties

The Keto Sage Sausage Patties is a unique recipe made with ingredients like ground pork, garlic, oregano, and sage. This is a delicious and flavorful

keto diet rich in taste and health benefits. It is one of those boring keto diets that people eat just to maintain ketosis. It is something to e savored and enjoyed.

Lunch: Cucumber Noodles with Tahini Sauce

The Cucumber Noodles with Tahini Sauce is a nutrient-packed, healthy, and high fat keto recipe created to provide the body with more keto fuel to burn. It is also rich in nutrients and minerals that help the body remain healthy and strong over long periods.

Dinner: Bebere Enchilada Stuffed peppers

The Berbere Enchilada Stuffed peppers recipe is a spicy meal that is high in protein and healthy fats, but low in carbs. It isn't the traditional Mexican enchiladas. However, it

is guaranteed that you'll have a good time consuming this keto diet.

Saturday

Breakfast: Feta Frittata

The Feta Frittata recipe is a healthy ketogenic diet made from ingredients such as avocados, feta cheese, and chopped tomatoes, etc. It is a special meal that can easily satisfy your appetite while delivering the desired result of the provision of high fats and low carbs. Enjoy!

Lunch: Salmon Poke Bowl

This is a healthy dish that contains high-fat dressing and low-carb vegetables – which is ideal for people that seek to lose weight and also reduce sugar content in their system.

Dinner: Keto Chili

The Keto Chili is an easy but extremely nutritious keto recipe. It is delicious, filling, and hearty, but the best of all is that it contains a meager 5g of carbohydrates only. It is a dinner recipe that will keep you satisfied and in good stead.

SundayBreakfast: Southwestern Omelet

The Southwestern Omelet is a flavor-rich, hearty egg dish that contains the right dietary supply of healthy fats, protein, carbs, and other nutrients that keep the body in good stead, and most importantly, in Ketosis. It is quick and easy to make, nutritious, tasty, and flavorful. Take out time to explore this southwestern recipe.

Lunch: Keto Ceasar Salad

The Keto Ceasar Salad is a simple but nutritious recipe made with healthy food ingredients like egg yolk, avocado oil, parmesan, apple cider vinegar, anchovy fillets, and others. It is a high-fat and low-carb diet that helps the body lose weight and fight diseases like diabetes, heart diseases, and others. Make out time to explore this rich recipe.

Dinner: Keto Meatballs

The Keto Meatballs is a delicious meal that unlocks different layers of nutrients and minerals. It is the perfect meal to keep you locked in ketosis. It also contains medical properties that control cholesterol, inflammation, and blood sugar levels.

Chapter 7: Types of Keto Diet Plans

A ketogenic or keto diet is one that contains a little number of carbohydrates, moderate proteins, and is high in dietary fats. The main aims of such foods are to burn body fat and reduce the levels of glucose circulating in the blood. These diets are particularly therapeutic to overweight people, people with epilepsy, and type 2 diabetics. Due to the low carbohydrates, the body learns to obtain its calories and glucose from other sources. Therefore, the liver breaks down fats into ketone bodies and fatty acids.

Dietary fats and the body's fat storage become the new sources of calories. The brain and other organs use ketone bodies as a substitute for glucose. For health reasons, the associated breakdown of fatty tissue leads to weight loss. As a result, ketogenic diets are beneficial to sufferers of obesity and other related weight loss programs. Beware of meager amounts of dietary carbohydrates and proteins since you may become underweight and stunted in growth, respectively.

Keto Starting Plan

For you to get started on a keto regimen, you need to adhere to some dietary instructions. The keto starting plan requires the creation of a food strategy based on specific guiding principles. The starting plan will act as a guideline on what to consume in your diet. It also contains details on how much you should eat, and how to manage the keto flu. The keto flu is a myriad of uncomfortable symptoms from which you may suffer when newly embarking on a ketogenic diet. Experiencing this type of flu is akin to having carbohydrate withdrawal symptoms. It is imperative to stick to specific foods for you to achieve a proper keto diet. Such keto-friendly diets will allow you to have an improved health status by enabling you to lose a significant amount of weight.

A basic rule involves keeping an eye on what you eat and knowing what to avoid. For instance, you need to cut down on starchy grains, cereals, and tubers such as potatoes. In addition, you must keep clear of sources of too much sugar, specifically honey, maple syrup, and sweet fruits. Try to seek whole foods while avoiding all forms of processed meals, as well. Your keto objectives are achievable by sticking to keto recipes when cooking meals and checking food labels for hidden carbs. Examples of the recommended foods include beef, fish, eggs, avocadoes, cheese, nuts, berries, poultry, and leafy vegetables.

The next rule concerns the quantity of food that you need to consume. After establishing the right type of keto meal, determining its precise amount is crucial in your planning. Calories are the leading indicators of weight gain or loss, hence the need to pay attention to them. For you to attain a balance in calories, an awareness of your food quotas in addition to sticking to the correct food is essential. Gaining weight is a result of a calorie surplus, while a deficit causes an associated weight loss.

Since all human bodies treat calories as an energy source, it is almost impossible to avoid caloric diets entirely. Hence, the need to pay attention to the number of calories that you consume. Weight loss is associated with a low risk of developing diabetes and heart diseases. Thus, your objective should be to lose weight healthily by keeping your carb intake levels below thirty-five grams daily. For you to achieve this aim, you need to consume a

lot of fat and an adequate amount of proteins. Both of these quotas allow you to maintain proper weight and muscle growth, respectively. In addition, you can keep track of your caloric intake by using a keto calculator or any mobile apps that can monitor calories.

Sufficient protein levels are essential for the repair and maintenance of muscle bulk. A complete lack of proteins in the diet usually leads to stunted growth and loss of muscle mass. However, too much protein is counter-productive since it can undergo gluconeogenesis, thereby impairing the much-needed ketosis. The recommended portion of your meals that are made up of protein is around twenty percent. A high-fat diet is the underlying principle of a ketogenic meal. It is the primary source of

calories in any keto regimen due to the low amounts of carbohydrates in such a meal. You should strive to allocate around seventy-five percent of your diet to fats. This portion should be enough to meet the target of losing one to two pounds of weight each week.

Such excellent sources of dietary fat include eggs, avocadoes, bacon, nuts, and seeds. Beef is a highly recommended source of both protein and fat as opposed to poultry or fish, which have a high protein but zero fat level. In addition to controlling the amount of food that you consume regularly, you should develop a habit of eating when you are hungry. Besides, although exercise is not necessary, it is highly recommended in a ketogenic lifestyle. However, the light practice has to be mild and not exhaustive since you lack the high number of calories that typically come from carbs.

In the case of keto flu, you should be aware of its related symptoms and the way to remedy it. Whenever you decide to enter into a keto regimen, flu-like signs may accompany the experience. These irritable feelings are the result of your body switching from carbs as a principle source of fuel to

fats. Symptoms typically develop within a few days of starting a keto diet. They include generalized fatigue, headaches, muscular cramps, and mental fogginess. Constipation and diarrhea are bowel symptoms that occur because of ketones and fat intolerance, respectively.

These last two symptoms are not necessarily part of the keto flu since poor fat tolerance is an inborn or, perhaps, a genetic condition. For you to get relief from the keto flu, you should maintain adequate hydration levels. In addition to drinking more water, you need to increase your intake of electrolytes, especially sodium, magnesium, and potassium. The high degree of ketones in the blood circulation that results from ketosis leads to constipation. However, the inclusion of leafy vegetables in your diet can remedy this condition.

Keto Basic Plan

A basic plan for a ketogenic diet involves the preparation of a sample meal that meets the targets set by a keto regimen. The objective is to have a low carb, adequate-protein, and high-fat diet. Drinking plenty of water for hydration is advisable, as well. A basic keto plan for a single week can include the following:

Monday

- Breakfast: cheese omelet, tomatoes, and eggs
- Lunch: peanut butter, almond milk, and chicken salad
- Dinner: salad, beef, and leafy vegetables **Tuesday**
- Breakfast: whole milkshake or dark chocolate

- Lunch: avocadoes and fish salad in olive oil
- Dinner: consume broccoli, pork chops, and salad **Wednesday**
- Breakfast: eggs, bacon, and tomatoes
- Lunch: cheese, leafy vegetables, and chicken fillet
- Dinner: asparagus, and salmon prepared in butter **Thursday**
- Breakfast: mushrooms, bacon, and fried eggs
- Lunch: cheeseburger and guacamole
- Dinner: you can eat eggs and steak with salad **Friday**
- Breakfast: tomatoes, cheese, and ham omelet
- Lunch: beef, vegetables, or salad with a helping of nuts and seeds
- Dinner: eggs, spinach, and whitefish **Saturday**
- Breakfast: stevia, cocoa powder, and sugarless yogurt
- Lunch: fried beef and vegetables
- Dinner: you can consume an egg sandwich with cheese and bacon **Sunday**
- Breakfast: avocado slices and omelet with onions
- Lunch: salsa, guacamole, celery sticks with nuts and seeds
- Dinner: cream cheese, vegetables, pork chops, and chicken salad

Keto Snack for your health

Keto snacks are useful in case you experience hunger pangs between mealtimes. The examples of keto snacks that are beneficial for your health include hard-boiled eggs, fat yogurt, strawberries, cheese, and a handful of seeds or nuts. A few pieces of fatty meat from the remaining portions of previous keto meals can function as snacks, as well.

Keto Fasting Plan

This plan involves employing intermittent fasting as a weight-loss strategy in addition to your keto diet. Skipping meals leads to a significant loss of body fat, especially during periods of weight stagnation. Other health benefits of periodic fasting include better muscle growth with strength, an enhanced level of metabolism, and increased cellular autophagy. The process of autophagy involves the cellular breakdown of unnecessary sections of itself, followed by protein recycling. Your cells, therefore, rid themselves of radical elements and toxic compounds that would otherwise accelerate the aging process or cause cancer eventually. Your mental focus and thought clarity will also show an overall improvement throughout the day. Any instances of mental fogginess and absent-mindedness disappear as well.

This strategy typically breaks down your eating habits into feeding and fasting periods. The main objective is to enable you to have a large meal in a single sitting after an extended period of hunger. A limit on your intake of calories results from intermittent fasting since the body can tolerate only a definite quantity of food at a go. Beware of snacking subconsciously during the fasting windows. After a period of adjustment to this new strategy, your body adapts to the cyclical sequence. A period of fasting

enhances the process of ketosis, leading to the breakdown of your fatty tissues. Rather than look for energy from dietary fat, your body will obtain its necessary fuel from the stored body fat instead.

A famous type of intermittent fasting involves splitting the day into two sections that contain either sixteen or eight hours each. In this strategy, you can allocate the first sixteen hours to fasting, followed by the consumption of all your recommended daily calories in the remaining eight hours. Another method that you can use involves allocating the fasting and eating periods into separate days, thereby resulting in twenty-four-hour alternating windows. Intermittent keto fasting is attainable by skipping both your lunch and breakfast every day, as well.

The overarching purpose is to refrain from eating any food for a specified period consciously while being mindful of your timing strictly. However, fasting may seem challenging at first, but it is possible with proper dedication and discipline. After all, its success depends on your efforts and willingness to attain your ketogenic and weight loss objectives. Remember that fasting leads to a state of caloric deficit, thereby assisting you in achieving your aims. Although it is not essential, fasting in regular cycles is always beneficial if you want to maintain a specific weight standard. It generally leads to a refreshed feeling afterward among most people who incorporate it into their keto lifestyle.

In addition, whenever you experience the periods of fasting, your metabolic state shifts into a fat-burning mode. The liver receives instructions from the brain to begin the process of lipolysis, which generally involves breaking down fatty tissue. From this breakdown, you will have ketone bodies and fatty acids. The ketone bodies serve as fuel for the brain activities in place of the deficient glucose. As a result, the health

of your nervous system gets a massive boost while preventing unwanted cases of epilepsy.

More so, fasting and the resulting ketones have an inhibitory effect on certain hormones that link to hunger. For instance, ketones inhibit the secretion and activity of the ghrelin hormone. This hormone is responsible for the sensation of hunger in humans. Its suppression eliminates the associated feelings of food cravings from your system. The inclusion of Keto-proof coffee or tea in your breakfast diet has the same hunger- suppressing effect as well as boosting your energy levels. Cortisol hormone rises in response to the increased levels of circulating ketones as well.

The high cortisol level enhances the process of muscle growth and repair. It also enables you to have a good night's sleep, especially when confronted with the keto flu. Therefore, overall, fasting led to fat breakdown and increased ketone production, which in turn, results in the suppression of hunger. All these actions and their corresponding effects give rise to a positive feedback loop that makes your intermittent fasting worthwhile eventually.

A keto calculator is a helpful tool with which you can estimate your daily macronutrient requirements. It comes in handy, especially during times of intermittent fasting. When you are still new to using the fasting strategy in your ketogenic lifestyle, you will need this calculator more than anyone will. In ketogenic fasting, you are bound to rely on hunches and guesswork on the amount of food to consume. The urge to overeat during your feeding periods may cause you to surpass the recommended daily caloric intake accidentally. A longer feeding cycle should precede your first fasting window to offset this high caloric temptation. The keto calculator uses

your relevant details and any information that you feed it to compute the ideal amount of calories needed during your next meal.

Since you will have all of your data at your fingers, you must use it to keep track of your progress in the initial phases of ketogenic fasting. Certain mobile apps, such as Chronometer and MyFitnessPal, also offer services that are similar to the keto calculator. The portability factor provided by such apps comes in handy, especially in situations that render you to somewhat unfamiliar surroundings. Another essential point to keep in mind is not to engage in any snacking. Snacks are meals too, albeit tiny amounts, and hence they will defeat the purpose of fasting.

A sample meal during the feeding phase of a regular keto fasting cycle could look like this:

- **Breakfast:** Keto-proof green tea or coffee. Remember that this drink contains a mixture of dietary fats and oils within it. This fatty mixture is justified as long as you can avoid any form of carbs.

- **Lunch:** Black coffee, water, and sugarless tea. This lunch is ideally a fasting period that allows you to consume lots of water and other fluids. The resulting improvement in hydration serves to mitigate any adverse effects from the keto flu.

- **Dinner:** Consume your meals as per the ketogenic diet and follow the dinner examples shown earlier within the basic plans.

Keto Vegetarian Plan

The combination of a vegetarian diet with a ketogenic one is often doubly beneficial to your overall health status. Both heart diseases and problems related to increased weight are preventable using this vegetarian keto diet.

You end up keeping conditions such as obesity and diabetes at bay effectively. Unlike the vegan keto diet, a vegetarian one allows you to consume animal products without the need for the real animal or its flesh. Your diet should have the usual limitation to its carbohydrate contents to below thirty-five grams daily. The incorporation of eggs and dairy is standard in such foods.

The widespread reasons for embarking on a vegetarian diet share a common thread. The common ground relates to environmental preservation, curbing climate change, sustainability, and eliminating cases of animal torture. Losing weight and attaining better health are often novelty reasons for including a ketogenic component to the diet. Restricting your animal products to free-range livestock is an extra step that you can take to ensure adherence to your ethos. Controlled animals are likely to face exposure to fattening hormonal injections and chemical treatments that are detrimental to your health in the end.

Remember that your keto diet should contain high-fat sources to make up for the low quantities of carbs while sticking to your vegetarian principles. Your sources of dietary fat are plenty in spite of a lack of fatty beef, pork chops, bacon, or steak. Eggs, high-fat dairy products, and plant-based fats can make up the difference. The inclusion of micronutrient and multivitamin supplements in your diet is advisable, too, since you may not get all the recommended nutrients from plant sources alone.

Consuming plenty of low-carb vegetables such as asparagus, celery, zucchini, and leafy spinach is also preferable. In case you run into challenges when trying to estimate the number of calories you need to include in the diet, use a keto calculator. It works in the same manner

across all forms of keto diets to keep your intake of calories within the recommended limits.

Keto Vegan Plan

A vegan diet is devoid of any animals or their products as the primary source of protein. Due to the highly restrictive nature of a vegan ketogenic diet, you will need tremendous willpower to pull it off successfully. In this case, you may have to combine a typical ketogenic diet with high-carb vegan sources to meet your daily caloric quota. Such a vegan keto diet contains many low-carb vegetables limited to thirty-five grams daily, as well as many plant-based fats and proteins. Multivitamin supplements are beneficial to account for the vitamin deficiency that is common in vegan bodies.

For you to know how much fats and proteins, you will require from the plant sources, you need to use the keto calculator as well. Keep in mind that your diet will be entirely void of fish, poultry, beef, eggs, dairy, and any other animal products. However, you can use meat substitutes such as tofu and soy products in some instances. Mushrooms, leafy vegetables, nuts, and seeds also provide a low-carb source of calories. Avocadoes and berries contained in the regular keto diet are safe within a vegan setting, as well. Dairy products in a particular vegan diet are replaceable with coconut milk and cream. In addition, coconut oil and butter are useful in cooking and frying specific foods within this category. Beware of the lower melting point of the coconut oil over its butter equivalent.

You can choose from a variety of vegan cheese in the market nowadays. Based on your preference, vegan cheese replaces the need for dairy sources efficiently. You can easily substitute ground flax seeds for poultry eggs to obtain a credible vegan keto diet. Other available substitutes for eggs

include silken tofu, baking soda, and vinegar. Examples of plant-based sources of fat include avocadoes, coconut oils, olive oils, seeds, coconut butter, and most nuts. This diet is often pointless for people who are unfortunate to suffer from neural ailments such as epilepsy, Alzheimer's, and Parkinson's diseases. The epileptic nature of these brain conditions is manageable using a ketogenic diet via the production of therapeutic ketones.

Chapter 8: The Information You Must Know About Keto Cycling

Keto diet is a low-carb, moderate protein, and high-fat diet, which has several variations. Keto cycling is one of the less restrictive keto diet variations that allow one to have a day of eating carbs. People who follow a keto diet eat under 50 grams of carbs per day. This enables their bodies to switch from using carbs as a primary source of fuel to using fat, a process known as ketosis.

What Is a Cyclical Keto Diet?

For a cyclical keto diet, an individual would need to follow a strict low- carb, high-fat diet for five to six days a week, and then have a high carb once or twice in a week, which is essentially a cheat day. When you follow a cyclical keto diet, it removes the body out of ketosis for one or two days and goes back into ketosis thereafter for the rest of the week until your next cheat day. The high-carb eating day also known as the refeeding day replenishes the body's glucose reserves. This helps improve muscle growth as well as exercise performance.

The Way to Equilibrate Cycles of Keto Diet

It is possible to cycle on and off a keto diet. Some people feel great eating a low-carb diet and can maintain it for a long period however; some give it a shot but find it hard to stick by it. Instead of quitting altogether, there are ways you can adjust to an on and off-cycle and still enjoy the health benefits. You can experiment and tweak your keto diet until you find what

works best for you. You can equilibrate cycles of the keto diet in the following three ways:

1. The moderate carb approach

This approach allows you to increase your daily carb approach from the normal 50 grams to about 150 grams per day and reduce your high fat intake. The extra carbs should be from healthy carb options like brown rice, baked yams, sweet potatoes, or fruits. The fats should also be from healthy sources like nuts, avocado, olive oil or seeds. This approach is perfect for people who prefer a slightly higher carb intake. The increase in carbs promotes a person's sleep pattern.

2. The weekly keto cycling approach

Another approach you can use to avoid going off keto entirely is to cycle your carb intake throughout the week. Follow a strict 50 grams low carb diet for five to six days then increase your carb intake up to 155 grams for one or two days and then go back to the low-carb keto diet. This approach works well for people who need help to jump-start their metabolism.

3. The seasonal keto approach

This approach works well for people who cannot follow a keto diet full time or those who need to adjust to in-season foods. Some people may want to follow a keto diet maybe once or twice a year to reap its benefits for a short period, and then go back to normal eating. Athletes cannot follow a keto diet full time but can follow it off-season.

Keto Cycle Program

To start on a cyclical keto diet,

1. It is best to follow a keto diet for at least a month before starting keto cycling.

Follow the standard keto diet for four to six weeks. That way your body gets time to adjust to the keto diet and you can drift on and off ketosis as you like. When your body is used to ketosis, it usually reverts to ketosis faster after having a high-carb day.

2. Follow the standard keto diet (SKD) for five to six days a week

During that period consumes less than 50 grams of carbs a day and increase the amount of healthy fats intake. Such fats include avocado, eggs, coconut oil, olive oil, nuts, and seeds. Choose healthy sources of protein like salmon, fish, poultry, or lean beef. Avoid processed meat like sausages and bacon. Ensure you follow a meal plan of 75% fat, 20% protein, and only 5% carbs. Avoid sugary foods, grains, fruits, root vegetables, and tubers.

3. Have a high carb cheat day

Choose a day or two when you can indulge in high carbs to get the body out of ketosis and replenish glucose levels. Don't have a whole pizza or burger and fries, stick to healthy carbs like brown rice, beans, quinoa, lentils, oats, or sweet potatoes. Pair the meal with moderate protein.

4. Go Back to Ketosis

After the refeeding days, go back to your standard keto diet. To achieve ketosis faster, you can either practice:

- **Intermittent Fasting -** This is time-restricted feeding where you have meals within a short period of six hours and fast for the remaining 18 hours of the day. Intermittent fasting helps the body transition smoothly in and out of ketosis.
- **High-Intensity Workouts -** On the days following refeeding, go for high-intensity workouts, which help burn the excess carbs consumed.

Benefits of Keto Cycling
1. Weight loss

When you reduce carbs and increase fat intake, the body enters a metabolic state called ketosis. Ideally, the body uses carbs as the main source of energy but during ketosis, because very little carbs are consumed, the body is forced to use fat as a source of energy. After a few days of following the diet, the body starts burning fat for fuel causing weight loss.

2. Muscle building

Some studies have revealed that going on Keto cycling can help those who want to lose weight and gain muscle. Healthy carbs are good for building muscles. The keto cycle usually prevents the production of muscle- building hormones like insulin. However, with the on and off ketosis days, you regulate insulin production, which promotes muscle gain.

3. Reduces full-on Keto side effects

When you follow any keto diet, you are likely to experience serious side effects. This may include headaches, nausea, weakness, fatigue and sometimes lack of sleep. When you break the full-on Keto diet with a day or two of indulging in a high carb, it decreases these symptoms because you are not in ketosis for so many days at once.

4. Makes the diet more sustainable

Keto diets cut down on all types of carbs, which normally account for at least 50% of what the majority of people eat. Because it is so restrictive, it is really hard to follow through the long term. When you use the cyclical keto diet, you have days you can eat carbs, therefore making the diet more sustainable.

5. Boostperformance

Studies have revealed that athletes who followed a cyclical keto diet performed better compared to those following a standard keto diet.

6. Reduces the negative effects

When on a full keto diet, people don't indulge in carbs and according to some studies, this carb restriction over a long period has a negative impact on hormones, cholesterol levels, and mood swings. But with regular replenishment using keto cycling, these problems are avoided.

7. BetterInsulinSensitivity

When you go for the five days on a low carb diet, your body becomes more sensitive to insulin. However, prolonged periods of a low carb diet can make the body insensitive to insulin and cause weight gain. Keto cycling ensures that you don't stay on a low carb diet for too long to cause such effects.

The Difference Between Keto Cycling and Carb Cycling

While both involve eating fewer carbs, keto cycling follows a high fat, moderate protein and lower carb diet and carb cycling follows a high- protein, moderate fat and just cuts down on carbs for a few days. With carb cycling, the body does not have to switch to burning fat for fuel.

Keto cycling allows one to have high carbs once or twice a week to replenish glucose levels while in carb cycling you alternate your carb intake on a daily, weekly, or monthly basis. The goal is to train the body not to rely solely on carbs for energy but also to use fat as an alternative source of fuel. Most people who follow carb cycling are athletes because it helps enhance their performance and maximize energy stores for competition.

In carb cycling, you can program your carb intake based on your routine. You can have high carbs on days you do high-intensity workouts and muscle building days and eat low carbs on your rest days. While in keto cycling, the high carb days are fixed. If you have carbs on Saturdays, you should have them on all other consecutive Saturdays. Carb cycling typically prevents the negative impacts of a low carb diet experienced on a keto cycling.

Is Keto Cycling Good for You? (Advantages and Disadvantages)

The jury is still out on whether keto cycling is good or bad. It all boils down to an individual's preferred dietary choices. If you feel keto cycling is helping you stay on track, then go for it and if you also feel like keto cycling is challenging and is making you overindulge on those refeeding days, then do not do it.

Women who are pregnant or nursing should not follow Keto cycling or any keto diet. Patients with type 2 diabetes need to consult their doctors beforehand but those with type 1 diabetes should not follow a keto diet.

Keto cycling is a good way to help you stick to the keto diet in the end

however; it is also too unbalanced and restrictive. It restricts a person from eating certain food items regularly, which are important.

Advantages

1. Losing weight

Many people follow keto cycling to lose weight. Research has shown that people lose weight faster when they go on keto diets. Without glucose from carbs, your body burns stored fat as fuel.

2. Curbs inflammations

You use fat as fuel as opposed to carbs it causes far less inflammation. The fat breaks down into ketones, which also reduces the inflammatory response.

3. Keeps you fuller for longer

A Keto cycling diet keeps you full for longer because ketones regulate the hormones responsible for hunger. When you are hungry, your body will just burn stored fat to keep you going.

4. Good for the brain

On the five or six days that you are on ketosis, the brain benefits a lot. It uses ketones for energy to make more mitochondria and with more mitochondria; your cells generate more energy.

Disadvantages

1. Difficult to Sustain

Even though Keto cycling allows for carbs intake once or twice a week, it still restricts too many important food groups and even though people do lose weight, the majority gains it back when they resume their carb intake.

2. Weight fluctuations

People experience weight fluctuations when they transition from a full-on keto diet to a cyclical keto diet. This is because their bodies retain excess water when high-carb foods are consumed. So, during refeeding, they will gain weight and when they are back to ketosis, the weight goes back down.

3. Binge Eating

People who follow the keto cycling will maintain a low-carb diet for the five or six days but on the refeeding day, they indulge in as many carbohydrates as they want which counteracts the weight loss benefits of any keto diet. That restriction on carbs can lead to bingeing.

4. Your body might store more fat

When you eat a high-fat diet and then switch to high carbs, you can be in danger of storing much of the consumed fat. The body might use the carbs as energy, stop converting fat to energy, and therefore store the fat.

5. Ketocanleadtohighcholesterol

Keto follows a high-fat diet. If a person does not avoid bad fats like saturated fats or Trans fats, they can lead to high cholesterol levels, heart diseases, and stroke. Fat consumed during keto should have good cholesterol levels. People on a keto diet should stick to plant-based unsaturated fats like avocados, nuts, and seeds.

Chapter 9:Weight Loss Quickly With Ketogenic Diet Recipes

Obesity is now one of the biggest health problems in the world today. Obesity-related diseases kill more than two million people annually, and in the quest to put an end to this trend, many diets have emerged. Most of these diets lack any research backing, but the Ketogenic diet has been backed by numerous scientific studies over the years.

There is enormous evidence backing the fact that ketogenic diets are extremely effective for weight loss. They are not only effective in burning fats, but they also help to fight diseases and preserve muscle mass.It must be stated that a low-fat diet is different from the Ketogenic diet, and numerous studies have shown that the Ketogenic diet is far superior, even with the same amounts of calories consumed.

A study showed that people on a keto diet lost about 2.2 times more weight than their counterparts on a low-fat, low-calorie diet, HDL cholesterol, and triglyceride levels were also boosted.

Mechanisms behind weight loss and ketogenic diets

This is exactly how ketogenic diets help to boost weight loss:

- **Improved insulin sensitivity**Keto diets are known to boost insulin sensitivity, and this results in improved metabolism and utilization of fuel.

- **Improved Protein consumption**Most keto diets boost the intake of protein, and this leads to several weight loss benefits.

- **Reduced fat storage**Several research findings have shown that ketogenic diets retain the ability to possibly reducing lipogenesis, the process that involves the conversion of sugar into fat.

- **Food elimination**The Ketogenic diet limits the intake of a carb, which in turn limits food options. When people's feeding options reduce, it results in the reduction of calorie intake, which is a major factor in fat burning.

- **Appetite-suppressant**One of the hallmarks of the ketogenic diet is its ability to make people feel full, and it is primarily supported by leptin and ghrelin – the hunger hormones.

- **Gluconeogenesis**Ideally, the human body converts protein and fats into carbs for fuel. Thus, additional calories can be burnt daily.

- **Improved burning of fat**With the Ketogenic diet, the body's ability to burn daily fat improves significantly, and it doesn't matter whether you are exercising or resting.

What all that has been said, it is obvious that a ketogenic diet is an effective tool for weight loss and fat burning.

Ketogenic Diet and Weight Loss Results

The keto diet is renowned for its weight loss ability due to the drastic reduction of carbon intake, leading to the body burning fats in place carbs for energy.Due to several factors, including peculiar body composition and insulin resistance, results different among different people. However, the keto diet, over the years, has resulted in weight loss in different situations including athletic performance, type 2 diabetes, and obesity.

In 2017, a study was conducted to ascertain the effects of a keto diet and CrossFit training on performance and body composition. The result showed that people who follow low-carb keto diets experienced reduced body fat percentage, body weight, and fat mass compared to others in the control bracket.

People that followed the keto diet experienced the following:

1. Improved CrossFit performance as those within the control bracket

2. Maintained lean body mass as those within the control bracket

3. Lost about 6.2 pounds of fat mass (the fat dominated areas of the body) compared to those within the controlled group who recorded zero loss of fat.

4. Lost about 2.6% body fat compared to those within the control bracket who recorded zero loss of body fat.

5. Lost about 7.6 pounds compared to those within the control bracket who recorded zero loss in total body weight.

In 2014, Dashti et al., who carried out a research that observed the long- term effects of a keto diet in obese patients, came out with the following findings;

- The amount of glucose in the blood reduced significantly.

- After 24 weeks of treatment, the number of triglycerides (fat) reduced significantly.

- From week one – week twenty-four, the total amount of cholesterol dropped significantly.o LDL cholesterol (bad cholesterol) concentration dropped significantly after treatmentso HDL cholesterol (good cholesterol) concentration increased significantly.

6. The body mass and weight index of the patients went down significantly.

In 2012 Partsalaki et al. undertook research that compared the effects of the keto diet with a hypocaloric diet in obese adolescents and children. The findings showed;

- Children on the keto diet experienced a significant reduction in waist circumference, fat mass, body weight, and fasting insulin levels.

- Children on the keto diet, to a greater degree, experienced a significant reduction in the homeostatic model assessment-insulin resistance

(HOMA-IR) than those on the hypocaloric diet.

- Children on the keto group showed an increase in high molecular weight (HMW) adiponectin – an important marker of insulin sensitivity and cardiovascular disease – compared to those in the hypocaloric diet group that showed none.

Furthermore, a study that explored the effects of low-carb keto diet vs. low-glycemic index diet in type diabetics was carried out in 2008. It was concluded in this study that those on the ketogenic diet had greater improvements in weight loss, high-density lipoprotein (HDL) cholesterol, and hemoglobin A1C, compared to those following the low-glycemic index diet.

The result of the ketogenic diet group:

1. Diabetes treatments were eliminated or reduced in 62% of participants in the low-glycemic index group as compared to 95.2% of those following the ketogenic diet.

2. Zero increase in HDL cholesterol in the low-glycemic index group versus an average of 5.6mg/dL increase in the Ketogenic diet group

3. 0.5% reduction of HbA1c levels on the low-glycemic index diet group versus 1.5% reduction of HbA1c on the ketogenic diet group

4. The low-glycemic index diet group lost on average 15.2 pounds, versus an average of 24.5 pounds by those on the ketogenic diet plan.

The reason why the ketogenic diet is efficient for weight loss is not rocket science. It works because it is centered on high fat, sufficient protein, and extremely low intake of carbs.

Breakfast Recipes

Breakfasts are an essential part of every diet plan because they set the tone for the rest of the day. If you get it right with your breakfast, you have

achieved half of your daily goal of eating healthy. The Ketogenic breakfast recipes in this section have been carefully selected to provide you with meals that are not only keto-friendly but also contribute many other essential nutrients and minerals to your body. They are meant to engage your taste bud, nourish, and supply your body with the required amount of good fats required to induce you into ketosis.

If you can be disciplined enough to prep these meals ahead of time and maintain a regimented keto eating plan, you will experience an upsurge in physical and mental performance, weight loss, and productivity.

With that said, the following breakfast recipes have been carefully selected for you to explore the ketogenic diet;

1. Pancakes with Almond Flour and Coconut Flour- Paleo

The pancake with almond flour and coconut flour-paleo recipe are quick and easy to prepare a low-carb diet that is gluten-free, delicious and fluffy. The ingredients that make up this recipe are healthy, and nutrient-packed, giving it a delicious flavor, as well as many other health benefits, including controlling cholesterol levels, mitigating blood pressure, and combating skin diseases, etc. You can kick off your day with this nutritious, high-fat, low-carb meal that will brighten your day and project you in a better state before consumption. Take out time to explore this rich recipe.

Prep time: 5 minutesCook time: 15 minutesTotal time: 20 minutes Servings: 2 3" –pancakes each

Ingredients:

- Sea salt, 1⁄4 teaspoon
- Blanched almond flour, 1 cup
- Vanilla extract, 1 1⁄2 teaspoon
- Coconut flour, 1⁄4 cup
- Avocado oil (or any other tasteless oil that remains in the liquid state at room temp), 1/4 cup
- Erythritol (or any substitute sweetener), 2-3 tablespoons
- Unsweetened Almond milk (or any other type of milk), 1 teaspoon
- Baking powder (gluten-free), 1 teaspoon
- Eggs, 5

Method:

1. In a bowl, stir all the ingredients together until smooth. The mixture shouldn't be too thick; it should be like a regular pancake batter. Thus, you can add more milk if it's too thick, but don't add too much.

2. Put an oiled pan on the burner set on low to medium heat. Empty the mixture on the preheated oiled pan and cook into circles. Cover the lid and cook for about one to two minutes until you notice the formation of bubbles. Then, flip and cook until each side turns brown. Do the same with the remaining batter.

Nutrition Facts:

Amount per serving

- Sugar 1g
- Fiber 3g
- Total Carbs 6g
- Protein 9g
- Fat 23g

2. Paleo Egg Muffins

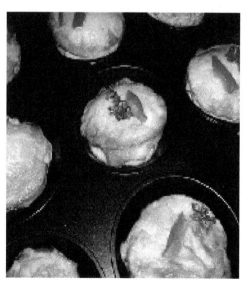

This is a quick and easy-to-make recipe that comes with different levels of flavor. In terms of looks, it is colorful, well-textured, and packed with nutritious elements that boost the overall wellbeing of the consumer. Enjoy this yummy keto diet that provides your body with a healthy dose of good fats and protein. The Paleo Egg Muffins is a ketogenic diet recipe that will boost your chances of eating a healthy and tasty meal, rich in good fats and low in carbs. Here is your chance of starting off your day with the right dietary requirements in your quest to attain and maintain ketosis. Enjoy this nutritious meal.

Prep time: 20 minutes Cook time: 20 minutes Total time: 40 minutes

Servings: 12

Ingredients:

- Ground pepper
- Fresh spinach, 1 1/2 cups
- Extra virgin olive oil, 1 tablespoon
- Salt, 3/4 teaspoon
- Eggs, 9
- Sweet onion, 1/2
- Fresh oregano (chopped or 1/2 t. dry oregano), 1 teaspoon
- Pork breakfast sausage, 8 oz
- Coconut milk (or regular milk), 1/4 cup
- Red bell peppers (thinly sliced or chopped, any color), 3/4 cup

Method:

1. Heat oven beforehand to 350 degrees Fahrenheit. Get a muffin tin and grease.

2. Set a frying pan over medium to high heat and add the ground sausage. While cooking, use a spatula and break the pork into crumbles.

3. After cooking the pork midway, add the pepper, olive oil, oregano, and onions. Fry until you notice that onion becomes translucent, then add the spinach and place a lid on the pan. Allow to cook for about thirty-five seconds, take off the lid, and mix the ingredients. Take off from the heat.

4. In a mixing bowl, add the eggs, milk, salt, and pepper, and stir until the eggs are completely beaten.

5. Add the vegetables and sausage to the egg batter and whisk until even.

6. Empty the mixture into twelve greased muffin tins and ensure that the ratio of each thin is consistent.

7. Place the muffin tins for about 18-20 minutes in the oven that has been heated beforehand. Allow to cool for a couple of minutes and take off from the tins, using a knife to loosen the edges.

Nutrition Facts:

Serving size: 1 muffin

- Sodium 335mg
- Saturated fat 3.3g
- Cholesterol 158.1mg
- Polyunsaturated fat 1.4g
- Total carbohydrate 4g

- Trans fat 0g
- Dietary fiber 1.6g
- Monounsaturated fat 3.9g
- Sugars 1.3g
- Total fat 9.8g
- Protein 10.4g
- Iron 2.7mg
- Vitamin C 24.1mg
- Riboflavin (B2) 0.3mg

3. Ham Egg & Cheese Roll-Ups

The Ham Egg and Cheese Roll-ups is a healthy and nutrient-rich recipe that takes only twenty minutes to prepare. It is the perfect meal for people that seek a healthy supply of protein, healthy fats, and a few carbohydrates. Make out time to make this meal that can help in maintaining ketosis.

Prep time: 20 minutes Total time: 20 minutes Servings: 5

Ingredients:

- Baby spinach, 1 cup
- Eggs, 10
- Butter, 1 1/2 cups
- Garlic powder, 2 teaspoons
- Ham, 20 slices
- Kosher salt
- Chopped tomatoes, 1 cup
- Butter, 2 tablespoons
- Black pepper (freshly ground)

Method:

1. Heat broiler. Crack eggs and empty in a bowl. Stir in the garlic powder, add pepper and salt to desired taste.

2. Add butter in a large frying pan set over medium heat. Add and scramble eggs for three minutes, stirring from time to time. Stir in cheddar until melted. Stir in tomatoes and baby spinach until properly mixed.

3. Put 2 slices of ham on a cutting board. Use a spoonful of eggs (scrambled) to top it and roll-up. Follow the same step with the remaining scrambled eggs and ham.

4. On a shallow baking dish, place the roll-ups and broil for five minutes, until ham is crispy.

Nutrition Facts:

- Fiber 1g
- Calories 410
- Sodium 1620mg
- Carbohydrates 6g
- Fat 26g
- Protein 38g
- Saturated fat 13g
- Sugar 4g

4. Keto French Omelet

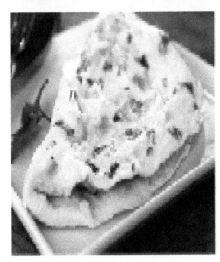

This hearty and flavorful Keto French Omelet is easy to make, a recipe that possesses the right dietary requirements needed to induce consumers into ketosis. It is rich in nutrients and contains elements that can help control blood sugar levels, prevent certain forms of cancer, and even reduce inflammation. Breakfasts are very important, and if you've decided to eat healthily, it presents you with the opportunity of making a huge statement early in the day. This recipe is healthy and nutritious, and its components will greatly further your goal of losing weight and staying healthy. Make out time to explore this meal, and you'll be thankful that you did. Enjoy

Prep time: 20 minutes Total time: 20 minutes Servings: 2

Ingredients:

- Green pepper (chopped), 1 tablespoon
- Eggs (large), 2
- Fully cooked and cubed ham, 1/4 cup
- White eggs (large), 4
- Shredded reduced-fat cheddar cheese, 1/4 cup
- Fat-free milk, 1/4 cup
- Chopped onion, 1 tablespoon
- Salt, 1/8 teaspoon
- Pepper, 1/8 teaspoon

Method:

1. Beat the eggs, white eggs, fat-free milk, salt, and pepper with a whisk.

2. Put a frying pan over low-medium heat (it should be coated with cooking spray). Add the egg batter. It will set towards the edges. Once the eggs begin to set, move the cooked areas to the middle, allowing the uncooked areas to move under.

3. When all areas of the eggs are fully cooked, use the unused ingredients as topping on one half. Bend omelet in half. Cut in half to serve.

Nutrition Facts:

- Protein 22g
- Fiber 0g
- Sugars 3g
- Carbohydrates 4g
- Sodium 648mg
- Cholesterol 207mg
- Saturated fat 4g
- Fat9g
- Calories 186

5. Keto Sage Sausage Patties

The Keto Sage Sausage Patties is a unique recipe made with ingredients like ground pork, garlic, oregano, and sage. It is a delicious and flavorful keto diet rich in different cadres of taste and many other health benefits. Besides, it isn't one of those boring keto diets that people eat just to maintain ketosis. This meal is something to be enjoyed and savored, even while you have one eye on eating right and chasing/ maintaining ketosis. It comes highly recommended, and I advise everyone on the ketogenic diet to incorporate it into their meal plans. Enjoy.

Prep time: 10 minutes Cook time: 15 minutes Total time: 25 minutes Servings: 8

Ingredients:

- Dried oregano, 1/8 teaspoon
- Ground pork, 1 pound
- Garlic powder, 1/8 teaspoon
- Cheddar cheese (shredded), 3⁄4 cup
- Pepper, 3⁄4 teaspoon
- Buttermilk, 1⁄4 cup
- Salt, 3⁄4 teaspoon
- Onion (finely chopped), 1 tablespoon
- Sage (rubbed), 3⁄4 teaspoon

Method:

1. Add all ingredients in a bowl and mix thoroughly. Make 8 different half-inch thick patties and store in the fridge for an hour.
2. Place a skillet over medium heat and cook patties for six to eight minutes on each side.

Nutrition Facts:

Serving Size: 1 patty

- Protein 13g
- Carbohydrate 1g
- Fiber 0g
- Sugar 0g
- Sodium 323mg
- Cholesterol 49mg
- Saturated fat 5g
- Fat 11g
- Calories 162

6. Feta Frittata

The Feta Frittata recipe is a healthy ketogenic diet made from ingredients such as avocados, feta cheese, and chopped tomatoes, etc. It is a special meal that can easily satisfy your appetite while delivering the desired result of the provision of high fats and low carbs. If you intend to start off the day by boosting your energy levels, this is the right recipe for you. Make no mistake about the taste; you'll be giving yourself a morning treat if you opt to have the Feta Frittata for breakfast. Enjoy

Prep time: 25 minutes Total time: 25 minutes Servings: 2

Ingredients:

- Reduced-fat sour cream, 2 tablespoons
- Thinly sliced green onion, 1
- Peeled avocado, 4 thin slices
- Small garlic clove (minced), 1

- Plum tomatoes (chopped), 1/3 cup
- Large eggs, 2
- Crumbled feta cheese (divided), 4 tablespoons
- Egg substitute, 1/2 cup

Method:

1. Set nonstick frying over medium heat, add garlic and onion, and saute until soft. Beat together three tablespoons feta cheese, egg substitute, and eggs. Add the mixture to the frying pan. Cover the lid and cook for about four to six minutes or until nearly set.

2. Spray the remaining feta cheese and tomatoes. Put the lid and allow cooking for another two to three minutes. Give it five minutes to cool. Then cut in 1/2 and serve with sour cream and avocado.

Nutrition Facts:

Serving Size: 1 wedge

- Protein 17g
- Fiber 3g
- Sugars 3g
- Carbohydrate 7g
- Sodium 345mg
- Cholesterol 224mg
- Saturated fat 4g
- Fat 12g
- Calories 203

7. Southwestern Omelet

The Southwestern Omelet is a flavor-rich, hearty egg dish that contains the right dietary supply of healthy fats, protein, carbs, and other nutrients that keep the body in good stead, and most importantly, in Ketosis. It is quick and easy to make, nutritious, tasty, and flavorful. Take out time to explore this southwestern recipe that will supply your body with the right nutrients and fuel to keep your body going all day. Enjoy! Prep time; 10 minutes Cook time: 10 minutes Total time: 20 minutes Servings: 4

Ingredients:

- Pepper and salt to taste
- Chopped onion, 1/2 cup
- Shredded Monterey Jack Cheese (divided), 1 cup
- Minced jalapeno pepper, 1
- Ripe avocado (cut into one-inch slices), 1
- Lightly beaten large eggs, 6
- Small tomato (chopped), 1
- Canola oil, 1 tablespoon
- Bacon strips (cooked and crumbled), 6
- Salsa (not compulsory)

Method:

1. Add oil, jalapeno, and onion in a frying pan and sauté until tender; use a slotted spoon to remove and keep aside. Set the same frying pan over

low heat, add eggs, and cool for three to four minutes.

2. Spray with the avocado, onion mixture, 1/2 cup cheese, tomato, and bacon. Add pepper and salt to taste.

3. Roll up the omelet in 1/2 overfilling. Cover the lid and cook until you see that the eggs are set or let say between three to four minutes. Then, spray with the leftover cheese. It is optional, but you can serve with salsa.

Recommendation:

Don't expose your skin; make sure you put on hand gloves before chopping the hot peppers; the oils can cause skin burn. Also, try your best not to use your hands on your face.

Nutrition Facts:

- Protein 22g
- Fiber 4g
- Sugar 2g
- Carbohydrate 8g
- Sodium 480mg
- Cholesterol 355mg
- Saturated fat 10g
- Fat 31g
- Calories 390

8. Broccoli Quiche Cups

The Broccoli Quiche cup is a tasty recipe that contains 16g of protein, 24g of fat, and 4g of carbs. It is a typical ketogenic diet that is crustless and cheesy but also tasty and healthy. Invest twenty minutes of your precious time to make this recipe, and you'll always come back for more. Prep time: 10 minutes Cook time: 15 minutes Total time: 25 minutes Servings: 1 dozen

Ingredients:

- Pepper, 1/4 teaspoon
- Fresh broccoli (fresh), 1 cup
- Salt, 1/4 teaspoon
- Shredded pepper jack cheese, 1 cup
- Shallot (minced), 1
- Large eggs (lightly beaten), 6
- Bacon bits, 1/2 cup
- Heavy whipping cream, 3/4 cup

Method:

1. Heat the oven beforehand to 350 degrees Fahrenheit. Share cheese and broccoli among twelve different muffin cups

2. Whisk all the other ingredients together and empty them into the muffin cups. Bake for fifteen to twenty minutes, or until it sets.

Nutrition Facts:

Serving Size: 2 cups

- Protein 16g
- Fiber 0g
- Sugars 2g
- Carbohydrate 4g
- Sodium 532mg
- Cholesterol 243mg

- Saturated fat 12g
- Fat 24g
- Calories 291

9. Cheesy Chive omelet

The cheesy Chive omelet is a fifteen minutes breakfast recipe made with eggs and other supporting nutrient-rich food ingredients. It is easy to prepare, delicious, and can be consumed by most people. Set aside one of these mornings to prepare the tasty Cheesy Chive Omelet.

Prep time: 7 minutes Cook time: 8 minutes Total time: 15 minutes Servings: 2

Ingredients:

- Shredded cheddar cheese, 1/4 - 1/2 cup
- Large eggs, 3
- Butter, 1 tablespoon
- Water, 2 tablespoons
- Fresh chives (minced), 1 tablespoon
- Salt, 1/8 teaspoon
- Dash pepper

Method:

1. Whisk pepper, salt, eggs, and water in a small bowl. Stirring, add the chives.
2. Cook butter in a frying pan over medium to high heat. Add the egg mixture. As usual, it'll set towards the edges. Once the eggs set, move the areas that are properly cooked to the middle, allowing the yet to be cooked side go underneath.

3. When eggs are fully cooked and thickened, sprays cheese on either side; roll omelet in half, cut in half, and serve in plates.

Nutrition Facts:

Serving Size: Half omelet

- Protein 13g
- Fiber 0g
- Sugars 0g
- Carbohydrate 1g
- Sodium 392mg
- Cholesterol 309mg
- Saturated fat 9g
- Fat 18g
- Calories 216

Broccoli and Ham Frittata

The Broccoli and Ham Frittata is a simple high-fat and low-carb recipe made with healthy ingredients that boost ketosis and provide other health benefits ranging from blood sugar control, anti-inflammation, and blood sugar control. It is also easy to make and tasteful! Prep time: 15 minutes Cook time: 15 minutes Total time: 30 minutes Servings: 4

Ingredients:

- Chopped broccoli (fresh), 1 cup
- Large eggs, 6· Butter, 1 tablespoon· Pepper, 1/4 teaspoon
- Cube and fully cooked ham, 1 cup
- Dash salt

- Shredded Swiss cheese (divided), 1-1/4 cups

Methods:

1. Heat broiler beforehand. Whisk salt, pepper, and eggs in a bowl. Stirring, add ham, and one cup of cheese.

2. Heat butter in a ten inches skillet (ovenproof) set over medium to high heat. Add broccoli and cook, while stirring until soft. Set heat on low, add egg mixture. Cover the lid and cook until almost set, or for four to six minutes. Spray the leftover cheese on it.

3. Broil 3-4in until eggs are set completely. Allow it stand for five minutes, then chop into wedges.

Nutrition Facts:

- Protein 26g
- Fiber 1g
- Sugars 2g
- Carbohydrate 4g
- Sodium 665mg
- Cholesterol 374mg
- Saturated fat 11g
- Fat 23g
- Calories 321

11. Spinach frittatas

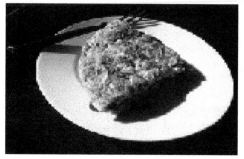

These crunchy mini frittatas are tasty and delicious. They are rich in protein and healthy fats but low on carbs. It is one of those recipes you just can't get over, after having a taste. Take out some time to explore it and feel the goodness of all that has been said about it. Enjoy!

Prep time: 30 minutes Total time: 30 minutes Servings: 2 dozen

Ingredients:

· Pepperoni, 24 slices· Whole milk ricotta cheese, 1 cup· Pepper, 1/4 teaspoon· Grated Parmesan cheese, 3/4 cup· Salt, 1/4 teaspoon· Fresh mushrooms (chopped), 2/3 cup· Dried oregano, 1/2 teaspoon· Frozen chopped spinach, thawed and squeezed dry, 1 package (10 ounces)· Large egg, 1

Method:

1. Heat the oven beforehand to 375 degrees Fahrenheit. Whisk everything except the slices of pepperoni. Then, get twenty four slightly greased mini-muffin cups and add a slice of pepperoni in each. Do the same with the cheese mixture.

2. Put in the preheated oven and bake until set completely- usually takes between twenty to twenty minutes.

Loosen the frittatas by running a knife on each side of the mini-muffin cups. Serve while warm.

Nutrition Facts:

Serving Size: One mini frittata

- Protein 10g
- Fiber 1g
- Sugars 2g
- Carbohydrate 4g
- Sodium 396mg
- Cholesterol 50mg
- Saturated fat 5g
- Fat9g
- Calories 128

Lunch Recipes

Lunch is one of the most important meals of the day because it helps to boost energy levels during the most productive part of the day. It also consolidates the achievements recorded by breakfast.

With that said, the Keto lunch recipes on this list have been carefully selected to add more healthy fats to your body, which in turn results in the production of more ketones, which are further used as fuel for the body. These meals are delicious, tasty, and enjoyable.

1. Keto Brunch Spread

This is a simple keto recipe rich in nutrients and minerals. It is filling and satisfying too. With only here ingredients, it is one of the easiest recipes you can think of. Set out time to enjoy this tasteful keto brunch spread.

Prep time: 10 minutes Cook time: 20 minutes Total time: 30 minutes Servings: 4

Ingredients:

- Pastured, sugar-free bacon, 12 slices
- Asparagus Spears,24
- Large eggs, 4

Method:

1. Heat the oven beforehand to 400 degrees Fahrenheit.

2. From the bottom, trim the asparagus. Then, wrap them in pairs with a single slice of bacon. Wind the slice of bacon from under, to the top of the spear. While winding, pull the bacon slowly so that it'll wrap tightly. Put it on a sheet pan.

3. Do the same thing with the other asparagus, thus making it twelve pairs wrapped in bacon.

4. Set in the oven for twenty minutes

5. While the oven is running, Boil water in a small pot. Add the four large eggs in boiling water. Wait for six minutes

6. Pour ice water in a bowl. Wait for six minutes, after the eggs must have been done, remove the eggs and immerse in ice water. Before peeling the eggs, allow them to sit in the water for two minutes.

7. Crack the tip of the egg on a solid surface and peel off the shell to access the tip.

8. Serve the asparagus on a cutting board or tray when they are ready. In other to hold the eggs up, you can use either an egg holder or espresso cups.

9. Using a small spoon, take off the top of the egg to reveal the yolk.

10. Finally, dip the asparagus spears into the eggs.

Nutrition Facts:

- Protein 17g

- Carbohydrate 3g

- Saturated fat 13g

- Fat 38g

- Calories 426

2. Turkey Sausage Frittata

The Turkey Sausage Frittata is a low-carb, high-fat diet that can help you maintain Ketosis, or aid your process of attaining Ketosis. It is not only made with healthy food ingredients, but it is also tasty and delicious. Enjoy this recipe today!

Prep time: 10 minutes Cook time: 30 minutes Total time: 40 minutes Servings: 8

Ingredients:

- Shredded Tillamook Cheddar (optional), 2oz.

- Ground breakfast sausage (turkey), 12 oz.

- Kerry Gold butter, 2 teaspoons

- Bell peppers, 2

- Black pepper, 1 teaspoon

- Eggs, 12

- Pink Himalayan salt, 1 teaspoon

- Sour cream (lactose-free), 1 cup

Method:

1. Heat oven beforehand to 350 degrees Fahrenheit.

2. Crack and empty all eggs into a blender, add pepper, salt, and sour cream. Blast for thirty seconds on high speed. Set aside.

3. Set a large frying pan on low-medium heat. Once it gets heated, add the butter.

4. Slice the bell peppers. Throw it in the frying pan. Fry for six minutes or until color turns brown.

5. Stirring, add the sausage, breaking up the meat for eight minutes until color turns brown. Flatten the sausage to the bottom of the pan. Then spray the peppers across (evenly). Add the egg mix.

6. Slot the pan in the oven and bake for thirty minutes. To add the cheese, spray it over the frittata immediately it comes out of the oven.

Nutrition Facts:

- Protein 16.7g

- Carbohydrate 5.5g

- Fat 16.7g

- Calorie 240

3. Keto Cloud Bread

The Keto Cloud Bread recipe takes forty minutes from start to finish, and it is made with healthy food ingredients like tomato, eggs, lettuce, and others. These ingredients do not only contain low carbs and high-fats, but they are also rich in elements that support the proper functioning of the human body. Also, the Cloud Bread is delicious and tasty and will become one of your favorite keto diets, only if you try it out just once. Enjoy! Prep time: 15 minutes

Cook time: 25 minutes Total time: 40 minutes Servings: 4

Ingredients:

Cloud bread

- Cream of tartar, 1/4 spoon
- Eggs, 3
- Baking powder, 1/2 teaspoon
- Softened Cream cheese, 4 1/2 ounces
- Ground Psyllium Husk powder, 1/2 tablespoon
- Salt, to taste

Toppings:

- Tomato (thinly sliced), 1
- Mayonnaise, 8 tablespoons
- Lettuce, 2 ounces
- Cooked bacon, 5 ounces

Method:

1. Heat the oven beforehand to 300 degrees Fahrenheit. As per the eggs, separate the yolks from the whites.
2. Add cream of tartar and salt to the egg whites. Use a hand mixer and whip
3. Mix the psyllium husk powder, egg yolks, and cream cheese.

4. Roll the egg whites into the yolks. Make sure you do not over mix because the whites will lose their whip.
5. Get some parchment paper and add it to the baking sheet. Shape the batter into eight rounds and bake until golden, or for twenty- five minutes.
6. Flip the cloud bread over, ensuring the top is facing downward.
7. Top the four bread pieces with tomato, lettuce, and bacon. Do the same with the other bread pieces to make the sandwiches.

Nutrition Facts:

1. Protein 19.75g
2. Carbs 4.83g
3. Fat 46.98g
4. Calories 527.93

4. Ketofied Chick-Fil-A-style Chicken

The Ketofied Chick-Fil-A-Style Chicken recipe is made with healthy food ingredients like avocado, eggs, paprika, parmesan and protein powder, etc. It is rich in nutrients and minerals, low in carbohydrates, and rich in healthy fats. This is one of the meals to prepare while on the ketogenic diet. Prep time: 10 minutes Cook time: 20 minutes Total time: 30 minutes Servings: 8

Ingredients:

- Avocado oil, 2 tablespoons
- Pickle jar, 24-ounces
- Eggs, 2

- Uncooked chicken breast tenders (medium), 8
- Paprika, 1 teaspoon
- Unflavored 100% whey protein powder, 2 scoops
- Pepper and salt
- Grated Parmesan, 1/4 cup

Method:

1. In a plastic bag, pour the pickle juice and add the chicken. Deposit in the refrigerator for at least one hour.

2. Mix the paprika, pepper, salt, grated parmesan, and protein powder in a plate. On a different plate, beat the eggs together.

3. Heat a saucepan over low-medium heat beforehand. Add the avocado oil and wait till it heats up while breading the chicken.

4. Immerse the chicken tenders into the egg, then; use the breading mixture to coat.

5. Fry until the tenders fully cooked and golden brown

Nutritional Facts:

- Protein 47.6g
- Carbohydrates 1.68g
- Fats 14.8g
- Calories 342.53

5. Shrimp Avocado Salad with Feta and Tomatoes

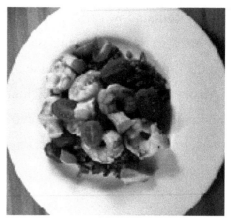

This is a simple and delicious keto recipe that contains elements that help to keep the body in ketosis. It is healthy and contains elements that aid human organs.

Prep time: 15 minutes Cook time: 5 minutes

Total time: 20 minutes Servings: 2

Ingredients:

- Black pepper, 1/4 teaspoon
- Shrimp (peeled, deveined, patted dry)
- Salt, 1/4 teaspoon
- Large avocado (diced), 1
- Olive oil, 1 tablespoon
- Small beefsteak tomato (diced and drained), 1
- Lemon juice, 1 tablespoon
- Crumbled feta cheese, 1/3 cup
- Salted butter (melted), 2 tablespoons
- Parsley or Cilantro (freshly chopped), 1/3 cup

Method:

1. In a bowl, add the melted butter with shrimp until well coated.

2. Set a saucepan over medium-high heat and wait till it gets hot. Add the

well-coated shrimps to the saucepan and sear until the edges turn pink. Flip and cook for about two minutes, until shrimp are thoroughly cooked.

3. When the shrimp are done, remove and put in a plate. Allow them to lose steam while you put other ingredients together.

4. Get a mixing bowl and add all other ingredients, including; pepper, salt, olive oil, lemon juice, cilantro, feta cheese, diced tomato, and diced avocado, and mix properly.

5. Stirring, add shrimp, and thoroughly mix. Add more pepper and salt to taste.

Nutrition Facts:

Per serving:

- Protein 24g
- Sugar 1.5g
- Fiber 6g
- Carbohydrate 12.5g
- Potassium 600mg
- Sodium 1250mg
- Trans Fat 0g
- Saturated Fat 12g
- Total Fat 33g
- Calories 430

6. Salmon Poke Bowl

This is a healthy dish that contains high-fat dressing and low-carb vegetables – which is ideal for people that seek to lose weight and also reduce sugar content in their system.

Prep time: 20 minutes Cook time: NATotal time: 20 minutes Servings: 1

Ingredients:

- Black sesame seeds, 1 teaspoon
- Fresh Salmon, Debone and skinless, 8 ounces
- Sesame seeds, 1 teaspoon
- Tamari Sauce, 1 teaspoon
- Keto Sesame Mayonnaise, 2 tablespoons
- Pinch salt
- Cilantro, 1/4 cup
- Shredded cabbage, 2 cups
- Avocado (diced), 1/2
- Small Radish (thinly sliced), 1
- Cucumber (sliced), 4 ounces

Method:

1. Start by cutting the salmon into cubes and placing them in a bowl.

2. Add the salt, tamari, and sesame oil, and allow it to marinate.

3. Get two bowls; combine the cilantro, avocado, radishes, cucumber, and cabbage.

4. Use the marinated salmon as a topping, spray with the sesame mayonnaise and sesame seeds.

Nutrition Facts:

- Iron 1/9mg
- Calcium 75mg
- Vitamin C 33mg
- Vitamin A 365IU

- Sugar 3g
- Fiber 6g
- Potassium 995mg
- Sodium 236mg
- Cholesterol 62mg
- Saturated Fat 6g
- Fat 34g
- Protein 26g
- Carbohydrate 11g
- Calories 446

7. Cucumber Noodles with Tahini Sauce

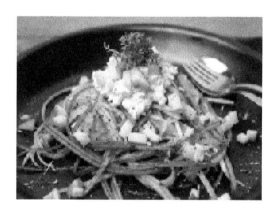

The Cucumber Noodles with Tahini Sauce is a nutrient-packed, healthy, and high fat keto recipe created to provide the body with more keto fuel to burn. It is also rich in nutrients and minerals that help the body remain healthy and strong over long periods.

Prep time: 10 Minutes Total time: 10 minutes Servings: 4

Ingredients:

- Tahini sauce, 1 recipe
- Cucumber, large (10 oz each), 2

Method:

1. Use a spiralizer to spiralize the cucumbers. Use some salt on it and drain.
2. Dry the cucumber noodles. Share on different plates. Top with tahini sauce.

Nutrition Facts:

Serving size: 1/4 total recipe

- Sugar 2g
- Fiber 1g
- Carbohydrate 7g
- Protein 3g
- Fat 18g
- Calories 202

8. Ham and Cheddar Calzones

The Ham and Cheddar Calzones recipe contains several nutrients with the ability to fight diseases such as morning sickness, common cold, skin irritation, and others. It is rich in healthy fats but low in carbs – making it a perfect ketogenic diet. Enjoy this recipe. Prep time: 15 minutes Cook time: 30 minutes Total time: 45 minutes Servings: 4

Ingredients:

- Egg yolk (whisked), 1
- Almond flour, 1/4 cup
- Diced ham,1 1/2 cups
- Plain whey protein powder, 1/3 cup
- Shredded Cheddar Cheese, 3 cups

- Coconut flour, 1/3 cup

- Large 3ggs, 3

- Baking powder, 1 tablespoon

- Butter (melted), 1/3 cup

- Garlic powder, 1 1⁄2 teaspoon

- Xanthan gum, 3⁄4 teaspoon

Method:

1. Heat the oven beforehand to 325 degrees Fahrenheit. Use parchment to line a baking sheet.

2. In a bowl, mix the xanthan, garlic powder, baking powder, coconut flour, protein powder, and almond flour.

3. Stirring, whisk in the eggs and melted butter until dough is formed.

4. Share dough in two and cover each piece between two pieces of parchment.

5. Fold each piece of dough into a twelve-inch circle, then take off the pieces of parchment at the top.

6. The top half of each dough circle ham and shredded cheese, save a 3/3- inch border.

7. Roll dough circles over the fillings and pinch the edges together, crimp to seal

8. Put the calzones on the parchment-lined baking sheet and brush with egg yolk.

9. Slot in the oven and bake for twenty five to thirty minutes, until they turn golden brown.

Nutrition Facts:

- Carbohydrates 7.5g

- Protein 268g

- Fat 43g

- Calories 545

9. Chicken Cucumber Avocado Salad

The Chicken Cucumber Avocado Salad is a simple keto recipe that is perfect for lunch and dinner. It is a nutritious meal that contains low- carbs, moderate protein, and high-fats. Apart from its ketogenic properties, this recipe also contains other medical properties that help reduce blood cholesterol, blood sugar, and inflammation. Enjoy this healthy recipe! Prep time: 10 minutes Cook time: NATotal time: 10 minutes Servings: 6

Ingredients:

- Large Roma tomatoes (sliced and chopped), 4-5

- Large cucumber (Continental or English), halved lengthways, sliced into 1⁄4-inch thick slices, 1

- Pepper and salt to taste

- Rotisserie chicken deboned and shredded (skin on or off), 1

- Lemon juice or juice of two limes, 2-3 tablespoons

- Thinly sliced red onion, 1⁄4

- Olive oil, 3 tablespoons

- Flat-leaf parsley (chopped), 1⁄2 cup

- Avocados (peeled, pitted and diced), 2

Method:

1. In a large bowl, add and mix the chopped parsley, avocados, onion, tomatoes, cucumbers, and shredded chicken.

2. Spray with lemon juice (or lime juice) and olive oil. Add pepper and salt to taste.

3. Slowly toss to mix the favors.

Recommendation:

- Instead of parsley, you can use cilantro or fresh basil.

Nutrition Facts:

- Iron 3mg
- Calcium 46mg
- Vitamin c 22.7mg
- Vitamin A 1050IU
- Sugar 2g
- Fiber 5g
- Potassium 868mg
- Sodium 127mg
- Cholesterol 121mg
- Saturated Fat 8g
- Fat 38g
- Protein 40g
- Carbohydrates 10g
- Calories 545

10. Keto Caesar Salad

The Keto Caesar Salad is a simple but nutritious recipe made with healthy food ingredients like egg yolk, avocado oil, parmesan, apple cider vinegar, anchovy fillets, and others. It is a high-fat and low-carb diet that helps the body lose weight and fight diseases like diabetes, heart diseases, and others. Prep time: 15 minutes Cook time: NATotal time: 15 minutes Servings: 4

Ingredients:

- Parmesan for garnish, 4 tablespoons
- Egg yolk, 1
- Pork rinds chopped in tiny pieces, 2 oz.
- Avocado oil, 8 tablespoons

Romaine hearts, 24 whole leaves Apple Cider Vinegar, 3 tablespoons Parmesan (grated), 4 tablespoons Dijon mustard, 1 teaspoon

Garlic cloves, 2 Anchovy fillets, 4

Method:

1. Place the mustard, ACV, and egg yolk inside the cup of an immersion blender. Slot the blender stick, and while standing on the egg yolk carefully pour the avocado oil on top.

2. Blast the blender (set on low), firmly in position.

3. At this point, the egg yolk will emulsify with the oil, resulting in a mayonnaise.

4. When you have your mayo, take off the blender; add grated parmesan, garlic, and anchovies to the cup.

5. Blend (on slow) again, and wait until a smooth mayonnaise is created.

6. Arrange the romaine leaves on four serving plates, but make sure you wash and dry them first.

7. Using a spoon, spray the dressing on the leaves.

8. Portion the pork rind between the four dishes.

9. Use the shaved parmesan for garnishing.

Nutrition Facts:

Serving size: 1

- Protein 13g
- Fiber 0.5g
- Carbohydrate 1.8g
- Fat 38.75g
- Calories 727

Dinner Recipes

Dinner is the last meal people eat before they retire to bed at night. Thus it is important to eat easily digestible meals that contain nutrients and minerals that enrich the body. The ketogenic dinner recipes on this list have been vetted, and are some of the best you will ever find anywhere. They are nutrient-packed, rich, and, most of all, filled with good fats and low carbs.

1. Keto Lasagna

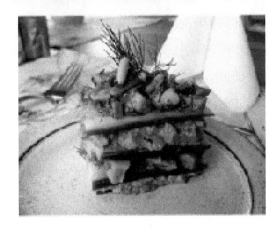

This tasty and delicious, low carbohydrate lasagna is a breadth of fresh air from the regular lasagna. It is contains everything in the regular lasagna minus carbohydrates. Explore this classic meal today and get a feel of the good life.

Prep Time: 10 minutes Cook Time: 45 minutes Total Time: 55 minutes

Servings: 6

Ingredients:

- Basil, 1/4 cup
- Butter, coconut oil, ghee, or lad, 1 tablespoon
- Red pepper flakes (depending on your desired level of spiciness),1/4 – 1/2 teaspoon
- Ricotta cheese, 15 oz.
- Mixed Italian herb seasoning, 1 tablespoon
- Coconut Flour, 2 tablespoons
- Rao's marinara sauce (low-carb), 16 oz.
- Whole egg, 1

- Large zucchinis (sliced long to 1/4" pieces), 4

- Salt, 1 1/2 cup

- Parmesan cheese, 1/3 cup

- Pepper 1/2 teaspoon

- Mozzarella cheese, 1 1/2 cup

- Garlic powder, 1 teaspoon

- Finely chopped garlic clove, 1

Method:

1. Wash the zucchini and slice. Add salt to it and wrap it with a paper towel for thirty minutes. After that, you have to remove any remaining water from the zucchini by squeezing with a paper towel.

2. Get a skillet and cook 1 tablespoon butter set over medium heat. Crumble and cook the sausage. Remove from heat and set aside to cool.

3. Use butter or cooking spray to coat a baking dish (preferably 9x9 baking dish); also, heat oven to 375 degrees Fahrenheit.

4. In a small bowl, add and mix pepper, garlic powder, 1 egg, garlic, salt, parmesan cheese, and coconut flour. When it is completely smooth, set aside. In a jar containing marinara, add red pepper flakes and Italian seasoning, stir and mix properly, and set aside.

5. On the greased dish, add one layer of sliced zucchini. Roll about 1/4 cup cheese mixture over the zucchini, spray 1/4 of the Italian sausage, then top with another layer of sauce. Add the leftover mozzarella cheese and spread the remaining parmesan cheese.

6. Place in a foil and slot in the oven for thirty minutes. Take off the foil and bake until the color becomes golden brown (usually takes fifteen minutes). Turn off the oven, remove the dish, and let it rest for five to ten minutes. Use oregano or fresh basil if necessary.

Nutrition Facts:

- Protein 32g

- Carbohydrates 12g

- Fat 21g

- Calories 364

9. Cauliflower Bake

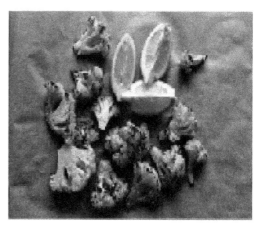

This is a high fat, low-carb keto recipe that can be truly enjoyed while maintaining your ketosis status. It is made from some of the most nutritious food ingredients around, and as such, it provides the body with the required supply of fat to keep burning, while also nourishing other areas of the body. Explore the recipe today and thank me later. Enjoy!

Prep time: 15 minutes Cook time 45 minutes
Total time: 1 hour Servings: 4

Ingredients:

- Green onions (chopped), 1⁄4 cup
- Large head cauliflower (cut into florets), 1
- Bacon slices (cooked and crumbled), 6
- Butter, 2 tablespoons
- Pepper and salt to taste
- Heavy cream, 1 cup
- Shredded sharp cheddar cheese (separated), 1 1⁄4 cup
- Cream cheese, 2 oz.

Method:

1. Heat oven beforehand to 350 degrees Fahrenheit.
2. Add cauliflower florets in a pot of boiling water for two minutes
3. Remove the cauliflower and then use paper towels to dry.
4. Cook butter, cream cheese, salt, heavy cream, pepper, and one cup of shredded cheddar cheese in a pot, until consistently combined.
5. Get a baking dish and add cheese sauce, green onions (remaining one tablespoon), shredded cheddar cheese, and crumbled bacon (remaining one tablespoon). Mix properly.
6. Use the remaining green onions, crumbled bacon, and shredded cheddar cheese as a topping.
7. Slot in the oven and bake for thirty minutes, or until the cauliflower becomes tender and cheese is golden.
8. Serve while warm.

Nutrition Facts:

Serving size: 1

- Protein 13.9g
- Carbohydrate 5.8g
- Fat 45g
- Calories 498

3. Keto Mayo

Keto Mayo is a delicious, healthy, and low-carb alternative of the traditional mayo dish. It contains zero sugar; it is dairy-free and gluten- free. Talking about versatility, you can use the Keto Mayo in every keto meal plan. In five minutes, a cup of mayo is prepared and ready to be

consumed. Thus it remains one of the easiest but most rewarding keto recipes around. Enjoy!

Prep time: 5 minutes Cook time: NATotal time: 5 minutes Servings: 1 cup

Ingredients:

- Pink Himalayan salt, 1⁄4 teaspoon • Egg,1
- Apple cider vinegar, 2 teaspoons
- Olive oil (light), 1 cup

Method:

1. Take out the egg from the fridge and leave it exposed at room temperature for two hours. Then, Separate the egg white from the yolk. The egg white isn't needed for this recipe, so you can do whatever you want with it.

2. Add salt, mustard, apple cider vinegar, olive oil, and egg yolk in a mason jar.

3. Position a blender (immersion) in the bottom of the jar, turn it on, and allow to blend for thirty to forty seconds or until the mixture is consistent (like mayonnaise).

4. Once that is done, turn off the blender and reposition it to the top of the mixture. Turn on and allow the blender to travel from top to bottom. Repeat the process about 3-4 times, making sure you turn off the blender once it reaches the bottom, and turning on once it reaches the top.5. When it is completely emulsified, you can store in the fridge or server alongside your delicious keto meals.

Nutrition Facts:

Serving size: 1 tablespoon

- Protein 0.6g
- Carbohydrates 0g
- Fat 14.3g
- Calories 124

4. Portobello Bun Cheeseburgers

These healthy and nutrient-packed burgers are designed to keep the body in ketosis. But that this not to say they're not tasty and delicious too. They are filling, nutritious, and high in healthy fats. Take out time to prepare this amazing recipe. Prep time: 5 minutes Cook time: 15 minutes Total time: 20 minutes Servings: 6

Ingredients:

- Sharp cheddar cheese, 6 slices
- Grassfed 80/20 ground beef, 1lb
- Portobello mushroom caps (stem removed, rinsed and dabbed dry), 6
- Worcestershire sauce, 1 tablespoon
- Avocado oil, 1 tablespoon
- Pink Himalayan salt, 1 teaspoon
- Black pepper, 1teaspoon

Method:

1. Mix pepper, salt, Worcestershire sauce, and ground beef in a bowl.

2. Mould beef into patties for the burger.

3. Steam avocado oil in a saucepan over medium heat. Then, throw in the portobello mushroom caps and cook for three to four minutes (flipping on each side). Take off from the heat.

4. Heat the burger patties in the same saucepan, four minutes on the first side and five minutes on the flips side, or until properly cooked. At the top of the burgers, add cheese, cover the lid

and wait for one minute for the cheese to thaw.

5. It should be in this format; Portobello mushroom, cheeseburger, garnishes, and portobello mushroom cap topping.

6. Serve and enjoy.

Recommendations:

You can use the following to garnish the burger

- Spicy brown mustard
- Sliced dill pickles
- Sugar-free barbecue sauce
- Romaine

Nutrition Fact:

Serving size: One

- Protein 29.1g
- Carbohydrate 5.8g
- Fat 22.8g
- Calories 336

5. Berbere Enchilada Stuffed peppers

The Berbere Enchilada Stuffed peppers recipe is a spicy meal that is high in protein and healthy fats, but low in carbs. It isn't the traditional Mexican enchiladas. However, it is guaranteed that you'll have a good time consuming this keto diet. Prep time: 10 minutes Cook time: 50 minutes Total time: 1 hour Servings: 5

Ingredients:

- Large bell peppers, 5
- 85% lean pastured ground beef, 2lb
- Berbere, 2 teaspoons
- Organic frozen cauliflower rice, 1 cup
- Smoked sea salt, 2 teaspoons
- Kerry Gold butter, 3 tablespoons
- Garlic cloves, 2
- Maui onion, 1⁄2
- Carrot (large), 1
- Organic, lactose-free sour cream, 5 dollops

Method:

1. Dice the garlic, onion, and carrot. Also, steam a frying pan over medium heat.

2. In the heated frying pan, add butter; when it melts completely, add the diced garlic, onion, and carrot.

3. Allow to fry while stirring from time to time (about eight minutes).

4. Add the berbere, salt, and beef, stir thoroughly, breaking up the beef until it turns brown and crumbly. Add the cauliflower rice, stirring until completely mixed. Take off the frying pan from the burner.

5. Heat oven beforehand to 450 degrees Fahrenheit. Cut open the peppers from the top; then take off the seeds and core. Add the mixture into the peppers. Use a casserole dish to arrange them.

6. Use sour cream as topping on each of them. Spray some extra spice on top.

7. Slot in the oven and bake for forty minutes. Don't allow to cool; serve while hot.

Recommendations:

- Use Green Valley as sour cream
- As for the spice mix, you can hot curry or any taco seasoning

Nutrition Facts:

- Protein 35g
- Carbohydrates 8.4g
- Fat 38.8g
- Calories 516

6. Low-carb Meatloaf

The low- carb meatloaf is a keto diet recipe that goes along with other low- carb side veggies like zucchini broccoli or cauliflower. With this nourishing meal, you are guaranteed to remain in ketosis. Prep time: 10 minutes Cook time: 50 minutes Total time: 1 hour Servings: 6

Ingredients:

- Garlic clove, 4
- 85% lean grass-fed ground beef, 2 pounds
- Chopped fresh oregano, 1/4 cup
- Fine Himalayan salt, 1/4 cup
- Black pepper, 1 teaspoon
- Chopped parsley
- Nutritional yeast, 1/4 cup
- Lemon zest, 1 tablespoon
- Large egg, 2

- Avocado oil, 2 tablespoons

Method:

1. Heat oven beforehand to 400 degrees Fahrenheit.
2. Mix nutritional yeast, ground beef, black pepper, and salt in a large bowl.
3. Mix the garlic, lemon, and herbs in a food processor or blender. Blast until the garlic, lemon, and herbs are completely mixed and mixed, and the eggs are frothy.
4. Mix the blend with the beef and combine properly.
5. Pour the mixture on a pan. Smooth and flatten out.
6. Bake until the top becomes brown, a process that normally takes between fifty to sixty minutes.
7. Turn off the oven and tilt the pan towards one edge so any remaining liquid can be discarded. Leave it in the open for five to ten minutes before slicing.
8. You can use fresh lemon to garnish before serving.

Nutrition Facts:

- Protein 33g
- Fiber 2g
- Carbohydrate 4g
- Fat 29g
- Calories 344

7. Keto Chili

The Keto Chili is an easy but extremely nutritious keto recipe. It is delicious, filling, and hearty, but the best of all is that it contains a meager 5g of carbohydrates only.

Prep time: 5 minutes Cook time: 30 minutes Total time: 35 minutes Servings: 6

Ingredients:

- Black pepper, 1 teaspoon
- Avocado oil, 1 or 2 tablespoons
- Salt, 1 teaspoon
- Ribs celery (chopped), 2
- Cumin, 1 tablespoon
- Chipotle chili powder, 1 teaspoon
- Garlic powder, 2 teaspoons
- 15 oz. can no-salt-added tomato sauce, 1
- Chili powder, 2 teaspoons
- 16.2 oz. container Kettle and Fire Beef Bone Broth, 1

Method:

1. Steam avocado in a large pot set on medium heat. Add celery and steam for three to four minutes, until soft and tender. Remove the celery and put in a different bowl, then move on to other things.

2. Add brown beef, spices, and beef in the same pot and cook thoroughly.

3. Reduce the heat to medium-low, add beef bone broth and tomato sauce to the steamed beef, cover with the lid and allow to simmer, stirring from time to time.

4. Add celery and stir until completely mixed.

5. Finally, you can garnish and serve.

Recommendation:

For garnishing, you can use green onion, cilantro, sliced jalapeno, cheddar cheese, or sour cream.

Nutrition Facts:

Serving size: 1 cup

- Protein 34.4g
- Carbohydrate 6.7g
- Ft 22.8g
- Calories 359

8. Keto Meatballs

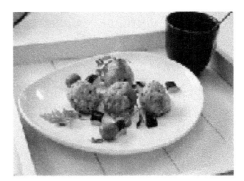

The Keto Meatballs is a delicious meal that unlocks different layers of nutrients and minerals. It is the perfect meal to keep you locked in ketosis.

Prep time: 10 minutes Cook time: 40 minutes Total time: 50 minutes Servings: 10

Ingredients:

- Olive oil
- 85% lean grass-fed ground beef, 1lb
- Garlic powder, 1 tablespoon

- Pastured Chicken livers, 1lb
- Dried thyme, 1 tablespoon
- Large shallot, 1
- Black pepper, 2 teaspoon
- Carrots (medium), 4
- Salt (separated), 3 teaspoons
- Garlic cloves, 3
- Coconut aminos (separated), 2 tablespoons
- Grass-fed butter, 2 tablespoons
- Oregano (dried), 1 teaspoon
- Apple cider vinegar, 1 tablespoon

Method:

1. Set a large frying pan on medium heat. While steaming, mince the garlic, carrots, and shallots. Once the frying pan gets to the desired temperature, add the vegetables and fry until soft and aromatic, while stirring. It often takes about eight minutes.

2. Add dried oregano, one teaspoon salt, and chicken livers. Steam (while stirring) until livers are thoroughly cooked. Add one tablespoon apple cider vinegar and one tablespoon coconut aminos and steam until reduced, and livers are thoroughly cooked.

3. Turn off the heat and allow cooling for some time. Empty in a food processor and pulse until it transforms into ground beef. Empty the mix in a large bowl, and give some time to cool.

4. Heat oven beforehand to 425 degrees Fahrenheit. Add the ground beef to the bowl with the remaining seasoning and salt. Combine properly. Make one and a half-inch size balls (approximately thirty).

5. On the sheet pan, sprinkle olive oil. Use the olive oil to coal each meatball and place it on the sheet pan. Then sprinkle the rest of the coconut aminos on them.

6. Place the sheet pan with the meatballs in the oven and roast at 425 degrees Fahrenheit for five minutes. Then reduce the temperature to 350 degrees Fahrenheit and roast for a further twenty minutes before turning off the oven.

7. You can use them with lemon tahini sauce, or any other desired food.

Nutrition Facts:

- Protein 31.8g
- Carbohydrates 4.3g
- Fat 21g
- Calories 323

9. Mushroom Bacon Skillet

This is an extremely easy and quick to make a keto recipe that provides the body with the required amount of fat to keep going. It is rich in protein and low in carbs. Enjoy!

Prep time: 10 minutes Cook time: 10 minutes Total time: 20 minutes Servings: 1-2

Ingredients:

- Garlic confit, 1 tablespoon
- Pastured pork bacon, 4 slices
- Sprigs thyme, 2
- Halved mushrooms, 2 cups
- Salt, 1/2 teaspoon

Method:

1. Set a frying pan over low – medium heat and prep the ingredients while it's getting heated.
2. Cut mushrooms in half, Slice bacon into half-inch pieces, and separate thyme stems from the leaves.
3. Add the bacon to the frying pan and steam until tender, then shifts towards one end and add the mushrooms. Fry, occasionally stirring, until tender and brown.
4. Add garlic, thyme, and salt. Continue steaming, occasionally stirring for five more minutes.
5. When the mushrooms are gleaming in fat, juicy and golden, remove from the heat.
6. You can serve with warm broth, boiled eggs, or greens.

Recommendations:

It is important to understand that garlic confits are garlic cloves slowly roasted and submerged in oil. For people that buy garlic in large amounts, it is one of the best ways to preserve them, plus it is very tasty. For a keto- friendly confit, it is best to use avocado oil.

Nutrition Facts:

- Protein 13.6g
- Fiber 0.3g
- Carbohydrates 8.4g
- Fat 8.5g
- Calories 213

10. Baked Cauliflower Rice with Shrimp Stir Fry

The Baked Cauliflower rice with shrimp stir fry is low carb, high fat keto recipe that is exceptionally tasteful and nutrient-packed. It is a highly recommended dish for newcomers and veterans alike, in the world of keto. Take out time to explore this meal and have a truly good time. Prep time: 8 minutes

Cook time: 15 minutes Total time: 23 minutes Servings: 3-4

Ingredients:

- MCT oil, 2 tablespoons
- Shrimp (peeled, tail on), 16oz (1lb)
- Frozen riced cauliflower, 12oz
- The nub of ginger root, 2 inch
- Bacon fat, 3 tablespoons
- Green onion, 4 stalks
- Pink Himalayan salt, more to taste, 2 teaspoon
- Garlic cloves, 2
- Lemon rind, 1-inch piece
- Bella mushrooms (baby), 4

Method:

1. Heat oven beforehand to 400 degrees Fahrenheit.

2. Get a sheet pan and spread the cauliflower rice on it. Sprinkle some salt and spray with MCT oil.

3. Deposit in the oven and bake for ten minutes.

4. Peel of the skin of the garlic cloves and ginger root. Chop the onion into one-inch pieces. Peel off a slice of lemon rind.

5. Steam large frying on low-medium heat. Add all the aromatics and bacon fat, fry until fragrant and tender.

6. Put the shrimp and fry, stirring from time to time until they are coiled and pink. Add salt and coconut aminos, stir for a further two to three minutes. Take off from the heat.

7. Garnish with chili flakes, sesame seeds, or with some more green onions. You can serve the shrimp over a foundation of baked cauliflower rice.

Nutrition Facts:

- Protein 24.7g

- Carbohydrates 9g

- Fat 24.8g

- Calories 357

Dessert Recipes

The Ketogenic dessert recipes are meant to help people in the keto world eat within the ambits of the ketogenic diet. These desserts further consolidate the breakfast, lunch, and dinner recipes; they provide the body with more healthy fats and moderate amounts of problems. The reason why people should embrace these ketogenic dessert recipes is the fact that any form of deviance will stall any all forms of progress achieved.

1. Low Carb Lemon Strawberry Cheesecake Treats

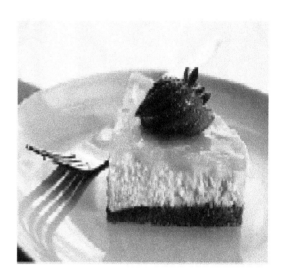

This is the low carb strawberry and lemon keto treat that is guaranteed to lighten up your day. It is tasty, nutritious, and easy to prepare.

Prep time: 15 minutes Total time: 15 minutes Servings: 2

Ingredients:

- Strawberries (large), 2

- Cream cheese (softened), 3 oz

- Zest of 1 lemon

- Heavy whipping cream, 3⁄4 cup

- Lemon extract, 2 teaspoons

- Swerve sweetener, ¾ cup

Method:

1. Mix the whipping cream, sweetener, and cream cheese in a mixing bowl until creamy and smooth

2. Add and mix the lemon extract. Depending on how you want it, you can add as much lemon zest as possible.

3. Chop one of the strawberries into tiny pieces. Slice the remaining one into little heart-shaped pieces.

4. Using the cream cheese mixture, fill two jars halfway.

5. In both jars, add the chopped strawberries.

6. Use the cream cheese mixture to top the strawberries.

7. In the middle of each flower, spray lemon zest.

Recommendation:

The type of sweetener to use optional, just ensure that the amount equals 1/3 cup sugar.

Nutrition Facts:

- Carbohydrates 5.7g
- Protein 4.5g
- Fiber 0.4g
- Fat 48.2g
- Calories 474

1. Vanilla Pound Cake

The Vanilla Pound Cake is quick and easy to make a dessert that comes with the right amounts of nutrients and flavor. It is tasty, sweet, and easy to preserve. Explore this recipe today. Prep time: 15 minutesCook time: 50 minutesTotal time: 1 hour and 5 minutes

Ingredients:

- Eggs (large), 4
- Almond Flour, 2 cups
- Cream cheese, 2 ounces
- Butter, ½ cup
- Sour cream, 1 cup
- Granular erythritol, 1 cup
- Vanilla extract, 1 teaspoon
- Baking powder, 2 teaspoons

Method:

1. Heat oven beforehand to 350 degrees Fahrenheit.

2. Grease a saucepan and set aside

3. In a large bowl, mix baking powder and almond flour set aside

4. In a different bowl, add cream cheese. Cut butter into tiny squares and add them into the same bowl.

5. Slot the bowl containing cream cheese and butter in the microwave for thirty seconds. Make sure you don't burn the cream cheese. Stir until completely mixed.

6. Add sour cream, vanilla extract, and erythritol to the mixture. Mix and stir thoroughly.

7. Empty the ingredients into a bowl containing baking powder and almond flour. Mix and stir properly.

8. Add egg. Mix and stir properly.

9. Empty the batter into the greased pan, slot in the oven, and set timer for fifty minutes.

10. After baking, allow the cake to rest and cool for at least two hours (overnight, preferably). Enjoy!

Recommendation:

- It is normal for the edges to turn dark brown very fast. However, it doesn't mean that it is burnt.

- It is also possible to use coconut flour in the making of the Vanilla Pound Cake.

- You can easily tweak the shape to create a loaf or cupcakes. It is also possible to change the flavor by introducing blueberries or strawberries to the cake batter, or the dish once it's finished.

Nutrition Facts:

- Fat 20.67g
- Protein 7.67g
- Net carbs 5.23g
- Sugar alcohols 16g
- Fiber 2g
- Calories 249

3. Vegan Coconut Macaroons

This is a sweetened recipe made from various fruits and other healthy ingredients that contain loads of healthy fats, for the sole purpose of ketosis.

Prep time: 5 minutes Cook time: 18 minutes
Total time: 23 minutes Servings: 24

Ingredients:

- Vegan far chocolate, melted (for dipping), 1⁄2 cup
- Unsweetened shredded coconut (divided), 2 1⁄2 cups
- Pinch salt
- Almond flour, 1⁄2 cup
- Almond extract, 1⁄2 teaspoon
- Monk fruit sweetener (or any sweetener of your choice), 1⁄2 cup
- Vanilla extract, 1 teaspoon
- Aquafaba, 1⁄2 cup

Method:

1. Heat oven beforehand to 350 degrees Fahrenheit. Use a silicone mat or parchment paper to line the baking dish.

2. Heat a cup of coconut for eight to ten minutes in the oven.

3. In a large bowl, add the toasted coconut and all the other ingredients and mix properly.

4. On the baking sheet, place 1 tablespoon round cookie scoops.

5. Bake for eighteen to twenty minutes.

6. Melt a half cup of vegan chocolate. When cookies cool a little, place the bottoms inside and place them on parchment paper. Refrigerate for five

to ten minutes. If you don't intend to dip them in chocolate, then you don't have to refrigerate.

7. You can have them with non-diary milk. Enjoy!

4. Grain-Free Maple Pecan Bars

This is a healthy keto dessert recipe that helps add further healthy fat content to your regular dishes. It is pro-ketosis.

Prep time: 20 minutes Cook time: 20 minutes Total time: 40 minutes Servings: 16

Ingredients:

Tart crust:

- Egg,1
- Almond Flour, 2 cups
- Swerve granulated, 1/3 cup
- Butter, 3 tablespoons
- Vanilla (optional), 1⁄2 teaspoon Tart Filling:
- Pecans, 1 cup + 2 tablespoons for garnish
- Full fat cream cheese, 8 ounces
- Maple extract, 1 teaspoon
- Sour cream (optional), 2 tablespoons
- Egg,1
- Swerve granulated, 1⁄2 cup

Method:

Almond Tart Crust:

1. Mix swerve, vanilla, and almond flour with melted butter.

2. Add egg yolk.

3. Empty in a pan, by using fingers to press

4. Heat oven to 350 degrees Fahrenheit and bake for ten minutes

5. Filling:1. Mix sour cream with cream cheese, egg, maple extract, and vanilla.

6. Begin with half teaspoon extract and taste. Tart:

7. Cut pecans

8. Add pinch sea salt

9. In a pan, add pecans with the tart crust

10. Add cheesecake

11. To garnish, add 2 tbsp chopped pecans

12. Use tin foil to protect the entire tart pan. This is to prevent the tart crust from burning.

13. Bake until the mixture is set. This takes about twenty minutes, and the oven has to be set at 350 degrees Fahrenheit.

14. Allow cooling.

15. Slot in the fridge for at least six-hour or overnight.

16. Cut into sixteen squares.

Recommendations:

- It is not compulsory to use the exact tart pan that was used in this recipe. Any other square pan will suffice. However, place the crust at the bottom and make sure you of parchment paper.

- It is good to use maple extract, but if you have none, you can skip it because they come out nice even without it.

5. Cacao Butter Keto Blondies

Prep time: 15 minutes Cook time: 20 minutes Total time: 35 minutes Servings: 20 blondies

Ingredients:

Primal Keto Blondies

- Powdered erythritol, 6 tablespoons
- Baking powder, 1 teaspoon of cream tartar 1/2 teaspoons + 1/4 teaspoon baking soda
- Butter (unsalted), room temp, 2 tablespoons
- Cacao butter (3 oz), 6 tablespoons

Fudgy

- Powder erythritol, 1/4 cup
- Cream of tartar, 1/2 teaspoons
- Coconut oil 1 oz, Soft, room tempt, 2 tablespoons
- Cacao butter 3 oz., 6 tablespoons Both Versions:
- Walnuts/any nuts/chia (optional), 2 tablespoons
- Dash salt

Keto Blondies alternative:

- Dark chocolate (chopped), 1/2 oz.
- Large eggs (room temp), 2
- Coconut Flour, 2 1/2 tablespoons
- Stevia extract, 1 pinch
- Almond flour, 1/4 cup
- Vanilla extract, 1 pinch
- Coconut cream, 2 tablespoons
- Vanilla bean seeds, 1 teaspoon
- Vanilla extract, 1 teaspoon

Method:

1. Heat oven beforehand to 360 degrees Fahrenheit. Use parchment paper and line an eight-inch square baking pan. Then, measure all the available ingredients.

2. In a bowl that can be used in the microwave, add cacao butter — slot in the microwave and heat for 1 1/2 minute. While stirring, make sure there are no lumps if there are lumps or inconsistencies, microwave for a further one minute. Set aside and allow it to get cool. When cooled, add (stir in) the coconut oil or butter.

3. Mix the vanilla extract, salt, vanilla seed beans, erythritol, and eggs, using a handheld automatic mixer. Add the coconut cream and combine properly.

4. Add the cooled butter and combine, stirring until the mixture becomes dense. The density is dependent on the temperature of the ingredients. Thus, you should endeavor to have all ingredients at room temperature.

5. Sieve and mix both flours and cream of tartar or baking soda. Combine this flour mixture to the cream. Using a spatula, mix properly. Stirring, add the chopped chocolate

6. It is optional, but you can add chia seeds or ground walnuts (two

tablespoons). Add either to the chopped chocolate or use it on its own.

7. On the prepared baking pan, use a spatula to spread out the mixture.

8. Bake in the oven for twenty minutes. By this time, the toothpick will come out neat when slotted into the middle, but the middle of the blondies will remain juicy. It is pertinent that you don't over bake it.

9. When you finish baking, Remove the batch from the pan along with the parchment paper and give some time to cool down. When cooled, slice into twenty equal-sized blondies. It is best served twenty-four hours later.

Nutrition Facts:

- Protein 2.1g
- Fiber 0.9g
- Carbohydrates 1.6g
- Monounsaturated fat 2.0g
- Saturated fat 4.6g
- Fat 7.6 g
- Calories 80

Snack Recipes

Snacks are an important part of every type of dieting plan known to man, and that is why dieticians advise people to put in the same amount of effort in snacks as they do while making regular meals. There are times when you really can't make proper meals, and it is in these times that snacks come in handy. They help to fill in the gaps in other to avoid hunger, and that's why they present

you with an excellent opportunity to consolidate on your dieting plan.

The snack recipes listed underneath are meant to help you eat within the recommended limits of the ketogenic diet plan.

1. Keto Mummy dogs

These savory and succulent bundles are tasty and delicious. They are nutrient-packed and, most of all, keto.

Prep time: 5 minutes Cooking time: 45 minutes Servings: 4

Ingredients:

- Egg, 1 (For brushing of dough)
- Almond flour, 1/2 cup
- Uncured hot dogs or sausages in links, 1lb
- Coconut Flour, 4 tablespoons
- Egg,1
- Salt, 1/2 teaspoon
- Shredded cheese, 6 oz.
- Baking powder, 1 teaspoon
- For the mummy eyes (optional), 16 cloves
- Butter, 2 1/2 oz

Method:

1. Heat the oven beforehand to 350 degrees Fahrenheit.

2. In a large bowl, combine the baking powder, coconut flour, and almond flour.

3. In a saucepan set on low heat, melt the cheese and butter. For a smooth and flexible batter, use a wooden spoon to stir comprehensively. Remove from heat after a few minutes.

4. Stirring, add the egg into the flour mixture, toss the cheese mixture, and combine until solid dough is formed.

5. Flatten into a rectangle

6. Cut into eight long strips, less than one inch wide.

7. Wrap the dough strips around the hot dog and brush with a whisked egg.

8. Use parchment paper and line a baking sheet. Place the dough on it and bake until golden brown (usually takes fifteen to twenty minutes). The hot dog will be thoroughly cooked too.

9. Serve

Recommendations:

- If you're using bigger hot dogs, make sure you pre-fry them for a few minutes before using them with the cheese dough.

Nutrition Facts:

- Serving size: Two
- Calories 759
- Protein 29g
- Fat 67g
- Fiber 4g
- Carbohydrate 7g

2. Salad Sandwiches

The salad sandwiches are extremely versatile snacks that can be consumed during dinner, lunch, or breakfasts. They are made with fresh veggies and are simple to make. Enjoy! Prep time: 5 minutes Cook time: NATotal time: 5 minutes Serving: 1

Ingredients:

- Cherry tomatoes, 1
- Baby gem lettuce or Romaine lettuce, 2 oz.
- Avocado, 1/2
- Butter, 1/2 oz.
- Edam cheese/any other cheese as desired, 1 oz.

Method:

1. Wash and rinse lettuce. Then, use as the foundation for toppings

2. On the lettuce leaves, smear butter. Slice the tomato, avocado, and cheese and use it as toppings.

Recommendations:

Egg salad and tuna salad are other delicious toppings you can also use. Allow your kids the option of choosing their topping because you might just stumble on something incredible.

Nutrition Facts:

- Calories 374
- Protein 10g
- Fat 34g

- Fiber 8g
- Carbohydrate 3g

3. Keto Roast Nuts

The spicy, salty, and crunchy nuts recipe is guaranteed to keep your whole household asking for more. It is tasty, flavorful, delicious, and rich in healthy monounsaturated fats. Besides, it contains health benefits that keep the body in good stead. Enjoy this delicious snack. Prep time: 5 minutes Cook time: 10 minutes Total time: 15 minutes Servings: 6

Ingredients:

- Chili powder or paprika powder, 1 teaspoon
- Walnuts, almonds or pecans, 8 oz.
- Ground cumin, 1 teaspoon
- Salt, 1 teaspoon
- Coconut oil or olive oil, 1 tablespoon

Method:

1. In a medium skillet, combine all the ingredients and steam on low-medium heat until almonds are warmed thoroughly.
2. Allow to cool and serve.
3. You can serve with water or drink. For storage; you can keep in a container at room temperature, and with the lid closed

Recommendations:

- You can use nuts such as pecan nuts as an alternative to almonds.

Nutrition Facts:

- Calories 285
- Protein 4g
- Fat 30g
- Fiber 4g
- Carbohydrate 2g

4. Keto Cheese Chips

This crunchy snack is a keto recipe that boosts the number of healthy fats in the body. It is nutrient-packed, tasty, and easy to prepare. Enjoy!

Prep time: 5 minutes Cook time: 10 minutes Servings: 4

Ingredients:

- Paprika powder, 1/2 teaspoon
- Edam cheese, or provolone cheese or cheddar cheese (shredded) 8 oz.

Method:

1. Heat oven beforehand to 400 degrees Fahrenheit.
2. In small heaps, add shredded cheese on a baking sheet lined with foil or parchment paper. Ensure that there is enough distance between them. They must not touch each other.
3. Spray Paprika powder on top and bake for eight to ten minutes (depending on the thickness). Be vigilant, so you don't end up burning the cheese because burnt cheese has a bitter taste.

4. After baking, remove and place on a cooling rack. Allow to cool and serve.

Nutrition Facts:

- Calories 231
- Protein 13g
- Fat 19g
- Fiber 0g
- Carbohydrate 2g

5. Keto Garlic Bread

The Keto garlic Bread is a crispy snack with an outstanding garlic flavor. It is healthy, nutritious, and tasty, and is perfect for people indulging in the keto lifestyle because it has only one gram of carbs per piece.

Prep time: 20 minutes Cooking time: 50 minutes Total time: 1 hour 15 minutes Servings: 20

Ingredients:

- Bread
- Egg whites, 3
- Almond flour, 1 1/4 cups
- Boiling water, 1 cup
- Ground Psyllium husk powder, 5 tablespoons
- White wine vinegar or cider vinegar, 2 teaspoons
- Baking powder, 2 teaspoons
- Sea salt, 1 teaspoon
- Garlic butter
- Salt, 1/2 teaspoon
- Butter (room temperature), 4 oz.
- Fresh parsley (finely chopped), 2 tablespoons
- Garlic clove (minced), 1

Method:

1. Heat oven beforehand to 350 degrees Fahrenheit. In a bowl, combine the dry ingredients.Heat water and bring to a boil. In a bowl, add the water, egg whites, and vinegar, and use a hand mixer to whisk for thirty seconds. Mix the dough minimally, because the consistency should be like that of Play-Doh.

2. With your moist hands, make ten pieces of hot dog buns. Place them on the baking sheet, but make sure there is enough space between each of them.Slot in the lower rack and bake for forty to fifty minutes. Tap on the bottom of the bun, to ascertain if there's a hollow sound. Once you hear the sound, it means it is done.

3. While the bread is baking, prepare the garlic butter by combining all the ingredients. Refrigerate.After removing the buns from the oven, allow them to cool. Remove the garlic butter from the fridge. When the buns are cooled, use a serrated knife to halve them and apply the garlic butter on each of them.

4. Set the oven to 425 degrees Fahrenheit and bake the garlic bread until golden brown or for ten to fifteen minutes.

Nutrition Fact:

- Calories 93

- Protein 2g
- Fat9g
- Fiber 2g
- Carbohydrate 1g

Conclusion

The Ketogenic lifestyle is a unique lifestyle pattern that aims to keep the body healthy by consuming low-carb, moderate protein, and high-fat diets. The idea is to push the body into ketosis – a state where the liver converts Ketones into fuel, as opposed to glucose.

There are several benefits linked to the ketogenic diet, but the primary reason most people indulge is to lose weight. Weight loss is a big issue in the world today; people ridicule other people that they consider to be fat; even people that feel they are overweight do not feel comfortable in their skin. Thus, the race for trimming down has reached a fever pitch, and one of the most popular ways of tackling it is by adopting the ketogenic diet lifestyle.

The Ketogenic diet plan has been around for decades, but its adoption and constant approval by celebrities and other influential people have made it one of the most sought after by people who intend to improve their eating habits and lose weight.

In Ketosis, instead of the body to use carbohydrates as its primary energy source, it changes focus to fats. The idea of stimulating the body into ketosis revolves around the concept of consuming insignificant amounts of carbohydrates, and high amounts of fats to make up for the shortage of

carbs. When this happens, the body realizes that there is a scarcity of glucose stored in the body. Thus it begins to convert fat into ketones, which are burnt down as fuel for the body to work with.

The ketogenic diet has several advantages; for example, it helps to reduce insulin levels to healthy thresholds. Resistance to insulin is one of the major causes of type II diabetes.

The ketogenic diet generally promotes foods that constitute low carbohydrates, and this, in turn, leads to lower amounts of blood sugar in the bloodstream. When blood sugar is controlled, the risk of being exposed to a myriad of diseases is reduced.

Other advantages of the ketogenic diet plan include improved skin, weight loss, mental alertness, protection against epilepsy, control cholesterol and blood pressure, increased energy, and normalized eating.

One of the major problems faced by people in the ketogenic lifestyle is the consumption of all sorts of fats, without knowing that there are good and bad fats. The keto diet plan restricts people from consuming bad fats because it negates the whole idea of the program. Thus, for optimum productivity, it is important to be able to identify the good fats from the bad fat and integrate only the good ones into your diet.

Good fats are mostly saturated fats, unsaturated fats, and naturally existing trans fats, whereas bad fats are mostly processed trans fats. While good fats will induce you into ketosis and boost other bodily functions, bad fats will jeopardize your overall wellbeing, e.g., they can increase

inflammation and also boost the occurrence of certain types of cancer like colon and prostate cancer.

The Ketogenic diet plan is effective and efficient; however, before kicking off the plan, it is advisable to get your whole body prepared because failure to do so might come with some negative impacts. Professionals advise that carbohydrate reduction should be made in phases because a radical change or implementation might negatively affect the functioning of the body and lead to serious health problems.

In terms of a shopping list, certain types of foods should be in abundance, especially foods that contain high fats (healthy fats), and low carbohydrates. Also, foods that contain high carbs must be boycotted.

As per the daily Ketogenic diet plan, the designated amounts of carb should stay under 25g per day. When you hit that target, coupled with high amounts of healthy fats, your body will naturally slide into ketosis, which is the stage where you get to unlock the numerous benefits of the ketogenic diet plan.

There are different ways to approach the ketogenic meal plan; for example, the way a man approaches the plan is not the way a woman should. Also, the ketogenic diet is known to work yield results faster in men than in women; however, it isn't tied to the diet itself, but on other naturally existing factors.

Thus, it is important for women to study themselves and how they react to certain phenomenon before they embrace the ketogenic diet.

Even for athletes, certain factors have to be taken into consideration before embarking on a ketogenic diet. It is important because fully understanding the workings of the diet might help to boost performance, whereas a lack of understanding can impede performance and progress.

This book covered the issue of the ketogenic diet and diabetes. Diabetes is triggered by excessive sugar content in the bloodstream, and though the keto diet rids the body of sugar content, it is not a good idea for persons with type 1 diabetes to indulge in the keto diet. However, there are numerous health benefits linked to type 2 diabetes and the keto diet plan. Some hospitals even have ketogenic diet plans that support diabetes patients, and the results have shown to reduce cholesterol, prevent heart diseases, and even control blood sugar.

In terms of recipes, their hundreds of ketogenic diet recipes out there, and many more are still being created daily. The keto diet is an amazing invention that has touched and continues to touch lots of lives globally.

In this book, there are loads of ketogenic diet breakfast recipes that newcomers and veterans alike can embrace and explore, in other to make healthy, low-carb, moderate protein, and high-fat meals. These recipes are simple, and the instructions are clearly stated for easy implementation.

There is a list of lunch recipes that showcases some of the best keto diet recipes available for people to consume to lunch hours. These recipes are not only keto-friendly; they also contain elements that support the general wellbeing of their consumers.

Lastly, there are dinner, snacks, and dessert ketogenic diet recipes that are easy to make, nutritious, and aimed at complementing each other. These recipes are some of the very best you can find anywhere, thus having them in your custody, will make your journey in the ketogenic world, easy and stress-free.

This is a well-thought-out book that explores the endless possibilities of the Ketogenic diet. It contains information that can transform your health, physical outlook, and life in general.

CLARA WILLIAMS

....

The Frugal
Renal Diet Cookbook
for Beginners

How to Manage Chronic Kidney Disease (CKD) to Escape Dialysis
21-Day Nutritional Plan for Progressive Renal Function Recovery
301 Kidney-Friendly Recipes.

Clara Williams

DEDICATION

Tthis book is dedicated to all the people who struggle to prevent their kidney disease from
getting worse by forcing them to dialysis or even a kidney transplant

Introduction

The two kidneys clear and filter the blood each day to eliminate waste and excess fluid left as urine by the body. About a billion small structures called nephrons reside within each kidney. Kidneys filter the blood. Kidneys maintain the blood composition healthy, which helps the body to perform optimally. The urine goes through tubules, ureters. It goes to your bladder, where the urine is stored before you go to the restroom. Many disorders of the kidneys target the nephrons. This injury will render the kidneys incapable of processing waste. Some reasons are hereditary problems, events, or medications. When you have obesity, elevated blood pressure, or a family history of kidney disease, you have a greater chance of kidney disease. Kidney disease affects the nephrons gradually for many years. Some complications with the kidneys include

Stones

Cancer

Infections

Cysts

Other health issues, such as heart disease, can result from kidney disease. It raises the risk of getting a stroke or heart attack because of kidney failure. High blood pressure may be both a source of kidney failure and a consequence. Your kidneys are weakened by high blood pressure, and damaged kidneys don't perform well enough to regulate your blood pressure better. People have a greater chance of having a sudden shift in kidney function caused by illness, injury, or certain medications if you have chronic kidney disease. This is considered acute kidney injury.

By managing and preventing health issues that can cause kidney damage, such as high blood pressure and diabetes, you can help shield your kidneys. You can still question the doctors about the health of your kidneys after an appointment. There might not be any early kidney failure signs, but being screened might be the best way to ensure if the kidneys are safe. Your doctor will help decide on how often to test you.

If you have a urinary tract infection (UTI), which, if left unchecked, will trigger kidney damage, you should seek medical advice right away. It's just as necessary to make adjustments to your lifestyle to take medication. It may help alleviate many of the root causes of kidney failure by following a healthier lifestyle and eating healthy.

You should

- Lower the consumption of high salt, high potassium, and phosphorous
- Control diabetes through insulin injections
- Should not eat foods high in cholesterol
- Consume heart-healthy diets such as whole grains, fresh fruits, low-fat dairy products, and vegetables
- Increase physical activity at least half an hour a day
- Leave smoking
- Limit your alcohol consumption
- Try to lose excess weight
- Control your fluid intake

Kidney disease ordinarily will not go away once it's diagnosed. The best way to keep your kidneys healthy is to acquire a healthy lifestyle and healthy eating habits. Over time, kidney disease can get worse. It could also contribute to the failure of the kidneys. If it is not treated on time, kidney failure may be life-threatening. When the kidneys are partially functioning or not functioning at all, kidney failure happens. This is monitored by dialysis. Using a pump to remove waste from your blood, your doctor may prescribe a kidney transplant in severe instances.

Hence, to keep your kidneys healthy, you must eat kidney-friendly healthy food less in potassium, phosphorous, and sodium, since kidneys filter out all the toxic waste from food.

Part 1: the introduction to the CKD and at the diet manage it.

Chapter 1: Kidney Diseases

There are two bean-shaped organs, situated at the rib cage base, approximately the size of a fist. Each side of the spine is kidneys. Kidneys clean out blood with excess water and waste, and they produce urine. Kidney failure means the kidneys are impaired, in the way they can't filter the blood. The kidneys control the amounts of pH, sodium, and potassium levels. They create hormones that stabilize blood pressure and monitor red blood cell development. The kidneys also trigger a source of vitamin D that lets the body absorb calcium. The human body's potential to disinfect blood, filter excess water out of blood, and help regulate blood pressure may be influenced by kidney disease. It may also affect the development of red blood cells and the required vitamin D synthesis for bone protection.

Per year, kidney failure impacts nearly 26 million people. High blood pressure, diabetes, and numerous other chronic conditions may trigger damage. Other health conditions, including nerve damage, weak bones, and starvation, can lead to kidney disease. Kidneys can stop functioning entirely if the situation worsens with time. This suggests that the work of the kidneys would require dialysis. Dialysis is a procedure that uses a machine to clean and purify the blood. It can't cure kidney failure, but your life can be prolonged.

1.1 What Your Kidneys Do

Healthy kidneys maintain a blood balance of fluids and minerals such as phosphorus, sodium, and potassium. After absorption, muscle function, exposure to toxins or drugs eliminate waste from the blood.

- Create renin, which is used by the body to regulate blood pressure better
- Create erythropoietin, a compound that helps the body to make red blood cells.
- Create vitamin D, an active form necessary for the health of the bone and teeth

As blood goes to the kidneys, advanced Sensors within kidney cells control how much fluids to excrete in the form of urine, with how much concentration of electrolytes. If someone is dehydrated from exercising or from a disease, the kidneys will retain as much liquid as possible, and the urine will be very concentrated. When The urine is even more diluted because enough water is available in the bloodstream, and the urine appears transparent.

The urine that each kidney generates passes through the ureter, a conduit that links the bladder to the kidney. Urine is contained inside the bladder, and it empties urine into a channel called the urethra as urination happens.

1.2 Symptoms of Chronic Kidney Disease

Kidney damage advances slowly, symptoms and signs of chronic kidney disease evolve. Kidney disease is a condition that can go undetected easily until the side effects get serious. An early indicator that you may be having kidney failure are the following symptoms

- Swelling around your eyes

- Swelling of the legs
- Bone pain
- Shortness of breath
- Vomiting, nausea, after eating or in the morning
- Mental cloudiness
- Brittle hair and nails
- Abnormally dark or light skin
- Numbness in hands and feet
- A urine-like odor to your breath
- An ashen cast to the skin
- Drowsiness
- Restless leg syndrome
- A loss of muscle mass
- Easy bruising and bleeding
- Blood in the stools
- Excessive thirst
- Muscle twitching and cramps
- Chest pain, if fluid builds up around the lining of the heart
- Sudden weight loss

If your chronic kidney disease is already more advanced, you may experience

- Itching or numbness
- Dry skin
- Headaches
- Increased or decreased urination
- Loss of appetite
- See "foam" in your urine
- Muscle cramping
- Nausea
- Malnutrition
- Sleep problems
- Weight loss
- Anemia

A child with chronic kidney disease may not be growing as anticipated, feel worn out, have less appetite than usual, and sleepier than usual.

1.3 Risk Factors

For adults older than 65 years, the incidence of chronic kidney disease rises. There is a greater chance of experiencing kidney failure in persons with diabetes. Diabetes, responsible for approximately 44 percent of new cases, is the primary source of kidney failure. If you have kidney failure, you will also be more likely to get other diseases. Some chronic kidney disease risk factors include

- Obesity
- High blood pressure
- Cigarette smoking
- Diabetes types 1 & type 2
- Obstructive kidney disease
- Liver failure
- High cholesterol
- When urine flows back into the kidneys (vesicoureteral reflux)
- A narrow artery that supplies the blood to the kidney
- Bladder cancer
- Heart and blood vessel (cardiovascular) disease
- Vasculitis
- Kidney cancer
- Being Asian-American, African-American, and native American
- Family history of kidney disease
- Autoimmune disease

- Abnormal kidney structure
- Older age
- History of chronic kidney disease in the family

1.4 Kidney Disease Causes

Causes of acute kidney disease: acute renal failure if your kidneys unexpectedly quit functioning.

The typical reasons are

- Obstruction in the blood flow to the kidneys
- Significant kidney damage
- Backed up urine in the kidneys
- Incidents that affect kidneys, when you:
- Extreme blood loss as a result of an injury,
- Muscle tissue starts to break down or is dehydrated, flowing too much protein into the bloodstream.
- A person is in shock because they have a serious infection called sepsis.
- An enlarged or swelled prostate which blocks the flow of urine
- Taking certain medicines or certain toxins directly harm the kidney.
- Have health problems such as preeclampsia or eclampsia during pregnancy
- Autoimmune disorders can also trigger acute kidney injury when the immune system attacks your body.

Individuals with severe liver failure or heart failure usually also experience acute kidney injury. Chronic kidney disease happens when kidney function is impaired by an illness or condition, causing kidney damage to deteriorate over several months or even years.

Polycystic kidney disease, the recurrent renal disease also referred to as pyelonephritis.

Kidney failure symptoms are caused by waste products that do not get excreted. Too much fluid can cause swelling, weakness, lethargy, breathing difficulty, and confusion. Too much potassium in the bloodstream may lead to uneven heart rhythms, even sudden death. Kidney failure does not cause any symptoms in the initial phases. There are multiple kidney failure factors, and the first step in attempting to correct the kidney abnormality to treat the underlying disease.

Some factors of kidney failure can be treated, and the kidney function can return to normal. Kidney loss may, sadly, be widespread in some cases and can be permanent.

1.5 How is Kidney Disease Diagnosed?

- **Filtration Rate of Glomerular (GFR)**

This assessment will measure how good kidneys are working and let you know about the kidney disease stage.

- **Ultrasound or Scan computed tomography(CT)**

Ultrasounds or CT scans produce crystal clear images of the urinary tract and kidneys. This will allow the doctor to examine if kidneys' sizes are too large or small. CT can see any structural problems or tumors that are present.

- **Kidney Biopsy**

During this procedure, the doctor will take out a small piece of tissue from the kidney while sedated. This tissue sample will help the doctor to know how much damage has happened and the type of kidney disease.

- **Urine test**

To check levels of albumin, a urine test is done. Albumin is a protein that is excreted into the urine when the kidneys are not working fully.

- **Creatinine Blood test**

Creatinine is an excretion product. When creatine breaks down, it's released into the blood. Creatinine amounts in your blood can rise if kidneys are not operating properly.

1.6 Chronic Kidney Diseases

Chronic kidney failure indicates that the kidneys are weakened, and they do not filter blood as they need to. Other health conditions may also be induced by chronic kidney disease.

- **Blood in Urine**

Blood in the urine may indicate that the kidneys or some urinary tract components are doing something different. Not generally, having blood in urine means you possess kidney disease, but kidney malfunction can lead to kidney disease.

- **Protein in Urine**

One of the early symptoms of kidney failure is finding protein in the urine. In the blood, everybody has protein. Healthy kidneys flush away fluid and toxins and blood and keep nutrients in blood that you use, such as protein. A protein, albumin, escape from your blood into the urine when the tiny filters in your kidneys are weakened. Treating this issue early will help avoid it from getting worse.

- **Kidney Stones**

One of the most serious kidney complications is kidney stones. Generally, they are caused by the buildup of certain minerals within kidneys that glues together. When they move through the urinary tract, big kidney stones trigger pain. If a tiny kidney stone passes easily through the urinary tract, you might not feel something. It is termed passing a kidney stone.

- **Infection of the Kidneys**

Bacteria transmit to kidneys from some other section of the urinary tract are typically responsible for kidney infections. Pain in your back, Fever, vomiting, or pain in the groin are common side effects of kidney infections.

- **Kidney Pain**

In the mid to upper back and on sides, kidney pain can be felt. Pressure in the sides or back does not always imply that the kidneys are not functioning properly Kidney infection.

- To reduce your risk of developing kidney disease.

- Follow instructions on prescribed medications.

- Lose excess weight and maintain a healthy weight

- Quit smoking

- Choose foods that are heart-healthy and also for the entire body

Chapter 2: Foods Elements & Chronic Kidney Disease

Fluid can accumulate in the body when the kidneys can be damaged and cannot work effectively, and waste can buildup in the blood. But eliminating or restricting items in the diet will help minimize the buildup of waste products in the blood, enhance the kidneys' efficiency, and prevent more damage.

By eating healthy foods and limiting foods high in phosphorus, sodium, and potassium. An individual may delay or prevent some health issues related to chronic kidney disease (CKD). a person with intensive chronic renal disease should learn about proteins, calories, fats, fluids is important. Protein-rich foods like dairy and meat products break up into waste products removed from the blood by healthy kidneys.

Nutritional preferences shift as progressive kidney disorder advances. A health care professional can prescribe that foods be selected carefully by a patient with impaired kidney function. To control chronic kidney illness, people may need to change what they eat. Work with a qualified dietitian to build a meal schedule that contains meals you love consuming while protecting your kidneys' health.

2.1 Food Elements in Chronic Kidney Disease

Here are some important elements that needs to be monitored if you are experiencing kidney diseases symptoms

2.2 Potassium

Potassium has multiple important functions in the body, and it is the task of the kidneys to regulate the balance of minerals in the body, such as phosphorus and potassium. In patients with renal impairment and those on dialysis, the kidneys don't work properly. Hence, it is also necessary to restrict their intake of some of these minerals. An erratic pulse or heart failure may occur if potassium concentration in the body become abnormal. In certain situations, in addition to reducing some potassium-containing diets, kidney patients need not taking potassium-containing nutrients, multivitamins, and heart vitamins, although people with kidney failure need to reduce potassium to prevent dangerously elevated blood levels. Limiting potassium to less than 2,000 mg a day is typically prescribed.

2.2 Phosphorus

It is a mineral that is more likely to be restricted in patients with renal failure. Phosphorus can accumulate in the blood, which will damage the bones, rendering them more frail and weak. Kidney patients ought to be mindful of foods rich in phosphorus and to monitor their nutritional consumption. Monitoring your phosphorus intake and talking to your doctor before taking any phosphorus-containing multivitamins or supplements is important. Large amounts may cause bodily harm, so dietary phosphorus is limited to less than 800-1,000 mg per day in most patients.

2.3 Calcium

Extra calcium is not necessary for all kidney patients. Calcium supplementation specifications can, however, be independently defined. For some patients, supplementation can be beneficial. Many people take calcium-containing supplements, and too much calcium can cause kidney stones or painfully high levels of calcium in the blood in kidney patients. Greater blood calcium levels for a long time may lead to damage to the kidneys. Always talk with your doctor about your calcium regimen.

2.4 Sodium

In many foods, sodium is found and is a critical element of table salt. Damaged kidneys, causing their blood levels to rise, cannot filter out excess sodium. Limiting sodium to less than 2,000 mg a day is often recommended.

2.5 Iron

Iron is essential for the formation of red blood cells and anemia. Low red blood cell count can be attributed to a decrease in iron levels. Kidney patients cannot ensure consistent iron stores, particularly those on dialysis, so they are at risk of developing anemia. The experts say to take regular iron supplements to achieve target iron levels to prevent anemia in kidney patients. For kidney and dialysis patients, a steady supply of iron in your multivitamin might be helpful.

2.6 Trace Elements

In patients with kidney failure and others on dialysis, reduced trace elements, zinc, copper, and selenium, are also observed. Elevated oxidative stress may result from the loss of such trace elements. As defined by the Guidelines, supplements for kidney patients must have sufficient amounts of trace minerals.

Chapter 3: Normal Diet & Chronic Kidney Disease

As chronic diet patients, you ought to know the most important aspect of your lifestyle is the food you eat. A normal or typical diet that everyone is accustomed to may not be ideal for people with Chronic Kidney Disease. It contains higher levels of potassium, sodium, and phosphate.

Hypertension, Obesity, smoking, and diabetes are all considered to raise the likelihood of kidney disease. A majority of scholars now know that phosphorus in our food should also be included in the list. Companies have also been introducing phosphorus-containing compounds to thousands of foods, including phosphoric acid and sodium phosphate.

A well-balanced diet supplies you every day with the proper levels of vitamins, protein, minerals, and calories. Staying physically active, eating a healthy diet, and taking all your medicines as prescribed are important parts of keeping you healthy and feeling well. Your kidneys help to preserve the body's correct balance of minerals and nutrients and. But your kidneys may not even be able to do such a job well if you have kidney disease. You may need to make some adjustments to your food.

Making healthy food choices is vital to all of us, but it is much more critical if you have kidney disease (CKD). Good nutrition can assist you, in

- Help maintain a healthy weight
- Provides you the energy to do daily tasks
- Prevent many infections
- Stop the loss of muscle mass
- Slow down the progression of kidney disease

Based on your diagnosis and personal lifestyle, a dietician can educate you to make the right food choices. Making improvements in the diet to manage diabetes properly and high blood pressure will also help prevent kidney failure from becoming worse.

There is not anyone meal pattern that is appropriate for everyone with kidney disease. Based on how much renal function someone has and other variables, what you can or cannot eat can alter over time. If you are trying to follow a specific diet for diabetes or cardiac problems, you will have to continue pursuing it.

People with kidney disease may need to monitor potassium, protein, sodium, calcium, and phosphorus in their diet. If kidney disease keeps getting worse, other nutrients may need to be limited as well.

3.1 Side Effects of Consuming High Calorie, High Sodium, Phosphorous Diet

If you keep count of how often you consume certain foods and liquids, you may know what to cut back on. Additional fluid may accumulate up in the body, if your kidneys are not working properly, and can cause

- Swelling in the hands, legs, face and weight gain, known as Edema
- Fluctuations in blood pressure
- Accumulation of fluid in the lungs, making it hard to breathe
- Heart failure: unnecessary accumulation of fluids in the blood can overburden your heart, making it weak and enlarged

- Difficulty breathing: fluid can accumulate in the lungs, making it difficult to breathe

So much phosphate in blood forces calcium out of your bones on consuming a regular diet. Losing calcium could weaken your bones and make them likely to break. Another side effect of too much phosphorus is it may make your skin itchy. It may be challenging to limit phosphorus because phosphorus-containing foods, such as milk and meat, often provide the protein you require. You ought to be careful not to eat that much protein but not get far too much phosphorus. Packaged and processed foods contain particularly high phosphorus levels. Hemodialysis patients should normally only have half a cup of milk each day.

It can be very hazardous to have too much or too little potassium in the blood. The concentration of potassium you require depends on your kidneys' activity and the medicines you are using.

Far too much sodium can provoke fluid buildup, higher blood pressure, swelling, and strain on the heart if your kidneys do not work well. A portion of salt is sodium. Sodium is present in fast foods canned, frozen, packaged. In many seasonings, flavorings, and meats. consuming much sodium makes you thirsty, which will lead you to drink excessive fluids

Continue to consume fresh meals that are naturally low-sodium. Take a look for "low sodium" labeled products, particularly in frozen foods and canned food. Do not use replacements for salt because they contain potassium.

3.2 Habits & Lifestyle That Can Effects Kidney

An everyday diet consumed without thinking through or the lifestyle habits that are not good for your mind and body can affect your kidneys in the long run.

- Eating too many Processed Foods
- Not being physically active
- Taking too many Painkillers
- Adding much salt in meals
- Disturbed sleeping schedule
- Consuming too much Red Meat
- Eating foods high in Sugar
- Not Drinking Enough fluids
- Smoking
- Drinking too much Alcohol

It is necessary to eat healthy fresh food and make healthy balanced life choices so you can avoid hypertension, obesity, and diabetes, which all will leads to the regression of kidney function

Chapter 4: The Renal Diet

To decrease the generation of waste in their blood, individuals with impaired kidney function must stick to a renal or kidney diet. Blood waste occurs from food and drinks that are ingested. As kidney activity is affected, the kidneys do not adequately remove or extract debris. It will adversely influence the electrolyte levels of a patient if the excess is left in the blood. It can even help improve kidney function and delay total kidney disease development by maintaining a kidney diet.

An integral aspect of every recovery regimen for a chronic kidney disorder is a healthy renal diet. One that is low in protein, phosphorous, sodium is a renal diet. A renal diet often highlights the value of eating high-quality protein and typically limiting liquid. Potassium and calcium will also need to be restricted to certain patients. The body of an individual is different, so it is important for each patient to collaborate with a renal dietitian to create a diet customized to the patient's needs. When you have serious kidney failure, you ought to have a kidney-friendly meal schedule. It can encourage you to be healthier by monitoring what you consume and drink.

Your well-being is influenced by what you consume and drink. It will help regulate your blood pressure and keep at a healthier weight and consume a nutritious diet low in salt and fat. You have to regulate your blood pressure if you have diabetes by consciously deciding what you consume and drink. A renal diet can help keep kidney disease from getting worse by managing high blood pressure and diabetes.

Depending on the level of kidney failure, how strict the meal schedule can be. You could have few to no limitations on what you consume and drink in the early stages of kidney disease. Your doctor may consider restricting your:

- Sodium
- Potassium
- Phosphorus
- Protein
- Fluids; If your kidney disease worsens.

4.1 Consume Foods with Less Sodium & Salt

Usually, there is a sodium reduction in the context of "No Added Salt." This is important because higher sodium consumption can result in improperly regulated blood pressure and increased thirst, which may contribute to difficulties adhering to your diet's fluid restrictions.

To reduce your sodium intake, you should not consume

1) Table salt or any flavoring that has salt in it
2) Salt alternative as they can have potassium in them
3) Salty meats such as ham, bacon, hot dogs, sausage, bologna, lunch meats, and canned meats,
4) Salty snacks such as salted crackers, cheese curls, Chips, salted nuts
5) Thoroughly wash canned meats, vegetables, fish, and beans
6) Do not eat instant noodles, canned soups, and frozen dinners
7) Consume fresh food often.
8) Cook foods at home instead of dining out, frozen dinners, canned foods, and fast foods it is better to control

ingredients when you make food yourself

9) Use sodium-free seasonings, spices, and herbs, instead of salt

10) Do not consume brined olives, sauces, MSG, and bottled pickles

4.2 Consume The Right Types of Proteins

To help in the development and preservation of body tissue, protein is necessary. Protein also serves a part in the battle against bacteria, wound healing, and allowing the body to supply energy. Per day, you can make sure to consume 7-8 ounces of protein. Protein-rich foods are meat, pork, turkey, beef, and chicken.

Fish, eggs, and seafood. One egg is equivalent to one ounce of protein; 3 ounces of protein is similar to a deck of cards in size. Eat small portions of protein foods on a renal diet

A cooked portion of fish, chicken, or meat is near 2-3 ounces, like to size of a deck of cards. A portion of dairy is one slice of cheese or half a cup of yogurt or milk.

Plant based-protein foods:

1. Grains
2. Nuts
3. Beans

Cooked beans' portion is about half cup. A portion of cooked noodles or cooked rice is a half cup. A serving of bread is a single slice.

4.3 Consume Drinks & Food with Less Phosphorus

Try to eat less of high phosphorus foods like:

1. Dairy, Meats, fish, and poultry (you can eat one serving)

2. Dairy products Milk and cheese (one 4 oz. serving)

Avoid this food or eat very less of

Black Beans, Lima Beans, Red Beans, White Beans, and Black-eyed Peas

Unrefined, Dark, whole grains

Refrigerated doughs

Vegetables and fruits that are Dried

- Dark-colored sodas
- Chocolate

You may take a phosphate binder if prescribed by your doctor. Choose those meats, fish, and pasta that are low in phosphorous. The daily limit is 1000mg/day.

4.4 Choose Heart-Healthy Foods

Rather than deep-frying, broil, grill, bake, stir-fry roast, foods. Rather than butter, cook with cooking spray or a tiny quantity of olive oil. Cut fat from meat before eating, remove the skin from the meat. Try to restrict trans fats and saturated fats and Read the nutrients of the food. Low-fat or fat-free milk, yogurt, and cheese

4.5 Consume Food with Less Amount of Potassium

High potassium may induce erratic heart rhythms, and if potassium levels get high, it may also cause the heart to stop. For those with a large amount of potassium, there are usually no signs. If Your potassium level is troubling, consult with your doctor

Patients can consume 2000 mg/day of potassium.

Foods that are Lower in Potassium

Peaches, apples, White pasta and bread, Carrots, Rice milk, green beans

White rice, Apple, or grape or cranberry juice, Cooked rice, grits, and wheat cereals.

4.6 Limit Intake of Fluids

Your doctor can tell you to restrict the amount of fluid based on kidney disease and recovery levels. You will have to ease up as to how much you drink fluids. Any items that include a lot of water will even need to be cut down on. There is a lot of water in soups or melting items, such as ice, ice cream, and gelatin. Many vegetables and fruits and even have strong water content too.

The daily limit is usually four cups of fluid each day for server kidney failure. or as your doctor has prescribed.

Chapter 5: The Benefits of Renal Diet

There are greater protein requirements for anyone with end-stage renal failure receiving dialysis, a procedure that filters and cleanses the blood. Dialysis continues to help you do more of the job that kidneys do before they were good. Yet dialysis can't replace good kidneys' function, and all that healthy kidneys function cannot be done. In your body, particularly in dialysis treatments, some waste and fluid can still build up. Over time, bone, heart, and other health issues can be triggered by excess waste and fluid in the blood. You must monitor the quantities of liquid and some nutrients you take per day if you have kidney failure / ESRD. This will help prevent waste and fluid from piling up and creating complications with your blood. There are various limitations for patients in the early phases of kidney disease instead of kidney impairment, commonly known as an end-stage renal disease (ESRD).

Kidney failure will no longer expel excessive potassium as the kidneys malfunction, so potassium levels build up in the body. High blood potassium is recognized as hyperkalemia, which may trigger:

- Heart attacks
- Muscle weakness
- Slow pulse
- An irregular heartbeat
- Even Death

Depending on your recovery strategy and other health issues, exactly how specific your food can be. The majority of people on dialysis individuals ought to restrict:

1. Fluids
2. Potassium
3. Phosphorus
4. Sodium

The accumulation of acids, sodium, potassium, water, phosphorus leads to unhealthy factors, including oxidative stress, inflammation, cardiac disease, hyperparathyroidism, and metabolic acidosis hyperphosphatemia. Renal diets theoretically decrease it. It can improve kidney function and delay the development of total kidney failure by maintaining a kidney friendly diet. One that is minimal in phosphorous, sodium, and protein is a renal diet. A renal diet often stresses the value of eating high-quality protein and typically limiting liquid.

In the renal diet, the nutritional alteration can have a cardiovascular preventive impact in patients with chronic renal disease by operating on both non-traditional and regular cardiovascular risk factors combined with the ketoacidosis supplementation and vegetarian aspect of the renal diet.

The regulation of blood pressure can be supported by reducing sodium consumption with the composition of the renal diet, which is therefore very critical for lowering serum cholesterol and enhancing the profile of plasma lipids. In patients with end-stage renal failure, fluid excess plays a significant part in the progression of hypertension. The latest findings show that hypertension induces harm to the target organ, such as renal oxidative stress. It helps boost kidney function while preventing further damage.

Every individual with renal disease has a different nutritional requirement, so it's important to speak about your particular dietary needs with your health professional.

5.1 Top 10 Renal Diet Foods

Luckily, several tasty and nutritious choices that are low in sodium, phosphorus, and potassium.

Cauliflower

1. Cauliflower is rich in B vitamin folate, vitamin C, and vitamin K. It's full of anti-inflammatory properties such as indoles and has lots of fiber.

2. 1 cup of cooked cauliflower (124 grams) has

3. Potassium: 176 mg| sodium: 19 mg| phosphorus: 40 mg

Blueberries

- It has antioxidants; it may protect against certain cancers, heart disease, diabetes, and cognitive decline.

- 1 cup of fresh blueberries (148 grams) contains:

- Sodium: 1.5 mg| phosphorus: 18 mg| potassium: 114 mg

Sea bass

- Sea bass is a top quality protein that has omega-3s that comprises extremely good fats.

- Omega-3s help minimize inflammation and can reduce the likelihood of cognitive loss, depression, and anxiety.

- 3 ounces of cooked sea bass (85 grams) contains:

- Potassium: 279 mg | sodium: 74 mg | phosphorus: 211 mg

Red grapes

- They are rich in vitamin C and include flavonoids, antioxidants that are shown to decrease inflammation.

- These kidney-friendly sweet fruits, a half-cup (75 grams) contains:

- Potassium: 144 mg | sodium: 1.5 mg| phosphorus: 15 mg

Egg whites

- While egg yolks are rather healthy, they produce large phosphorus levels, rendering egg whites a healthier option for individuals who adopt a renal diet.

- Egg whites are a kidney-friendly, high-quality protein source.

- Two large (66 grams) egg whites contain

- Potassium: 108 mg | sodium: 110 mg| phosphorus: 10 mg

Garlic

1) It has high levels of manganese, vitamin B6, vitamin C, and sulfur. Garlic offers a perfect substitute for salt, bringing flavor to meals and offering health benefits.

2) Three cloves of garlic (9 grams) contain:

3) Potassium: 36 mg | sodium: 1.5 mg | phosphorus: 14 mg

Buckwheat

- Buckwheat is a healthy gluten-free whole grain, good magnesium, B vitamins, and fiber iron.

- A half-cup of cooked buckwheat (84 grams) contains:

- Potassium: 74 mg | sodium: 3.5 mg | phosphorus: 59 mg

Olive oil

- Olive oil is an important source of phosphorus-free monounsaturated fat, anti-inflammatory properties

- One tablespoon of olive oil (13.5 grams) contains
- Potassium: 0.1 mg | sodium: 0.3 mg| phosphorus: 0 mg

Cabbage

- From a family of cruciferous vegetables and rich in vitamin C, vitamin K, and vitamin B. With insoluble fiber, low in phosphorus, sodium, and potassium.
- One cup of shredded cabbage (70 grams) containing
- Potassium: 119 mg |sodium: 13 mg | phosphorus: 18 mg

Chicken (Skinless)

1. Skinless chicken breast has less sodium, potassium, and phosphorus.
2. 3 ounces of skinless chicken breast (84 grams) contains
3. Potassium: 216 mg |sodium: 63 mg | phosphorus: 192 mg

   Besides this, other good foods are beneficial for people practicing a renal diet

Part 2: The Methodology of Clara Williams

Chapter 1: Foods to Avoid in Chronic Kidney Disease

The kidneys do not sufficiently remove surplus phosphorus, sodium, and potassium, in people with a severe kidney disorder. As a consequence, increased blood levels of these minerals are at greater risk.

There will also be differing dietary requirements for people with end-stage renal failure that need dialysis. To prevent the concentration of such contaminants or nutrients in the blood, the vast majority of people with late- to end-stage kidney failure will need to adopt a kidney-friendly diet. Restricting potassium sodium to 2,000 mg a day and reducing phosphorus to 800-1,000 mg each day typically involves a kidney-friendly diet or renal diet.

Damaged kidneys could also be having difficulty removing protein metabolism leftover waste. People with renal disease in stages 1-4 will also choose to restrict the number of proteins in their diets. However, those undertaking dialysis with end-stage renal disease has an elevated protein demand.

To hold you on track, here are some tips

- Eat a good portion of protein in meals, including poultry, meat, fish, eggs, and fresh pork.
- Cut off phosphorus and potassium.
- Avoid dried beans, peanut butter, lentils, seeds, and nuts. They are high in protein phosphorous and potassium.
- Eat less salty foods. This will help to regulate your blood pressure.
- Use spice, herbs with low-salt
- Do not eat high fiber foods and whole grain.
- Restrict intake of cheese, yogurt, milk as they are high in phosphorus.
- As the majority of the fruits have some potassium. Restricting potassium will protect the heart. Choose berries, apples over bananas, and oranges.
- Choose cabbage, broccoli over asparagus, and potatoes.

Here is food on a renal diet that you can probably avoid

- Pickled foods
- Chips
- Nuts
- Ham
- Sausage
- Monosodium glutamate (MSG)
- Too much cheese
- Chocolate
- Instant rice
- Melons
- Brewer's yeast
- Offal
- Instant mixes
- Sweet relish pickles
- Yolk
- Raisins
- Oranges
- Legumes

- Dried fruit
- Nuts
- Bananas
- Water chestnuts
- Lima beans
- Bran

Kiwi, coconut and Chestnuts

- Apricots
- Pre-packaged fruit juice
- Vegetables: potatoes, spinach, and artichokes
- Potassium salt
- Bouillon cubes
- Cocoa
- Cod and sardines
- Meats like the goose, lamb, duck, and wild animals
- Baking Soda
- Black-Eyed Peas
- Cheese
- Dates
- Dill Pickles
- Tomato Soup
- Mango
- Orange Juice
- Tomato Paste
- Prunes
- Tomatoes
- Tomato Juice
- Tomato Sauce
- Shrimp, to be eaten less due to higher protein content

Dark-colored soda

- They produce phosphorus in its added form, which is easily absorbable by the human body and should be prevented on a renal diet.

Avocados

- In a renal diet, avocados could be limited because of their high potassium content. Almost 37 percent of the 2,000-mg potassium limitation is provided by one cup of avocado.

Canned foods

- Sometimes, packaged foods are rich in sodium. It is generally safer to stop, ban, or purchase low sodium varieties to reduce sodium intake.

Whole wheat bread

- Due to the lower amounts of phosphorus and potassium, white bread is usually preferred over whole wheat bread on a renal diet. All bread includes salt, but comparing product labeling and picking a smaller variety of salt is best

Brown rice

- Brown rice has a higher level of potassium and phosphorus content and is likely to be reduced on a renal diet. Bulgur, White rice, buckwheat couscous and are also healthy substitutes.

Dairy

High levels of potassium, phosphorus, and protein are present in dairy products and should be restricted to a renal diet. Although the strong calcium content of milk, the phosphorus content among those with kidney failure may damage bones.

Processed Meats

Processed meat is high in protein. Salt should be eaten on a renal diet in controlled amounts

Pickles, Olives, & Relish

- As they are fermented and cured to taste less acidic, dried olives often tend to be high in salt.

Tomatoes

- One high potassium fruit that should probably be restricted to a renal diet is tomatoes.

Crackers, Pretzels, and Chips

- In wide portions, crackers, pretzels, and chips are readily eaten and appear to include heavy salt concentrations. Also, a large quantity of potassium is provided by chips produced from potatoes.

- Reducing the phosphorus, potassium, and sodium consumption will be an essential part of treating the condition if you have kidney problems. Based on the degree of kidney function, dietary restrictions, and nutrient consumption guidelines can differ.

Chapter 2: Kidney Friendly Food in Renal Diet

Researchers are making more and more associations between inflammation, chronic illnesses, and foods that can inhibit or defend against excessive fatty acid oxidation. This phenomenon happens as the body's oxygen responds to fat in the cells and blood. Oxidation is a common mechanism in the body for the processing of energy and certain chemical processes. Still, excessive cholesterol and fat oxidation produce free radicals, damaging the proteins, genes, and cell membranes. Oxidative disruption has been correlated with heart attack, Parkinson's disease. Stroke, Alzheimer's disease, and other debilitating and degenerative diseases.

Foods that produce antioxidants, though, may help neutralize free radicals and safeguard the organs. Many oxidation-protective foods are included in the renal diet and make excellent choices for patients with dialysis or people with chronic kidney disease.

Here are kidney-friendly foods that should be included in your diet

- Fish: Swordfish, Salmon, Tuna
- Olive oil
- Bread without salt
- Meat such as Chicken, Pork, Beef, and Turkey
- Pasta
- Rice
- Spices
- Bell peppers
- Vegetables: Sweet potatoes, Carrots, Cabbages, Broccoli, Zucchini
- Garlic, Ginger Onion, Beets, Peas, & Cauliflower
- Pear, Strawberries, Apple, Blueberries,
- Raspberries, Cherries, and Lemon
- Egg white
- Honey

Bell peppers

- half cup of bell pepper: 88 mg potassium |1 mg sodium |10 mg phosphorus.
- Red bell peppers are high in taste and low in potassium, but that's not the only purpose they're suitable for the renal diet. Such delicious vegetables, with folic acid, vitamin B6, and fiber, are also an outstanding source of vitamin A and vitamin C. Since they have lycopene, an antioxidant that defends against some tumors, red bell peppers are healthy for you.

Cauliflower

- Half a cup of boiled cauliflower provides 88 mg potassium |9 mg sodium| 20 mg phosphorus. Cauliflower produces large amounts of vitamin C and is a healthy source of fiber and folate.
- Compounds that enable the liver neutralize harmful compounds that could destroy cell membranes and DNA are also filled with thiocyanates, indoles, and glucosinolates

Onions

- Half a cup of onion provides 116 mg potassium |3 mg sodium| 3 mg phosphorus

- In several cooked dishes, onion, a part of the Allium family and a simple flavoring, contains sulfur compounds that give it its musky fragrance. But onions are also abundant in flavonoids, particularly quercetin, a strong antioxidant that works to protects against many cancers to decrease heart disease, in addition to making some people weep. Onion is low in potassium and is a strong chromium source, a mineral that assists in the digestion of sugars, fats, and proteins.

Apples

- One apple with skin provides 158 mg potassium |0 sodium|10 mg phosphorus

- It is understood that apples lower cholesterol, suppress constipation, reduce cancer danger. Eliminate heart disease an apple a day, which is rich in fiber and anti-inflammatory compounds, can keep the doctor away. It is Good news for kidney disease patients who have their fair share of doctor visits.

Cranberries

- Half cup of cranberry juice cocktail provides 22 mg potassium |3 mg sodium| 3 mg phosphorus

- 1/4 cup of cranberry sauce provides 17 mg potassium |35 mg sodium| 6 mg phosphorus

- half cup of dried cranberries provides 24 mg potassium |2 mg sodium| 5 mg phosphorus

These tangy, delicious berries are believed to safeguard against bladder infections by keeping bacteria from clinging to the bladder wall. Cranberries prevent the stomach from ulcer-causing bacteria and, supporting GI health, protecting the lining of the gastrointestinal (GI) tract. It has also been shown that cranberries guard heart failure and against cancer and

Fish

- 3 ounces of wild salmon provides 368 mg potassium| 50 mg sodium| 274 mg phosphorus

- Fish has high-quality protein and includes fats called omega-3s that are anti-inflammatory. The good fats in fish will help combat diseases such as heart disease and cancer. Omega-3s often support lower LDL cholesterol of low level, poor cholesterol, and boost HDL cholesterol of high density, which is healthy cholesterol.

Chapter 3: Kidney Friendly Grocery List

Being on a renal diet is tough but not impossible, as many of the foods are restricted, but some delicious healthy foods are encouraged to be eaten. Here is a food list to narrow it down for you and save time while grocery shopping.

- Beef
- Chicken
- Bagels
- Egg whites
- Berries, strawberries, apples, pineapples
- Fish
- Beansprout
- Turkey
- Beets
- Bread (white, French Caution for sugar intake)
- Tofu
- Coleslaw
- Couscous
- Cauliflower
- Unsalted crackers
- Chives
- Chili peppers
- Spices (no salt added)
- Cucumber
- Eggplant
- English Muffins
- Coffee
- Green Beans
- Kale
- Oyster Crackers
- Limeade
- Cherries
- Leeks
- Pita Bread
- Mushrooms
- Rice (white)
- Onions
- Rice Cakes
- Nondairy Creamers
- Vegan cheese
- Mixed Vegetables
- Parsley
- Spaghetti
- Tea
- Butter(plant-based)
- Cream Cheese (low fat)
- Turnips
- Peas
- Vegetable Oils
- Olive oil
- Onions
- Garlic
- Ginger
- Sweet potatoes
- Potatoes (leached)
- Mineral Water

3.1 Leaching Potatoes & Vegetables

By leaching the potassium out of certain vegetables, then high potassium foods should be prepared for eating. Typically, this requires about 2-4 hours.

The following method includes carrots, rutabagas potatoes, sweet potatoes.

- Add the vegetables to a cold pot of water enough to cover the vegetables.

- Peel and slice them as you like and put them in cold water.

- Drain the cold water, then wash with warm water

- Add 10 cups of water to one cup of potatoes, submerge all the cut vegetables in 10:1 water.

- Soak for 2-3 hours. If soaking for more, change the water.

- After soaking, get the vegetables out and cook as usual. Or cook them in 5:1. one cup of soaked potatoes to cook in 5 cups of water.

- Mushrooms, squash, frozen greens and, cauliflower can also be leached

Chapter 4: 21-Day Kidney Friendly Meal Plan

This meal plan is designed to provide you with the best healthy food for your kidneys. All these recipes are with clear instructions ahead. Try to eat one serving of these foods, but remember not to starve yourself. Enjoy.

Week 1

Monday (Day 1)

Breakfast: One Blueberry Muffin with Coffee or Tea

Lunch: Green Pesto Pasta

Snack: Half A Cup of Leached Broccoli

Dinner: Turmeric Lime Chicken

Tuesday (Day 2)

Breakfast: Two Maple Pancakes

Lunch: Quinoa Burger

Snack: A Few Slices of Apples

Dinner: Garlic Roasted Salmon & Brussels Sprouts

Wednesday (Day 3)

Breakfast: Blood Orange, Carrot, and Ginger Smoothie

Lunch: Cleansing Detox Soup

Snack: Half A Cup of Fresh Berries

Dinner: Turkey & Noodles

Thursday (Day 4)

Breakfast: One or two egg muffins

Lunch: Slow Cooker Cabbage Soup

Snack: 2,3 baby carrots with tea or coffee

Dinner: One Pot Greek Chicken and Lemon Rice

Friday (Day 5)

Breakfast: Loaded Veggie Eggs

Lunch: Chicken and Rice Soup

Snack: Few slices of pineapples

Dinner: Green Falafels

Saturday (Day 6)

Breakfast: Dilly Scrambled Eggs

Lunch: Vegan Meatloaf

Dinner: Turkey New Orleans style

Sunday (Day 7)

Breakfast: Homemade Buttermilk Pancake

Lunch: Pasta Soup

Snack: One Blueberry Muffin

Dinner: Roast Chicken with Turmeric and Fennel

Week 2

Monday (Day 8)

Breakfast: Easy Turkey Breakfast Burritos

Lunch: Capers pasta salad

Dinner: One-Pot Chicken and Dumplings

Tuesday (Day 9)

Breakfast: Diet Breakfast

Lunch: Cauliflower Soup

Dinner: Juicy Turkey Burgers with Zucchini

Wednesday (Day 10)

Breakfast: Egg Muffins

Lunch: Butternut Squash and Apple Soup

Snack: Half A Cup of Cherries

Dinner: Baked Pork Chops

Thursday (Day 11)

Breakfast: Quick and Easy Apple Oatmeal Custard

Lunch: Tofu Parmigiana

Snack: Low-Sodium Crackers

Dinner: Easy one-pot pasta

Friday (Day 12)

Breakfast: Microwave Coffee Cup Egg Scramble

Lunch: Pasta with Cauliflower

Snack: A Few Breadsticks

Dinner: Turmeric Lime Chicken

Saturday (Day 13)

Breakfast: Southwest Baked Egg Breakfast Cups

Lunch: Yucatan Lime Soup

Dinner: Turkey Chili

Sunday (Day 14)

Breakfast: Stuffed Breakfast Biscuits

Lunch: Healthy Pizza Pasta Salad

Snack: One Bagel with Coffee or Tea

Dinner: Spaghetti Squash Parmigiano

Week 3

Monday (Day 15)

Breakfast: Two Maple Pancakes

Lunch: Garlic Shells

Snack: Low Sodium Crackers

Dinner: Beef Stew

Tuesday (Day 16)

Breakfast: Mushroom & Red Pepper Omelet

Lunch: Broccoli Balls

Snack: Unsalted Pretzels

Dinner: Swordfish with Olives, Capers Polenta

Wednesday (Day 17)

Breakfast: Beach Boy Omelet

Lunch: Cauliflower Steaks

Snack: Few slices of apples

Dinner: Green Chili Stew

Thursday (Day 18)

Breakfast: Apple onion omelet

Lunch: Garbanzo Stir Fry

Snack: Animal crackers

Dinner: Seasoned Pork Chops

Friday (Day 19)

Breakfast: Quick and Easy Apple Oatmeal Custard

Lunch: Vegan Minestrone Soup

Dinner: Turmeric Lime Chicken

Saturday (Day 20)

Breakfast: No-Fuss Microwave Egg White French Toast

Lunch: Salmon with Lemon Caper Sauce

Snack: One blueberry muffin

Dinner: Pork Fajitas

Sunday (Day 21)

Breakfast: Apple Muffins

Lunch: Honey Garlic Chicken

Snack: One Bagel

Dinner: Vegan Minestrone Soup

Part 3: 301 Kidney-Friendly recipes

Chapter 1: Kidney-Friendly Breakfast Recipes

- Fluffy Homemade Buttermilk Pancake

Ingredients

- Olive oil: ¼ cup
- Low-fat buttermilk: 2 cups
- All-purpose flour: 2 cups
- Lemon juice: 1 teaspoon
- Sugar: 2 tablespoons
- 2 large eggs white
- Baking powder: one and a half teaspoons

Instructions

- Put a pan over medium flame.
- In a large bowl, add all the dry ingredients. In another bowl, add oil, buttermilk, and egg whites mix and mix with dry ingredients.
- Mix it well.
- Spray oil on the pan. Pour the batter into the pan in a pancake shape.
- Cook until brown on both sides.
- Repeat with the rest of the batter, enjoy.

Nutrition Per Serving: Calories 217| Total Fat 9 g| Saturated Fat 1 g| Cholesterol 44 mg| Sodium 330 mg| Carbohydrates 27 g| Protein 6 g|Phosphorus 100 mg|Potassium 182 mg| Fiber 1 g| Calcium 74 mg

1.2 Blueberry Muffins

Ingredients

- 2 and a half cups fresh blueberries
- Half cup low-fat unsalted butter
- One and 1/4 cups of artificial sweetener
- Soy milk: 2 cups
- All-purpose flour: 2 cups
- Half teaspoon of salt
- Three eggs' white
- Baking powder: 2 teaspoons

Instructions

- In a food mixer, add sugar alternative and margarine, blend it on low until smooth.
- Add eggs, mix until combined well.
- Add dry ingredients after sifting, and add milk.
- Take half a cup of berries and mash them. Mix in the mixture with your clean hands. Add the rest of the berries.
- Spray oil on the muffin cups.
- Pour muffin mixture into muffin cups.
- Bake in the oven for half an hour at 375° F.

Nutrition Per Serving: Calories 275| Total Fat 9 g| Saturated Fat 5 g| Cholesterol 53 mg| Sodium 210 mg| Carbohydrates 44 g| Protein 5 g| Phosphorus 100 mg| Potassium 121 mg| Dietary Fiber 1.3 g| Calcium 108 mg

1.3 Easy Turkey Breakfast Burritos

Ingredients

- ¼ cup of chopped bell peppers

- 4 cups of ground turkey
- ¼ cup of olive oil
- 8 egg whites, whisked
- ¼ cup of chopped onions
- Half teaspoon of chili powder
- Jalapeño peppers(seeded): 2 tablespoons
- Eight pieces of flour burrito shells
- Scallions: 2 tablespoons, diced
- Half teaspoon of smoked paprika
- 1 cup shredded vegan cheese

Instructions

- In a pan over medium heat, sauté peppers, cilantro, turkey, scallions, and onions. Until translucent.
- In another pan, cook the whisked eggs.
- In burrito, add turkey and vegetable mix, eggs, and cheese.
- Fold and serve.

Nutrition Per Serving: Calories 407| Total Fat 24 g| Saturated Fat 7 g| Trans Fat 0 g| Cholesterol 237 mg| Sodium 513 mg| Carbohydrates 23 g| Protein 25 g| Phosphorus 359 mg |Potassium 285 mg| Dietary Fiber 2 g| Calcium 209 mg

1.4 Loaded Veggie Eggs

Ingredients

1. 1/4 cup of diced onion
2. 6-7 whites of eggs
3. 3 cups of fresh kale
4. One clove of pressed garlic
5. Oil: 1 tbsp.
6. 1/4 cup of diced bell pepper
7. One cup of cauliflower

8. Black pepper: 1/4 tsp
9. Spring onion for garnish

Instructions

- Whisk the egg whites.
- In a pan, over medium flame, add peppers and onions in the pan and sauté for three minutes.
- Then add garlic and cauliflower— Cook well on low heat for five minutes.
- Add egg whites, mix with vegetables.
- When eggs are cooked, garnish with spring onion, black pepper.
- Serve hot.

Nutrition Per Serving: Calories 240| Total Fat 16.6g| Cholesterol 372mg| Sodium 195mg| Total Carbohydrate 7.8g| Dietary Fiber 2.7g| Protein 15.3g| Potassium 605.2mg| Phosphorus 253.6mg

1.5 Diet Breakfast

Ingredients

1. 3 egg whites
2. Garlic: 1/4 tsp, minced
3. Bell pepper: 2 tbsp. Chopped
4. Cabbage: 1/4 cup, chopped
5. Mushrooms: 1/4 cup
6. Black pepper
7. Jalapeno: 2 tbsp. chopped

Instructions

- In a saucepan, sauté all ingredients, add the mushroom in the last.
- Do not overcook vegetables.
- Then add pepper and garlic to eggs.
- Scramble on Low Heat.
- Sprinkle with basil and serve

Nutrients per serving: Calories 176 | Protein 7.3 g |Carbohydrates 9.2 g |Fat 8.2 g |Cholesterol 132 mg |Sodium 162 mg | Potassium 211 mg| Phosphorus 115 mg | Calcium 17.4 mg |Fiber 3 g

1.6 Breakfast Burrito

Ingredients

- 2 flour tortillas
- 4 egg whites
- Green chilies: 3 tablespoons chopped
- Half tsp. Of hot pepper sauce
- Ground cumin: 1/4 teaspoon

Instructions

- In a skillet over medium flame, spray cooking oil.
- In a mixing bowl, add eggs, cumin, green chilies, hot sauce, and whisk well.
- Add whisked eggs into skillet. Let it cook for two minutes until eggs are cooked.
- Now, lay burritos on a hot skillet and or microwave them and place egg mixture on them.
- Roll and fold on sides.
- Serve hot

Nutrients per serving: Calories 366|Protein 18 g| Carbohydrates 33 g| Fat 18 g| Cholesterol 372 mg| Sodium 394 mg| potassium 215 mg| Phosphorus 254 mg| Calcium 117 mg| Fiber 2.5 g

1.7 Maple Pancakes

Ingredients

- 1% low-fat milk: 1 cup
- All-purpose flour: 1 cup
- Honey: 1 tablespoon
- Salt: two pinches
- Maple extract: 1 tablespoon
- Egg whites: 2 large
- Baking powder: 2 teaspoons
- Olive oil: 2 tablespoons

Instructions

- In a mixing bowl, mix flour, baking powder, salt. Mix well.
- Set it aside.
- In a big mixing bowl, mix egg whites, oil, maple extract, honey, and milk.
- Now mix dry ingredients and wet ingredients. Do not over mix. It should be lumpy.
- Put a skillet over medium flame, spray cooking oil and pour the batter and cook pancakes until brown on both sides.
- Serve hot

Nutrients per serving: Calories 178|Protein 6 g| Carbohydrates 25 g| Fat 6 g| Cholesterol 2 mg| Sodium 267 mg| Potassium 126 mg| Phosphorus 116 mg| Calcium 174 mg| Fiber 0.7 g|

1.8 Mini Frittatas

Ingredients

- Low fat shredded cheese: ¼ cup
- Red bell pepper: ⅓ cup chopped
- Zucchini: ⅓ cup chopped
- Broccoli: ⅓ cup diced
- Fresh basil: 2-3 tbsp.
- Pepper: ¼ tsp
- Seasoning(salt-free): half tbsp.
- 10-12 eggs' whites and 3 yolks

Instructions

- Let the oven Preheat to 375 degrees.

- Spray the muffin pan with oil.
- In a mixing bowl, mix zucchini, basil, red bell pepper, and broccoli.
- In another bowl, mix pepper, cheese, seasoning (salt-free), eggs, and salt.
- Mix the egg mix to vegetables.
- Pour the egg mixture into muffin cups, at least 1/3 cup.
- Bake for 18-20 minutes at 375 F or until cooked.
- Serve right away.

Nutrients per serving: Calories 245 | Protein 11 g |Carbohydrates 9.2 g |Fat 7.7 g | Cholesterol 121 mg |Sodium 99.2 mg | Potassium 201 mg| Phosphorus 109 mg | Calcium 27.9 mg |Fiber 2 g

1.9 Dilly Scrambled Eggs

Ingredients

- Dried dill weed: 1 teaspoon
- Three large egg white
- Crumbled goat cheese: 1 tablespoon
- Black pepper: 1/8 teaspoon

Instructions

- In a bowl, mix eggs.
- Pour the egg mixture into the skillet over medium flame.
- Sprinkle dill weed and black pepper to eggs.
- Cook until eggs are done.
- Garnish with goat cheese.
- Serve right away.

Nutrients per serving: Calories 194|Protein 16 g| Carbohydrates 1 g| Fat 14 g| Cholesterol 334 mg| Sodium 213 mg| Potassium 162 mg| Phosphorus 50 mg| Calcium 214 mg| Fiber 0.2 g

1.10 Start Your Day Bagel

Ingredients

- 1 bagel
- Two red onion slices
- Low fat cream cheese: 2 tablespoons
- Lemon-pepper seasoning(low-sodium): 1 teaspoon
- Two small tomato slices

Instructions

- Slice the bagel and toast to your liking
- Spread cream cheese on each half bagel.
- Add tomato slice, onion slice.
- Sprinkle with lemon pepper.

Nutrients per serving: Calories 134|Protein 5 g| Carbohydrates 19 g| Fat 6 g| Cholesterol 15 mg| Sodium 219 mg| Potassium 162 mg| Phosphorus 50 mg| calcium 9 mg| Fiber 1.6 g

1.11 Egg Muffins

Ingredients

- Ten large eggs whites
- bell peppers: 1 cup
- 2 cups ground pork
- Onion: 1 cup
- Garlic minced: half teaspoon
- Half teaspoon of herb seasoning
- Poultry seasoning (no salt): 1/4 teaspoon
- Salt: two pinches or to taste
- Milk substitute: 2 tablespoons

Instructions

- Let the oven preheat to 350° F and spray cooking oil on the muffin tin
- Chop the vegetables finely.

- In a bowl, mix garlic pork, herb seasoning, poultry seasoning to make sausage.

- In a skillet, cook the sausage until done and drain the liquid if any

- Whisk the eggs with salt and milk.

- Add vegetables and sausage crumbles, mix well.

- Add egg mixture into muffin tins, leave some space on top.

- Bake for 18 to 20 minutes or until done.

- Serve hot.

Nutrients per serving: Calories 154|Protein 12 g| Carbohydrates 3 g| Fat 10 g| Cholesterol 230 mg| Sodium 155 mg| Potassium 200 mg| Phosphorus 154 mg| Calcium 37 mg| Fiber 0.5 g

1.12 Quick & Easy Apple Oatmeal Custard

Ingredients

- Half cup of almond milk

- Quick-cooking oatmeal: 1/3 cup

- Cinnamon: 1/4 teaspoon

- Half apple

- Two egg white

Instructions

- Finely diced the half apple.

- In a large mug, add almond milk, egg, and oats. Mix well with a fork.

- Add apple and cinnamon. Mix well.

- Microwave for two minutes, on high.

- Fluff it with a fork.

- Cook for another sixty-second if required.

- Add in little milk or water if the consistency is too thick.

Nutrients per serving: Calories 248|Protein 11 g| Carbohydrates 33 g| Fat 8 g| Cholesterol 186 mg| Sodium 164 mg| Potassium 362 mg| phosphorus 240 mg| Calcium 154 mg| Fiber 5.8 g

1.13 Microwave Coffee Cup Egg Scramble

Ingredients

- 1% low-fat milk: 2 tablespoons

- 1 large egg+ 2 whites

Instructions

- Spray the coffee cup with oil. Add eggs and milk and whisk.

- Put the coffee cup in the microwave, let it cook for 45 seconds, then remove and fluff with a fork.

- Cook for an additional 30-45 seconds, until eggs are almost done.

- Add pepper and enjoy.

Nutrients per serving: Calories 117|Protein 15 g| Carbohydrates 3 g| Fat 5 g| Cholesterol 188 mg| Sodium 194 mg| Potassium 226 mg| Phosphorus 138 mg| Calcium 72 mg| Fiber 0 g

1.14 No-Fuss Microwave Egg White French Toast

Ingredients

1. Half cup of egg whites

2. One slice of bread

3. Sugar-free syrup: 2 tablespoons

4. Unsalted butter: 1 teaspoon, softened

Instructions

- Add bread to slice. Cut into cubes.

- Add cubed slices into a bowl.

- Add egg whites over bread pieces
- Add syrup on top. Microwave for 60 seconds or more until eggs are set.

Nutrients per serving: Calories 200 | Protein 15 g|Carbohydrates 24 g|Fat 5 g| Cholesterol 11 mg|Sodium 415 mg| Potassium 235 mg|Phosphorus 54 mg| Calcium 50 mg|Fiber 0.7 g

1.15 Easy Turkey Breakfast Burritos

Ingredients

- 8 flour burritos
- 4 cups of ground turkey
- Olive oil: ¼ cup
- Diced onions: ¼ cup
- Bell peppers: ¼ cup chopped
- Fresh scallions: 2 tablespoons, chopped
- 9 whisked egg white
- Jalapeño peppers(seeded): 2 tablespoons
- Fresh cilantro
- Smoked paprika: half teaspoon
- Chili powder: half teaspoon
- Vegan shredded cheese: 1 cup

Instructions

- In a skillet, sauté scallions, turkey, cilantro, peppers, and onions. Add in spices and mix well. turn off the heat
- In another pan, on medium flame, add oil and eggs. Cook well
- In a burrito shell, add vegetables and meatloaf mix, add eggs and cheese in burrito shells.
- Fold on sides and serve.

Nutrition Per Serving: Calories 407 Cal| Total Fat 24 g|Saturated Fat 7 g| Trans Fat 0 g|Cholesterol 237 mg|Sodium 513 mg| Carbohydrates 23 g| Protein 25 g| Phosphorus 359 mg|Potassium 285 mg| Dietary Fiber 2 g| Calcium 209 mg

1.16 Tofu Scrambler

Ingredients

1. Onion powder: 1 teaspoon
2. Olive oil: 1 teaspoon
3. Green bell pepper: ¼ cup diced
4. Red bell pepper: ¼ cup diced
5. Turmeric: ⅛ teaspoon
6. Firm tofu: 1 cup (less than 10% calcium)
7. 2 clove garlic, minced

Instructions

- In a non-stick pan, add bell peppers and garlic in olive oil.
- Rinse the tofu, and add in skillet break it into pieces with hands.
- Add all the remaining ingredients.
- Stir often, and cook on medium flame until the tofu becomes a light golden brown, for almost 20 minutes.
- Serve warm.

Nutrition Per Serving: Calories 213 Cal| Total Fat 13 g| Saturated Fat 2 g| Trans Fat 0 g|Cholesterol 0 mg|Sodium 24 mg| Carbohydrates 10 g |Protein 18 g|Phosphorus 242 mg|Potassium 467 mg|Dietary Fiber 2 g| Calcium 274 mg

1.17 Southwest Baked Egg Breakfast Cups

Ingredients

- Rice: 3 cups, cooked
- Half cup of shredded cheddar cheese

- Half cup of chopped green chilies
- 1/4 cups of cherry peppers diced
- Half cup of skim milk
- 3 egg whites whisked
- Ground cumin: half teaspoon
- Black pepper: half teaspoon

Instructions

- In a bowl, mix chilies, cherry peppers, eggs, cumin, 2 ounces of cheese, rice, black pepper.
- Spray the muffin tins with oil
- Pour mix into muffins tin. Garnish with cheese.
- Bake for 15 minutes at 400° F or until set.

Nutrition Per Serving: Calories 109 cal| Total Fat 4 g|Saturated Fat 2 g| Trans Fat 0 g|Cholesterol 41 mg|Sodium 79 mg| Carbohydrates 13 g|Protein 5 g|Phosphorus 91 mg|Potassium 82 mg|Dietary Fiber 0.5 g| Calcium 91 mg

1.18 Stuffed Breakfast Biscuits

Ingredients

- Baking powder: half teaspoon
- Honey: 1 tablespoon
- Lemon juice: 1 tablespoon
- Softened unsalted butter: 8 tablespoons
- Milk: ¾ cup
- Flour: 2 cups

Filling

- Cheddar cheese: 1 cup shredded
- Five egg white
- Scallions: ¼ cup, thinly sliced

- 1 cup chopped bacon (reduced-sodium)

Instructions

- Let the oven Preheat to 425° F.

For Filling

- Cook the eggs, scrambled
- Cook bacon to crisp.
- Mix filling ingredients and set it aside

The Dough

- In a big bowl, add all the dry ingredients.
- Add in butter and cut with a fork, and add in lemon juice and milk. Knead well.
- Spray muffin tin with oil generously.
- Pour ¼ cup of mixture into the muffin tins.
- Bake for 10-12 minutes at 425° F until golden brown.

Nutrition Per Serving: Calories 330 cal| Total Fat 23 g|Saturated Fat 11 g| Trans Fat 0.6 g|Cholesterol 105 mg|Sodium 329 mg| Carbohydrates 19 g|Protein 11 g|Phosphorus 170 mg|Potassium 152 mg|Dietary Fiber 1 g| Calcium 107 mg

1.19 Cheesesteak Quiche

Ingredients

- Olive oil: 2 tablespoons
- 2 cups of trimmed sirloin steak, roughly chopped
- Onions: 1 cup, chopped
- Cheese: Half cup, shredded
- Six egg white whisked
- Ground black pepper: half teaspoon
- Low-fat Cream: 1 cup
- Par-cooked prepared piecrust

Instructions

- In a pan with oil, Sauté onions, and chopped steak. Cook until meat is cooked. Let it cool for ten minutes. Mix in cheese set it aside.

- In a bowl, whisk cream eggs with black pepper, mix it well.

- Add cheese mix and steak on pie crust, then add the egg mixture on top and half an hour bake at 350° F.

- and turn off the oven and Cover the quiche with foil.

- Let it sit for ten minutes, then serve.

Nutrition Per Serving: Calories 527 cal| Total Fat 19 g|Saturated Fat 17 g| Trans Fat 1 g|Cholesterol 240 mg|Sodium 392 mg| Carbohydrates 22 g|Protein 22 g|Phosphorus 281 mg|Potassium 308 mg|Dietary Fiber 1 g| Calcium 137 mg

1.20 Chocolate Pancakes with Moon Pie Stuffing

Ingredients

Moon Pie Stuffing

- Heavy cream: ¼ cup

- Cocoa powder(unsweetened): 1 tablespoon

- Half cup of low fat softened cream cheese

- Honey: 2 tbsp.

Chocolate Pancakes

- One large egg white

- Flour: 1 cup

- Cocoa powder(unsweetened): 3 tablespoons

- Half teaspoon baking powder

- Olive oil: 2 tablespoons

- Lemon juice: 1 tablespoon

- Honey: 3 tablespoons

- Vanilla extract: 2 teaspoons

- Almond milk: 1 cup

Instructions

Moon Pie Filling

- Beat cocoa and heavy cream together until stiff peaks are formed.

- Whip in cream cheese, marshmallow cream, and whey protein powder for about a minute or until well blended, but don't overbeat. Cover and set aside in the fridge.

Pancakes

- Mix all the dry ingredients in a large bowl and set aside.

- Mix all the wet ingredients in a medium-size bowl.

- Slowly fold in wet ingredients to the dry ingredients just until wet, but don't over mix.

- Cook the pancakes on a lightly oiled griddle on medium heat or 375° F.

- Use about 1/8 cup of batter to form 4-inch pancakes, flipping when they start to bubble.

Nutrition Per Serving: Calories 194 Cal | Total Fat 9 g|Saturated Fat 4 g|Trans Fat 0 g| Cholesterol 36 mg|Sodium 121 mg| Carbohydrates 22 g| Protein 7 g| Phosphorus 134 mg|Potassium 135 mg|Dietary Fiber 1 g| Calcium 67 mg

1.21 Apple Muffins

Ingredients

1. One and a half tsp of cinnamon

2. One and a half cup of raw apple

3. Half cup of water

4. 1 cup honey

5. Half cup olive oil
6. 2 large egg white
7. Vanilla: 1 tbsp.
8. One and a half cup all-purpose white flour
9. Baking powder: 1 tsp

Instructions

- Let the oven preheat to 400 F. add muffin papers in a muffin tin.
- Peel and chop the apple into small pieces.
- In a bowl, whisk eggs with water, honey, oil, vanilla and mix well
- In another bowl, mix baking powder, one teaspoon cinnamon, flour.
- Sift the flour mixture into the egg mix.
- The batter should be lumpy. Add in the apple pieces.
- Pour batter into muffin cups, sprinkle cinnamon on top.
- Enjoy warm.

Nutrition per serving: Sodium 177 mg| Protein 3 g|Potassium 46 mg|Phosphorus 34 mg |Calcium 10 mg|Calories 162 kcal|Fat 10 g| Water 60 g |Carbohydrates 15 g

1.22 Breakfast Casserole

Ingredients

1. 1% low-fat milk: 1 cup
2. One cup of pork sausage (reduced-fat)
3. Five large egg whites
4. Half teaspoon dry mustard
5. One cup of cream cheese (low fat)
6. Half chopped onion
7. White bread, cut into cubes: 4 slices

Instructions

- Let the oven preheat to 325 F
- Break the sausage and cook in a pan, set it aside
- In a blender, pulse the rest of the ingredients. Do not add bread yet.
- Add the cooked sausage to the mix.
- In a 9 by 9 dish, add the bread, and add sausage mix on top
- Bake for 55 minutes.
- Serve hot and enjoy.

Nutrients per serving: Calories 224 | Protein 11 g| Carbohydrates 9 g| Fat 16 g| Cholesterol 149 mg| Sodium 356 mg| Potassium 201 mg| Phosphorus 159 mg| Calcium 97 mg |fiber 0.4 g|

1.23 Apple Onion Omelet

Ingredients

- Butter: 1 tablespoon
- Three large egg whites
- Water: 1 tablespoon
- Black pepper: 1/8 teaspoon
- 1% low-fat milk: 1/4 cup
- Shredded cheddar cheese: 2 tablespoons
- Sweet onion: 3/4 cup
- One big apple

Instructions

1. Let the oven Preheat to 400º F.
2. Peel and clean apple. Thinly slice the onion and apples
3. In a bowl, whisk the egg with milk, pepper, water. Set it aside.
4. In a pan, over a low flame, melt the butter.

5. Add apple and onion to the butter, cook for five minutes.

6. Add egg mix on top cook on medium flame until the edges are set.

7. Add the cheese on the top.

8. Put the skillet in the oven and bake for 10-12 minutes, or until set.

9. Serve hot

Nutrients per serving: calories 284 | Protein 13 | Carbohydrates 22 | Fat 16 | Cholesterol 303| Sodium 169| potassium 341|Phosphorus 238 |Calcium 147 |Fiber 3.5

1.24 Beach Boy Omelet

Ingredients

- Green bell pepper: 2 tablespoons, chopped
- Canola oil: 1 teaspoon
- Hash browns: 2 tablespoons (shredded)
- Soy milk: 2 tablespoons
- One egg and two egg whites
- Onion: 2 tablespoons, chopped

Instructions

- In a pan, heat oil over medium flame. Sauté green pepper and onion for two minutes
- Then add hash browns, cook for five minutes.
- Whisk eggs with non-dairy creamer or soy milk
- In another pan, cook the eggs until set.
- Add the hash brown mixture in the center of eggs, wrap with eggs and serve

Nutrients per serving: Calories 228 | Protein 15 g |Carbohydrates 12 g |Fat 13 g | Cholesterol 165 mg |Sodium 180 mg |

Potassium 307 mg|Phosphorus 128 mg | Calcium 38 mg |Fiber 0.9 g

1.25 Mushroom & Red Pepper Omelet

Ingredients

- Half cup raw mushroom
- 3 large egg white
- Onion: 2 tablespoons
- Red peppers: 1/4 cup
- Whipped cream cheese: 2 tablespoons
- Butter: 2 teaspoons
- Black pepper: 1/4 teaspoon

Instructions

- Chop up the red peppers, onion, and mushroom
- In a pan, melt the butter (one tsp.). Sauté red peppers, onion, and mushroom. Set it aside.
- Melt another tsp. of butter in a pan. Cook eggs. When eggs are half cooked, pour vegetable mix with cream cheese on top. Cook eggs until set
- Continue cooking until eggs are set.
- Fold the half omelet on top of the cream cheese mix. Add black pepper and serve

Nutrients per serving: Calories 178 | Protein 8.8 g |Carbohydrates 8.2 g |Fat 6.7 g |Cholesterol 132 mg |Sodium 156 mg | Potassium 201 mg|Phosphorus 121 mg | Calcium 21 mg |Fiber 0.4 g

Chapter 2: Kidney-Friendly Soup Recipes

2.1 Spring Vegetable Soup

Ingredients

- Vegetable broth(low-sodium): 4 cups
- Fresh green beans: 1 cup
- Half cup carrots
- Celery: 3/4 cup
- Garlic powder: 1 teaspoon
- Half cup onion
- Half cup mushrooms
- Olive oil: 2 tablespoons
- Dried oregano leaves: 1 teaspoon
- 1/4 teaspoon salt
- Half cup frozen corn

Instructions

- Trim the green beans and chop into two-inch pieces
- Chop up the vegetables.
- In a pot, heat olive oil, sauté the onion and celery, till tender.
- Then add the remaining ingredients.
- Let it boil. Lower the heat, let it simmer.
- Cook for almost an hour.

Nutrients per serving: Calories 114| Protein 2 g| Carbohydrates 13 g| Fat 6 g| Cholesterol 0 mg| Sodium 262 mg| Potassium 365 mg| Phosphorus 108 mg| Calcium 48 mg| Fiber 3.4 g|

2.2 Kidney Diet Friendly Chicken Noodle Soup

Ingredients

- One cup cooked Chicken Breast
- Unsalted Butter: 1 tbsp.
- Half cup of Chopped Celery
- Chicken Stock: 5 cups
- Half tsp Ground Basil
- Half cup of chopped Onions
- Ground Black Pepper: 1/4 tsp
- Egg Noodles: 2 cups, Dry
- Sliced Carrots: 1 cup
- Half tsp Ground Oregano

Instructions

- Chop up all the vegetables.
- In a Dutch oven (5 quarts), melt butter over low heat—Cook celery and onion for five minutes. Add in the carrots, oregano, chicken stock, basil, pepper, chicken and, noodles.
- Let it boil. Lower the heat and let it simmer for 20 minutes.
- Serve hot.

Nutrition per serving: Calories: 186| Protein: 15.8 g| Carbohydrate: 19.7 g| Dietary Fiber: 1.461 g| Phosphorus: 178.8 mg| Potassium: 478.9 mg| Sodium: 327.2 mg|

2.3 Renal-Friendly Cream of Mushroom Soup

Ingredients

- Minced mushrooms: 1/4 cup
- Unsalted butter: 3 tbsp.
- All-purpose flour: 2 and a half tbsp.
- Sea salt, pepper to taste
- Low sodium chicken broth: half cup
- Finely chopped onion: 1/4 cup
- Unsweetened almond milk: half cup

Instructions

- In a skillet, melt the butter and sauté onions till tender

- Add mushrooms and cook for five minutes. Add flour and cook for one minute or a few seconds more

- Add in milk and broth mix continuously.

- Let it simmer until it becomes thick for five minutes.

Nutrition per serving: Total Fat 18.2g| Cholesterol 45.8mg| Sodium 162.8mg| Total Carbohydrate 10.2g| Dietary Fiber 0.9g| Protein 2.1g| Iron 1mg| Potassium 123.7mg

2.4 Rotisserie Chicken Noodle Soup

Ingredients

- Carrots: 1 cup, sliced

- One cooked rotisserie chicken

- Half cup of onion, chopped

- Celery: 1 cup, sliced

- Chicken broth(low-sodium): 8 cups

- Fresh parsley: 3 tablespoons

- Wide noodles: 6 ounces, uncooked

Instructions

- Take the bones out of the chicken and cut into one-inch pieces. Take four cups of chicken pieces.

- In a large pot, add chicken broth let it boil.

- Add noodles, chicken, and vegetables to the broth.

- Let it boil, and cook for 15 minutes. Make sure noodles are tender.

- Serve with chopped parsley on top.

Nutrients per serving: Calories 185| Protein 21 g| Carbohydrates 14 g| Fat 5 g| Cholesterol 63 mg| Sodium 361 mg|

Potassium 294 mg| Phosphorus 161 mg | Calcium 22 mg| Fiber 1.4 g

2.5 Quick & Easy Ground Beef Soup

Ingredients

- Frozen mixed vegetables: 3 cups

- Half cup of onion, chopped

- Beef broth(reduced-sodium): 1 cup

- White rice: 1/3 cup, uncooked

- Lemon pepper (no salt): 2 teaspoons, seasoning

- 4 cups of lean ground beef

- Sour cream: 1 tablespoon

- Water: 2 cups

Instructions

- In a pot, sauté onion, brown the beef. Drain the fat.

- Add all the remaining ingredients and seasoning.

- Let it boil. Lower the heat, cover it, and cook for half an hour.

- Turn off the heat, add sour cream.

Nutrients per serving: calories 222 | Protein 20 g| Carbohydrates 19 g| Fat 8 g| Cholesterol 52 mg| Sodium 170 mg| Potassium 448 mg| Phosphorus 210 mg| Calcium 43 mg| Fiber 4.3 g

2.6 Chicken & Dill Soup

Ingredients

- One chicken whole

- Carrots, 1 pound, sliced

- Low-sodium veggie stock for 6 cups

- One cup of yellow, diced onion

- A pinch of black pepper and Salt

- Two dill teaspoons, diced

- Half cup red, minced onion

Instructions

- Place the chicken in a saucepan, add the water to coat it. Let it simmer for 1 hour.

- Take chicken out, remove the bones, strip the meat, strain the soup, put everything back in the saucepan, hot it over a moderate flame, and add the chicken.

- Add the carrots, red onion, a pinch of Salt, yellow onion, black pepper, and dill, roast for fifteen minutes, and put in bowls.

Nutrients per serving: Calories 295| Protein 21 g| Carbohydrates 28 g| Fat 11 g| Cholesterol 45 mg| Sodium 385 mg| Potassium 312 mg| Phosphorus 252 mg| Calcium 183 mg | Fiber 3.3 g

2.7 Maryland's Eastern Shore Cream of Crab Soup

Ingredients

- 1 cup non-dairy creamer
- Unsalted butter: 1 tablespoon
- Old bay seasoning: 1/4 teaspoon
- 2 cups crab meat
- Chicken broth(low-sodium): 4 cups
- One medium onion
- Cornstarch: 2 tablespoons
- Black pepper: 1/8 teaspoon
- Dill weed: 1/8 teaspoon

Instructions

- In a large pot, melt butter over medium flame.
- Add chopped onion to the pot. Cook until tender.

- Add crab meat   Cook for 2 to 3 minutes. Stir often.

- Add chicken broth, let it boil. Turn heat down to low.

- Mix starch and creamer in a bowl. Mix well.

- Add the mixture to the soup, increase the heat, stir until the soup thickens and gets to a boil.

- Add Old Bay, dill weed, pepper to soup.

Nutrients per serving: Calories 130 | Protein 12 g| carbohydrates 7 g| Fat 6 g| Cholesterol 53 mg| sodium 212 mg| Potassium 312 mg| Phosphorus 80 mg| Calcium 86 mg|Fiber 0.4 g

2.8 Old Fashioned Salmon Soup

Ingredients

- Chicken broth, reduced-sodium: 2 cups
- Unsalted butter: 2 tablespoons
- Half cup of onion, chopped
- Sockeye salmon: 1 pound, cooked
- One medium carrot, chopped
- 1% low-fat milk: 2 cups
- Half cup of celery, chopped
- Black pepper: 1/8 teaspoon
- Water: 1/4 cup
- Cornstarch: 1/4 cup

Instructions

- In a large pot, melt the butter and cook the vegetables on low, medium flame until tender.

- Add the cooked salmon chunks. Add in the milk, broth, pepper.

- Let it simmer on low heat.

- Mix water and cornstarch. Keep stirring and slowly add the corn starch mix. Cook until soup becomes thick.
- Simmer for 5 minutes and serve.

Nutrients per serving: Calories 155| Protein 14 g| Carbohydrates 9 g| Fat 7 g| Cholesterol 37 mg| Sodium 113 mg| Potassium 369 mg| Phosphorus 218 mg| Calcium 92 mg| Fiber 0.5 g

2.9 Turkey, Wild Rice, & Mushroom Soup

Ingredients

- Turkey: 2 cups, cooked, shredded
- Half cup of onion, chopped
- Half cup of carrots, chopped
- Two garlic cloves, minced
- Chicken broth, low-sodium: 5 cups
- Half cup of red bell pepper, chopped
- Half cup of uncooked wild rice,
- Olive oil: 1 tablespoon
- Half teaspoon salt
- Two bay leaves
- Herb seasoning: 1/4 teaspoon
- Dried thyme: 1-and half teaspoon
- Black pepper: 1/4 teaspoon
- Half cup of sliced mushrooms

Instructions

- In a pot, boil the one and ¾ broth over medium flame. Add rice to the broth and cook. Let it boil. Turn the heat down. Cover it and let it simmer until all broth is absorbed.
- In a Dutch oven, heat oil, add garlic, bell pepper, onion, and carrots. Sauté them.

- Add the mushroom to the vegetables, then add the broth, turkey, herb seasoning, salt, pepper, thyme, and bay leaves. Cook until it is well heated. Stir often.
- Before adding the rice, take out the bay leaves. Cook for a minute and serve.

Nutrition per serving: Calories 210| Protein 23 g| Carbohydrates 15 g| Fat 5 g| Cholesterol 35 mg| Sodium 270 mg| Potassium 380 mg| Phosphorus 200 mg| Calcium 32 mg| Fiber 2.3 g

2.10 Slow Cooker Kale & Turkey Meatball Soup

Ingredients

- 4 cups of ground turkey
- Bread: 2 slices
- Kale: 4 cups
- ¼ of a cup milk
- 2 cloves of garlic pressed
- One medium shallot finely diced
- ½ of a teaspoon freshly grated nutmeg
- One teaspoon of oregano
- 1/4 of a teaspoon red pepper flakes
- Italian parsley chopped: 2 tablespoons
- 2 carrots cut into slices
- One egg white
- One tablespoon of olive oil
- Chicken or vegetable broth: 8 cups
- Half yellow onion finely diced
- Half of a cup Parmigiano-Reggiano grated, extra for garnish
- Kosher salt and freshly ground pepper

Instructions

- In a large mixing bowl, add milk, cut the bread into pieces, and let it soak in milk. Add the garlic, turkey, nutmeg, shallot, red pepper flakes, salt, oregano, pepper, egg, cheese, and parsley. Mix carefully with your hands. Use a scooper to make half-inch balls.

- Put a wide skillet on medium flame, heat the olive oil, then sear the meatballs gently on every side for two minutes. Turn off the heat and set it aside.

- Add the onion, stock, kale, and carrots to a 5 to 7 quarter slow cooker.

- Add meatballs the kale, and cook for four hours at low or until the meatballs start floating to the top.

- Garnish the soup with Parmesan grated cheese, red pepper flakes, and fresh leaves of parsley.

Nutrition per serving: 250 calories| total fat 23g |carbohydrates 20.3g | protein 14.4g| Cholesterol 25 mg| Sodium 214 mg| Potassium 276 mg| Phosphorus 198 mg| Calcium 28.8 mg| Fiber 2.8 g

2.11 Greek Lemon Chicken Soup

Ingredients

- Boneless: 4 cups of skinless chicken thighs, cut into bite-size pieces

- Chicken broth: 8 cups

- Kale: 4 cups

- Extra-virgin olive oil: 2 tablespoons, divided

- Freshly ground black pepper and Kosher salt

- Three carrots peeled, finely diced

- 2 stalks of celery finely chopped

- 4 cloves of pressed garlic

- Half teaspoon of dried thyme

- Two bay leaves

- Sliced fresh dill: 2 tablespoons

- One cup cubed sweet potatoes

- One onion finely chopped

- Squeezed lemon juice: 2 tablespoons(fresh)or more, if needed

- Sliced fresh parsley leaves: 2 tablespoons

Instruction

- Put a large saucepan or Dutch oven over medium flame and add one tablespoon of olive oil.

- Season the chicken thighs with black pepper and fine salt to your liking. Add the seasoned chicken things to the pan and cook for about three minutes; until golden brown, set it aside.

- Add the remaining one tablespoon of olive oil in the separate pan, with celery, garlic, onion, and carrots, stir frequently, and let it cook for about four minutes.

- Add in thyme, cook for about one minute, until fragrant.

- Then stir in the bay leaves and chicken stock, let it boil. Add in chicken and potatoes, stir and cook for 15 minutes, till soup is thickened.

- Add in the kale, cook for two minutes, till wilted. Add in parsley, dill, and lemon juice

- Season with salt and black pepper, to your taste.

- Serve hot, and enjoy

Nutrition per serving: Calories 243 g| Total Fat 9.0g|Carbohydrate 18.0g|Protein 19.0g | Cholesterol 18.2 mg| Sodium 198 mg| Potassium 213 mg| Phosphorus 187 mg| Calcium 29.2 mg| Fiber 2.5 g

2.12 Lemon Chicken Soup

Ingredients

- Eggs: 3 large whites
- Chicken broth: 6 cups
- Shredded and cooked chicken breast: 1 cup
- Fresh lemon juice:1/4 cup
- Kosher Salt and freshly ground black pepper (to taste.)
- Orzo:1 cup

Instructions

- Add chicken stock to a big saucepan and let it boil.
- Add in orzo, cook until soft to your liking.
- Mix eggs and lemon juice.
- When orzo is cooked to your liking, take out one cup of chicken broth and add in egg mix one tablespoon at a time. Mixing constantly
- Then add this egg mixture back into the broth, constantly stirring.
- Add the cooked shredded chicken in the broth, let it simmer until the soup becomes thick, often stirring, for about five minutes.
- Add salt and freshly ground black pepper to taste.

Nutrition per serving: Calories 451|Carbs: 42g| Protein: 32g |Fat: 15g

2.13 Vegan Minestrone Soup

Ingredients

- Cubed bread: one cup
- Low-sodium vegetable broth: 3 cups
- Garlic: 5 cloves
- Leek: one cup (chopped)
- Olive oil: 3 tbsp.
- Carrots: one cup(chopped)
- Water: three cups
- Small pasta: one cup
- Kosher salt: 3/4 tsp.
- Beans: 15 ounces
- Baby kale: 3 cups
- Zucchini: 10 ounces (thinly sliced)
- Peas: 1 cup
- Ground pepper: half teaspoon

Instructions

- Let the oven Preheat oven to 350 F.
- Cook the garlic in two tablespoons of oil over medium heat in a medium skillet, stirring continuously for three minutes until the garlic is softened.
- Add bread; toss it to coat. Spread the combination uniformly on a baking dish. Bake, for ten minutes, until toasted.
- In the meanwhile, heat the leftover one tablespoon oil over medium flame in a big pan. Add the leek and carrots; simmer for five minutes, stirring frequently until softened.
- Add salt, broth, and water, cover it and bring to a simmer over a high flame.
- Add the pasta on low flame; cook uncovered for five minutes, stirring regularly. Then add zucchini, stirring regularly, for around five minutes, until the pasta is al dente.

- Stir in kale, beans, peas, and seasoning. Cook for around two minutes, stirring regularly until the kale is wilted.
- Pour the soup into six bowls, evenly garnish with the croutons.

Nutrition per serving: 267 calories| total fat 8.6g |carbohydrates 8.7g | protein 9.7g

2.14 Lemon Chicken Orzo Soup with Kale

Ingredients

- Chicken broth: 4 cups
- Chicken breasts: 4 cups (1-inch pieces)
- Dried oregano: 1 tsp.
- Olive oil: 2 tbsp.
- Salt: 1 and ¼ tsp.
- Diced onions: 2 cups
- One bay leaf
- Orzo pasta: 2/3 cup
- Diced celery: 1 cup
- Chopped kale: 4 cups
- Two minced cloves of Garlic
- Diced carrots: 1 cup
- One lemon juice and zest
- Black pepper: ¾ tsp.

Instructions

- Heat one tbsp. Of oil over medium flame in a big pot. Add the chicken, oregano (half teaspoon), salt, pepper. Cook for five minutes till light brown. move the chicken to the plate
- Add the remaining one spoonful of oil, carrots, onions, celery, and carrots in the same pot. Cook for five minutes until the vegetables are tender. Add the bay leaf, Garlic, and oregano (half teaspoon) cook for around 30 to 60 seconds,
- Add broth and let it boil over a high flame. Adding orzo. Then lower the heat for five minutes to let it simmer, cover, and let it cook. Add the chicken and kale and any leftover juices. Continue cooking for ten minutes until the orzo is soft and the chicken is cooked.
- Remove from flame. Throw away the bay leaf. Add lemon zest and lemon juice, 3/4 tsp, salt, and 1/4 tsp. of pepper.
- Serve right away.

Nutrition per serving: Calories 245|Net carbs 20g| protein 12 g|fat12 g| Cholesterol 17.6 mg| Sodium 214 mg| Potassium 220 mg| Phosphorus 187 mg| Calcium 29.2 mg| Fiber 2.4 g

2.15 Slow-Cooker Chicken & Chickpea Soup

Ingredients

- 8 cups bone-in, trimmed skin removed, chicken thighs,
- Dried chickpeas: 1 and a ½ cups (soaked overnight)
- Chopped red bell pepper: 1 and a half cup
- One large yellow onion, thinly sliced
- Tomato paste: 2 tablespoons
- 4 cups of water
- 4 cloves of garlic, minced
- One bay leaf
- Paprika: 4 teaspoons
- Ground cumin: 4 teaspoons
- ¼ of a teaspoon freshly ground black pepper

- ¼ of a cup halved pitted olives(oil-cured)
- Half of a teaspoon salt
- ¼ of a cup of chopped fresh parsley
- ¼ of a teaspoon cayenne pepper

Instructions

- Rinse and drain the chickpeas, put them in a large slow cooker, add four cups of water, chopped red pepper, bay leaf, tomato paste, and paprika cayenne, freshly ground black pepper, garlic, cumin.
- Mix well then, add the chicken.
- Cover it and cook on High for four hours or on low for at least 8 hours.
- Take out the chicken to a cutting surface and let it cool a little.
- Throw away the bay leaf. Then add olives, salt to the cooker and mix well.
- With forks, shred the chicken, set aside the bones. You would not need them.
- Add the shredded chicken into the soup.
- Garnish with cilantro and parsley.
- Serve hot.

Nutrition per serving: 446 calories| total fat 15.3g |carbohydrates 43g |protein 21.6g | Cholesterol 22.3 mg| Sodium 221 mg| Potassium 332 mg| Phosphorus 187 mg| Calcium 24 mg| Fiber 2.8 g

2.16 Ravioli & Vegetable Soup

- **Ingredients**
- One package of fresh ravioli
- Red chopped bell pepper: one and a half cups

- Extra-virgin olive oil: 1 tablespoon
- Onion: 2 cups diced
- One can of 15 ounces' low sodium chicken broth or vegetable broth
- 1 and ½ cups of hot water
- Dried basil: 1 teaspoon
- 2 cups chopped zucchini
- 2 cloves of minced garlic
- Freshly ground black pepper, to taste
- 1/4 of a teaspoon crushed red pepper(optional)

Instructions

1. Heat the oil over medium flame in a big saucepan or Dutch oven. Add the onion-pepper mixture, ground red pepper, garlic, and cook for one minute, stirring. Add water, red bell pepper, stock, basil over a high flame, let it boil.
2. Add the ravioli and cook less than three minutes than the box instructs. Add the zucchini, let it boil again.
3. Cook for about three minutes until the zucchini is soft, and adjust the taste by adding freshly ground black pepper

Nutrition per serving: 261 calories| total fat 8.3g | carbohydrates 32.6g |protein 10.6g

2.17 Hearty Chicken Soup

Ingredients

- Chicken broth, reduced-sodium: 4 cups
- 4 cups of chicken breasts, uncooked (skin and boneless), cubes
- 1 and a half cups celery
- Olive oil: 1 tablespoon
- Carrots: 1 cup, sliced
- 1 and a half cups onion, chopped

- Green beans: 1 cup, cut in 2 inch
- All-purpose white flour: 3 tablespoons
- Frozen green peas: 2 cups
- Dried basil: 2 teaspoons
- Nutmeg: 1/4 teaspoon
- Dried oregano: 1 teaspoon
- 1% low-fat milk: half cup
- Black pepper: 1/4 teaspoon
- Thyme: 1 teaspoon

Instructions

- In a skillet, cook the chicken for 5-6 minutes. Turn off the heat.
- In another pan, sauté celery and onion in heated olive oil.
- Add carrots, chicken pieces, flour, green beans, nutmeg, thyme, oregano, and basil—Cook for three minutes.
- Add milk; broth, let it boil.
- Add peas in. cook for five minutes.
- Add pepper and serve.

Nutrients per serving: Calories 131| Protein 14 g| Carbohydrates 12 g| Fat 3 g| Cholesterol 32 mg| Sodium 343 mg| Potassium 467 mg| phosphorus 171 mg| Calcium 67 mg| Fiber 2.8 g

2.18 Low Sodium Chicken Soup

Ingredients

- Onion: 1 tablespoon
- Mixed vegetables: 1 cup
- 4 cups of chicken breast cooked, shredded
- Four stalks of celery, chopped
- Carrots: 1 cup, chopped
- Butter: 1 tablespoon
- Chicken broth, low-sodium: 5 cups

- Fresh parsley: 2 tablespoons
- Seven and a half cups water
- Black pepper: 1/8 teaspoon

Instructions

- In a large pot, sauté onion in butter for five minutes.
- Add chicken broth and water let it boil.
- Add parsley, chicken, pepper, celery, cover it and let it simmer for half an hour.
- Add carrots, simmer for 20 minutes, then add frozen vegetables cook for another 20 minutes.
- Serve hot.

Nutrients per serving: Calories 97| Protein 13 g| Carbohydrates 5 g| Fat 3 g| Cholesterol 31 mg| Sodium 301 mg| Potassium 274 mg| Phosphorus 116 mg| Calcium 27 mg| Fiber 1.6 g

2.19 Barley & Beef Stew

Ingredients

- All-purpose white flour: 2 tablespoons
- Pearl barley: 1 cup, uncooked
- Black pepper: 1/4 teaspoon
- Half cup of onion, chopped
- Half teaspoon of salt
- 4 cups of stew meat, lean beef, cut into cubes
- Olive oil: 2 tablespoons
- 2 carrots, chopped
- One large stalk of celery, chopped
- One clove of garlic, minced
- Onion herb seasoning: 1 teaspoon

Instructions

- Soak barley in two cups of water for 60 minutes

- In a zip lock bag, add black pepper, stew meat, flour. Mix it well

- In a large pot, brown the meat in heated oil. Set it aside.

- Sauté garlic, onion, celery in meat residue for two minutes.

- Add 8 cups of water. Let it boil.

- Add bay leaf, salt, meat to the pot. Let it simmer.

- Drain barley, and add to the pot. Cover it let it cook for one hour. Stir occasionally.

- After one hour, add herb seasoning, carrots. Let it simmer for 60 minutes.

- Add more water if needed.

Nutrients per serving: Calories 246| Protein 22 g| Carbohydrates 21 g| Fat 8 g| Cholesterol 51 mg| Sodium 222 mg| Potassium 369 mg| phosphorus 175 mg| Calcium 30 mg| Fiber 6.3 g

2.20 Beef Stew with Carrots & Mushrooms

Ingredients

- Beef broth, low-sodium: 4 cups

- Onion chopped: 2 cups

- 3 cloves of garlic, minced

- Carrots, 2 cups diced

- Potato: 1 cup(leached)

- Stew meat, lean beef: 2 pounds

- Olive oil: 2 tablespoons

- Dry red wine: 1 cup

- Shitake mushrooms: 1 cup, sliced

- Dried thyme: half tablespoon

- All-purpose white flour: 1/3 cup

- One bay leaf

- Half teaspoon black pepper

- Herb seasoning: 3/4 teaspoon

Instructions

- In a Dutch oven, over medium flame, heat 2 tsp. of olive oil

- Sauté onion, add thyme, mushrooms cook for five minutes. Add garlic and cook for one minute.

- Add red wine and stir.

- Coat the beef in flour. In a large pan, over medium flame, heat two teaspoons of oil.

- Brown the beef and add herb seasoning. Add beef into mushroom mix.

- Add the broth and bay leaf. Let it boil.

- Cover it, turn the heat low, simmer for one hour.

- Add carrot, potatoes with beef. Simmer uncovered for 1 hour, stir as the soup thickens.

- Add black pepper. Take out the bay leaf and serve.

Nutrients per serving: Calories 282| Protein 33 g| Carbohydrates 15 g| Fat 10 g| Cholesterol 88 mg| Sodium 110 mg| Potassium 534 mg| Phosphorus 252 mg| Calcium 39 mg| Fiber 2.5 g|

2.21 Mediterranean Soup Jar

Ingredients

- Red pepper flakes: 1/8 teaspoon

- Black olives, reduced-sodium: 3 large

- Half cup of bell pepper & onion strips

- Half tablespoon of garlic & herb seasoning

- Canned chickpeas, no salt added: 1/3 cup
- Half teaspoon of black pepper
- Extra virgin olive oil: 1 teaspoon
- Half cup of coleslaw mix
- Cheese: 1 tablespoon

Instructions

- Wash the chickpeas and Slice the olives.
- Layer all ingredients in a big jar.
- Keep in Refrigerate until ready to serve.
- Take out from the fridge at least 15 minutes before serving.
- Add a half cup and a little more boiling water to the jar and shake the jar with a closed lid. Let it rest for two minutes. Then open and serve.

Nutrients per serving: Calories 222| Protein 7 g| Carbohydrates 26 g| Fat 10 g| Cholesterol 8 mg| Sodium 184 mg| Potassium 396 mg| Phosphorus 118 mg| Calcium 91 mg| Fiber 6.0 g

2.22 Green Chili Stew

Ingredients

- 1.75 cups of chicken broth, low-sodium
- Six flour tortillas
- Half cup of all-purpose flour
- One teaspoon of black pepper
- 4 cups of lean pork chops
- One cup of canned green chili peppers
- Olive oil: 1 tablespoon
- One tablespoon of garlic powder
- Iceberg lettuce: 3/4 cup
- One clove of garlic
- Cilantro: 1/4 cup

Instructions

- In a zip lock bag, add garlic powder, black pepper, and flour and mix. Add pork (bite sizes) pieces in the bag and coat well
- In a pot, brown the pork in olive oil.
- In a slow cooker, add minced garlic, chicken broth, browned pork, diced chili peppers—Cook for ten hours on low.
- Add ¾ cup stew on tortilla and serve with cilantro and lettuce. Or eat as it is.

Nutrients per serving: Calories 420| Protein 25 g| Carbohydrates 44 g| Fat 16 g| Cholesterol 45 mg| Sodium 552 mg| Potassium 454 mg| Phosphorus 323 mg| Calcium 90 mg| fiber 3.2 g

2.23 Kidney-Friendly Vegetable Soup

Ingredients

- Olive oil: 1 tablespoon
- 1 medium onion
- 2 sticks celery
- 2 large cloves of garlic
- Six large carrots
- One cube of chicken or vegetable low sodium
- 1 medium turnip
- Water: 1 and 1.2 l
- Fresh thyme
- One bay leaf
- Black pepper

Instructions

- Chop all the vegetables

- In a pot, add carrots and turnip, add water four times of their volume

- Let it boil until tender

- in a heavy-based pan, heat the olive oil.

- Add the celery, onion, and garlic— Cook for a few minutes.

- Cover it and cook on low heat for 15 minutes. Make sure it is not burning.

- After 15 minutes, add boiled turnip and carrots. Dissolve cube in water.

- Pour the stock into the vegetable mix, add thyme and bay leaf, pepper

- Let it boil and simmer for half an hour, take out the bay leaf

- Puree the soup in a blender. Add more water if too thick

Nutrition per serving: Calories: 42kcal| Carbohydrate Content: 5.7g|Fat Content: 1.6g|Protein Content: 1g|Salt: 0.1g|Sugar Content: 4.6g|Potassium: 3.3mg|Phosphate: 23mg

2.24 Yucatan Lime Soup

Ingredients

- Eight cloves of garlic, minced

- Chicken breast: 1 and a half cups cooked, shredded

- Two serrano chili peppers, chopped

- Chicken broth, low-sodium: 4 cups

- One small tomato

- Cilantro: 1/4 cup, chopped

- Half cup of onion, diced

- Two tortillas, cut into strips

- Olive oil: 1 tablespoon

- 1/4 teaspoon of salt

- Black pepper

- 1 bay leaf

- Lime juice: 1/4 cup

Instructions

- Let the oven preheat to 400° F.

- place tortilla strips on a baking tray and spray with oil. Bake for three minutes or till slightly toasted. Take out from the oven and set it aside.

- In a pot, sauté chili, garlic, and onion in olive oil, till translucent

- Add salt, chicken, tomato, bay leaf, and chicken. Simmer for ten minutes.

- Add black pepper, cilantro, lime juice.

- Serve with toasted strips.

Nutrients per serving: Calories 214| Protein 20 g| Carbohydrates 12 g| Fat 10 g| Cholesterol 32 mg| Sodium 246 mg| Potassium 355 mg| Phosphorus 176 mg| Calcium 47 mg| Fiber 1.6 g

2.25 Sausage Egg Soup

Ingredients

- 4 egg whites

- 2 cups of ground beef

- Half teaspoon of ground sage

- Olive oil: 2 tablespoons

- Half teaspoon of dried basil

- Day-old 4 slices bread

- Half teaspoon of black pepper

- Herb seasoning: 1 tablespoon

- Half teaspoon of garlic powder

- Grated parmesan cheese: 2 tablespoons

- Two cloves of garlic

- Chicken broth, low-sodium: 3 cups

- 1 and a half cups water
- Fresh parsley: 4 tablespoons

Instructions

- Let the oven preheat to 375° F.

- In a bowl, mix black pepper, ground beef, garlic powder, sage, and basil. Set it aside

- Cut bread into cubes and add herb seasoning, olive oil. Bake for 8 minutes or until golden brown. Set aside.

- Fry the sausage (beef mix) until it's done. Take out from the pan and drain.

- Sauté the garlic in 2 tbsp. Of drippings. Add parsley, water, broth

- Cover it and let it boil, simmer for ten minutes.

- Turn the heat to low. Gently add egg whites.

- Serve with croutons and cheese.

Nutrients per serving: Calories 335| Protein 26 g| Carbohydrates 15 g| Fat 19 g| Cholesterol 250 mg| Sodium 374 mg| potassium 392 mg| Phosphorus 268 mg| Calcium 118 mg| Fiber 0.9 g

2.26 Chicken Corn Soup

Ingredients

- Water: 14 cups

- 4 pound of roasting chicken

- Dried parsley: 1 tablespoon

- Half cups and a little more uncooked flat noodles

- 2 cans of unsalted corn

- Black pepper: 1/4 teaspoon

Instructions

- In a pot, cook chicken in 8 cups of water. Reserve the broth and cooked chicken separately.

- Cook the noodles as per instructions, without salt. Set it aside.

- Take the fat out from chicken broth. Chop the chicken into pieces.

- In a big pot, add 6 cups of broth, 6 cups of water, chopped chicken.

- Add parsley, corns, pepper, cooked noodles. Let it simmer and then serve

Nutrients per serving: Calories 222| Protein 25 g| Carbohydrates 17 g| Fat 6 g| Cholesterol 67 mg| Sodium 240 mg| Potassium 303 mg| Phosphorus 212 mg| Calcium 21 mg| Fiber 1.4 g

2.27 Moroccan Chicken Soup

Ingredients

- Spaghetti pasta: 2 cups

- 4 cups of skinless chicken legs,

- One cup of zucchini

- Cilantro: 1 tablespoon

- Seven and a half cups of water

- Half teaspoon of cumin

- Half teaspoon of turmeric

- Couscous: 1 cup, dry

- Chickpeas: 1/3 cup

- Black pepper: 1 teaspoon

- Half teaspoon of salt

Instructions

- In a pot, add chicken legs with six cups of water, simmer for almost one hour or until cooked.

- Add spaghetti and chickpeas to the soup and simmer for 15 minutes.

- Add chopped cilantro, zucchini, spices to the soup. Cook for another 15 minutes.
- Prepare couscous as you like. Serve with hot soup.

Nutrients per serving: Calories 224| Protein 18 g| Carbohydrates 29 g| Fat 4 g| Cholesterol 42 mg| Sodium 313 mg| potassium 296 mg| Phosphorus 148 mg| calcium 42 mg| Fiber 3.0 g

2.28 Italian Wedding Soup

Ingredients

- 1 cup uncooked pasta
- 4 cups of ground beef (extra-lean)
- Dried bread crumbs: 1/4 cup
- Grated cheese: 2 tablespoons
- Cooked chicken: 2 cups, diced
- 2 large egg whites
- Dried basil: 1 teaspoon
- Fresh kale leaves: 1 cup
- Carrots: 3/4 cup, diced
- Low-sodium chicken broth: 10 cups
- Chopped onion: 3 tablespoons

Instructions

- In a bowl, add eggs, cheese, onion, beef, basil, bread crumbs. mix well
- Make small meatballs.
- In a pot, add chicken broth, heat it. Add pasta, kale, meatballs, carrots.
- Let it slow boil for ten minutes, then turn the heat down low.
- Add chicken. Make sure meats balls and pasta is cooked before serving.

Nutrients per serving: Calories 165| Protein 21 g| Carbohydrates 11 g| Fat 6 g| Cholesterol 73 mg| Sodium 276 mg|

Potassium 360 mg| phosphorus 176 mg| Calcium 42 mg| Fiber 1.0 g

2.29 Vegan Chickpeas & Mushroom Soup

Ingredients

- Half onion chopped
- Dried Italian seasoning: 1 tablespoon
- 2 cloves garlic minced
- 2 cups of sliced mushrooms
- 1 can of chickpeas
- Olive oil: 1 tbsp.
- Salt & pepper to taste
- Vegetable broth: 3 cups
- Dried rosemary: 1 teaspoon
- Pinch, hot pepper flakes

Instructions

- In a pan, sauté onion, garlic in olive oil until slightly brown.
- Add mushrooms after a minute or two, add chickpeas and spices. Add salt and pepper.
- Cook for 3 to 5 minutes, add broth and let it boil. Add chili flakes, and let it simmer for half an hour.
- Then blend it in a blender. Pour back in pot heat it through.

Nutrition per serving: Calories: 197kcal | Carbohydrates: 31g | Protein: 11g | Fat: 4g | Sodium: 790mg | Potassium: 879mg | Fiber: 7g | Sugar: 4g | Vitamin A: 415IU | Vitamin C: 3.9mg | Calcium: 107mg | Iron: 4.2mg

2.30 Carrot Soup

Ingredients

- 1 cup carrot, shredded
- 1 teaspoon curry paste
- 1 tablespoon olive oil

- 1 yellow onion, diced
- ½ teaspoon chili flakes
- 1 tablespoon lemon juice
- 2 cups low-sodium chicken broth

Instructions

- Heat olive oil in the saucepan and add the onion. Cook it until light brown.
- Add grated carrot, curry paste, chili flakes, and chicken broth.
- Close the lid and cook the soup for 25 minutes.
- Then blend it with the help of the immersion blender until smooth.
- Add lemon juice and cook the soup for 5 minutes more.

Nutrition per serving: 92 calories|2.2g protein|8.3g carbohydrates| 5.7g fat|1.7g fiber| 0mg cholesterol| 74mg sodium, | 178mg potassium.

2.31 Pasta Soup

Ingredients

- 2 oz. whole-grain pasta
- ½ cup corn kernels
- 1 oz. carrot, shredded
- 3 oz. celery stalk, chopped
- 2 cups low-sodium chicken stock
- 1 teaspoon ground black pepper

Instructions

- Bring the chicken stock to boil and add shredded carrot and celery stalk. Simmer the liquid for 5 minutes.
- After this, add corn kernels, ground black pepper, and pasta. Mix the soup well.

- Simmer it on the medium heat for 8 minutes.

Nutrition per serving: Calories: 140 kcal| Protein: 4 g| Carbohydrates: 21 g| Dietary Fiber: 2 g| Phosphorus: 79 mg| Potassium: 224 mg|Sodium: 52 mg

2.32 Chicken & Rice Soup

Ingredients

- Two chicken breasts, cubed cooked, boneless and skinless
- 3 cup chopped mixed vegetables
- Celery: 1 cup, diced
- Black pepper
- Baby carrot: 1 cup chopped
- Onion: 1 cup, diced
- Extra virgin oil: 2 tbsp.
- Four thyme sprigs
- Lime juice: 2 tbsp.
- One bay leaf
- Instant white rice: ¾ cup uncooked
- Vegetable/chicken broth, no salt added: 10 cups

Instructions

- In a pot, in olive oil, sauté celery, carrots, and onion. Until tender.
- Add fresh thyme, pepper, stock, bay leaf, and rice. Let it boil.
- Lower the heat and let it simmer for 12-15 minutes
- Add cooked chicken. Let it Simmer for ten minutes.
- Take out bay leaf, add lime juice serve hot

Nutrient per serving: Calories: 160 g| Protein: 14 g| Carbohydrates: 19 g| Fiber: 2

g| Total Fat: 3 g| Sodium: 221 mg| Phosphorus: 90 mg| Potassium: 251 mg|

2.33 Beef Stew

Ingredients

- Five chopped carrots
- stew meat, Lean beef: 8 cups
- 3 celery stalks, diced
- One onion, diced
- 3 cloves of minced garlic
- Sliced mushrooms: 1 cup
- One potato diced (leached)
- Salt-free table seasoning: 1 teaspoon
- One can of beef broth, low sodium
- All-purpose flour: 5 tablespoons
- Dry red wine: 1 cup
- Olive oil: 2 tablespoons

Instructions

- Coat the beef in seasoning and flour mix. In a pot, in olive oil, brown the beef, take the meat out, add all vegetables, do not add carrots, and cook until onions are translucent.
- Lower the heat, add in the red wine. Let it simmer for five minutes, add in the cooked beef.
- Add broth, let it boil. Lower the heat, let it simmer, covered, for 60 minutes. Add in the carrots and potatoes.
- Let it Simmer uncovered for 60 minutes. Add spices, salt-free seasonings, and herbs to your taste.

Nutrient per serving: Calories: 193 g| Protein: 14.4 g| Carbohydrates: 18.2 g| Fiber: 2 g| Total Fat: 3.4 g| Sodium: 227 mg| Phosphorus: 111 mg| Potassium: 198 mg|

2.34 Tuscan Vegetable Soup

Ingredients

- Chicken broth, low sodium: 8 cups
- Olive oil: 1 tablespoon
- Thyme: 1 and a half teaspoons, dried
- Garlic: 3 teaspoons, minced
- Onion: 1 and a half cups, finely chopped
- Green cabbage: 4 cups, roughly chopped
- 1 can chickpeas: 15 ounce
- Celery: 2 cups, sliced
- Baby carrots: 2 cups, diced
- One cup of bell pepper
- Parmesan cheese: 1 tablespoon shredded
- Half cup basil, chopped fresh
- Zucchini: 3 cups, sliced

Instructions

- In a pot, sauté garlic, onion, and thyme for 3 to 5 minutes
- Add in the chickpeas, bell peppers, cabbage, carrots, celery, sauté for ten minutes
- Add in zucchini, chicken broth, basil, let it boil.
- Then lower the heat, let it simmer, cover it saucepan, let it simmer for 40 minutes or more
- Add cheese on top while serving.

Nutritional per serving: Calories 137| protein 7.6 g| Carbohydrates 24 g| Dietary fiber 5.3 g| fat 2.7 g| Saturated fat0.6 g| cholesterol 0.3 mg| Sodium 272 mg| Calcium79.6 mg| Iron 2.1 mg| Potassium 718 mg

2.35 Healthy Chicken Wild Rice Soup

Ingredients

- Chicken broth or water: 9 cups
- 6 cups of chicken pieces
- 2 cloves of minced garlic
- 2 cups sliced mushrooms
- Two carrots, roughly chopped
- Cauliflower: one and a half cups
- 3 celery stalks, chopped
- One large onion, finely diced
- Almond milk: 2 cups
- Wild rice: 1 and a half cups
- Mustard: 1 tbsp.
- Garlic powder: 2 tsp
- Ground black pepper, to taste
- Half tsp dried thyme
- 2 tsp of salt

Instructions

- In a slow cooker, add garlic, chicken, celery, onion, carrots, mushrooms, cauliflower, pepper, wild rice, salt, water, and thyme. Cover it and cook for 8-10 hours on Low or for 5-6 hours on High.
- Take chicken out and shred it. in the slow cooker, add garlic powder, milk, and mustard
- Blend the soup and return to the pot.
- Add the shredded chicken, serve hot

Nutrition per serving: Calories 251 kcal | Sodium 123 mg| Protein 13.2 g| Potassium 292 mg| phosphorus 131 mg| Calcium 25.4 mg| Fat 8.9 g| | Carbohydrates 8.6 g

2.36 Beef & Vegetable Soup

Ingredients

- Carrots: ½ cup, diced
- 4 cups of beef stew
- Sliced onions: 1 cup
- Basil: ½ tsp
- Green peas: ½ cup
- 3 ½ cup of water
- Black pepper: 1 tsp
- Corn: ½ cup
- Okra: ½ cup
- Thyme: ½ tsp

Instructions

- In a pot, add black pepper, beef stew, water, onions, thyme, and basil
- Cook for 45 minutes.
- Add all vegetables let it simmer on low heat till meat is tender. Enjoy.

Nutrition per serving: Calories 190 kcal | Sodium 56 mg| Protein 11 g| Potassium 291 mg| phosphorus 121 mg| Calcium 31 mg| Fat 13 g| Water 130 g| Carbohydrates 7 g

2.37 Healing Cauliflower Holiday Soup

Ingredients

- Vegetable broth, low sodium: 4 cups
- Olive oil: 1 tablespoon
- 3 cloves of minced garlic
- 6 cups of cauliflower, chopped
- Leeks sliced: 2 cups
- Nutmeg: 3/4 teaspoon
- Red pepper flakes: half teaspoon
- Half teaspoon pepper
- 2 cups of water
- Half teaspoon salt

- 1/4 cup cashews

Instructions

- In a pot, sauté garlic, leeks, cook for about two minutes
- Add spices and cauliflower, sauté for five minutes.
- Add the broth, water, let it boil, then let it simmer, covered, for at least 20 minutes. Longer if you need it.
- Add cashews, and blend the soup. Add water if too thick
- Transfer soup back in the pot. Season and taste with pepper and salt.

Nutrition per serving: Calories: 187 kcal | Carbohydrates: 21.5 g | Protein: 10g | Fat: 5g | Sodium: 645 mg | Potassium: 345 mg | Fiber: 4.5 g | Sugar: 5g | Calcium: 65 mg | Iron: 3.8mg

2.38 Vegetarian Cabbage Soup

Ingredients

- 2 cloves of minced garlic
- 4 cups of cabbage, shredded
- 2 cups of cauliflower, cut into cubes
- One large onion, chopped
- Vegetable broth, low sodium: 4 cups
- 2 big carrots, cut into cubes
- Olive oil: 1 tbsp.
- 2 cups of diced bell pepper
- 2 stalks of sliced celery
- Two pinches of chili flakes
- 3-4 bay leaves
- Paprika: 1 tsp
- Salt & pepper, to taste

Instructions

- In a pot, sauté celery, paprika, onion, bay leaves, carrots, chili flakes, garlic in hot olive oil.
- Cook for five minutes.
- Add shredded cabbage and keep stirring for one minute.
- Add red peppers, cauliflower florets, broth, and a pinch of salt.
- Increase the heat and let it boil, then cover it, and let it simmer for 25 minutes.
- Then, remove the bay leaves.
- Blend the soup in the blender. Return soup to the pot, season with salt and pepper.

Nutrition per serving: Calories: 146kcal | Carbohydrates: 25g | Protein: 5g | Fat: 4g | Saturated Fat: 1g | Sodium: 117mg | Potassium: 846mg | Fiber: 9g | Sugar: 12g | Calcium: 125mg | Iron: 2mg

2.39 Slow Cooker Cabbage Soup

Ingredients

- Two cloves of minced garlic
- Carrots: 1 cup, diced
- One onion diced
- Cabbage: 4 cups, chopped
- Green beans: 1 cup trimmed into one-inch pieces
- 2 celery stalks diced
- 2 bell peppers diced
- Tomato paste: 2 tablespoons
- 2 bay leaves
- Fresh kale: 2 cups roughly chopped
- Low sodium stock vegetable: 6 cups
- Italian seasoning: 1 and a half tsp.
- Pepper

- Basil: 1 tablespoon
- Parsley: 1 tablespoon

Instructions

- In a pot, add vegetables. Add tomato paste, Italian seasoning, broth, pepper, bay leaves. Mix well
- Cook on high for five hours or slow on 8 hours in a slow cooker.
- After its cooked, add basil, parsley, kale, and cook for five minutes and serve.

Nutrition per serving: Calories: 40| Carbohydrates: 6g| Protein: 2g|Sodium: 64mg| Potassium: 158mg| Fiber: 1g| Sugar: 2g| Vitamin A: 2230IU| Vitamin C: 32.5mg| Calcium: 28mg|Iron: 0.7mg

2.40 Healthy Mushroom Soup

Ingredients

- Vegetable broth: 2 cups
- 4 cups of mushrooms, roughly chopped
- 3 garlic cloves, minced
- Soya sauce, low sodium: 1 tbsp.
- Olive oil: 2 tbsp.
- One onion, chopped
- Thyme leaves: half tsp
- All-purpose flour: 1/4 cup
- Soy milk: 1 cup
- Salt & black pepper to taste

Instructions

- In a large pot, sauté garlic, onions in olive oil for 3 minutes. Add thyme, mushrooms, salt, pepper. Cook until the mushroom starts to turn brown for five minutes. Take out three tbsp. of mushroom and set them aside

- Add in the one tbsp. of oil, flour cook for half a minute.
- Now add broth and mix well. Let the mixture boil. Then let it simmer and lower the heat. Add milk
- Simmer again, often stirring, for 15-20 minutes.
- Add the soya sauce and stir for one minute
- Add salt if required.
- Serve with sautéed mushrooms on top.

Nutrition per serving: Calories: 213kcal | Carbohydrates: 22g | Protein: 10g | Fat: 11g | Saturated Fat: 2g | Cholesterol: 4mg | Sodium: 379mg | Potassium: 656mg | Fiber: 3g | Sugar: 9g | Calcium: 110mg | Iron: 1mg

2.41 Green Beans Soup

Ingredients

- ½ onion, diced
- 1/3 cup green beans, soaked
- 3 cups of water
- ½ sweet pepper, chopped
- 2 potatoes, chopped
- One tablespoon fresh cilantro, chopped
- 1 teaspoon chili flakes

Instructions

- In the saucepan, put all the ingredients and close the lid.
- On medium heat, cook the soup for 40 minutes or until the ingredients are all tender
- Serve.

Nutrients Per serving: 87 calories|2.3g protein|19.8g carbohydrates| 0.2g fat| 3.4g fiber|0mg cholesterol|13 mg sodium| 132 mg potassium.

2.42 Pureed Broccoli Soup

Ingredients

- 1tbsp. unsalted Butter
- Olive Oil: 1tbsp.
- Chicken Broth low-sodium 4cups
- Onion: one (chopped).
- 2 cloves of minced garlic
- Fresh Thyme
- Broccoli 8 cups chopped
- Celery stalk: one, chopped
- Water 2cups
- Non-dairy creamer half cup, optional
- Freshly Ground Pepper to taste
- Salt: ½ tsp

Instructions

- In a large pot, sauté celery, onion in butter until tender for 5-6 minutes
- Add thyme and garlic, cook for ten seconds.
- Add in broccoli. Add broth and water, let it simmer for 8 minutes.
- Blend the soup in a blender. Add creamer and black pepper

Nutrition Per Serving: Calories 69| protein 4g.| Carbohydrate 7g.|Total Fat 4g.| Cholesterol 4mg.| Potassium 230mg.| Sodium 258mg.| Phosphorus 45mg.|

2.43 Zucchini Curry Soup Recipe

Ingredients

- Extra virgin olive oil: 2 tbsp.
- A large onion
- Red curry powder: 2 tbsp.
- Chicken broth: 3 cups

- Plain Greek yogurt
- Five large zucchini
- Salt and pepper, to taste

Instructions

- Cut zucchini, onion into pieces.
- In a pan, sauté vegetables, with curry, pepper, and salt in olive oil, until tender
- Add the broth. Cover it and let it cook for 20 minutes.
- Blend the soup in a blender till smooth.
- Taste salt and pepper and adjust.
- Garnish with tablespoon plain Greek yogurt

Nutrition per serving: Calories: 89kcal | Carbohydrates: 8g | Protein: 2g | Fat: 5g | Saturated Fat: 0g | Cholesterol: 0mg | Sodium: 445mg | Potassium: 579mg | Fiber: 2g | Sugar: 4g | Vitamin A: 345IU | Vitamin C: 39mg | Calcium: 47mg | Iron: 1.5mg

2.44 Butternut Squash & Apple Soup

Ingredients

- 2 red apples diced
- one peeled butternut squash, cut into cubes
- one fennel bulb nicely chopped
- 4 – 5 cloves of garlic cloves
- Olive oil: 1/4 cup
- Rosemary: 1 tablespoon
- One white onion chopped
- Vegetable broth: 4 cups
- Ground cinnamon: half teaspoon
- Dried thyme: 1 teaspoon
- Nutmeg: 1/4 teaspoon

- Salt & pepper
- Water as needed
- Ginger: 1/4 teaspoon

Instructions

- Let the oven preheat to 400 F.
- Mix all the spices and oil. Pour over onion, squash, garlic, fennel, and apples. Mix it well and roast the vegetables for 30 to 40 minutes. Shake vegetables halfway, so they do not burn.
- Add the roasted vegetables to the pot, add broth and let it boil.
- Turn down the heat and let it simmer for 10-12 minutes, or until everything is tender.
- Blend the soup, in a blender, until creamy and smooth
- Add water as required. Serve warm

Nutrition per serving: Calories: 200kcal | Carbohydrates: 30g | Protein: 2g | Fat: 9g | Saturated Fat: 1g | Sodium: 412 mg | Potassium: 423 mg | Fiber: 5g | Sugar: 11g | Calcium: 99mg | Iron: 1.7mg

2.45 Lemon & Garlic Wild Rice Soup

Ingredients

- Italian seasoning, low sodium: 1 tablespoon
- Olive oil: 1 tablespoon
- Lemon zest: 1 tablespoon
- Chopped carrots: 1 cup
- Sliced celery: 1 cup
- Five garlic of minced cloves
- Half cup white onion
- Lemon juice: 1/4 cup
- Salt & pepper

- Half cup of wild rice
- Almond milk: 1 cup
- Fresh kale: 1 cup
- Vegetable broth, low sodium: 4 cups

Instructions

- In a large pot, sauté carrots, garlic, onion, celery, in olive oil, until tender for five minutes. Add all the seasonings, zest, and cook for three minutes.
- Add in the rice, vegetable broth and let it boil. Cover it and let it simmer until rice has cooked for half an hour or more.
- Add in the milk, lemon juice, kale once the rice is cooked. Cook until kale is wilted.
- Serve immediately.

Nutrition per serving: Calories: 162kcal | Carbohydrates: 27g | Protein: 4g | Fat: 4g | Sodium: 245 mg | Potassium: 370mg | Fiber: 4g | Sugar: 5g | Calcium: 139mg | Iron: 1.3mg

2.46 Gingered Carrot Bisque

Ingredients

- Diced celery: half cup
- Olive oil: 1 tablespoon
- One-piece (1-1/2) of ginger, finely diced
- Vegetable broth: 4 cups
- Diced onion: 3/4 cup
- Salt
- No salt curry powder: 1 and 1/2 teaspoons
- No salt cashew cream: 1/3 cup, optional
- One carrot diced

Instructions

- In a pot, sauté ginger, celery, and onion until translucent.
- Add in curry powder, broth, potato, carrots, let it boil.
- Lower the heat and let it simmer. Stir occasionally, for 25 minutes.
- Blend the soup in a blender. Pour it back into the pot.
- Cook on low heat until heated through.
- Add in the cashew cream if you want.
- Serve hot.

Nutrition per serving: Calories: 261 kcal | Carbohydrates: 35g | Protein: 10g | Fat: 22g | Saturated Fat: 3g | Sodium: 256 mg | Potassium: 213mg | Fiber: 5g | Sugar: 5 g | Calcium: 29.9 mg | Iron: 3.8mg

2.47 Roasted Garlic Cauliflower Chowder

Ingredients

- Vegetable broth, low sodium: 2 cups
- Cashews soaked: half cup
- One small potato(leached) chopped
- One garlic bulb
- One head of cauliflower, cut into florets
- Oil: 2 tablespoons
- Half cup of garlic hummus, low sodium
- Water: 2 cups
- Miso paste: 2 teaspoons
- Half cup cooked quinoa
- Salt and pepper to taste

Instructions

- Let the oven preheat to 425°F.

- Put cauliflower and potato, cut the garlic bulb in two-three pieces but wrap in foil, on a baking tray. Add one tbsp. of oil, add pepper and salt
- Roast for 20 to 25 minutes till cauliflower starts to brown, and the potatoes become soft. Check the garlic after 15 minutes. It should not be burning.
- Cook the vegetables for 5-10 minutes, then blend it. Take the skin of garlic and mix it also.
- Add cashew to a blender, with quinoa and hummus. Add in miso, liquids, pepper, and salt. Blend on high until creamy.
- Adjust seasoning to your taste.

Nutrition per serving: Calories: 284kcal | Carbohydrates: 25g | Protein: 9g | Fat: 17g | Saturated Fat: 2g | Sodium: 794mg | Potassium: 536mg | Fiber: 5g | Sugar: 2g| Calcium: 47mg | Iron: 4.1mg

2.48 Golden Soup

Ingredients

- Cauliflower, 5 cups of florets
- Oil: 2 tablespoons olive
- Half onion, chopped
- 2 cloves of garlic, minced
- Water: 7–8 cups
- Turmeric: 1 tablespoon
- One tsp. Of salt
- Lemon juice

Instructions

- In a pot, sauté garlic, turmeric, onion, cauliflower in oil for ten minutes.

- Add water and salt let it simmer. Transfer the soup to a blender till it becomes creamy.

- Take the blended soup into the pot again. Add more water if required. Season with salt if needed. Add lemon juice.

Nutrition Per Serving: Calories 180| Total Fat 13.3g| Cholesterol 0mg| Sodium 213.3mg| Total Carbohydrate 13.2g| Dietary Fiber 3.1g|sugars 3.6g| Protein 5.7g

2.49 Anti-Inflammatory Thai Pumpkin Soup

Ingredients

- 4 cloves of sliced garlic
- Pumpkin: 600 g
- Soy milk: ½ cup
- Olive oil: 1 tablespoon
- Vegetable stock: 3 cups
- Lemongrass: 1 tablespoon (white part), diced
- Two shredded kaffir lime leaves
- One turmeric sliced
- Coriander seeds: 1 teaspoon
- One small red chili de-seeded, thinly sliced
- Cumin seeds: 1 teaspoon
- One onion, diced
- Black pepper
- One-inch ginger minced

Instructions

- Let the oven preheat to 350 F. Add baking paper on a tray.

- Chop the peeled pumpkin, coat with soy milk, and roast until golden.

- In a pot, heat oil, sauté onion till golden, add coriander seeds, cumin

- Cook for a few minutes

- Add garlic, lemongrass, chili, ginger, kaffir leaves, turmeric, cook for another minute. Do not overcook

- Add broth and pumpkin, cover it and let it boil. Let it simmer for t10 minutes. Add milk, increase the heat.

- Cook for 5-10 minutes.

Nutrition per serving: Calories: 349kcal | Carbohydrates: 35g | Protein: 11g | Fat: 21g | Saturated Fat: 17g | Sodium: 225mg | Fiber: 3g | Sugar: 11g | Calcium: 130mg | Iron: 5.8mg

2.50 Turkey Vegetable Soup

Ingredients

- Two medium onions, diced
- 2 tablespoons of flour
- Unsalted butter: 1/4 cup
- Low-sodium curry powder: 1 and a half teaspoons
- Lean ground turkey: 2 pounds, cooked
- Half cup of carrots, diced
- Low-sodium chicken broth
- Half cup celery, diced
- Parsley: 2 tablespoons
- Half teaspoon sage, diced
- One and a half cups of soy milk
- Frozen chopped kale: 1 and ¼ cups
- 1 cup potatoes, leached and diced
- Black Pepper

Instructions

- In the pot, melt butter over medium flame

- Sauté onions cook until translucent, for ten minutes

- Stir in curry powder and flour, cook for 2-3 minutes

- Add potatoes, broth, parsley, carrots, sage, and celery

- Let it boil. Turn the heat low. cover it and simmer for ten minutes

- Add kale, turkey, and milk

- Cover it and simmer until all heated through

- Add black pepper.

Nutrition per serving: Calories 245| Fat 13.8 g| Carbohydrates 8 g| protein 24 g| Dietary Fiber 1.5 g| Calcium 49 mg| Phosphorous 270 mg| Sodium 125 mg| Potassium 498 mg

2.51 Cauliflower Soup

Ingredients

- Margarine: 1 Tbsp.

- Three cups of water

- Chicken bouillon, low-sodium: 1/4 cube

- Low-fat mayonnaise: 1 Tbsp.

- Half onion, diced

- 1/4 cup celery, diced

- 1 cup of cauliflower, diced

- Three baby carrots, sliced

- 1 Tbsp. Flour

- Pepper: 1/4 tsp.

- Dried basil: 1/8 tsp

- Cream cheese: 3 Tbsp.

- Half tsp. of salt

- 2 minced garlic

Instructions

- In a pot, add the bouillon cube, water, celery, onion, and carrots. Let it boil over low heat.

- Add cream cheese, salt, mayonnaise, pepper, herbs, and one tbsp. of margarine.

- Add cauliflower to soup and cook for five minutes.

- Add cornstarch to water and add in the soup. Stir until thickens, and serve

Nutrition per serving: Calories: 57 | protein 2 g |Sodium 212 mg | Phosphorus 32 mg| Calcium 36 mg | Potassium 156 mg|

Chapter 3: Kidney-Friendly Pasta Recipes

3.1 Pasta Primavera

Ingredients

- All-purpose white flour: 2 tablespoons

- One and a half cup of uncooked pasta,

- 2 cups of chicken broth, low-sodium

- Non-dairy creamer: 1/4 cup

- One and a half cup of frozen mixed vegetables

- Grated Parmesan cheese: 1/4 cup

Instructions

- Cook vegetables and pasta separately, as per instruction on boxes. Set them aside.

- In a pot, add chicken broth on low flame

- Add flour to the chicken broth keep whisking, so lumps will not form

- Add garlic powder, creamer, and mix.

- Let it simmer for 5 -10 minutes or until it thickens.
- Stir sometimes, while it is simmering.
- Add cooked pasta and vegetable and cook till all heated through.
- Sprinkle with cheese.

Nutrients per serving: Calories 273|Protein 13 g| Carbohydrates 48 g| Fat 3 g| Cholesterol 6 mg| sodium 115 mg| Potassium 251 mg| Phosphorus 154 mg| Calcium 93 mg| Fiber 4.5 g

3.2 The Best Pasta Ever

Ingredients

- 4 oz. of uncooked Spaghetti Noodles
- Extra-virgin olive oil: 2 Tbsp.
- Half small minced Onion
- Dried Cranberries: 1/4 cup
- Kale: 4 cups
- Crumbled Feta Cheese: 2 Tbsp.
- Six cloves of sliced Garlic
- Water: 1/4 cup

Instructions

- In a skillet, sauté garlic in olive oil, over medium flame, until slices are lightly golden brown. Take out the slices and set it aside.
- Lower the heat, add onion, add pepper and salt for three minutes
- Add kale; cranberries add more pepper, salt if required. Add water, cover it, and let it cook for five minutes.
- Cook spaghetti as per instructions.
- Add spaghetti to the skillet, then toss everything. Add 1/4 cup pasta water if required. Sprinkle cheese and serve

Nutrients Per Serving: 271 Cal| Total Fat 18.4g| Cholesterol 8.3mg| Sodium 226.9mg| Total Carbohydrate 27.5g| Dietary Fiber 3.6g| Protein 3.9g|Iron 1.4mg| Potassium 268.6mg| Phosphorus 88.5mg

3.3 Linguine with Garlic & Shrimp

Ingredients

- 2 and a half quarts of water
- Peeled and cleaned, Raw shrimp: 3/4 pound
- Linguine: 12 ounces, uncooked
- Olive oil: 2 tablespoons
- Chopped flat-leaf parsley: 1 cup
- Lemon juice: 1 tablespoon
- 2 whole heads of garlic
- Black pepper: 1/4 teaspoon

Instructions

- Cook pasta as per instructions.
- Separate cloves of garlic leave the skin on.
- Heat the garlic cloves in a pan over medium flame, continuously stirring till it becomes soft and darkens. Skin will come off easily. Peel off the skin and set it aside
- Now fry the garlic in olive oil till light golden brown
- Add shrimp, parsley, and cook for two minutes, until shrimp is cooked.
- Add one cup of pasta water and all pasta to the pan. Mix it all up. Add more pasta water if required.
- Add black pepper, lemon juice. Serve.

Nutrients per serving: Calories 322| Protein 20 g| Carbohydrates 47 g| Fat 6 g| Cholesterol 86 mg| Sodium 106 mg|

Potassium 298 mg| Phosphorus 220 mg|
Calcium 87 mg| Fiber 2.4 g

3.4 Spicy Lemon Pasta

Ingredients

- Lemon zest: 1 teaspoon
- Chopped onion: 1/4 cup
- Butter: 2 teaspoons
- Chopped green bell pepper: 1/4 cup
- Cooked pasta: 3/4 cup
- Fresh lemon juice: 2 tablespoons
- Chopped celery: 1/4 cup
- Onion herb seasoning: 1 teaspoon

Instructions

- In a pan, sauté celery, green bell pepper, and onion in butter.
- Add the sautéed vegetables into hot pasta.
- Add herb seasoning, lemon zest, and lemon juice to the pasta.

Nutrients per serving: Calories 140|
Protein 4 g| Carbohydrates 22 g| Fat 4 g|
Cholesterol 10 mg| Sodium 44 mg|
Potassium 156 mg| Phosphorus 76 mg|
Calcium 24 mg| fiber 2.9 g

3.5 Pesto Pronto

Ingredients

- Half cup Mushrooms, thick slices
- White Pasta: 16 oz.
- 1 Yellow Squash, half-moons slices
- Pesto Sauce: 2/3 cup
- 1 Red Bell Pepper, chopped
- 2 Zucchini, half-moons slices
- Olive Oil: 2 tbsp.
- 2 cloves of minced Garlic

Instructions

- Let the oven preheat to 425. Add bell pepper, zucchini, mushrooms, squash, and onion, and a baking sheet. Pour olive oil, coat in an olive oil well. Roast until vegetables are tender. Cook pasta as per instruction.
- In a bowl, add cooked pasta and pesto and roasted vegetable. Coat evenly
- Serve warm.

Nutrition Per Serving: Cal 492| total Fat 18.8g| Cholesterol 5.6mg| Sodium 336.3mg| Total Carbohydrate 66.9g| Dietary Fiber 4.3g| Protein 13.4g| Iron 3.3mg| Potassium 476mg| Phosphorus 237mg

3.6 Pasta with Cheesy Meat Sauce

Ingredients

- Half cup onions, chopped
- Half box pasta, large-shaped
- 4 cups ground beef
- Beef stock: 1 and a half cups, no sodium
- Worcestershire sauce: 2 tablespoons, reduced-sodium
- Beef bouillon: 1 tablespoon, no salt added
- Onion flakes: 1 tablespoon
- Tomato sauce: 1 tablespoon, no salt added
- Pepper jack cheese: ¾ cup shredded
- Half tsp. of Italian seasoning
- Half tsp. of ground black pepper
- One cup of cream cheese softened

Instructions

- Cook pasta as per instructions

- In a pan, cook onions, onion flakes, and ground beef until meat is browned. Drain.

- Add tomato sauce, stock, and bouillon.

- Let it simmer. Add in cooked pasta.

- Turn off the heat, add cheese, cream cheese, and seasonings. Mix pasta until cheese melts.

Nutrition Per Serving: Calories 502 | total Fat 30 g| Saturated Fat 14 g| Trans Fat 1 g| cholesterol 99 mg| Sodium 401 mg| carbohydrates 35 g| Protein 23 g| Phosphorus 278 mg| Potassium 549 mg| Dietary Fiber 1.7 g| Calcium 107 mg

3.7 Spaghetti & Broccoli Carbonara

Ingredients

- Canola oil: 2 teaspoons

- Onions: 1 cup, diced

- One egg whisked

- Non-dairy creamer: 1 cup

- Chicken stock, low-sodium: ¼ cup

- Cooked pasta: 3 cups (spiral noodle)

- 2 cups broccoli, chopped

- Black pepper: 1 teaspoon

- Scallions: ½ cup, chopped

Instructions

- In a pan, sauté onions in oil over medium heat

- In a bowl, add creamer and egg, whisk together.

- Reduce the heat and add the egg mixture into onions, constantly mix until thickens

- Add the broccoli, stock, black pepper, pasta, keep mixing until all heated through.

Nutrition Per Serving: Calories 304 | Total Fat 19 g| Saturated Fat 10 g| Trans Fat 0.5 g| Cholesterol 78 mg| Sodium 141 mg| Carbohydrates 27 g| Protein 9 g| Phosphorus 143 mg| Potassium 287 mg|Dietary Fiber 5.4 g| Calcium 65 mg

3.8 Mediterranean Pasta Salad

Ingredients

- Chopped walnuts: 1 tablespoon(toasted)

- Plain hummus: 2 tablespoons

- Half of a cup diced red bell pepper

- Water: 1 tablespoon

- One cup lightly packed baby kale

- One can unsalted, light tuna in water(drained)

- Half of a cup cooked farfalle (whole-wheat)

- Crumbled feta cheese: 1 tablespoon

- Extra-virgin olive oil: 2 teaspoons

- Juice from ¼ of a lemon

Instructions

- In a mixing bowl, mix water and hummus and set it aside.

- Take a nonstick medium skillet, add extra virgin olive oil and turn the heat on medium.

- Add the chopped bell pepper let it cook for one minute. Then, add kale. Carefully add in the tuna, do not break large fish pieces. Let it warm through for one minute.

- Then add the pasta. Turn off the heat, and add in hummus sauce. Garnish with walnuts, feta. On top of it, drizzle with lemon juice.

Nutrition per serving: 345 calories| total fat 24.5g |carbohydrates 28.3g |protein 33.4g

3.9 Herb Fish with Penne

Ingredients

- Herb Seasoning: 2 teaspoons
- 4 cups of fish cubes
- Small broccoli florets: 2 cups (fresh or frozen)
- Half-and-half: 1 cup(fat-free)
- One cup of penne pasta
- Half teaspoon of Sea Salt
- ½ cup of cheese cubed

Instructions

- In a large saucepan, add pasta and cook as instructed on the packaging. In the last three minutes, add broccoli and fish. Drain it well.
- In the meantime, add half-and-half to a small saucepan on medium flame and let it simmer.
- Lower the heat after, add seasoning, sea salt, and cream cheese. Mix with a whisker until cheese is melted. The sauce is well combined.
- In a bowl, add pasta, broccoli, and fish
- Pour cheese over, lightly coat.
- Serve right away.

Nutrition per serving: 291 calories| total fat 8g |carbohydrates 36g| protein 24g

3.10 Pasta Salad Mediterranean Style

Ingredients

- One pint of cherry tomatoes

- Chinese eggplants: 2 mediums, chopped into small cubes
- Extra virgin olive oil
- One teaspoon of salt
- Pinch of freshly ground black pepper
- 1/4 teaspoon of ground cumin
- 1/4 teaspoon of red pepper flakes
- 1/4 teaspoon of granulated garlic
- 1 package brown of 16 ounces' rice spaghetti, cooked and cooled

Lemon Dressing

- Finely sliced dill: 1 tablespoon
- Finely sliced mint: 1 tablespoon
- Finely sliced parsley: 1 tablespoon
- Finely sliced cilantro: 1 tablespoon

Instructions

- Let the oven pre-heat to 400F, put parchment paper on a rimmed baking sheet
- Add diced eggplant, three tablespoons of extra virgin olive oil, black pepper, red pepper flakes, salt, cherry tomatoes, granulated garlic, and cumin. Mix it well.
- Put this vegetable mix onto the parchment-lined baking tray.
- Bake for about half an hour, until all vegetables, are soft and lightly golden.
- Take out from the oven, and let it cool slightly.
- In a serving bowl, add the cooked, cooled brown rice pasta, drizzle the lemon dressing and mix keep tasting, add as much as to your liking, start slow, then add eggplant mixture/ cherry tomato mix, herbs, and carefully mix everything.

- Taste it and season with additional pepper and salt if required.
- Serve right away or chill in the refrigerator and serve later.

Lemon Dressing

- Half cup of extra virgin olive oil
- 4-6 cloves of garlic minced or press them
- ¼ of teaspoon granulated sugar
- Zest of one lemon
- 1/4 of teaspoon salt
- Freshly ground black pepper
- 1/4 of a cup lemon juice
- Half teaspoon of Dijon mustard

Instructions

- Add all ingredients in a big jar with a lid, cover the top with lid and mix until emulsified.
- Use right away, or store in the fridge to keep cool.
- This dressing works well with other salads and pasta.

Nutrition per serving: 284 calories| total fat 10g | carbohydrates 23g |protein 14g.

3.11 Renal-Friendly Macaroni Salad

Ingredients

- 2 cloves of pressed garlic
- 4 cups, elbow macaroni, cooked
- 1⁄4 cup onion, chopped
- 1 sweet bell pepper, chopped
- Half cup celery, sliced
- 1 and 1⁄2 cups low fat mayonnaise

- Apple cider vinegar: 1 teaspoon
- Dijon mustard: 2 teaspoons
- 1 teaspoon honey
- Half teaspoon of black pepper

Instructions

- In a bowl, add bell pepper, macaroni, onions, and celery, mix.
- In another bowl, add mustard, honey, salt, mayonnaise, vinegar mix it well
- Mix these two bowls' ingredients
- Serve chilled.

Nutrient per serving: Calories: 171 g| Protein: 7 g| Carbohydrates: 20.1 g| Fiber: 2.9 g| Total Fat: 2.1 g| Sodium: 101 mg| Phosphorus: 89 mg| Potassium: 98 mg|

3.12 Pasta & Kidney Bean Soup

Ingredients

- One cup chopped onion
- One cup of chopped red bell pepper
- Butter: 1 tablespoon
- 2 cans of red kidney beans
- 4 cups of low-sodium chicken broth
- Six cloves of minced garlic,
- Dried oregano: Half teaspoon
- Olive oil: 2 tablespoons
- Red pepper flakes: half teaspoon
- 1 cup small pasta
- 2 bay leaves
- Salt and black pepper

Instructions

- In a pan, heat butter and olive oil and sauté garlic, red pepper flakes, onion, and oregano, until onion is tender

- Add bell peppers, broth, bay leaves, and beans. Bring it to a boil, then let it simmer for 20 minutes.
- Add pasta to the soup in the last ten minutes. Add salt and pepper.
- Take out bay leaves, and serve.

Nutrient per serving: Calories: 214 g| Protein: 12 g| Carbohydrates: 22 g| Fiber: 2.2 g| Total Fat: 6.5 g| Sodium: 204 mg| Phosphorus: 132 mg| Potassium: 245 mg|

3.13 Healthy Kidney Bean Pasta

Ingredients

- One Tablespoon of olive oil
- Cooked penne pasta: 2 cups
- Peas: 1 cup
- Chopped one onion
- Kidney beans: 2 cups
- Sea salt
- Three cloves of pressed garlic
- One Tablespoon of white wine vinegar

Instructions

- Cook pasta as per instructions. Set it aside.
- In a pan, sauté olive oil, onion, vinegar, garlic, cook for five minutes
- Add the kidney beans; peas continue to cook for three minutes, stirring continuously.
- Add the pasta and mix well.
- Serve immediately.

Nutrient per serving: Calories: 234 g| Protein: 14 g| Carbohydrates: 18.5 g| Fiber: 1.9 g| Total Fat: 4 g| Sodium: 109 mg| Phosphorus: 98 mg| Potassium: 145 mg|

3.14 Chilled Veggie & Shrimp Noodle Salad

Ingredients

- Mushrooms chopped: 2 cups
- One pound of cooked spaghetti
- Chili oil: 2 teaspoons
- Sliced scallions: 1 cup
- Broccoli florets: 2 cups
- Carrots: 1 cup
- 4 cups of cooked shrimp
- Sesame oil: 2 tablespoons
- Garlic: 2 tablespoons chopped
- Half cup of rice wine vinegar
- Zest of lime: 1 tablespoon
- Ginger: 1 tablespoon, chopped
- Soy sauce, low-sodium: ¼ cup
- ¼ cup fresh lime juice

Instructions

- Mix all ingredients in a bowl.
- Toss everything together and serve

Nutrition Per Serving: Calories 254 | Total Fat 11 g| Saturated Fat 2 g| Trans Fat 0 g| Cholesterol 84 mg| Sodium 433 mg| Carbohydrates 27 g| Protein 13 g| Phosphorus 229 mg| Potassium 325 mg| Dietary Fiber 3 g| Calcium 73 mg

3.15 Macaroni & Cheese

Ingredients

- Unsalted butter: 2 tablespoons
- Rotini pasta: 1 cup uncooked
- Low-fat milk: half cup
- Grated parmesan cheese: 3 tablespoons

- Half cup and a little more of cream cheese, reduced-fat
- Crushed red pepper flakes: 1/8 teaspoon
- Black pepper: 1/4 teaspoon
- One clove of pressed garlic

Instructions

- Cook pasta as per instructions, without salt.
- In a pan, sauté garlic for one minute in butter. Add cream cheese, milk, whisk well.
- Simmer the sauce on low heat.
- Add black pepper, red pepper flakes to taste.
- Add cooked pasta to the sauce.

Nutrients per serving: Calories 266| Protein 9 g| Carbohydrates 26 g| Fat 14 g| Cholesterol 43 mg| Sodium 237 mg| Potassium 222 mg| Phosphorus 188 mg| Calcium 147 mg| Fiber 2.3 g

3.16 Easy Pantry Pasta

Ingredients

- Canned cannellini beans: 1 cup
- One and a half cup of dried pasta
- Half cup of tuna packed in water, low-sodium
- Tomato sauce: half cup (no salt added)
- Chicken broth: half cup, low-sodium
- Olive oil: 2 tablespoons
- Roasted red peppers jarred: 1/3 cup
- Onion powder: half teaspoon
- Garlic powder: half teaspoon
- Dried basil: half teaspoon
- Green peas: half cup

- Parmesan cheese: 1 tablespoon
- Dried oregano: 1/4 teaspoon

Instructions

- Cook pasta as per instructions, without salt. Reserve half a cup of pasta water.
- Slice the red peppers.
- In a pan, add remaining ingredients, do not add cheese and peas.
- Add pasta to the sauce and mix well. Add pasta water to the sauce. If the sauce is too thick
- Add parmesan cheese and green peas mix well. Enjoy

Nutrients per serving: Calories 344| Protein 18 g| Carbohydrates 50 g| Fat 8 g| Cholesterol 13 mg| Sodium 290 mg| Potassium 542 mg| Phosphorus 230 mg| Calcium 76 mg| Fiber 5.4 g

3.17 Pasta with Cauliflower

Ingredients

- One and a half cups of chicken broth, low-sodium
- Olive oil: 2 tablespoons
- One onion, chopped
- One cauliflower, medium head, chopped
- 3 cloves of garlic, minced
- Black pepper: 1/4 teaspoon
- 2 cups of linguine, uncooked
- Fresh parsley: 2 tablespoons
- Crushed red pepper: 1/4 teaspoon

Instructions

- In a pan, sauté garlic and onion in oil until translucent

- Add red pepper, cauliflower, and black pepper and sauté for five minutes.
- Add broth and let it boil. Lower the heat to simmer till cauliflower is tender.
- Cook pasta as per instructions, without salt
- Put the drained pasta back in the pot add cauliflower broth to the pasta so it will not stick
- Add pasta in a serving bowl, add cauliflower broth and serve.

Nutrients per serving: Calories 298| Protein 12 g| Carbohydrates 49 g| Fat 6 g| Cholesterol 4 mg| Sodium 133 mg| Potassium 420 mg| phosphorus 231 mg| calcium 89 mg| Fiber 8.6 g

3.18 Creamy Orzo & Vegetables

Ingredients

- Olive oil: 2 tablespoons
- Frozen green peas: half cup
- One clove of minced garlic
- One zucchini, chopped
- One carrot, shredded
- Curry powder: 1 teaspoon
- Chicken broth, low-sodium: 3 cups
- One diced small onion
- Black pepper: 1/4 teaspoon
- Salt: 1/4 teaspoon
- Fresh parsley: 2 tablespoons
- Orzo pasta: 1 cup, uncooked
- Grated Parmesan cheese: 1/4 cup

Instructions

- In a pan, sauté onion, carrots, garlic, and zucchini for five minutes.
- Add broth, curry powder, and salt. Let it boil.
- Add pasta and bring to a boil. Cover it and let it simmer. Cook, often stirring for ten minutes, till pasta is cooked.
- Add chopped parsley, cheese, and frozen peas.
- Heat until all vegetables are heated through. Add more broth if required. Add black pepper and serve.

Nutrients per serving: Calories 176| Protein 10 g| carbohydrates 25 g| Fat 4 g| Cholesterol 4 mg| Sodium 193 mg| Potassium 170 mg| Phosphorus 68 mg| Calcium 53 mg| Fiber 2.6 g

3.19 Lemon Orzo Spring Salad

Ingredients

- Olive oil: ¼ cup+ 2 tbsp.
- Orzo pasta: ¾ cup
- Green peppers: ¼ cup, chopped
- Parmesan cheese: 3 tablespoons
- Yellow peppers: ¼ cup, chopped
- Half cup onion, chopped
- Fresh lemon juice: 3 tablespoons
- Lemon zest: 1 teaspoon
- Zucchini: 2 cups, cubed
- Red peppers: ¼ cup, chopped
- Rosemary: 2 tablespoons, chopped
- Black pepper: half teaspoon
- Red pepper flakes: half teaspoon
- Dried oregano: Half teaspoon

Instructions

- Cook pasta as per instructions, without salt

- In a pan, sauté zucchini, onions, peppers, until translucent, with two tbsp. of oil

- In a bowl, mix lemon zest, juice, red pepper flakes, rosemary, oregano, ¼ cup olive oil, pepper, and cheese.

- Add pasta and vegetables and coat well

- Serve at room temperature.

Nutrition Per Serving: Calories 330 | Total Fat 22 g| saturated Fat 4 g| trans Fat 0 g| Cholesterol 3 mg| sodium 79 mg| Carbohydrates 28 g| Protein 6 g| Phosphorus 134 mg| Potassium 376 mg| Dietary Fiber 5 g| Calcium 67 mg

3.20 Garlicky Penne Pasta with Green Beans

Ingredients

- 2 tablespoons olive oil

- Butter: 2 tablespoon

- Red pepper flakes: 1/8 teaspoon

- Tabasco hot sauce: 1/4 teaspoon

- Shredded parmesan cheese: 1/4 cup

- 4 cups green beans

- Six garlic cloves, minced

- Black pepper: half teaspoon

- Lemon juice: 2 teaspoons

- One cup of uncooked penne pasta

Instructions

- Cook pasta as per instructions, without salt

- In a pan, sauté red pepper flakes, garlic in butter and olive oil for 2 to 3 minutes.

- Add green beans, lemon juice, black pepper, tabasco sauce, and cook for six minutes until tender crispy.

- Add pasta. And toss.

Nutrients per serving: Calories 258| Protein 9 g| Carbohydrates 33 g| Fat 10 g| Cholesterol 13 mg| Sodium 93 mg| Potassium 258 mg| Phosphorus 168 mg| Calcium 83 mg| Fiber 4.8 g

3.21 Italian Style Vegetables & Pasta with Chicken

Ingredients

- One cup of cooked pasta twists

- Olive oil: 1 tablespoon

- Chopped onion: 1/4 cup

- Half teaspoon of garlic powder

- Half cup of chopped green bell pepper

- Half cup broccoli florets

- ¼ cup of chicken, cooked, diced

- Fresh basil: 1 tablespoon

- Dried rosemary: 1 teaspoon

- Red pepper flakes: 1/4 teaspoon

- Cornstarch: 2 teaspoons

- Salt: 1/8 teaspoon

- Chicken broth, low-sodium: 1/4 cup

Instructions

- In a pan, fry onion, broccoli, bell pepper. Add basil, garlic powder, rosemary, salt, red pepper flakes.

- Add in the cooked chicken.

- Mix cornstarch with chicken broth, and add to chicken and vegetable mix. Cook till slightly thickened. Add in the hot cooked pasta.

- Serve.

Nutrients per serving: Calories 250| Protein 15 g| Carbohydrates 28 g| Fat 9 g| Cholesterol 22 mg| Sodium 265 mg|

Potassium 329 mg| Phosphorus 140 mg| Calcium 72 mg| Fiber 3.7 g

3.22 Green Pesto Pasta

Ingredients

- Fresh basil leaves: 2 cups
- Half cup and a little more of uncooked spaghetti
- 4 cloves of garlic
- Extra virgin olive oil: 1/4 cup
- Black pepper: 1/4 teaspoon
- Grated Parmesan cheese: 2 tablespoons

Instructions

- Cook pasta as per instructions, without salt. Drain.
- In a food processor, add Parmesan cheese, basil leaves, and garlic, chop them. Slowly add olive oil and pulse.
- Add black pepper. Add basil sauce to pasta and coat evenly.

Nutrients per serving: Calories 303| Protein 8 g| Carbohydrates 34 g| Fat 15 g| Cholesterol 2 mg| sodium 47 mg| Potassium 170 mg| Phosphorus 145 mg| Calcium 92 mg| Fiber 5.5 g

3.23 Classic Beef Stroganoff with Egg Noodles

Ingredients

- One egg whisked
- Onions: 1 cup, finely chopped
- Low-fat mayonnaise: 1 tablespoon
- Worcestershire sauce: 2 tablespoons, reduced-sodium
- Tomato sauce: 1 tablespoon, no salt added
- 4 cups of ground beef

- Breadcrumbs: ¼ cup
- Bouillon beef: 4 teaspoons, reduced-sodium
- Olive oil: 3 tablespoons
- Sour cream: ¼ cup
- Flour: 2 tablespoons
- Rosemary: 1 tablespoon, chopped
- Water: 3 cups
- Wide egg noodles, cooked
- Ground black pepper: 1 teaspoon
- Cubed butter: 2 tablespoons unsalted, cold
- 2 tablespoons chives
- Parsley: ¼ cup

Instructions

- In a bowl, add beef, egg, and spices, half of the black pepper mix well and make small meatballs.
- In a pan, brown the meatballs.
- In another pan, add flour, oil, and mix, add black pepper, bouillon, water, mix till thickened.
- Mix this sauce with chives, sour cream, and meatballs. Serve with egg noodles/.

Nutrition Per Serving: Calories 490 | total Fat 32 g| saturated Fat 11 g| trans Fat 1 g| Cholesterol 120 mg| sodium 598 mg| Carbohydrates 30 g| Protein 20 g| Phosphorus 230 mg| Potassium 423 mg| Dietary Fiber 1.8 g| Calcium 56 mg

3.24 Easy Chicken & Pasta Dinner

Ingredients

- Half cup of chicken breast, cooked, cut into strips
- Olive oil: 1 tablespoon

- One cup sliced zucchini
- Half cup of sliced red bell pepper
- Italian dressing, low-sodium: 3 tablespoons
- Cooked pasta: 2 cups

Instructions

1. In a skillet, sauté peppers, zucchini in olive oil until tender. Set it aside

2. In another pan, heat the chicken and pasta. Add Italian dressing and vegetables, mix well and serve.

Nutrients per serving: Calories 400| Protein 30 g| Carbohydrates 45 g| Fat 11 g| Cholesterol 60 mg| Sodium 328 mg| Potassium 455 mg| Phosphorus 270 mg| Calcium 33 mg| Fiber 3.5 g

3.25 Alfredo Sauce Pasta

Ingredients

- Unsalted butter: 1/4 cup
- Half cup of cream cheese, cut into cubes
- Soy milk: 3/4 cup
- White pepper: 1/4 teaspoon
- Garlic powder: 1/8 teaspoon
- Half cup grated Cheese

Instructions

- In a pan, mix all the ingredients on low heat until well combined.
- Add in the cooked pasta and coat well.
- Enjoy.

Nutrients per serving: Calories 124| Protein 3 g| Carbohydrates 3 g| Fat 12 g| Cholesterol 36 mg| Sodium 153 mg| Potassium 65 mg| Phosphorus 70 mg| Calcium 87 mg| Fiber 0 g

3.26 Roasted Vegetable & Chicken Pasta

Ingredients

Vegetables

- One pint sliced mushrooms
- One chopped zucchini
- Half sliced onion
- One cup cherry tomatoes
- 1 chopped yellow squash
- One small broccoli, chop into small pieces
- Olive oil: ¼ cup
- Garlic powder: ¼ teaspoon
- One red pepper, diced
- Onion powder: ¼ teaspoon
- Coarse kosher salt: 1 teaspoon
- Half teaspoon of pepper

Pasta

- Extra virgin olive oil: ¼ cup
- Salt and pepper to taste
- 1 box of pasta, cooked
- Cheese: ⅔ cup shredded

Chicken

- Extra virgin olive oil: 1 tablespoon
- 6 cups of chicken breasts
- Half teaspoon of pepper
- One full hand kale
- Half teaspoon of coarse kosher salt

Instructions

Vegetables

- Let the oven preheat to 350.
- On a baking sheet, place mushrooms, zucchini, broccoli, squash, red pepper,

onion, and tomatoes. Sprinkle onion powder, pepper, garlic powder, olive oil, and salt. Mix well

- Roast for half an hour, stirring every ten minutes.

Chicken

- Cut the chicken into cubes

- In a pan, sauté chicken with pepper and salt in olive oil

- Cook chicken for six minutes or till its cooked.

- Add kale to the chicken pan and cook for 20 seconds till kale has wilted.

Pasta

- Add salt, pepper, cheese to hot pasta and mix well

Assemble

- In a big bowl, add chicken, roasted vegetables, and pasta

- Taste and adjust seasoning.

- Serve right away

Nutrient per serving: Calories 282 g| Protein: 15 g| Carbohydrates: 21.4 g| Fiber: 2.7 g| Total Fat: 5 g| Sodium: 209 mg| Phosphorus: 145 mg| Potassium: 189 mg|

3.27 Roasted Red Pepper Pesto

Ingredients

- 2 cloves of garlic, cut in half

- 1 tsp. balsamic vinegar

- One jar of red bell peppers, roasted, drained

- Fresh basil: ¼ cup

- Pepper to taste

- Olive oil: ¼ cup

- One packet of Ravioli, low sodium

Instructions

- In a food processor, add all ingredients, except pasta. Pulse on high for 30 seconds, till smooth. Adjust seasoning

- Cook ravioli as per instruction.

- Coat the cooked ravioli with sauce and enjoy.

Nutrition per serving: Calories 526 kcals| Sodium 487 mg| Protein 17 g| Potassium 294 mg| Fat 37 g| calcium 66 mg | Carbohydrates 31 g| Phosphorus 186 mg| Fiber 2 g| Cholesterol 130mg

3.28 Chicken and Bow-Tie Pasta

Ingredients

- Cayenne pepper: 1/4 teaspoon

- Cooked bow-tie pasta: 3 cups

- Chicken broth, low sodium: 1 cup

- 2 cloves of minced garlic

- Olive oil: 1/4 cup

- Chopped red pepper: 1 cup

- One and a half cups chopped broccoli

- One cup of chicken breast, cut into strips

- Half cup of chopped green onions

- White wine: 3/4 cup

- Ground basil: 1 teaspoon

Instructions

- In a skillet, sauté garlic.

- Add chicken and brown it.

- Add all the remaining ingredients and let it simmer for 15 minutes

- Mix with cooked pasta.

Nutrition per serving: Calories 258 kcals| Sodium 50 mg| protein 13 g| Potassium 338 mg| Fat 10 g| Calcium 43 mg| Carbohydrates 25 g| phosphorus 173 mg| Fiber 5 g| cholesterol 22 mg|

3.29 Chicken Fusilli Salad

Dressing

- White pepper: half teaspoon
- Half cup of olive oil
- Vinegar: 1/4 cup
- Honey: 1 teaspoon
- Basil: 1/4 teaspoon

Salad

- Half cup of chopped red pepper
- Fusilli pasta cooked: 3 cups
- Shredded lettuce: 2 cups
- Half cup of cooked peas
- 1 carrot, thin slices
- Sliced zucchini: 1 cup
- One cup of diced cooked chicken

Instructions

- In a jar, add ingredients of dressing, shake and mix well, chill in the fridge for two hours.
- In a bowl, add zucchini, pasta, carrot, chicken, red pepper, and peas, mix well
- Add dressing, and mix well

Nutrient per serving: Calories 477 kcals| Sodium 65 mg| Protein 18 g| Potassium 446 mg| Fat 29 g| Calcium 31 mg| Carbohydrates 39 g| Phosphorus 239 mg| Fiber 8 g| Cholesterol 33 mg

3.30 Pad Thai

Ingredients

- Vegetable oil: 3 tablespoons
- Honey: 2 tablespoons
- 2 cloves of minced garlic
- Chinese chives: 6 tbsp.
- Half cups of extra-firm tofu
- Carrot & cabbage slaw mix: 1 cup
- One lime
- 4 tbsp. Of unseasoned rice vinegar
- Reduced-sodium soy sauce: 1 tablespoon
- Dried noodles, rice stick: 7 ounces
- Red chili sauce: 1 tablespoon
- One and a half cups of bean sprouts
- 2 eggs

Instructions

- Chop all the vegetables and tofu.
- In a boiled pot of water, turn off the heat, add rice noodles, separate them, soak for five minutes, drain and set it aside.
- In a small bowl, mix honey, chili sauce, vinegar, soy sauce. Set it aside
- In a wok, sauté tofu until it begins to brown for two minutes. Set it aside
- Add one tbsp. of oil and garlic in the wok fry a few seconds, add the noodles and chives, fry for few seconds. Add in the honey mix, add slaw mix, bean sprouts. Cook for two minutes.
- Cook eggs and coat with noodles, add tofu, and mix.
- Serve immediately.

Nutrients per serving: Calories 436| Protein 9 g| Carbohydrates 64 g| Fat 16 g| Cholesterol 93 mg| Sodium 430 mg|

Potassium 445 mg| Phosphorus 163 mg| Calcium 81 mg| Fiber 2.8 g

3.31 Spaghetti Squash Parmigiano

Ingredients

- 2 cloves of minced garlic
- One small spaghetti squash
- 1 onion
- Red chili flakes: 1/8 teaspoon
- Olive oil: 4 tablespoons
- Parmigiano-Reggiano cheese, grated: 3/4 cup
- Black pepper: 1/4 teaspoon

Instructions

- Let the oven preheat to 375° F.
- Stab squash with a fork—microwave for five minutes. Cut in half and remove seeds.
- Pour olive oil over the squash, and bake for 50 minutes.
- Take out squash. Let it cool down.
- In a skillet, sauté onion and garlic for 2 to 3 minutes. Turn off the heat.
- With a fork, pulp the squash and add to skillet. Add cheese, red flakes, and black pepper. Mix to combine

Nutrients per serving: Calories 138| Protein 5 g| Carbohydrates 7 g| Fat 10 g| Cholesterol 11 mg| Sodium 200 mg| Potassium 160 mg| Phosphorus 110 mg| Calcium 162 mg|Fiber 1.7 g

3.32 Pancit

Ingredients

- Carrots: 2 cups, shredded
- 3 cloves of minced garlic
- Half cup of onion, minced
- 4 cups of shredded cabbage
- 2 chopped green onions
- olive oil: 1 tablespoon
- 3 stalks of celery
- 1 cup cooked chicken
- 2 cups of frozen snow peas
- Chicken broth, low-sodium: 4 cups
- Rice sticks(noodles) of 16 ounces
- Half teaspoon of black pepper
- Soy sauce, reduced-sodium: 1 tablespoon

Instructions

- In a skillet, sauté onion, garlic in olive oil until tender
- Add in the chicken and soy sauce. Add three cups of broth and let it boil
- Add noodles, cook for 15 minutes, until translucent but do not overcook
- Add the vegetables, cook until cabbage becomes tender.
- Serve right away and add lemon juice.

Nutrients per serving: Calories 255| Protein 12 g| Carbohydrates 41 g| Fat 5 g| cholesterol 59 mg| Sodium 220 mg| Potassium 373 mg| Phosphorus 141 mg| calcium 49 mg| Fiber 2.7 g

3.33 Garlic Shrimp Zoodles

Ingredients

- Medium shrimp 3/4 pounds, deveined
- Olive oil: 1 tablespoon
- Garlic minced: 3-4 cloves
- Two medium zucchini
- Red chili flakes

- Chopped parsley
- Salt & pepper, to taste
- One lemon: Juice and zest

Instruction

- First off, spiralizer the zucchini and set it aside
- Add lemon juice, the olive oil, zest of lemon to a skillet on medium flame. Then add the shrimp until the pan is hot. Cook 1 minute per side of the shrimp.
- Add red chili flakes, garlic. Cook for a full minute, always stirring.
- Add the zoodles and toss for 2-3 minutes until cooked and warmed thoroughly
- Sprinkle with the sliced parsley and season with pepper and salt. Serve hot.

Nutrition per serving: Kcal 276| Fat 10g| Carbohydrates 9g|Protein 12g

3.34 Zucchini Noodles with Roasted Halibut

Ingredients

- Wild halibut of 6 ounces
- Olive Oil
- Red curry paste: 1 tablespoon
- One package of zucchini noodles
- Salt, pepper to taste
- Two minced cloves of garlic
- Four sliced scallions, sliced
- Half of cup of cilantro
- Two inches of ginger root(grated)
- Red pepper flakes: 1/4 teaspoon

Instructions

- Put a skillet over medium flame and heat the coconut oil.
- Add the zoodles, curry paste, ginger and, garlic. Cook for about four minutes until the noodles are tender, keep stirring—season taste.
- Put another skillet over medium flame and heat the coconut oil. Place skin-side down the fish. Season with red pepper flakes and salt.
- Turn on the broiler.
- Cook for seven minutes, then move to the broiler. Broil for five minutes or until the fish is completely cooked
- Add the noodles with scallions and cilantro and stir to combine.
- Place on a plate, top with fish, and serve.

Nutrition per serving :196 calories| total fat 1.1g |carbohydrates 24.6g |protein 23.5g

3.35 Red Bell Pepper Basil Garlic Chicken

Ingredients

- One pound of skinless chicken breasts
- Olive oil: 2 tablespoons
- Half onion, diced
- Three minced garlic cloves
- Red bell peppers: one and a half cups
- Basil: 1 cup
- Red chili flakes: 1/4 teaspoon
- Four zucchini and courgette: spiralizer into noodles

- Salt & pepper, to taste

Instructions

- Pound, the chicken breast to achieve the same overall thickness. When finished, sprinkle a touch of salt and pepper on either side.

- In a wide skillet, add one tablespoon of olive oil, warm it. stir in the chicken and fry each side for a few minutes until golden brown

- When the chicken has been cooked completely and browned, remove it from the skillet and put aside for the time being, on a separate dish.

- Using the same skillet, add olive oil and sauté the onion until it becomes translucent for around five minutes. Then add the garlic and Sautee for about another minute.

- Add the basil and tomatoes in the pan and add salt, pepper, and then red pepper flakes to season.

- Simmer for ten minutes until the sauce thickens. Please make sure you mix regularly.

- Send the chicken back to the skillet together with the zoodles for a couple of minutes so they can soak up the sauce. Serve hot

Nutrition per serving: Kcal 251| Fat: 8 g| Carbs 12g |Protein: 27g

3.36 Mac Stuffed Sweet Potatoes

Ingredients

- One sweet potato (leached)

- ¼ cup whole-grain penne pasta

- 1 tsp tomato paste, no salt added

- Olive oil 1 tsp

- ¼ teaspoon minced garlic

- 1 tbsp. soy milk

Instructions

- Cut the sweet potato in two and holes it 3-4 times with fork.

- Spray the sweet potato halves with olive oil and cook in the Preheated to 375 F oven for about 25-30 minutes or when the vegetables are tender.

- In the meantime, cook penne pasta, tomato paste, minced garlic, and soy milk.

- When the sweet potatoes are baked, spoon out the vegetable meat and spice it up with a penne pasta combination.

- Cover the sweet potatoes with the pasta mix.

Nutrition per serving: 105 calories| 2.7g protein|17.8g carbohydrates|2.8g fat|3g fiber|0mg cholesterol

3.37 Pasta Soup

Ingredients

- 2 oz. whole-grain pasta

- ½ cup corn kernels

- 1 oz. carrot, shredded

- 3 oz. celery stalk, chopped

- 2 cups low-sodium chicken stock

- 1 teaspoon ground black pepper

Instructions

Bring the chicken stock to boil and add shredded carrot and celery stalk. Simmer the liquid for 5 minutes.

After this, add corn kernels, ground black pepper, and pasta. Stir the soup well.

Simmer it on the medium heat for 8 minutes.

Nutrition per serving: 263 calories|11.8g protein|29.6g carbohydrates| 2.6g fat|9.4g fiber|0mg cholesterol| 200mg sodium|273mg potassium.

3.38 Lunch Tuna Salad

Ingredients

- Five ounces of dried, soaked tuna in water
- 1 spoon of red vinegar
- Olive oil for 1 tbsp.
- 1⁄4 cup green, minced onions
- Arugula two cups
- 1 tbsp. low-fat, grated parmesan
- A squeeze of black pepper
- Half cup of pasta, cooked

Instructions

- Mix the tuna and the vinegar, oil, arugula, pasta, green onions, and black pepper in a bowl. Mix.
- Split into Three pans, spray on top with parmesan and serve for lunch.

Nutrition per serving: calories 200| fat 4 g| fiber 4mg| carbs 14 g| protein 7g | potassium 217 mg| phosphorous 113 mg

3.39 Veggie Soup

Ingredients

- Two olive oil teaspoons
- 1 and 1⁄2 carrot cups, shredded
- Six cloves of garlic, minced
- 1 cup of yellow, chopped onion
- 1 cup of diced celery

- Low-sodium chicken stock: 4 cups
- Four Cups of Water
- 1 and 1⁄2 cups pasta
- two tablespoons of parsley
- 1⁄4 cup low-fat, grated parmesan

Instructions

- Over medium-high warm, warm a pan with the oil, add garlic, mix and simmer for 1 minute.
- Add the onion, celery, and carrot, stir, and roast for 7 minutes.
- Add onion, water and pasta, stir, bring to a boil and simmer for Eight more minutes over moderate flame.
- Split into cups, top, and serve each with parsley and parmesan.

Nutrition per serving: calories 212| fat 4 g| fiber 4 g| carbs 13 g| protein 8 g| potassium 198 mg| phosphorous 109 mg

3.40 Italian Pasta

Ingredients

- One pound penne pasta, cooked
- Three cloves of garlic, diced
- Olive oil, Two tablespoons
- Three carrots, cut
- One bell pepper red, diced
- 1 bell pepper purple, chopped
- One cup of cherry tomatoes halved
- black pepper
- 2/3 cup soy milk
- Two teaspoons low-fat, grated parmesan

Instructions

- Over medium-high heat, warm a skillet with the oil, add the garlic, stir and simmer for 2 minutes.

- Add the vegetables, stir and simmer for an additional four minutes.

- Add the bell peppers, yellow and red, and combine and roast for 5 minutes.

- Add black pepper, cherry tomatoes, milk, parmesan, pasta, mix, and serve

Nutrition per serving: calories 221|fat 7.8 g| fiber 2.2mg|carbs 15 g| protein 12 potassium 121 mg| phosphorous 108 mg

3.41 Creamy Garlic Pasta with Roasted Tomatoes

Ingredients

- 3 cups cherry tomatoes (halved)

- One and ¼ cup of pasta

- Olive oil

- Two medium shallots

- 8 large cloves minced garlic

- Sea salt and black pepper

- 3-4 Tbsp. all-purpose flour

- 2-1/2 cups of broth

Instructions

- Preheat oven to 400 degrees F (204 C) and toss tomatoes in a bit of olive oil and sea salt. Place cut side up on a parchment-lined baking sheet and bake for 20 minutes while preparing the rest of the dish. Then set aside.

- Bring a large pot of water to a boil and cook pasta according to package Instructions, and set aside.

- In the meantime, prepare the sauce. In a large skillet over medium-low heat, add 1 Tbsps. Olive oil and the garlic and shallot. Add a pinch of salt and black pepper and frequently stir, cooking for 3-4 minutes until softened and fragrant.

- Stir in flour and mix with a whisk. Once combined, slowly whisk in the almond milk a little at a time, so clumps don't form. Add another healthy pinch of salt and black pepper, bring to a simmer and continue cooking for another 4-5 minutes to thicken. Taste and adjust seasonings as needed,

- If you want an ultra-creamy sauce, transfer the sauce to a blender to blend it until creamy and smooth. Place back in the pan and reduce heat to a low simmer until the desired thickness is achieved.

- Once the sauce is to your desired thickness, taste and adjusts seasonings as needed, then add pasta and roasted tomatoes and stir.

- Serve immediately and garnish with extra black pepper, fresh basil, or vegan parmesan cheese. Best when fresh, but will keep for up to 2 days in the fridge.

Nutrition per serving: Calories: 379| carbohydrates: 64 g| Protein: 11.5 g| Fat: 9 g| saturated Fat: 0.8 g| trans Fat: 0 g| sodium: 360 mg| fiber: 8.5 g

3.42 Ratatouille-Stuffed Shells

Ingredients

- 2 cups of uncooked jumbo pasta shells

- One tablespoon olive oil

- 3/4 cup chopped onion

- One tablespoon minced garlic

- 1 and a half cups diced eggplant

- 1 cup diced red bell pepper

- 3/4 cup diced zucchini
- 3/4 cup chopped plum tomato
- 1 3/4 cups, Low-Sodium marinara sauce
- Half cup plus 2 Tbsp. torn fresh basil, divided
- 3/4 teaspoon freshly ground black pepper
- Half teaspoon kosher salt
- One cup shredded vegan cheese

Instructions

- Preheat 450 ° F oven.
- Cook spaghetti, omitting salt and fat in compliance with product instructions.
- Heat oil medium-high in a large skillet. Add onion and garlic. Cook for 4 minutes, stirring regularly. Add aubergine and pepper.
- Cover and prepare the courgettes, tomatoes, cook for 4 min. Stir in 1 cup of marinara, half cup of basil, black pepper, and salt and remove the pan from the sun.
- Spray oil on ceramic baker. Place marinara over the bottom of the dish remaining 3/4 cup. Spoon into pasta around two tablespoons of the vegetable blend. Sprinkle with cheese; place the shells complete in the dish—Bake 12 minutes at 450 ° F. Top with basil.

Nutrition per serving: Calories 370 | fat 11.8g | sat fat 4.1g | Mono fat 4.3g|Poly fat 1.4g | Protein 16g | Carbohydrate 30g|Fiber 6g | Cholesterol 20mg | iron 4mg |Sodium 486mg | calcium 275mg | Sugars 11g |

3.43 Capers Pasta Salad

Ingredients

- 2 cups rotini pasta
- ⅓ cup extra-virgin olive oil
- 2 pints' cherry or grape tomatoes
- ½ teaspoon fine sea salt
- One cup of mozzarella "pearls,"
- Several sprigs of fresh basil

Instructions

- Bring a big pot of water to a boil and prepare the pasta until ready for use. Set it aside.
- When the pasta has cooked, mix oil, tomatoes, salt on medium-high heat, in a Dutch oven. Cover the pot. Cook till the most tomatoes has soften, and also the olive oil has a faint red shade (around 6 to 12 minutes).
- Take off the heat and add in the pasta you have prepared. let the mixture to cool when chopping basil for a few minutes. We do not want to melt the cheese when in touch so wait until the next phase is mild (not hot) for your pasta.
- Drop from the pasta the mozzarella balls as well as basil. Taste the vinegar and apply extra vinegar or salt if it is not amazing yet. Let the combination sit for about 20 minutes of better taste so that the pasta will handle more sauce.

Nutrition per serving: Calories 552|Total Fat 33.9g | saturated Fat 11.5g| Monounsaturated Fat 16.7g |Cholesterol 50.6mg |Sodium 681.8mg |Total Carbohydrate 47.1g |Dietary Fiber 8.4g | Sugars 8.3g | protein 20g

3.44 Lemony Collard Greens Pasta

Ingredients

- One cup of fresh collard greens

- ⅓ or more of a package of whole wheat thin spaghetti or "spaghetti."
- Three tablespoons pine nuts
- Olive oil
- Two small cloves garlic, pressed
- Big pinch red pepper flakes
- Sea salt and black pepper
- 2 tbsp. of Parmesan cheese
- ½ or more of a lemon, cut into wedges

Instructions

- Carry a large pot of salted water and cook the pasta as instructed.
- Take the middle rib out of a green leaves. Place some greens together and roll them into the form of a cigar. As small as practicable (1⁄8″ to 1/4″), break through the pin. Give them a good chopping, so the branches aren't too fat. Shake the greens up.
- Heat a heavy-bottom pot over moderate flame and roast the pine nuts till they are golden and scented.
- Switch to medium heat and mix in an olive oil tablespoon. Sprinkle the garlic and whisk in red pepper. When the oil is dark enough to shine, pour it onto the greens. Add salt to the greens. Mix regularly, sauté the greens for around three minutes, and not to make them clump.
- Let the fire of the pan. Shift the vegetables into the pasta pot and add pasta water if necessary, with a second drizzle of olive oil.
- Separate into plates and put two larger citrus wedges, an individual on top of pine nuts and paramedic shavings.

Nutrition per serving: Calories 584| Total Fat 29.2g |Saturated Fat 6.1g |Trans Fat 0g | polyunsaturated Fat 8.5g | cholesterol 9.7mg |Sodium 238.1mg | Total Carbohydrate 68.1g |Dietary Fiber 14.3g | Sugars 2.8g | Protein 22.1g

4.45 Easy One-Pot Pasta

Ingredients

- One cup dry pasta
- 2 garlic cloves, minced
- Half yellow onion, thinly sliced
- 1 small zucchini, chopped and quartered
- 1/4 cup of mushrooms, sliced
- Half teaspoon red pepper flakes
- Half teaspoon kosher salt
- 1 and 1/4 cup pasta sauce of choice, no salt added
- 2 half cups of water
- ¼ cup kale

Instructions

- In a large pot (or pan with deep surfaces), incorporate the uncooked pasta. In addition to the kale, combine the remaining ingredients well. Blend well. Take the pot to a high heat boil.
- Reduce heat to a medium-low until cooked and cook pasta until al-dente for 10-14 minutes. Add the blend to the bottom of the pan after 2 minutes to avoid sticking.
- Turn off the heat and bring it into the pasta, the kale. When the kale has cooled, add the pasta into cups.

Nutrition per serving: Calories 378|Fat 5g | Sodium 272mg|Potassium 245 mg|

Carbohydrates 72g|Fiber 11g|Sugar 6.7 g| Protein 15g| Calcium 164mg|Iron 4.9mg

3.46 Scampi Linguine

Ingredients

- 1 clove of garlic, minced
- One tbsp. of olive oil
- Dry white wine: ¼ cup
- 1 tbsp. of lemon juice
- 1 tsp of basil
- Half cup of dry linguine
- 2 cups of shrimp, peeled, cleaned
- Chopped fresh parsley: 1 tbsp.

Instructions

- In a skillet, cook shrimp and garlic until shrimp turns pink
- Add basil, wine, parsley, and lemon juice. Cook for five minutes
- Cook pasta as per instructions, without salt
- Coat pasta with shrimp and serve

Nutrition per serving: Calories 208 kcal | Sodium 86 mg| Protein 15 g| Potassium 189 mg| Phosphorus 167 mg| Calcium 140 mg | Fat 5 g| Water 40 g| Carbohydrates 26 g

3.47 15-Minute Sesame Ginger Noodles

Ingredients

- One sliced green onion
- Baby bock choy: 3 cups, quarters
- Half pack rice noodles

Sauce

- 3 tbsp. low sodium soy sauce
- 2 cloves of garlic, chopped
- Maple syrup: 2 tbsp.
- Sesame oil: 2 tsp

- Crushed red chili: 2 tsp
- 2 tbsp. of ginger, chopped

Instructions

- In a bowl, mix all the ingredients of the sauce, set aside
- Boil rice noodles as per package instructions set it aside.
- In a pan, add sauce and cook for two minutes. Add green onions, bock choy. Mix well.
- Turn heat down and add in rice noodles
- Mix and serve.

Nutrition per serving: calories: 446 |fat: 2.6g |fiber: 4.8g |protein: 8.1g

3.48 Kidney Bean Pasta Salad

Ingredients

- Half chopped cucumber
- Pasta cooked: 2 cups
- 1 can of kidney beans
- Feta cheese: ¾ cup
- Half cup parsley, fresh
- One spring onion
- Half can sweet corn

Instructions

- In a big bowl, add all ingredients and mix well
- Add light sodium soy sauce on top if you want
- Enjoy

Nutrient per serving: Calories: 160 g| Protein: 14 g| Carbohydrates: 19 g| Fiber: 2 g| Total Fat: 3 g| Sodium: 189 mg| Phosphorus: 88 mg| Potassium: 176 mg|

3.49 Tuna Pasta Salad

Ingredients

- Chopped red onion: 1 cup
- Light tuna: 2 cans, packed in water
- Chopped celery: 1 cup
- Elbow pasta: 3 cups, cooked
- Low-fat mayonnaise: half cup.
- Frozen peas: 1 cup
- Red wine vinegar: 1 tbsp.
- Salt and pepper to taste

Instructions

- Cook pasta as per instructions, without salt, wash under cold water.
- In a bowl, add celery, pasta, peas, onion, tuna, mayonnaise, pepper, salt, and vinegar.
- Mix well and enjoy it.

Nutrition per serving: Calories: 355kcal | Carbohydrates: 59g | Protein: 17g | Fat: 5g | Saturated |fat: 1g | Cholesterol: 11mg | Sodium: 114mg | Potassium: 364mg | Fiber: 4g | Sugar: 5g | Calcium: 56mg | Iron: 2mg

3.50 Healthy Pizza Pasta Salad

Ingredients

- 16 oz. pasta
- ⅔ cup of low sodium Italian dressing
- 1 can chickpeas, drained
- One large green bell pepper, chopped
- One cup of sun-dried tomatoes, julienned
- Dried oregano leaves: 2 tsp

Instructions

- Cook pasta as per instructions, without salt

- In a bowl, add all ingredients, including cooked and washed pasta
- Mix well

Nutrition per serving: Calories: 257 |Fat: 4g |Saturated fat: 0g |Carbohydrates: 50g | Sugar: 6g| Sodium: 359mg |Fiber: 8g| Protein: 8g |Cholesterol: 0mg

3.51 Mediterranean Zucchini Noodle Salad

Ingredients

- Two zucchinis
- 1 onion peeled
- 2 cloves of crushed garlic
- One cup of bock choy quarter
- 1 cup: chickpeas
- Red wine vinegar: 2 tablespoons
- Half cup of crumbled feta cheese
- Olive oil: 1/4 cup
- 1 cup of red bell pepper
- Lemon juice: 1 tablespoon
- Dijon mustard: 1 teaspoon
- Salt and pepper to taste
- Dried oregano: 1 teaspoon

Instructions

- In a big jar, add all ingredients and mix.
- Spiralizer the zucchini.
- Spiralizer half the red onion.
- Mix these two noodles
- Add bock choy, chickpeas, feta cheese in the bowl.
- Add the dressing over vegetables and mix.

- Drizzle the salad dressing over the veggies and gently stir everything together. Serve and enjoy.

- **Nutrient per serving**: Calories: 151 g| Protein: 7.8 g| Carbohydrates: 12.1 g| Fiber: 3.4 g| Total Fat: 2.9 g| Sodium: 103 mg| Phosphorus: 87 mg| Potassium: 92 mg|

Chapter 4: Kidney-Friendly Chicken & Pork Recipes

4.1 Herb-Roasted Chicken Breasts

Ingredients

- One onion
- 4 cups of chicken breasts (boneless and skinless)
- 1–2 cloves of garlic
- Ground black pepper: 1 teaspoon
- Olive oil: ¼ cup
- Garlic & Herb Seasoning: 2 tablespoons (no salt added)

Instructions

- In a bowl, chop garlic, onion, add herb seasoning, olive oil, and pepper.
- Add chicken to this mix, cover with plastic wrap, then chill in the fridge for four hours.
- Let the oven preheat to 350 F
- Place marinated chicken on foil on a baking tray
- Add the marinade over chicken and bake for 20 minutes
- For browning, Broil for five minutes.

Nutrition Per Serving: Calories 270 | total Fat 17 g| Saturated Fat 3 g| Trans Fat 0 g| Cholesterol 83 mg| Sodium 53 mg| Carbohydrates 3 g| Protein 26 g| Phosphorus 252 mg| Potassium 491 mg| Dietary Fiber 0.6 g| Calcium 17 mg

4.2 Zesty Chicken

Ingredients

- Olive oil: 2 tablespoons
- Balsamic vinegar: 2 tablespoons
- Green onion: 1/4 cup
- Paprika: 1/4 teaspoon
- 8 ounces of chicken breast (skinless and boneless)
- Black pepper: 1/4 teaspoon
- Fresh oregano: 1 teaspoon
- Half teaspoon of garlic powder

Instructions

- In a mug, whisk olive oil and balsamic vinegar. Add chopped green onion, herbs, and seasoning, mix well. Cut chicken into two pieces.
- In a zip lock bag, add chicken and pour marinade over. Let it chill in the fridge for half an hour to 24 hours.
- Grease the pan, cook chicken until chicken's internal temperature reaches 170 F

Nutrients per serving: Calories 280| Protein 27 g| Carbohydrates 4 g| Fat 16 g| Cholesterol 73 mg| Sodium 68 mg| Potassium 280 mg| Phosphorus 205 mg| Calcium 26 mg| Fiber 0.3 g

4.3 Slow-Cooked Lemon Chicken

Ingredients

- One pound of chicken breast, skinless, boneless
- Dried oregano: 1 teaspoon
- Chicken broth: ¼ cup, low sodium
- 2 cloves of pressed garlic
- Black pepper: ¼ teaspoon
- Fresh basil: 1 teaspoon, chopped
- Butter: 2 tablespoons, unsalted
- Lemon juice: 1 tablespoon
- Water: ¼ cup

Instructions

- In a bowl, mix black pepper, oregano. Rub this mix on chicken.

- In a skillet, melt butter, brown the chicken in butter, then place in the slow cooker.

- Add garlic, water, broth, and lemon juice in the skillet. Let it boil, then pour over chicken

- Cook on low for five hours, high for two and a half hours.

- Baste chicken and add basil.

- Cover it, cook on high for half an hour minutes.

Nutrition Per Serving: Calories 197 | Total Fat 9 g| saturated Fat 5 g| Trans Fat 0 g| Cholesterol 99 mg| sodium 57 mg| carbohydrates 1 g| Protein 26 g| Phosphorus 251 mg| potassium 412 mg| Dietary Fiber 0.3 g| Calcium 20 mg

4.4 Turmeric Lime Chicken

Ingredients

- Vegetable oil: 4-5 TBSP

- Three minced garlic cloves

- Turmeric: one tablespoon

- Cilantro: two tablespoon

- Two beaten egg whites

- Boneless chicken breasts: six (not thick)

- Four halved juicy limes

- Bread crumbs: 2 cups

- Salt and pepper to taste

Instructions

- Make four tiny cuts on top of each chicken breast, then season on both sides with pepper and salt. This scoring will help the marinade flavors absorb the meat quicker and enable

the chicken breasts to cook quicker and more evenly.

- In a large bowl, combine fresh lime juice, minced garlic, and chopped cilantro and put the mixture's chicken breasts. Cover it up, and let stay at room temperature for half an hour.

- Whisk the eggs. Combine the turmeric powder and the panko or bread crumbs in another container

- Put each breast of chicken in the beaten egg bowl and switch to cover with egg. Then cover the turmeric/ bread crumb mixture on both sides of each chicken breast.

- Pan-fry the chicken breasts in a wide pan, use oil to coat the pan. Around 6-10 minutes per side, if required, after that, clean the pan. Repeat the process with each chicken breast.

- If the chicken is completely cooked. Serve in a sandwich or with a delicious mango salsa, steamed or sautéed vegetables of your choosing.

Nutrition per serving: 326 kcal | Carbohydrates: 20g | Protein: 29g | Fat: 14g | Potassium 181 mg| Phosphorus 102 mg

4.5 Grilled Moroccan Chicken

Ingredients

- Olive oil: one tbsp.

- Chicken breasts: 1 and ½ pound

- Coriander: 1/8 tsp

- Cumin: 2 tsp.

- Sea salt: ¾ tsp.

- Ginger: half tsp.

- Cinnamon: one tsp.

- Turmeric: half tsp.

- Cayenne: optional

- Paprika: one tsp.
- Lemon juice: two tbsp.

Instructions

- Drizzle lemon juice and olive oil all over the chicken
- Mix the salt and spices in a big bowl. evenly coat chicken in spices mixture
- Let it cool in refrigerate for two hours or overnight
- Heat the barbecue grill to a medium to high temperature. Add chicken and leave for around 5 minutes or until you have created grill lines.
- Shift the chicken away from heat and cook for 15-25 minutes on a lower level,
- Remove from flame, and allow to settle before serving or cutting for 5 minutes.

Nutrition per serving: Kcal 204 | Carbohydrates: 20g | Protein: 36g | Fat: 8g | Potassium 162 mg| Phosphorus 103 mg

4.6 Honey Turmeric Chicken

Ingredients

- Honey: 1 and half tbsp.
- Two minced cloves garlic
- Four chicken thighs (skin on but deboned)
- Turmeric powder: 3/4 tsp
- Salt, to taste
- Oil: 1 tablespoon
- One pinch of cayenne pepper
- Soy sauce: one tbsp.

Instructions

- Combine the chicken with the honey, oyster sauce, garlic, turmeric powder,

salt, and cayenne pepper, mix well to combine.

- Put the skillet on medium flame, add the oil. Move the chicken to the skillet and fry on both sides until the skin side becomes light brown, crispy at the bottom and wonderfully browned and crispy. Serve hot.

Nutrition Per Serving: Kcal315| Total Fat 45g | Carbohydrates 16g | Protein37g| Potassium 198 mg| Phosphorus121 mg

4.7 One-Pan Roasted Chicken with Turmeric

Ingredients

- Bone-in; skin on chicken: six pieces
- One sweet onion sliced
- Virgin olive oil: half cup
- Orange juice: half cup
- One juice of a lime
- Honey: 3 tbsp.
- Dry white wine: half cup
- Yellow mustard: 2 tablespoon
- Ground turmeric: 3/4 tbsp.
- Ground coriander: one teaspoon
- Sweet paprika: one teaspoon
- Garlic powder: 1 tbsp.
- Two oranges (sliced)
- One lime, thinly sliced
- One fennel bulb (sliced)
- Pepper and salt, to taste

Instructions

- Combine the orange juice, olive oil, lime juice, white wine, honey, and mustard in a big dish.
- Mix the spices in a bowl: paprika, turmeric, coriander, powdered garlic,

black pepper, and salt. To the liquid marinade, add approximately half of the spice blend. combine well

- Dry the chicken pieces with a paper towel and season well with the remaining spice mix. Make sure to season under the chicken skins and add some of the spice blends

- In the large bowl of marinade, add the chicken and the remaining ingredients. Mix it well. Cover and refrigerate for almost two hours. After marination, let the oven pre-heat to 475 F.

- Move the chicken to a large baking pan and the marinade and everything else, so that it is arranged in one layer. Make sure the skin of the chicken faces upwards. Sprinkle with a splash of salt and brown sugar, if needed.

- Roast for almost 45 mints, or until the chicken is completely cooked and the chicken's skin has browned well. The internal temperature of the chicken should be 170 degrees F.

Nutrition Per Serving: Kcal 382|Fat 14g| Protein 35g|Carbohydrate 38g| Potassium 164 mg| Phosphorus 103 mg

4.8 Anti-Inflammatory Chicken Quinoa

Ingredients

- Olive oil divided: 4 tbsp.

- Boneless, skinless chicken breasts: one pound

- Finely chopped red onion: ¼ cup

- Roasted red peppers: 2 cups

- One minced garlic clove

- Paprika: 1 tsp.

- Crushed red pepper: ¼ tsp(optional)

- Cooked quinoa: two cups

- Ground cumin: half tsp.

- Olives, chopped: ¼ cup

- Diced cucumber: one cup

- Almonds: ¼ cup

- Crumbled feta cheese: ¼ cup

- Salt: ¼ teaspoon

- Ground pepper: ¼ teaspoon

- Fresh parsley: 2 tbsp.

Instructions

- In the upper third of the oven, put a rack; let the broiler preheat to heavy. Place foil on a rimmed baking dish.

- Put salt and pepper on the chicken, and put on the prepared baking sheet. Broil it for 14 to 18 min, rotating once, till a thermometer instant-read added in the thickest section registers 165 degrees F. Move the chicken and slice on a cutting board.

- Meanwhile, put two spoons of oil, cumin, peppers, almonds, crushed red pepper in a food processor. Pulse it until creamy

- In a medium dish, mix olives, quinoa, two spoons of oil, and red onion. mix it well

- Divide the quinoa mixture into four bowls and finish with similar quantities of red pepper sauce, cucumber, and tomato to eat. Sprinkle with parsley and feta.

- Enjoy

Nutrition Per Serving: 219 calories| total fat 26.9g |carbohydrates 31.2g |protein

34.1g | Potassium 187 mg| Phosphorus 132 mg

4.9 Chicken& Quinoa Buddha Bowls

Ingredients

- Salt: ¼ tsp.
- Skinless chicken thighs: five boneless pieces' black pepper: half tsp.

Quinoa

- Light chicken broth: 3 cups
- Olive oil: 1 tbsp.
- Quinoa one and ½ cups
- Salt: ¼ tsp.

Italian Dressing

- Cloves of garlic: one large
- Olive oil: 1and ¾ cups
- Red-wine vinegar: ¾ cups
- Dijon mustard: one tbsp.
- Dried basil: 2 tsp.
- Honey: 1 and ½ tbsp.
- Dried oregano: 2 tsp.
- Ground pepper: ½ tsp.
- Water: 5 tbsp.
- Salt: ½ tsp.

Toppings

- 1 Can of chickpeas (15 ounces), rinsed
- Six radishes, sliced
- Toasted seeds /chopped nuts: ¼ cups
- Sprouts: one cup

Instructions

- For chicken preparation: Preheat oven to 425 degrees F. Put the chicken on a baking tray to roast with a half teaspoon of ground pepper and half a teaspoon of salt.
- Roast the chicken for 14 to 16 minutes, until the thickest section by an instant-read thermometer, registers 165 degrees F.
- Slice four thighs cooking quinoa: in a large saucepan, add broth, one tablespoon of oil, and 1/4 teaspoon of salt. Let it simmer on high heat.
- Switch to a boil and mix in the quinoa. Reduce heat and boil for 15 to 20 minutes, until the quinoa and the grains burst have drained all the moisture.
- Remove from heat, cover for 5 minutes, and let it sit. (Reserve two cups for further use.)
- For making dressing: In a mixer, add honey, vinegar, mustard, water, garlic, oregano, basil, pepper, and salt. Pulse till completely combine. Slowly add oil and puree until smooth, while the blender is still running.
- To make bowls: take four bowls and divide three cups worth of quinoa in them. Cover with chickpeas, chicken, and sprouts scatter with nuts—drizzle dressing of 3/4 cups.

Nutrition Per Serving: 250 calories| total fat 23g |carbohydrates 20.3g | protein 14.4g| Potassium 199 mg| Phosphorus 134 mg

4.10 Skillet Lemon Chicken & Potatoes with Kale

Ingredients

- Chopped tarragon: one tbsp.
- Boneless, skinless chicken thighs: one pound(trimmed)
- Ground pepper: half tsp. Divided

- Olive oil: 3 tbsp.

- Salt: half tsp. divided

- Light chicken broth: half cup

- Baby kale: 6 cups

- One lemon; sliced

- Four cloves of garlic(minced)

- Baby Yukon Gold potatoes: one pound; halved lengthwise(leached)

Instructions

- Let the oven pre-heat till 400 F

- In a large skillet, heat one tbsp. Of oil.

- Sprinkle with 1/4 teaspoon of salt and pepper on chicken. Cook, rotating once, before browning on both sides, a total of about 5 minutes. Move into a tray.

- Add 1/4 tsp. of salt and pepper to the pan with the remaining two teaspoons of oil, with potatoes.

- Cook potatoes, cut-side down, for around 3 minutes, until browned. Add lemon, broth, garlic, and tarragon. Bring the chicken back into the pan.

- Switch the frying pan to the oven.

- Roast, about 15 minutes, before the chicken is completely cooked and the potatoes are soft.

- Stir the kale into the mixture and roast for 3 to 4 minutes until it has wilted.

Nutrition per Serving: 347 Kcal| total fat 19.3g |carbohydrates 25.6g | protein 24.7g | Potassium 171 mg| Phosphorus 151 mg

4.11 Chicken Souvlaki Kebabs with Couscous

Ingredients

- Four minced garlic cloves

- Boneless, skinless chicken: one pound (breast halves, cut into half-inch strips)

- Dry white wine: 1/3 cup

- Lemon juice: ¼ cup

- Wedges of lemon

- Sliced fennel: 1 cup

- Olive oil: 3 tbsp.

- Salt: half tsp.

- Black pepper: ¼ tsp.

- Dried oregano: 2 tsp.

Couscous

- Large pearl couscous: half cup

- Water: 1 cup

- Dried tomatoes: half cup

- Olive oil: 1 tsp.

- Red sweet pepper: ¾ cup

- Chopped red onion: half cup

- Plain Greek yogurt: 1/3 cup

- Chopped cucumber: half cup

- Salt: ¼ tsp.

- Basil leaves: ¼ cup

- Fresh parsley: ¼ cup

- Lemon juice: one tbsp.

- Black pepper: ¼ tsp.

Instructions

- Making kabobs: In a resalable plastic bag, put the chicken and sliced fennel in a baking dish. For marinade, mix the white wine, lemon juice, oil, garlic, oregano, salt, and pepper mix in a cup. Remove the marinade about 1/4 cup, and put aside.

- Pour over the chicken mixture, the remaining marinade. Mix it in the bag. Marinate for 1 and half hours in the refrigerator, turning bag over, once.

- Meanwhile, soak eight 10- to 12-inch wooden skewers in water for half an hour. Drain the chicken and remove fennel and marinade—thread chicken on skewers, accordion-style.

- Grill skewers of chicken, covered, over medium-high heat for eight minutes or until the chicken is no longer pink keep turning 2, 3 times.

- With the reserved 1/4 cup of marinade, brush it on kabobs.

- Preparing the couscous: Pour one teaspoon of olive oil over medium heat in a saucepan. Cook and mix until light brown for about 4 minutes. Then add 1 cup of water. Let it boil on low flame.

- Simmer and cover for ten minutes, until couscous is soft and all the liquid is absorbed, adding the last 5 minutes of half cup snipped dried tomatoes; cool it down. The couscous is moved to a large bowl.

- Stir in the 3/4 cup of chopped red pepper, half cup of each chopped cucumber and chopped red onion, 1/3 cup simple fat-free Greek yogurt, 1/4 of a cup each sliced basil leaves and fresh parsley, one tablespoon of lemon juice, and 1/4 teaspoon of each fresh ground black pepper and salt

- Serve with couscous, lemon wedges, and basil leaves.

Nutrition Per Serving: 332 Kcal|total fat 9.4g |carbohydrates 27 g| protein 32.1g | Potassium 198.9 mg| Phosphorus 112 mg

4.12 Chicken and Snap Peas Stir Fry

Ingredients

- Skinless chicken breast: 1 and ¼ cups (sliced)

- Vegetable oil: 2 tbsp.

- Two minced garlic cloves

- Snap peas: 2 and ½ cups

- Black pepper and salt

- Cilantro: 3 tbsp. and for garnish

- One bunch of scallions (thinly sliced)

- Soy sauce, low sodium: 3 tbsp.

- One red bell pepper(sliced)

- Sriracha: 2 tsp.

- Sesame seeds:2 tbsp.

- Rice vinegar: 2 tbsp.

Instructions

- Heat the oil over medium flame in a large pan. Stir in the garlic and scallions, then sauté for around one minute until fragrant. Stir in the snap peas and bell pepper, then sauté for 2 to 3 minutes until soft.

- Add the chicken and cook for 4 to 5 minutes until golden and thoroughly cooked, and the vegetables are tender.

- Add the sesame seeds, soy sauce, rice vinegar, Sriracha, mix well to blend. Allow boiling the mixture for two minutes.

- Add the cilantro and garnish with coriander and sesame seeds. Serve hot

Nutrition Per serving: 228 calories|11g fat| 11g carbs|20g protein| Potassium 210 mg| Phosphorus 105 mg

4.13 Sheet-Pan Chicken Fajita Bowls

Ingredients

- Chicken tenders: 1 and ¼ pounds
- Chili powder: 2 tsp.
- Salt divided: ¾ tsp.
- Chopped steamed kale: 4 cups
- Ground pepper: ¼ tsp.
- Ground garlic: half tsp.
- Smoked paprika: half tsp.
- Ground cumin: 2 tsp.
- Olive oil: 2 tbsp.
- One red bell pepper, sliced
- One Can of black beans(15 ounces)
- Greek yogurt: ¼ cup
- Juice of lemon: 1 tsp.
- One green bell pepper, sliced
- Water: 2 tsp.
- One onion, sliced

Instructions

- Let the oven pre-heat till 425 F
- put the baking sheet in the oven
- in a big bowl, Combine half tsp of salt, chili powder, garlic powder, cumin. Paprika and pepper.
- Transfer 1 teaspoon from a mixture of spices to a small bowl, put it away. Stir one tablespoon of oil into the remaining spice blend.
- Add onion, bell peppers (red and green) to the chicken, stir to mix.
- Remove the pan from the oven cover with oil spray.
- Lay the chicken mixture into the pan in one layer—roast 15 minutes.
- In the meantime, mix the remaining 1/4 tsp of salt, oil with the kale and black beans. In a wide bowl, swirl to coat.
- Remove the frying pan from the oven. Stir the vegetables and chicken spread the beans kale uniformly.
- Roast 5 to 7 minutes more before the chicken is cooked through and the vegetables are ready.
- Add lime juice, water, and yogurt to the rest of the spice blend, mix well
- Take four bowls. Add the vegetables and chicken to bowls.
- Add yogurt dressing and serve hot.

Nutritional Per Serving: 243 calories| total fat 9.9g |carbohydrates 23.7g | protein 42.7g | Potassium 121 mg| Phosphorus 109 mg

4.14 Chicken with Red Bell Pepper Olive, & Feta Topping

Ingredients

- Half of a cup olive oil
- Four, skinless chicken breasts
- Half of a cup lemon juice
- Two tsp. of chopped garlic
- One cup of chopped red bell pepper
- 2 tsp. fresh oregano
- 1/3 of a cup sliced olives
- Black pepper and salt, to taste
- Half of a cup crumbled Feta cheese

Instructions

- Score the chicken breast from the top. But not to cut too far.

- Combine lemon juice, olive oil, oregano, and garlic.

- Take 1/4 cup of the mixture and then put aside

- Put chicken breast into a Ziploc bag and let it marinate in the refrigerator for at least an hour or as long as the whole day.

- Take the chicken out of the fridge when you are about to serve, and let it come to room temperature when cutting the olives and bell pepper.

- Mix the sliced pepper and olives, crumbled Feta, and the remaining marinade.

- Heat one teaspoon olive oil in a skillet over medium flame

- Take the chicken from the marinade and prepare for it to be cooked, scored side down in the skillet.

- Cook each side for about four minutes or completely cooked through

- Season the chicken with salt and black pepper fresh-ground to compare.

- Place chicken over the feta, tomato, and olive, on a platter. serve hot.

Nutrition Per Serving: 243 calories| total fat 9.9g |carbohydrates 23.7g | protein 42.7g | Potassium 129 mg| Phosphorus 98.9 mg

4.15 Roast Chicken with Turmeric & Fennel

Ingredients

- Six pieces of bone-in, skin-on chicken

- Half cup of olive oil

- Half cup of orange juice

- One lime juice

- Half-cup dry white wine

- honey: 3 tablespoon

- One tablespoon of garlic powder

- Yellow mustard: 2 tablespoon

- Turmeric: 3/4 tablespoon powder

- One teaspoon of ground coriander

- One teaspoon of sweet paprika

- One onion: sliced

- Fennel bulb: sliced

- 2 Oranges, peel on, sliced

- Salt and Pepper, to taste

- Lime slices(optional)

Instructions

- To make the marinade combine the white wine, olive oil, orange juice, honey, lime juice, and mustard in a bowl.

- Mix the spices in a small bowl: garlic powder, turmeric, paprika, coriander, pepper, and salt. To the liquid marinade, add approximately half of the spice blend. Mix it well

- With a paper towel, pat the chicken dry and season well with the remaining spice mix, rub the spice mix under the skin.

- In the large bowl of marinade, add the seasoned chicken and the remaining ingredients. cover with plastic wrap and refrigerate for two hours

- Let the oven pre-heat to 475F. Move the chicken to a large baking pan and the marinade and everything else; make sure the chicken's skin faces upwards. Sprinkle with a splash of salt and brown sugar,

- Let it bake for 45 minutes until the chicken is cooked through
- Serve hot

Nutrition per serving: Kcal 243| fat 18 g| Carbs 20.8 g| Protein 22 g| Potassium 150 mg| Phosphorus 111 mg

4.16 Roasted Pork Tenderloin with Vegetables & Quinoa

Ingredients

- Italian Dressing
- Olive oil: 1 and ¾ cup
- Sugar: 1 and ½ tbsp.
- Dried basil: 2 tsp.
- Dijon mustard: 1 tbsp.
- Clove garlic: one large
- Dried oregano: 2 tsp.
- Red-wine vinegar: ¾ cup
- Salt & ground pepper: half tsp. each
- Water: 5 tbsp.

Pork & Vegetables

- Olive oil: 3 tbsp.
- Pork tenderloin: one pound
- Parsnips: 2 medium
- Broccoli crown: 1 medium
- Carrots: four small
- Salt: ¾ tsp.
- Ground pepper: ¾ tsp.
- Italian seasoning: 2 tsp.
- Balsamic glaze: 4 tbsp.
- Quinoa: cooked in chicken broth and cooled

Instructions

- For making dressing: in a mixer, add sugar, vinegar, water, mustard, basil, garlic, oregano, pepper, and salt. Pulse till creamy.
- Slowly add oil and pulse until smooth, while the processor is running. reserve 2 tbsp. of dressing aside
- To cook pork & vegetables: In a wide sealable container, put pork and 1/4 cup of dressing. Take out air and seal rub the sauce all over the pork.
- Keep cool in the refrigerator for as long as you like.
- In the upper and lower thirds of the oven, put racks; let the oven preheat to 425F
- Peel the carrots, then parsnips, then cut into one-inch pieces.
- Cut the broccoli into florets. Add 2 tsp of oil, Italian seasoning, and half tsp. Each and salt and pepper to the vegetables. Place over a broad baking sheet,
- Take out the pork from the marinade and use paper towels to pat dry. Sprinkle the pork with and pepper. Heat one tablespoon of oil over medium flame.
- Add the pork and roast for 3 to 5 minutes, until browned. Switch over the pork and then move the pan to the upper rack. Place the vegetables on the shelf below.
- Roast the pork roughly for 20 minutes with an instant-read thermometer added into the thickest section registers145 degrees F.
- Roast the vegetables for 20 to 25 minutes, turning once or twice, until soft and browned in patches.

- Move the pork to a clean cutting board, and give 5 minutes to rest. Toss away the vegetables with the remaining two spoons of dressing.
- Slice the pork and serve with the quinoa, grilled vegetables, and over balsamic glaze drizzled.

Nutrition Per Serving: Kcal 490 | total fat 21.7g |carbohydrates 44.3g | protein 31g| Potassium 280 mg| Phosphorus 205 mg

4.17 Grilled Lemon Herb Chicken Salad

Ingredients

- Lemon-Herb Chicken
- Boneless, chicken breasts: 6 cups(skinless)
- Chopped fresh dill: 1 tablespoon
- Extra-virgin olive oil: 3 tablespoons
- Chopped fresh oregano: 1 tablespoon
- Kosher salt and freshly ground black pepper
- Juice of 2 lemons, and zest
- Chopped fresh parsley: 3 tablespoons

Salad

- Chicken broth: 2 and a ½ cups
- Barley: 1 cup
- Juice of 1 lemon and zest
- ⅓ of a cup extra-virgin olive oil
- One halved red onion, thinly sliced
- mustard: 1 tablespoon
- 2 heads of red-leaf lettuce, diced
- Dried oregano: 1 teaspoon
- Kosher salt and freshly ground black pepper

Instructions

- To make Lemon Herb Chicken Put the chicken inside a large plastic sealed plastic bag. In a bowl, add lemon juice, olive oil, dill, lemon zest, parsley, and oregano and mix well.
- Then pour this marinade into the sealed bag, seal, and chill for almost half an hour.
- To make the salad: in the meantime, put the chicken broth and barley over medium flame in a saucepan and let it simmer.
- Cover the pot and steam until the barley is soft for almost 30- 45 minutes. Drain and set it aside.
- Mix the oregano lemon juice, lemon zest, and mustard in a bowl, then slowly drizzle in the olive oil and mix properly. Add salt and pepper to taste.
- Let your grill pre-heat at high. Take chicken out from marinade and sprinkle with freshly ground black pepper and salt.
- Grill chicken on each side until charred and completely cooked through, cook for almost ten minutes, flipping as required, take the chicken from the grill and set it aside.
- In a big bowl, mix the onion, and lettuce, drizzle the dressing and coat well.
- Cut the chicken into slices, and serve

Nutrition per serving: 309 calories|15g fat |4g carbs|31g protein| Potassium 134 mg| Phosphorus 121 mg

4.18 Greek Chicken & Rice Skillet

Ingredients

- Green olives: 1 cup
- 6 pieces of chicken thighs
- Chicken broth: 2 and a ½ cups
- Long-grain rice: 1 cup
- Dried oregano: 1 teaspoon
- Garlic powder: 1 teaspoon
- Three lemons
- Extra-virgin olive oil: 2 tablespoons
- Half red onion, chopped
- 2 cloves of minced garlic
- ⅓ of a cup fresh chopped fresh parsley
- Chopped fresh oregano: 1 tablespoon (more for garnishing)
- Kosher salt and freshly ground black pepper

Instructions

- Let the oven pre-heat to 375°F.
- Add salt and pepper to chicken thighs, adjust the seasoning. mix garlic powder, dried oregano, zest of one lemon in a small mixing bowl, rub this mixture on chicken thighs generously
- In a wide skillet, heat the olive oil over medium flame. Put the meat, skin side down, then sear for nine minutes until the meat turns light brown. Move to the plate and set aside.
- Add the garlic and onion in the pan, and sauté for around five minutes until opaque. Add the rice and sauté for one minute; then season with salt.
- Add the broth and let it boil then slow to simmer. Add the zest and lemon juice, oregano. Cut two slices for later.

- Put the chicken skin side down into the rice. Put the skillet to pre-heated oven till all the broth is absorbed, and chicken is thoroughly cooked, for almost 25 minutes.
- Now turn the broiler, and put the lemon slices on the chicken. Broil until the lemons are finely crispy, and the chicken skin is also crispy, flor almost three minutes.
- Then add the olives over the lemon slices, top with parsley leaves, and serve hot.

Nutrition per serving: 703 calories|34 g fat|32 g carbs|38g protein| Potassium 183 mg| Phosphorus 111 mg

4.19 Pesto Chicken Salad

Ingredients

- Packed coarsely chopped arugula: One cup
- Half of a cup nonfat plain Greek yogurt
- Lemon juice: 2 teaspoons
- Half of a teaspoon salt
- ⅓ of a cup mayonnaise
- Chopped or shredded cooked chicken: 3 cups
- Half of a cup cherry tomatoes halved
- Pesto: 2 tablespoons
- Toasted pine nuts: 3 tablespoons
- Half of a teaspoon freshly ground black pepper
- Minced shallot: 2 tablespoons

Instructions

- In a big mixing bowl, add yogurt, shallot, mayonnaise, freshly ground black pepper, salt pesto, and lemon juice.

- Then add in the chicken, tomatoes, and arugula.

- Garnish with pine nuts.

- Chill in refrigerator until cold for two hours. Or serve at room temperature.

Nutrition per serving: 209 calories| total fat 15.7g |carbohydrates 3.4g | protein 13g

4.20 Edamame & Chicken Greek Salad

Ingredients

- One and half cups of frozen shelled edamame thawed

- Boneless skinless(trimmed)chicken breast: one piece

- ¼ of a cup red-wine vinegar

- Chopped romaine: 8 cups

- ¼ of a cup sliced red onion

- Extra-virgin olive oil: 3 tablespoons

- ¼ of a teaspoon salt

- Half of a European cucumber, sliced

- Half of a cup crumbled feta cheese

- ¼ of a cup sliced fresh basil

- ¼ of a teaspoon freshly ground black pepper

Instructions

- In a large saucepan, add chicken and add cover it by water by 2 inches. Let it boil. Lower the heat and let it simmer and cook. Check with an instant-read thermometer add into the chicken. It should show 165 degrees F after cooking for 15 minutes.

- Move the chicken to a clean cutting surface and cool it for five minutes. With a fork, shred it, or chop into pieces.

- In the meantime, add kosher salt, freshly ground black pepper, vinegar, oil in a big mixing bowl. Then Add romaine, edamame, feta, onion, cucumber, basil, and the chicken. Toss well.

- Serve right away.

Nutrition per serving: 336 calories| total fat 21.6g |carbohydrates 14.2g |protein 22.3g| Potassium 111 mg| Phosphorus 78 mg

4.21 One Pot Greek Chicken and Lemon Rice

Ingredients

- Chicken marinade

- Lemon juice: 4 tbsp.

- Five pieces of chicken thighs, bone-in, skin-on: one kg

- Zest of 2 lemons

- 4 cloves of minced garlic

- Half tsp of kosher salt

- Dried oregano: 1 tbsp.

Rice

- Chicken broth or stock: 1 and half cups

- Olive oil: 1 and half tbsp. separated

- Long-grain rice: 1 cup, uncooked

- Freshly ground Black pepper

- 3/4 of a cup water

- Dried oregano: 1 tbsp.

- One small onion, finely chopped

- ¾ of a tsp kosher salt

For Garnish

- Finely chopped parsley or oregano

- Lemon zest should be fresh

Instructions

- In a reseal able plastic bag, add the chicken and marinade ingredients and mix well. Set it aside for 20 minutes, for the minimum or preferably overnight.

- Let the oven preheat to 350°F.

- Heat half tbsp. Of olive oil over medium-high heat in a deep skillet.

- Put the chicken skin side down, cook till golden brown, and then flip and cook on the other side. Take chicken out from skillet and set it aside.

- Clean the skillet and put skillet again on the flame.

- Heat one tbsp. of extra virgin olive oil over medium flame in the skillet. Add onion and cook until transparent, for three minutes.

- Add the remaining ingredients for Rice and the Marinade reserve.

- Let the liquid boil and then let it simmer for 30 seconds.

- Put the chicken on top of the rice, then cover the skillet. Let it bake for 35 minutes after removing the cover and bake for another ten minutes, or until all the moisture is absorbed and the rice is soft.

- Remove from the oven and, if necessary, allow to rest for ten minutes before serving, garnished with oregano parsley and fresh lemon zest.

Nutrition per serving: Calories 323|fat 21g| carbs 33g|protein 18g| Potassium 220 mg| Phosphorus 105 mg

4.22 Greek Cauliflower Rice Bowls with Grilled Chicken

Ingredients

- Boneless, skinless: 4 cups of chicken breasts

- Cauliflower rice: 4 cups

- Extra-virgin olive oil: 7 tablespoons divided

- ⅓ of cup diced red onion

- Feta cheese(crumbled) :2 tablespoons

- Half cup of sliced fresh dill, divided

- Lemon juice: 3 tablespoons

- Oregano: 1 teaspoon (dried)

- ¾ of teaspoon kosher salt, divided

- Diced cucumber: One cup

- For garnish Lemon wedges

- Half teaspoon freshly ground black pepper, divided

Instructions

- Let the grill preheat on high.

- In a wide skillet over medium flame, add extra virgin olive oil (two tbsp.), add 1/4 teaspoon of salt, cauliflower, and onion. Stir often and let it cook. Cauliflower will become tender after cooking for five minutes. Turn off the heat and add 1/4 cup of dill. Set it aside.

- Rub one tbsp. of olive oil all over the chicken. Add 1/4 teaspoon of freshly ground black pepper and 1/4 teaspoon of salt over chicken.

- Grill it for about 15 minutes, and add an instant-read thermometer into the thickest part of the chicken should read 165 degrees F.

- Then, in a medium mixing bowl, add four tablespoons of oil, oregano, lemon juice, and 1/4 teaspoon of each salt and pepper and mix well.

- In four serving bowls, add cauliflower rice and add chicken slices, feta, cucumber, and 1/4 cup of dill.
- Garnish with lemon wedges, serve right away and enjoy.

Nutrition per serving: 411 calories| total fat 27.5g |carbohydrates 19.5g |protein 29g| Potassium 145 mg| Phosphorus 106 mg

4.23 Zucchini Noodles with Pesto & Chicken

Ingredients

- Boneless, skinless: 4 cups of chicken breast, cut into bite-size pieces
- 1/4 cup extra-virgin olive oil and two tablespoons more
- Four pieces of trimmed medium-large zucchini
- ¼ of cup shredded Parmesan cheese
- Fresh basil (packed) leaves: 2 cups
- Lemon juice: 2 tablespoons
- One large clove of chopped garlic
- ¼ of cup toasted pine nuts
- Half teaspoon of freshly ground black pepper
- ¾ of teaspoon kosher salt, divided

Instructions

- Cut the zucchini in length into big, thin strands, utilizing a spiral vegetable slicer. Chops these long noodles so the strands would not be very long. Put the zucchini in a colander, and add 1/4 teaspoon of salt. Let it drain for almost half an hour, then press gently to extract any remaining moisture.
- In a food processor bowl, add Parmesan, basil, 1/4 teaspoon of salt, pine nuts, 1/4 cup of olive oil, black pepper, lemon juice, and garlic, and pulse on high until smooth
- Put a wide skillet over medium flame, add one tbsp. of oil. Add chicken in an even layer then add 1/4 teaspoon of salt.
- Let it cook, often stirring, for about 5 minutes. Then Transfer to a bowl and stir in three tablespoons of the pesto.
- To the pan, add the remaining one tablespoon of olive oil. Then Add the dried zucchini noodles mix carefully for two-three minutes.
- Add these noodles to the bowl with the cooked chicken. Add the leftover pesto and toss lightly to coat.

Nutrition per serving: 430 calories| total fat 31.6g | carbohydrates 9.4g |fiber 2.5g | protein 28.6g| Potassium 187 mg| Phosphorus 143 mg

4.24 Slow Cooker Mediterranean Chicken

Ingredients

- Boneless skinless chicken breasts: 4 pieces' medium to large
- Kosher salt, to taste
- Freshly ground black pepper, To taste
- Italian seasoning: 3 teaspoons
- Juice of one large lemon: 2 tablespoons approx.
- Minced garlic: one tbsp.
- One medium onion, diced
- Roasted red peppers: 1 cup (roughly chopped)
- Capers: 2 tablespoons

- Fresh basil, thyme, and oregano for garnish

Instructions

- Put a wide skillet over medium flame, add chicken seasoned with salt and ground black pepper, and cook for two minutes. Both sides will be browned. Then add chicken to the slow cooker. Make sure to grease it before adding chicken.

- Add red peppers, capers, and onions to slow cooker. Put them on the side of chicken, not over chicken.

- In the meanwhile, mix lemon juice, garlic, and Italian seasoning. Pout it all over the chicken.

- Cover it and cook for two hours on high and four hours on low.

- Garnish with oregano, fresh thyme, and basil.

- Serve right away and enjoy.

Nutrition per serving: 304 calories| total fat 20.9g |carbohydrates 23.6g | |protein 19.9g| Potassium 187 mg| Phosphorus 121 mg

4.25 Spiced Pan-Roasted Chicken with Olives, Figs, and Mint

Ingredients

- Chicken broth: 1 cup

- Chicken: one whole

- Ground coriander: 1 tablespoon

- ⅛ of a teaspoon cayenne

- Fresh lemon juice: 2 tablespoons

- Kosher or sea salt: 1 tablespoon

- Eight figs: dried, roughly diced

- Extra-virgin olive oil: ¼ cup

- ¼ of teaspoon ground cinnamon

- Roughly chopped green olives: 2 tablespoons (roughly diced)

- Chopped mint: 1 tablespoon, extra more for garnish

Instructions

- Remove the backbone of chicken with kitchen shears and flatten with your hands

- In a mixing bowl, add coriander, salt, two tablespoons of olive oil, cayenne, and cinnamon.

- Rub this spice blend all over the chicken and put the chicken skin side up in the fridge, do not cover, for 4-24 hours.

- Let the oven pre-heat to 400F.

- To an oven-safe sauté pan add two tablespoons of olive oil and heat over medium flame until hot. Then add chicken. It should be skin side down and cook until golden brown.

- Put in the preheated oven, and cook for half an hour.

- Flip the chicken, then add mint, lemon juice, both types of olives, chicken broth, and figs to the oven-safe pan and let it cook in the oven for an hour an hour more internal temperature with instant-read thermometer reaches 165°.

- When chicken is cooked through, top with thinly sliced mint.

- Transfer the chicken to a clean surface and cut in slices

- To a serving plate, put the chicken and put pan drizzling on top, garnish with olives, figs mix.

- Serve right away and enjoy.

Nutrition per serving: 501 calories| total fat 36g| protein 34g.| carbs 23 g| Potassium 145 mg| Phosphorus 102 mg

4.26 Chicken Caprese Sandwich

Ingredients

- Extra virgin olive oil: 4 tablespoons, or more, divided
- Half lemon juiced
- ¼ cup of sliced fresh basil leaves
- Kosher salt and freshly ground black pepper
- One log of fresh mozzarella cheese of 8 ounces, sliced into rounds (1/4 thickness)
- Skinless: 2 pieces of boneless chicken breasts
- Fresh parsley: 1 teaspoon(sliced)
- One loaf of ten ounces, sourdough bread, cut in half lengthwise
- Balsamic glaze or balsamic vinegar, to taste

Instructions

- In a big mixing bowl, add parsley, black pepper, two tablespoons of extra virgin olive oil, salt, lemon juice, mix it well. Pour this over chicken breasts and toss lightly to coat well and let the chicken rest at room temperature.
- Put a grilling pan over medium heat. Add the chicken breast to the grilling pan, without the marinade, and add black pepper and salt. Flip the chicken after four minutes.
- Cook for three minutes more, till grill marks, appear.
- Lower the flame, and cover the chicken and cook till the instant-read thermometer reads 185 degrees.
- Turn off the heat and slice the chicken, and set it aside.
- Pour one tablespoon of extra-virgin olive oil to each side of the bread and grill it until golden brown.
- Slice the bread into three slices for each half. Add 3-4 slices of chicken, few slices of mozzarella cheese to each slice. Pour balsamic vinegar, extra virgin olive oil on top. Add basil leaves on top.
- Season with more salt and black pepper.
- Serve hot

Nutrition per serving: calories 321 g| Fat 32.06g|Carbohydrates 46.88g|Protein 34.42g| Potassium 210 mg| Phosphorus 125 mg

4.27 Smothered Pork Chops & Sautéed Greens

Ingredients

Smothered Pork Chops

- Flour: 1 cup + 2 tablespoons
- Six pork loin chops
- Paprika: 2 teaspoons
- Half cup of olive oil
- Onion powder: 2 teaspoons
- Half cup fresh scallions
- Black pepper: 1 tablespoon
- Garlic powder: 2 teaspoons
- Beef stock, low-sodium: 2 cups
- 1 and a half cups of sliced onions

Sautéed Greens

- Unsalted butter: 1 tablespoon
- Fresh collard greens: 8 cups, blanched and chopped

- Onions: ¼ cup, diced

- Garlic: 1 tablespoon, diced

- Black pepper: 1 teaspoon

- Crushed red pepper flakes: 1 teaspoon

- Olive oil: 2 tablespoons

Instructions

- Let the oven preheat to 350° F.

- For Pork Chops, Mix onion powder, black pepper, garlic powder, and paprika. Rub half of the mixture on both sides of the pork chops and combine the other half with one cup of flour.

- Coat the pork chops with the flour mix

- In a Dutch oven, heat oil on medium-high

- Brown the pork chops for 2 to 4 minutes on every side.

- Take out from pan and reserve two tbsp. Of oil,

- Sauté onions 4–6 minutes or until translucent. Add in two tbsp. of flour and mix with onion for one minute

- Gradually add the stock and mix until thickened.

- Add pork chops to the pan and coat with sauce. Cover with foil and cook in the oven at 350° F for 30-45 minutes.

- Take out from the oven and let rest for ten minutes

- For Sautéed Greens, In a pan, melt butter on medium-high heat. Add garlic and onions for 4 to 6 minutes

- Add greens and sprinkle with red pepper and black and cook for 5 to 8 minutes on high flame. Keep mixing.

- Serve right away

  Nutrition per serving: Cal 464|fat 28g|cholesterol 71 mg| protein 27 g| phosphorous 289 mg| potassium 604 mg

4.28 One-Pot Chicken & Dumplings

Ingredients

- Parsley: 1 tablespoon

- Cold unsalted butter: 5 tablespoons, divided

- One stalk of celery sliced

- Two carrots, diced

- One onion, minced

- All-purpose flour: 1 and 1/4 cup, divided

- Diced cooked chicken: 1 to 2 cups

- Green beans: 1/3 pound, cut into one-inch pieces

- Half tsp of thyme

- One bay leaf

- Chicken broth, low sodium: 3 cups

- Celery seed: 1/4 tsp

- Half tsp of rosemary

- Baking powder substitute: 1 teaspoon

- Three drops of sriracha sauce

- Pepper to taste

- Half cup of almond milk

- Chopped parsley: 2 tablespoons

Instructions

- In a pan, melt three tbsp. of butter sauté carrots, onion, and celery, cook until translucent for four minutes.

- Add 1/4 cup of flour cook for one minute. Add broth, keep mixing, let it boil, lower the heat and simmer for five minutes. Add in spices, chicken, and green beans.

- Take 2 tablespoons parsley, baking powder, one cup of flour, ½ tsp. of salt(optional), add two tbsp. of butter, almond milk mix.

- Add this mixture to the chicken, cover it, and let it simmer for 12 minutes.

- Serve right away

Nutrients Per Serving: Calories 230| Total Fat 10.3g| Cholesterol 27.1mg| Sodium 145.8mg| Total Carbohydrate 30.2g| Dietary Fiber 4.3g| Protein 5.2g| Iron 2.6mg| Potassium 455.3mg| Phosphorus 226.6mg

4.29 Easy Crispy Lemon Chicken

Ingredients

- Herb seasoning blend: 1 teaspoon

- Cooked white rice: 4 cups

- Half cup of all-purpose white flour

- One-pound chicken breasts (skinless and boneless), cut into slices

- Black pepper: 1/4 teaspoon

- One large egg white

- Salt: 1/4 teaspoon

- Half cup of lemon juice

- Water: 2 teaspoons

- Olive oil: 2 tablespoons

Instructions

- Season the chicken with herbs, pepper, and salt.

- In a bowl, whisk the egg white with water

- Coat chicken in egg white mix then in flour.

- Fry chicken in olive oil until light brown, but do not overcook the chicken

- Add lemon juice on top and serve.

Nutrients per serving: Calories 316| protein 22 g| Carbohydrates 39 g| Fat 8 g| Cholesterol 82 mg| sodium 144 mg| Potassium 234 mg| Phosphorus 201 mg| Calcium 28 mg| Fiber 0.8 g

4.30 Grilled Pineapple Chicken

Ingredients

- Chicken breast: 1-1/4 pound, skinless and bone-in

- Dry sherry: 1 cup

- Soy sauce, reduced-sodium: 1 tablespoon

- Four rings of pineapple

- Pineapple juice: 1 cup

Instructions

- In a zip lock bag, add all ingredients except for pineapple.

- Marinate it overnight in the refrigerator.

- Grill the marinated chicken for 15-20 minutes until cooked.

- In the last few minutes of cooking, grill pineapple for two minutes on each side. Serve with chicken breast.

Nutrients per serving: Calories 211| Protein 26 g| Carbohydrates 20 g| Fat 3 g| Cholesterol 67 mg| Sodium 215 mg| Potassium 376 mg| Phosphorus 198 mg| Calcium 21 mg| Fiber 0.5 g

4.31 Sheet Pan Chicken with Green Beans & Cauliflower

Ingredients

- One and 1/3 cups of frozen green beans
- Cauliflower floret: one and a half cups
- 2 cups of chicken strips, raw
- Italian dressing: 1 tablespoon
- Olive oil: 1 teaspoon
- Unsalted butter: 4 tablespoons

Instructions

- Let the oven preheat to 400° F.
- Toss cauliflower in one tsp. of olive oil.
- Spray a baking tray with cooking spray.
- Add the strips of chicken on 1/3 of the tray. Place the cauliflower down on the other 1/3 of the pan. Add frozen beans to the tray also.
- Melt butter and pour over the cauliflower, green beans, and chicken. Add Italian seasoning over all the tray.
- Bake for 20-30 minutes. Check them after 20 minutes and serve.

Nutrients per serving: Calories 330| Protein 25 g| Carbohydrates 19 g| Fat 17 g| Cholesterol 102 mg| Sodium 308 mg| Potassium 545 mg| Phosphorus 280 mg| Calcium 47 mg| Fiber 2.5 g

4.32 Pulled Pork

Ingredients

- Oil: 1 tablespoon
- One cup of minced onion
- 3 cloves of minced garlic
- 4 pounds of pork shoulder roast (boneless), cut in cubes, trimmed fat
- Worcestershire sauce: 2 and a half tablespoons
- Ketchup: half cup, no salt added
- Honey: 3 tablespoons
- Red wine vinegar: 3 tablespoons
- Liquid smoke: 1 teaspoon
- Half teaspoon of black pepper
- Orange-flavored drink, sugar-free: 1 cup

Instructions

- In a skillet in oil, cook onion, garlic, and pork for five minutes. Keep stirring.
- Add the rest of the ingredients and mix well. Let it boil, then simmer on low flame while being covered for one hour.
- Uncover it and cook for half an hour, till the liquid has evaporated.
- Shred the pork with two forks. Serve.

Nutrients per serving: Calories 233| Protein 22 g| Carbohydrates 7 g| Fat 13 g| Cholesterol 77 mg| Sodium 104 mg| Potassium 365 mg| phosphorus 197 mg| Calcium 21 mg| Fiber 0.1 g

4.33 Roast Pork with Apples

Ingredients

- Tart apple: 5 cups, sliced and peeled
- 3-pound of boneless, trimmed pork loin roast
- One slice of diced maple bacon
- Cider vinegar: 2 tablespoons
- Onion: 2 cups, chopped
- Black pepper: 1/4 teaspoon
- Green cabbage: 3 cups, sliced
- Four carrots, cut into large chunks

- Dry white wine: 3/4 cup
- Maple syrup: 2 tablespoons

Instructions

- Let the oven preheat to 375° F.
- In a Dutch oven, spray with cooking spray over medium-high heat, cook pork for 15 minutes, brown it on all sides. Take the pork out.
- Add bacon and onion to the pan, sauté for five minutes, or until tender.
- Add the pork to the pan, then add carrots, apples, and cabbage, the rest of the ingredients, let it simmer. Put the pan in the oven.
- Cook uncovered for 45 minutes at 375 F
- Turn the pork over, cook for half an hour.
- The internal temperature of pork should be 155° F.

Nutrients per serving: Calories 244| Protein 30 g| Carbohydrates 13 g| Fat 8 g| Cholesterol 68 mg| Sodium 99 mg| Potassium 538 mg| Phosphorus 185 mg| Calcium 48 mg| Fiber 3.1 g

4.34 Lemon Rosemary Pork

Ingredients

- Chicken broth, low-sodium: 1/4 cup
- All-purpose white flour: 2 tablespoons
- 1 pound of pork cutlets
- Half teaspoon of pepper
- Olive oil: 2 teaspoons
- Fresh rosemary: 1 tablespoon, chopped
- One cup lemon juice

Instructions

- In a zip lock bag, mix pepper and flour. Add pork and coat well
- Heat oil, cook pork for 2-3 minutes, on each side over medium-high heat.
- It should not be pink in the middle. Check with a sharp knife.
- Take out in plate keep warm with foil.
- In a skillet, add chicken broth, rosemary, and lemon juice. Let it boil for 3-4 minutes.
- Pour sauce over pork and serve.

Nutrients per serving: Calories 228| Protein 24 g| Carbohydrates 8 g| Fat 10 g| Cholesterol 69 mg| Sodium 51 mg| Potassium 378 mg| Phosphorus 160 mg| Calcium 18 mg| Fiber 0.5 g

4.35 Baked Pork Chops

Ingredients

- Unsalted margarine: 2 tablespoons
- Half cup of all-purpose flour
- Water: 1/4 cup
- Cornflake crumbs: 3/4 cup
- One large egg white
- Six pork chops: center cut
- Salt: 1/4 teaspoon
- Paprika: 1 teaspoon

Instructions

- Let the oven preheat to 350 °F.
- In a bowl, add flour.
- In a bowl, whisk water and egg. Add cornflake crumbs to another plate
- Coat pork chops in flour, then in egg, then in cornflakes.

- Put pork on a baking sheet, spray with oil, pour melted margarine
- Season with salt and paprika, chill in the fridge for one hour or more.
- Bake for 40 minutes or until cooked.
- Serve.

Nutrients per serving: Calories 282| Protein 23 g| carbohydrates 25 g| Fat 10 g| Cholesterol 95 mg| Sodium 263 mg| Potassium 394 mg| Phosphorus 203 mg| Calcium 28 mg| Fiber 1.4 g

4.36 Pork Fajitas

Ingredients

- Dried oregano: 1 teaspoon
- One green bell pepper, sliced
- One onion, sliced
- Pineapple juice: 2 tablespoons
- 2 cloves of garlic
- 4 flour tortillas
- Olive oil: 1 tablespoon
- Boneless pork: 1 pound, lean, cut into strips
- Half teaspoon of cumin
- Hot pepper sauce: 1/4 teaspoon
- 2 tbsp. of vinegar

Instructions

- In a big zip lock bag, add pineapple juice, hot sauce, oregano, vinegar, garlic, and cumin. Add pork into it and marinate for 10-15 minutes
- Let the oven preheat to 325° F.
- Heat the tortillas in foil.
- In a skillet, sauté green pepper, onion, pork in oil until pork is no longer pink for five minutes
- Serve with warm tortillas.

Nutrients per serving: Calories 406| Protein 26 g| Carbohydrates 34 g| Fat 18 g| cholesterol 64 mg| Sodium 376 mg| Potassium 483 mg| Phosphorus 267 mg| Calcium 57 mg| Fiber 2.4 g

4.37 Herb-Rubbed Pork Tenderloin

Ingredients

- One and a half tablespoons vegetable oil
- Dried rosemary: 1 teaspoon
- Dried parsley: 1 teaspoon
- Dried thyme: 1 teaspoon
- 2 cloves of minced garlic
- Dried basil: 1 teaspoon
- Black pepper: 2 teaspoons
- 2 pork tenderloins
- Dijon mustard: 2 tablespoons

Instructions

- In a bowl, add spices, garlic, mustard, mix well.
- Rub this mix over tenderloins—marinade for two hours.
- Let the oven preheat to 400° F.
- In a skillet in oil, brown the tenderloins, then place it on a baking dish.
- Bake t for 20 minutes or until the meat thermometer shows 160° F.
- Let it rest for 10-15 minutes before serving.

Nutrients per serving: Calories 178| Protein 24 g| Carbohydrates 1 g| Fat 8 g| Cholesterol 67 mg| Sodium 160 mg| Potassium 401 mg| Phosphorus 230 mg| Calcium 20 mg| Fiber 0.4 g

4.38 Dumplings Divine

Ingredients

Filling

- Ginger: 1 Tbsp., chopped
- 2 cups of ground pork
- Soy sauce, low-sodium: 2 Tbsp.
- Cabbage: 1 cup, thinly sliced
- Dough
- All-purpose flour: 2 cups
- Water: 3/4 cup

Sauce

- Balsamic vinegar: 1 Tbsp.
- Green onion: 1 Tbsp.
- Olive oil: 1 Tbsp.

Instructions

- To prepare the filling, mix pork, cabbage, ginger, and soy sauce. Keep in the fridge.
- In another bowl, mix flour with water. Knead until dough forms.
- Make one inch balls from the dough, flatten them and add one tbsp. of filling.
- Seal the edges with water. Pinch them as you like.
- In a large pot, boil the water and add dumplings. Cook for 10 to 15 minutes. And serve with sauce

Nutrients per serving: (5 dumplings): Cal 310| Total Fat 17.2g| Cholesterol 52.4mg| Sodium 142.8mg| Total Carbohydrate 20.5g| Dietary Fiber 0.9g|Protein 16.9g| Iron 2.1mg| Potassium 411.3mg| Phosphorus 196.2mg

4.39 Sweet N' Sour Meatballs

- 1.5 cups of chopped vegetables
- 8 cups of ground meat pork
- 1/4 tsp of nutmeg
- 2 cups of cooked rice
- Low sodium soy sauce: 1 Tbsp.
- Worcestershire sauce, low sodium: 1 Tbsp.
- 1/4 cup of unsweetened almond milk
- 2 tsp of garlic powder
- Half cup of finely diced onion

Sweet and Sour Sauce

- Pineapple juice: 2 cups
- Soy sauce, reduced-sodium: 2 tablespoons
- Half tsp sesame seed oil
- Vinegar: 1/3 cup
- Cornstarch: 6 tablespoons
- 5 cups of pineapple chunks, canned
- Water: 2/3 cup
- Honey: half and a little more cup

Instructions

- Let the oven preheat to 375° F.
- Chop the vegetables.
- Mix chopped vegetables, meat, rice, pepper, garlic powder, soy sauce, Worcestershire sauce, nutmeg. Mix well. Do not over mix.
- Make one inch balls and put them on a baking sheet
- Bake for 10-15 minutes.
- Pour the juice out of pineapple cans, add water in the juice to make two cups.
- Mix starch with sesame seed oil, honey, pineapple juice, soy sauce, water, and vinegar.
- Heat until becomes thick, mix constantly. Turn off the heat.

- Add pineapple chunks, bell peppers, meatballs, and sauce, heat on low until serving time.

Nutrient per serving (2 meatballs): Calories: 123 g| Protein 11.2 g| Carbohydrates: 15.3 g| Fiber: 1.8 g| Total Fat: 3 g| Sodium: 105 mg| Phosphorus: 78 mg| Potassium: 77 mg| 3

4.40 Honey-Garlic Low Sodium Marinated Kebabs

Ingredients

- Bragg's Liquid Amino: 1/4 cup
- 1/4 cup of olive oil
- 3 cloves of crushed garlic cloves
- Four medium chicken breast cut into cubes
- 1/3 cup of honey
- Four small onions, cut into cubes
- Black pepper: 1/4 tsp
- Three peppers, cut into cubes

Instructions

- In a zip lock bag, add all ingredients except for onion, peppers.
- Marinate for half an hour or more (overnight)
- Add on skewers alternate with pepper and onion.
- Grill until done.

Nutrients per serving: Calories 143| Total Fat 2.1g| Cholesterol 41.4mg | Sodium 137.4mg| Total Carbohydrate 17.9g| Dietary Fiber 1.4g| Protein 13.9g| Iron 0.5mg| Potassium 447.7mg| Phosphorus 145.5mg

4.41 Hawaiian-Style Slow-Cooked Pulled Pork

Ingredients

- Half teaspoon of garlic powder
- 4 pounds of pork roast
- Half teaspoon of paprika
- 2 tablespoons of liquid smoke
- Onion powder: 1 teaspoon
- Half teaspoon of black pepper

Instructions

- In a bowl, add garlic powder, black pepper, onion, and paprika.
- Run this spice mix on pork. Add pork in a slow cooker. Add liquid smoke
- Add water to half of the slow cooker. Cook on high for 4 to 5 hours.
- Shred with fork and serve

Nutrition Per Serving: Calories 285 | total Fat 21 g| Saturated Fat 7 g| Trans Fat 0 g| Cholesterol 83 mg| Sodium 54 mg| Carbohydrates 1 g| Protein 20 g| Phosphorus 230 mg| Potassium 380 mg| Dietary Fiber 0 g| Calcium 9 mg

4.42 Spicy Grilled Pork Chops with Peach Glaze

Ingredients

- Smoked paprika: 1 teaspoon
- 8 pork chops, center-cut
- Cilantro: 2 tablespoons
- Lime juice: ¼ cup
- Peach preserves: 1 cup
- Zest of one lime
- Half teaspoon of black pepper
- Dried onion flakes: 2 teaspoons
- Soy sauce, low-sodium: 1 tablespoon
- Half teaspoon of red pepper flakes
- Olive oil: ¼ cup

Instructions

- Heat the grill on high.

- In a bowl, add all ingredients except for pork chops, mix well.

- Take out a quarter of the mix and add the rest of it in a zip lock bag with pork chops overnight.

- Grill them for 6 to 8 minutes on each side.

- Glaze with reserved mix and serve.

Nutrition Per Serving: Calories 357 | Total Fat 18 g| Saturated Fat 5 g| trans Fat 0 g| Cholesterol 64 mg| Sodium 158 mg| Carbohydrates 27 g| Protein 23 g| Phosphorus 188 mg| Potassium 363 mg| Calcium 40 mg

4.43 Slow-Cooked Cranberry Pork Roast

Ingredients

- One cup of diced cranberries

- Ground cloves: ⅛ teaspoon

- Brown sugar: 1 tablespoon

- 4 pounds of center-cut pork roast

- Black pepper: 1 teaspoon

- Honey: ¼ cup

- Nutmeg: ⅛ teaspoon

- Zest of orange peel: 1 teaspoon

- Half teaspoon of salt

Instructions

- Season pork roast with pepper and salt. Put in a slow cooker.

- Mix remaining ingredients and pour over the pork.

- Cook on low for 8 to 10 hours.

- Take out from cooker, slice it, and serve with dipping.

Nutrition Per Serving: Calories 287 | Total Fat 14 g| Saturated Fat 5 g| Trans Fat 0 g| Cholesterol 85 mg| Sodium 190 mg|

Carbohydrates 8 g| Protein 30 g| Phosphorus 240 mg| Potassium 406 mg| Dietary Fiber 0.4 g| Calcium 40 mg

4.44 Herb-Crusted Pork Loin

Ingredients

- One pork loin roast, boneless

- Fennel seed: 2 tablespoons

- Low sodium soy sauce: 2 tablespoons

- Caraway seed: 2 tablespoons

- Dill seed: 2 tablespoons

- Anise seed: 2 tablespoons

Instructions

- Pour soy sauce on roast and coat well.

- In a baking pan, mix fennel, dill seed, caraway, and anise seed. Coat the pork in this mixture.

- Pack foil around pork and refrigerate for at least two hours or more

- Let the oven preheat to 325 F.

- Remove foil, put pork's fat side up on a rack in a shallow pan, and bake for 35 to 40 minutes each pound. Until the meat thermometer reads 145 F.

- Let rest for three minutes. Slice and serve

Nutrition Per Serving: Calories 224 | Total Fat 13 g| Saturated Fat 5 g| Trans Fat 0 g| Cholesterol 70 mg| Sodium 134 mg| Carbohydrates 2 g| Protein 24 g| Phosphorus 225 mg| Potassium 405 mg| Dietary Fiber 1.0 g| Calcium 53 mg

4.45 Roast Pork Loin with Sweet and Tart Apple Stuffing

Ingredients

- Marmalade Cherry Glaze:

- Half cup of orange marmalade, sugar-free
- Cinnamon: 1/8 teaspoon
- ¼ cup of apple juice
- Nutmeg: 1/8 teaspoon
- ¼ cup of dried cherries

Apple Stuffing

- Half cup of chicken stock, low-sodium
- Canola oil: 2 tablespoons
- Half cup of diced honey crisp apple
- Unsalted butter: 2 tablespoons
- Cubed Hawaiian rolls: 2 cups packed
- Chopped onions: 2 tablespoons
- Fresh thyme: 1 tablespoon
- Chopped celery: 2 tablespoons
- Black pepper: 1 teaspoon

Roast pork loin

- One pound of pork loin, boneless
- Butcher twine: 2 pieces

Instructions

- In a pan, combine all ingredients on medium flame until all is melted and well combined, bring it to simmer. Turn off the heat.
- Let the oven preheat to 400 F
- In a pan, fry all ingredients in oil, do not add chicken stock for 2 to 3 minutes.
- Gradually add a stick until it's only moist, not wet.
- Turn off the heat and let it come to room temperature.
- Cut slits, lengthwise, of one inch in pork, like pockets.

- Add two tbsp. of stuffing to every pocket.
- Tie the pork with twine so that stuffing will remain in place.
- Put the rest of the stuffing on the baking tray, put tied pork on stuffing.
- Bake at 400 F for 45 mints, or until internal temperature is 160 F
- Drizzle over the glaze shut the oven off, and let it rest for 10 to 15 minutes.

Nutrition Per Serving: Calories 263 | Total Fat 14 g| Saturated Fat 4 g| Trans Fat 0 g| Cholesterol 50 mg| Sodium 137 mg| Carbohydrates 22 g| Protein 14 g| Phosphorus 154 mg| Potassium 275 mg| Dietary Fiber 1 g| Calcium 68 mg

4.46 Kidney-Friendly Chicken Salad

Ingredients

- Onion: 1⁄4, diced
- Half cup of chicken breasts, skinless and boneless
- Spicy brown mustard: 1⁄4 teaspoon
- One celery stalk, diced
- Half teaspoon of vinegar
- Miracle whip: 1 tablespoon
- Half tsp. of garlic powder

Instructions

- Boil the chicken.
- Shred the cooled chicken
- Add mustard, whip, onions, vinegar, onion powder, celery and mix well.
- Serve.

Nutrient per serving: Calories: 198 g| Protein: 15.3 g| Carbohydrates: 15.4 g| Fiber: 1.9 g| Total Fat: 3.1 g| Sodium: 222

mg| Phosphorus: 101 mg| Potassium: 121 mg|

4.47 Honey Garlic Chicken

Ingredients

- Half cup of honey
- 4 pound of roasting chicken
- Garlic powder: 1 teaspoon
- Olive oil: 1 tablespoon
- Half teaspoon of black pepper

Instructions

- let the oven preheat to 350 F.
- Add olive oil to the pan.
- Add chicken in pan, do not overlap. Coat chicken with all the ingredients
- Bake for one hour or until done. Flip halfway through.
- Serve.

Nutrients per serving: Calories 279 kcals| Sodium 40 mg| Protein 13 g| Potassium 144 mg| Fat 10 g| Calcium 11 mg| carbohydrates 36 g| Phosphorus 99 mg| Fiber 0 g| Cholesterol 40mg

4.48 Seasoned Pork Chops

Ingredients

- 4 lean pork chops fat trimmed
- Vegetable oil: 2 tablespoons
- Black pepper: 1 teaspoon
- Half teaspoon of thyme
- Half teaspoon of sage
- All-purpose flour: ¼ cup

Instructions

- Let the oven preheat to 350°f.
- Add oil to baking pan.
- Mix sage, flour, thyme, and black pepper.

- Coat pork chops in flour mix and place in the pan.
- Bake for 40 minutes, or until cooked
- Serve hot.

Nutrition per serving: 434 calories| 60 mg sodium|19 g protein |79 mg cholesterol |332 mg potassium| 34 g total fat| 12 g carbohydrate |199 mg phosphorus| 10 g saturated fat |35 mg calcium

4.49 Homemade Pan Sausage

Ingredients

- Granulated sugar: 2 teaspoons
- 1 pound of fresh lean ground pork
- Ground black pepper: 1 teaspoon
- Half teaspoon of ground red pepper
- Ground sage: 2 teaspoons

Instructions

- Mix all ingredients to make sausage.
- Make patties of mixture 2 tbsp. each.
- Fry in oil and serve.

Nutritional per serving: 96 calories | 22 mg sodium|6 grams' protein| 43 mg cholesterol |87 mg potassium| 7 grams' total fat| 1-gram carbohydrate |53 mg phosphorus| 2 grams saturated | fiber 72 mg calcium

4.50 Salisbury Steak

Ingredients

- Vegetable oil: 1 tablespoon
- 1 pound of ground pork
- Half cup of diced green pepper
- 1 egg white
- Black pepper: 1 teaspoon
- One diced onion
- Corn starch: 1 tablespoon
- Half cup of water

Instructions

- In a bowl, add green pepper, meat, egg, onion, and black pepper.

- Make patties

- Cook patties in a pan until cooked completely

- Add water and simmer for 15 minutes. Take patties out

- Add the rest of the water, mix with corn starch, let it simmer to thicken.

- Serve the patties with gravy

Nutrition per serving: 249 calories| 128 mg sodium|22 grams' protein| 149 mg cholesterol |366 mg potassium| 57 grams' total fat| 7 grams' carbohydrate| 218 mg phosphorus|3 grams saturated fat| 1-gram fiber| 33 mg calcium

4.51 Jalapeno Pepper Chicken

Ingredients

- Chicken: 2-3 pounds, cut up skinless

- Vegetable oil: 3 tablespoons

- One onion, cut into rings

- 1 and a half cups of chicken stock, low-sodium

- Jalapeño peppers: 2 teaspoons, chopped without seeds

- Half teaspoon of ground nutmeg

- Black pepper: ¼ teaspoon

Instructions

- Brown chicken pieces in oil set it aside

- Sauté onion and add the stock, let it boil.

- Take chicken back to the pan, add pepper and nutmeg. Cover it and simmer for 35 minutes.

- Add in jalapeño peppers.

Nutrition per serving: 143 calories | 45 mg sodium|17 grams' protein| 46 mg cholesterol| 160 mg potassium|7 grams' total fat| 2 grams' carbohydrate |127 mg phosphorus|1 gram saturated fat| 12 mg calcium

Chapter 5: Kidney-Friendly Beef & Turkey Recipes

5.1 Rice with Beef

Ingredients

- 1 cup diced onion
- Vegetable oil: 2 tablespoons
- Rice: 2 cups, cooked
- Half teaspoon sage
- 1 and a half tsp. Seasoning of chili con carne powder
- Black pepper: ⅛ teaspoon
- 4 cups of lean ground beef

Instructions

- Sauté onion and brown the meat in the skillet
- Add seasoning and rice, mix well.
- Turn off the heat and cover it.
- Let it rest for ten minutes, then serve.

Nutrition per serving: 360 calories |1 g trans-fat |78 mg sodium| 23 g protein| 65 mg cholesterol |427 mg potassium|14 g total fat | 26 g carbohydrate| 233 mg phosphorus|4 g saturated fat| 2 g fiber| 34 mg calcium

5.2 Cilantro Burger

Ingredients

- Cilantro: 3 tablespoon
- 4 cups of lean ground turkey
- Oregano: ¼ teaspoon
- Black pepper: ¼ teaspoon
- Ground thyme: ¼ teaspoon
- Lemon juice: 1 tablespoon

Instructions

- In a bowl, mix all ingredients.
- Make into patties.
- Fry on a lightly greased skillet and broil for 10 to 15 minutes. Turning halfway once

Nutrition per serving: 171 calories |0 g trans-fat |108 mg sodium|20 g protein |90 mg cholesterol| 289 mg potassium|10 g total fat |0 g carbohydrate |180 mg phosphorus|3 g saturated |fat 0 g| fiber 21 mg calcium

5.3 Borscht

Ingredients

- Cubed beets: 1 and ½ cups(steamed)
- Olive oil: 2 tbsp.
- Light beef broth/vegetable broth: 2 cups
- One onion, diced
- Half teaspoon of salt
- ¼ tsp. of black pepper
- One potato, chopped, leached
- Red-wine vinegar: 2 tsp.
- Fresh parsley
- Sour cream: ¼ cup

Instructions

- Pour the oil on medium flame in a big saucepan. Add onion and fry for four minutes before browning starts.
- Add stock, potato, pepper, and salt; carry to a boil. Lower the heat to a simmer, let it cover, and cook for eight minutes until it is soft.
- Add vinegar and beets go to boil again. Cover and cook until the broth is red, and the potato is tender for almost three minutes.
- In a dish, mix the sour cream. Top the soup with the sour cream blend. enjoy

Nutrition per Serving: 160 calories| total fat 9g |carbohydrates 17.1g |fiber 2.4g | protein 3.7g

5.4 Turkey Apple Breakfast Hash

Ingredients

For(meat)

- Salt to taste
- Minced Turkey: 1 lb.
- Dried thyme: ½ teaspoon
- Cinnamon: ½ teaspoon
- Olive oil: 1 tbsp.

For(hash)

- Cubed frozen butternut squash: 2 cups
- Kale: 2 cups
- Carrots: ½ cup shredded
- Olive oil: 1 tablespoon
- One small onion
- One large zucchini
- Powdered ginger: ¾ teaspoon
- One apple chopped
- Cinnamon: 1 teaspoon
- Turmeric: ½ teaspoon
- Dried thyme: ½ teaspoon
- Salt to taste
- Garlic powder: ½ teaspoon

Instructions

- Heat a tablespoon of oil over medium flame in a skillet. Add turkey and stir until brown. Season with cinnamon, thyme, and sea salt. Set aside.
- Add remaining oil into the same skillet and sauté onion until softened for 2-3 minutes.

- Add the carrots, zucchini, frozen squash, and apple—Cook for around 4-5 minutes, or until veggies soften.
- Add and mix in kale until wilted.
- Add cooked turkey, seasoning, salt and remove from heat, and serve.

Nutrition Per serving: Kcal 156| Fat: 14g| Net Carbs: 13g| Protein: 15.5g

5.5 Baked Turkey Meatballs

Ingredients

- One egg beat
- Minced turkey: 1 pound
- Grated Parmesan cheese: ½ cup
- Fresh breadcrumbs: ½ cup
- Chopped parsley: 1 tablespoon
- Milk: 2-3 tablespoons
- Chopped fresh basil: ½ tablespoon
- Pinch of grated nutmeg
- Chopped oregano: ½ tablespoon

Instructions

- Let the oven pre-heat to 350F.
- Put parchment paper on two baking sheets.
- In a big bowl, add the turkey, breadcrumbs, cheese, herbs, egg, nutmeg, cinnamon, pepper, and milk. The amount of milk you can use needs to be changed depending on how dry your bread. The mixture should be moist that it binds together.
- Roll parts of the meat into roughly 1-inch balls using a teaspoon and put them onto a baking sheet. You should finish off with 25-30 meatballs.

- Bake the meatballs for around 30 minutes, frequently rotating, causing the meat to be cooked through and brown gently.

Nutrition per serving: Cal 216|Fat 3g| Sodium 17mg|Protein 22g|Carbohydrates 32g

5.6 Goat Cheese Pizza

Ingredients

- Olive oil: 1 tsp.
- Turkey breast (one ounce) shredded
- Whole wheat pizza crust: 7 inches - one piece
- Roma tomato: one(sliced)
- Kale: 1 cup
- Crumbled goat cheese:1/4 cup
- Snipped fresh basil: 2 tbsp.
- Red onion: ¼ cup thinly sliced

Instructions

- Take one spoonful of olive oil and brush it on the pizza crust.
- Add chicken breast, kale, turkey tomato, goat cheese, and red onion. Bake according to the Instructions on the crust package.
- For serving, sprinkle with basil.

Nutrition Per Serving: 219 calories| total fat 10g | carbohydrates 23g |protein 14g.

5.7 White Turkey Chili with green beans

Ingredients

- Chicken broth: 4 cups
- Ground turkey: 1 pound
- One onion, diced
- Four minced garlic cloves
- Olive oil: 2 tbsp.
- One cup of small cut beans
- Ground cumin: 2 tsp.
- White beans: one and a half cups
- Cayenne pepper: 1 tsp.
- Salt pepper, to taste
- Ground coriander: 1 tsp.

Instructions

- Heat the olive oil in a big pot over low flame. Stir in the onion and sauté for 6 to 8 minutes until translucent. Add the garlic and proceed to cook for one minute, until fragrant.
- Stir in the turkey and cook for 5 to 7 minutes until browned and thoroughly cooked. Stir in the coriander, cumin, and cayenne pepper. Add salt and pepper, and cook for two minutes until fragrant.
- Add the broth. Bring the soup over medium flame to a boil. Reduce heat to low and simmer for half an hour, until tastes develop
- Add the beans and cook for three minutes.
- Spoon the chili in bowls and finish with two teaspoons of green beans. Serve hot.

Nutrition Per serving: 144 calories|14g fat| 22g carbs|21g protein

5.8 Greek Turkey Burgers with Tzatziki Sauce

Ingredients

Turkey Burgers

- One pound minced turkey
- Olive oil: one tbsp.
- Half cup parsley
- Two minced garlic cloves

- One large egg
- One minced sweet onion
- Half teaspoon of dried oregano
- Bread crumbs: ¾ cup
- Salt & pepper to taste
- Half teaspoon of red chili flakes

Tzatziki Sauce

- One tbsp. of olive oil
- Half cucumber, diced
- ¼ cup of parsley
- 2 tbsp. of lemon juice
- One cup of Greek yogurt
- Garlic powder: 1 pinch
- Pepper and salt, to taste

Burger Topping

- Half onion, sliced
- Four whole-wheat buns
- Lettuce leaves
- Six slices of tomatoes

Instructions

- Heat olive oil over medium flame in a skillet. Add the onion and fry, for 3 to 4 minutes, until translucent. Add the garlic and sauté for one minute more, until fragrant. set it aside
- Mix the cooled onion mixture with the egg, parsley, oregano, red-pepper flakes with ground turkey in a bowl. Add the crumbs, season with pepper and salt, and whisk until combined.
- Let the oven Preheat to 375 ° F.
- Form four modest size patties of the meat mixture. spray oil on a skillet and place it on medium flame
- Put the burgers in the skillet and fry for five minutes per side until golden

brown. Move the skillet to the oven and cook for fifteen more minutes till the burgers are thoroughly cooked.

- Sauce: In a medium dish, mix the cucumber with yogurt, add the olive oil, garlic powder, and lemon juice.
- Using salt and pepper to season, then whisk in the parsley.
- Topping: Put each burger on the bottom half of a bun and cover it with around 1⁄4 cup of tzatziki sauce, two leaves of lettuce, two slices of tomatoes, and the top half of the bun. Serve hot.

Nutrients per serving: 226 calories|14g fat| 22g carbs|27g protein

5.9 Ground Turkey Sweet Potato Stuffed Peppers

Ingredients

- 2 cups of minced turkey
- Two minced cloves of garlic
- Half cup of chopped onions
- One tbsp. of olive oil
- Half of a cup tomato sauce, no salt added
- One and 2/3 cups of diced sweet potatoes, leached
- Two cuts in half, bell peppers
- Salt and pepper, to taste
- Red chili flakes (optional)
- Parsley

Instructions

- Let the oven pre-heat till 350F
- Heat the olive oil in a skillet over medium flame.
- Place the turkey and garlic in the skillet. Stir from time to time, and

cook for around 10 minutes or until the meat is brown. break any lumps of meat

- Stir in the onions and cook until light brown.

- Put the sweet potatoes on top, cover the pan, and cook until soft. It takes about eight minutes to finish.

- Add the chili flakes, tomato sauce, pepper, and salt. Add more olive oil or a bit of water if needed to cook the potatoes.

- Grease the pan and arrange the peppers. inner side up

- Add the ground turkey-sweet potato mixture in each half of the bell pepper.

- Bake for around half an hour uncovered, or until the peppers are soft, take out from the oven, then garnish with parsley.

Nutrition per serving: Kcal 324| Fat: 13.9g| Saturated Fat: 4.4g, |Carbohydrates: 25.6g|Protein: 26.3g

5.10 Mediterranean Bento Lunch

Ingredients

- One pita bread(whole-wheat) quartered

- 1 and a half cup of grilled turkey breast tenderloin

- ¼ of a cup rinsed chickpeas

- ¼ of a cup chopped tomato

- Chopped olives: 1 tablespoon

- Grapes: one cup

- ¼ of a cup chopped cucumber

- Chopped fresh parsley: 1 tablespoon

- Extra-virgin olive oil: half teaspoon

- Red-wine vinegar: 1 teaspoon

- Hummus: 2 tablespoons

Instructions

- In a mixing bowl, add tomato, feta, cucumber, olives, vinegar, oil, chickpeas, and parsley and toss well until well combined.

- Put this mixture in a dish.

- Put turkey or chicken (if using) in another dish.

- Add pita, hummus, and grapes side by side in small containers.

- Serve all these together in a lunch box or a box with different containers.

- Pack it away and enjoy it later.

Nutrition per serving: 497 calories| total fat 13.8g |carbohydrates 60.5g |protein 36.7g

5.11 Turkey Meatball Soup

Ingredients

- 4 cups of lean ground turkey

- Bread: 2 slices

- Kale: 4 cups

- ¼ of a cup of almond milk

- 2 cloves of garlic pressed

- One medium shallot finely diced

- ½ of a teaspoon freshly grated nutmeg

- One teaspoon of oregano

- 1/4 of a teaspoon red pepper flakes

- Italian parsley chopped: 2 tablespoons

- 2 carrots cut into slices

- One egg beat

- One tablespoon of olive oil

- Chicken or vegetable broth: 8 cups
- One can of 15- ounce white Northern beans rinsed, drained
- Half yellow onion finely diced
- Kosher salt and freshly ground pepper

Instructions

- In a large mixing bowl, add milk, cut the bread into pieces, and let it soak in milk. Add the garlic, turkey, nutmeg, shallot, red pepper flakes, salt, oregano, pepper, egg, cheese, and parsley. Mix carefully with your hands. Use a scooper to make half-inch balls.
- Put a wide skillet on medium flame, heat the olive oil, then sear the meatballs gently on every side for two minutes. Turn off the heat and set it aside.
- Add the onion, stock, beans, kale, and carrots to a 5 to 7 quarter slow cooker.
- Add meatballs the kale, and cook for four hours at low or until the meatballs start floating to the top.
- Garnish the soup with Parmesan grated cheese, red pepper flakes, and fresh leaves of parsley.

Nutrition per serving: 250 calories| total fat 23g |carbohydrates 20.3g | protein 14.4g

5.12 Steak & Onion Sandwich

Ingredients

- Vegetable oil: 1 tablespoon
- Four chopped steaks
- Italian seasoning: 1 tablespoon
- Black pepper: 1 tablespoon
- 4 sliced rolls
- Lemon juice:1 tablespoon

- One onion, sliced in rings

Instructions

- In a bowl, mix meat with Italian seasoning, black pepper, and lemon juice
- In a pan, brown the steaks until tender over medium flame.
- Turn the heat down, add onions, cook until tender.
- Serve on a sliced bread roll with onion rings.

Nutrition per serving:345 calories | 247 mg sodium|14 g protein| 40 mg cholesterol |200 mg potassium|21 g total fat |26 g carbohydrate |115 mg phosphorus|7 g saturated fat |2 g fiber | 98 mg calcium

5.13 Taco Stuffing

Ingredients

- Half tsp. of Tabasco sauce
- Vegetable oil: 2 tablespoon
- Italian seasoning: 1 teaspoon
- Lean ground beef: 1 and ¼ pounds
- Half tsp. Of teaspoon black pepper
- Garlic powder: 1 teaspoon
- Half tsp. Of ground red pepper
- Onion powder: 1 teaspoon
- One medium taco shells
- Half head of shredded lettuce
- Half tsp. of nutmeg

Instructions

- In a skillet, add all ingredients except lettuce and taco. Cook until well mixed.
- Add cooked meat in taco shells with shredded lettuce.

Nutrition per serving: 176 calories |124 mg sodium|14 g protein| 56 mg cholesterol| 258 mg potassium|9 g total fat| 9 g carbohydrate |150 mg phosphorus |2 g saturated fat |0 g fiber |33 mg calcium

5.14 Stuffed Green Peppers

Ingredients

- Vegetable oil: 2 tablespoon
- 2 cups of ground lean beef or turkey
- Onions: ¼ cup, Diced
- Celery: ¼ cup, Diced
- Lemon juice: 2 tablespoons
- Celery seed: 1 tablespoon
- Italian seasoning: 2 tablespoons
- Black pepper: 1 teaspoon
- Half tsp. Of honey
- Paprika
- 1 and a half cups of cooked rice
- Six small green peppers, seeds removed

Instructions

- Let the oven preheat to 325 F
- Sauté celery, meat, and onion, until meat is brown
- Add rest of the ingredients, do not add paprika green peppers.
- Mix well and turn off the heat
- Add the mixture into peppers. Wrap with foil and place in a dish.
- Bake for half an hour.
- Sprinkle with paprika and serve.

Nutrition per serving: 131 calories | 36 mg sodium|9 g protein |28 mg cholesterol |160 mg potassium|4 g total fat |15 g carbohydrate |83 mg phosphorus|1 gram saturated fat| 1-gram fiber |38 mg calcium

5.15 Curried Turkey & Rice

Ingredients

- Cooked white rice: 2 cups
- Vegetable oil: 1 teaspoon
- Chicken broth, low-sodium: 1 cup
- One diced onion
- Unsalted margarine: 1 tablespoon
- 1-pound of turkey breast, cut into cutlets
- Curry powder: 2 teaspoons
- Honey: 1 teaspoon
- Flour: 2 tablespoon
- Half cup of non-dairy creamer

Instructions

- In a skillet, cook the turkey for ten minutes, until no longer pink.
- Turn off the heat and keep warm on another plate.
- In the same skillet, add margarine, curry powder, and onion. Stir for five minutes. Then add flour, mixing continuously
- Add in honey, creamer, and broth. Mix until it becomes thick.
- Add turkey back to skillet—Cook for two minutes.
- Serve with rice.

Nutrient per serving: Calories 154 |Sodium 27 mg| Protein 8 g| Potassium 156 mg| Fat 5 g| calcium 25 mg| Carbohydrates 20 g| Phosphorus 88 mg| fiber 1 g| Cholesterol 14 mg

5.16 Tasty Beef Ribs

Ingredients

- Chili powder: 2 teaspoons
- 4 pounds of large beef ribs

- Paprika: 1 tablespoon
- Half tsp. Of garlic powder
- Pineapple juice: 1/4 cup
- Red pepper: 1/8 teaspoon
- Mustard powder: 1/4 teaspoon

Instructions

- In roasting pan, put ribs, meat side down in racks, roast for half an hour at 450 F. drain it
- Pour pineapple juice on ribs.
- Mix the rest of the ingredients, and sprinkle on ribs.
- Turn the temperature to 350 F. then roast for 45 to 60 minutes, with meat side up.

Nutrient per rib: Calories 187 kcals| Sodium 41 mg| Protein 19 g| Potassium 233 mg| Fat 11 g| Calcium 11 mg| carbohydrates 2 g| Phosphorus 149 mg| Cholesterol 56 mg

5.17 Roasted Turkey

Ingredients

- Poultry seasoning: 1 teaspoon
- 12-pound turkey
- Four sprigs of sage
- Turkey stock, low-sodium: 1 cup
- Four sprigs of rosemary
- Half cup of unsalted butter
- Four sprigs of parsley
- Four sprigs of thyme

Instructions

- Let the oven preheat to 425 F.
- look at the cooking time on the plastic wrapping of the turkey.
- Clean the turkey cavity of the giblet, neck. Rinse the turkey and pat dry
- Loosen the skin around drumsticks and breast with fingers.
- Rub seasoning on turkey under the skin.
- Add rosemary, parsley, thyme, sage between flesh and turkey skin.
- Insert a thermometer in the fleshy part.
- Drench turkey in melted butter, place in roasting pan breast side up.
- Cover with aluminum foil, loosely.
- Cook for half an hour, then turn the temperature to 325° F.
- Baste turkey after 15-20 minutes with stock and pan liquid.
- In the last half, an hour remove foil. Cook for 3-4 hours until the meat thermometer shows 165 F.
- Let it rest for half an hour before slicing.

Nutrients per serving: Calories 144| Protein 25 g| Carbohydrates 0 g| Fat 4 g| Cholesterol 64 mg| Sodium 57 mg| Potassium 256 mg| Phosphorus 182 mg| Calcium 22 mg

5.18 Turkey Vegetable Chili

Ingredients

- Cayenne pepper: 1/4 teaspoon
- Olive oil: 1 tablespoon
- Half cup of chopped onion
- 2 cloves of garlic minced
- 1-pound of lean ground turkey
- Diced zucchini: 2 cups
- Chili powder: 2 teaspoon
- Paprika: 1 and a half teaspoons

- 14 ounces of tomatoes canned, crushed, no salt added
- Black pepper: 1/4 teaspoon
- Ground cumin: 1 and a half teaspoons

Instructions

- Sauté the onion, turkey, zucchini, and garlic until tender.
- Drain the excess fluids. Add spices and tomatoes. Cover it and simmer for 30 minutes

Nutrients per serving: Calories 164| Protein 17 g| Carbohydrates 6 g| Fat 8 g| Cholesterol 47 mg| sodium 214 mg| Potassium 517 mg| Phosphorus 189 mg| Calcium 56 mg| Fiber 2.0 g

5.19 Mama's Meatloaf

Ingredients

- Low-fat mayonnaise: 2 tablespoons
- One egg whisked
- Half cup of bread crumbs
- 1-pound lean ground turkey

Seasonings

- Worcestershire sauce, low-sodium: 1 tablespoon
- Garlic powder: 1 teaspoon
- Beef Bouillon: 1 teaspoon low sodium
- Half teaspoon of red pepper flakes
- Onion powder: 1 teaspoon

Instructions

- Let the oven preheat to 375° F.
- In a bowl, add all ingredients, do not add the meat, mix until well combined.
- Add the meat and mix.

- Add meat to meatloaf pan. Cover with the foil—Bake for 20 minutes.
- Remove the aluminum foil and cook for five minutes.
- Turn off the oven, let it rest for ten minutes before serving.

Nutrition Per Serving: Calories 367 | Total Fat 23 g| Saturated Fat 8 g| Trans Fat 1 g| cholesterol 127 mg| sodium 332 mg| carbohydrates 14 g| Protein 25 g| Phosphorus 273 mg| Potassium 460 mg| Dietary Fiber 0.7 g| Calcium 32 mg

5.20 Turkey Soup

Ingredients

- 1 potato, diced(leached)
- 1 cup ground turkey
- 1 teaspoon cayenne pepper
- 1 onion, diced
- 1 tablespoon olive oil
- ¼ carrot, diced
- 2 cups of water

Instructions

- In a saucepan, heat the olive oil and add the chopped onion and carrot.
- For 3 minutes, prepare the vegetables. Then stir them well and add the cayenne pepper and ground turkey.
- Add the diced potato and stir well with the spices. Cook them for an extra 2 minutes.
- Add water, Cover the lid and simmer for 20 minutes to make the broth.

Nutrients Per serving: 317 calories|31.8g protein|14.2g carbohydrates| 16.9g fat| 2.3g fiber|112mg cholesterol| 131mg sodium| 319mg potassium.

5.21 Turkey Bolognese with Zucchini Noodles

Ingredients

- 2 tbsp. of Olive Oil
- 1 lb. of ground turkey
- one Onion, chopped
- Four Zucchini, spiralized
- Chicken stock: 4 cups, no salt added
- Red bell peppers, chopped: 1 cup
- Garlic Cloves Minced: 2 tbsp.
- Half tsp of Red Pepper Flakes
- Cayenne: 1/4 tsp
- 1/4 lb. of Spaghetti
- Nutmeg: 1/4 tsp
- Ground Bay Leaves: 1/4 tsp
- One tsp. of Oregano
- Dried Basil: 1/4 cup

Instructions

- In a pan, sauté onion, turkey, garlic until meat is browned.
- Add stock and all herbs and seasoning (do not add basil), bell peppers. Let it simmer for almost two hours.
- Cook pasta as per instructions, and add zucchini noodles halfway through.
- Add olive oil to pasta so it won't stick.
- When almost all the liquid is absorbed, add basil and noodles. Cook for 2 to 3 minutes, and serve

Nutrients per serving: Cal 212 |calcium 59 mg| potassium 253 mg| phosphorous 249 mg| protein 19 g| carbs 24 g

5.22 Turkey Gravy

Ingredients

- Pan juices of turkey: 1 cup
- Turkey fat: 4 tablespoons, pan drippings
- Giblet stock: 2 cups
- All-purpose white flour: 4 tablespoons
- Half teaspoon of salt

Instructions

- In a saucepan, heat the fat. Add in flour, whisk and let it boil.
- Add pan juices, salt, and stock.
- Keep mixing until it thickens. Lower the heat and simmer for ten minutes.

Nutrients per serving: Calories 87| Protein 2 g| Carbohydrates 4 g| Fat 7 g| Cholesterol 25 mg| Sodium 146 mg| Potassium 43 mg| Phosphorus 19 mg| Calcium 6 mg

5.23 Easy Turkey Sloppy Joes

Ingredients

- One and a half pounds of ground turkey with less fat
- Half cup of red onion, chopped
- Grilling Blend seasoning: 1 tablespoon
- Honey: 2 tablespoons
- Half cup of green bell pepper, chopped
- Tomato sauce, low-sodium: 1 cup
- Worcestershire sauce, low sodium: 1 tablespoon
- Six buns

Instructions

- In a skillet, cook turkey over medium flame until cooked through. Don't drain
- In a bowl, mix all seasoning with tomato sauce.
- Add seasoning mix to turkey. Turn the heat low and cook for ten minutes.
- Place in buns and serve.

Nutrients per serving: Calories 290| protein 24 g| Carbohydrates 28 g| Fat 9 g| cholesterol 58 mg| Sodium 288 mg| Potassium 513 mg| Phosphorus 237 mg| calcium 86 mg| Fiber 1.8 g

5.24 Roasted Turkey Breast with Salt-free Herb Seasoning

Ingredients

- Three pounds of half turkey breast, with skin and bone-in
- 1/4 cup of butter
- 1/4 cup of onion, minced
- Herb seasoning blend, salt-free: 1 tablespoon

Instructions

- Let the oven preheat to 350° F.
- Melt butter, sauté onion with herb seasoning blend.
- Separate the mixture into two bowls.
- In a roasting pan, put turkey breast skin side down. Add one tbsp. of seasoning and coat it.
- Turn over turkey and loosen skin. Add three tbsp. of seasoning between skin and flesh. Secure with toothpicks.
- Put in the oven and cook for 60 minutes.

- Take out from the oven and spread the rest of the seasoning over the turkey's skin.
- Cook for 15-20 minutes, until the thermometer, inserted reads 160° F.
- Rest the turkey breast for 10 to 15 minutes before serving.

Nutrients per serving: Calories 203| Protein 25 g| carbohydrates 1 g| Fat 11 g| Cholesterol 76 mg| Sodium 88 mg| Potassium 265 mg| Phosphorus 184 mg| Calcium 20 mg| Fiber 0 g

5.25 Turkey and Beef Meatballs

Ingredients

- one egg
- 1 pound of ground chuck beef
- Onion & Herb seasoning: 1 tablespoon
- Soft bread crumbs: 1 cup
- 1 pound of ground turkey
- Ground pepper: 1 teaspoon
- Worcestershire sauce, low sodium: 1 teaspoon
- Half cup of beef broth, reduced-sodium
- Dried parsley: 1 tablespoon

Instructions

- Let the oven preheat to 350° F.
- Add parchment paper on two baking sheets
- In a big bowl, mix both meats with dry ingredients, set it aside
- In another bowl, combine egg, broth, and low sodium Worcestershire sauce
- To the meat, add the wet ingredients. Mix well.

- Make one-inch meatballs and put on a baking sheet
- Bake for half an hour, turning halfway through.
- Serve hot with sauce

Nutrients per serving: Calories 175| Protein 16 g| Carbohydrates 3 g| Fat 11 g| Cholesterol 69 mg| Sodium 120 mg| potassium 236 mg| Phosphorus 142 mg| calcium 18 mg| Fiber 0.1 g

5.26 Turkey Bowtie Pasta

Ingredients

Pasta

- One sliced red pepper
- Cooked bowtie pasta: 4 cups
- Diced zucchini: 1 cup
- Black pepper
- Raw mushrooms: 1 cup
- 1 lb. of ground turkey

Sauce

- White flour: 4 tbsp.
- Margarine: 5 tbsp.
- Hot water: 2 cups
- Lemon juice: 1 tsp
- 1 tsp any seasoning no salt added
- Garlic powder: 1 tsp
- 1/4 tsp of red pepper flakes
- Sour cream: 4 tbsp.

Instructions

- In a pan, melt margarine, add flour, and mix. Slowly add hot water.
- Add sour cream and mix well, then add red pepper flakes, seasoning, lemon juice, garlic powder, mix for 1

to 3 minutes. Turn off heat and mix until cools slightly

- Cook the turkey in a pan sauté mushroom and zucchini till tender. Add peppers but do not soften them. Add black pepper, pasta, sauce, and turkey to vegetable mix well.

Nutrient per serving: Calories 516 g| Protein: 28 g| Carbohydrates: 43 g| Fiber: 3 g| Total Fat: 25 g| Sodium: 257 mg| Phosphorus: 257 mg| Potassium: 430 mg

5.27 Lime Grilled Turkey

Ingredients

- ⅔ lb. of turkey breast, boneless & skinless
- ¼ cup of vegetable oil
- 2 tbsp. of honey
- Half cup of lime juice
- 1 tsp of dried thyme
- 1 tsp of dried rosemary

Instructions

- In a bowl, mix all ingredients except for the turkey.
- Take out two tbsp. from marinade and set it aside
- Cut the turkey in half lengthwise so the pieces will be thinner.
- Add turkey in marinade, coat well, and chill in the fridge for 1 to 2 hours.
- Let the oven broiler preheat to 500 F
- Broil turkey on each side for four minutes.
- Baste turkey in 2 tbsp. of marinade while cooking.
- Serve hot.

Nutrient per serving: Calories: 245 g| Protein: 17.1 g| Carbohydrates: 11.5 g| Fiber: 0.4 g| Total Fat: 15 g| Sodium: 35 mg| Phosphorus: 131 mg| Potassium: 200 mg

5.28 Curried Turkey Casserole

Ingredients

- Broccoli florets: 3 cups
- Olive oil: 1/4 cup+ 2 tbsp.
- 2 cloves of minced garlic
- All-purpose flour: 1/4 cup
- One diced onion
- 2% milk: 1 cup
- Chicken broth, no salt: 2 cups
- Curry powder: 2 teaspoons
- 1 cup chopped bell peppers
- White bread: 3 cups, cut into cubes
- Black pepper
- Turkey: 4 cups, sliced into pieces

Instructions

- Let the oven preheat to 400 F
- In a pot, add oil sauté garlic, onion until tender for seven minutes.
- Add in flour and mix for one minute. Gradually add broth and milk, mixing continuously until it simmers.
- Add in black pepper, curry powder, peppers, broccoli cook for five minutes until softened. Add in cooked turkey.
- Place mixture in baking dish.
- In a bowl, add bread and oil, coat well. Add bread to the turkey mix.
- Bake for 15 minutes, until brown and bubbles.

Nutrient per Serving: Calories: 380 g| Protein: 26 g| Carbohydrates: 23 g| Fiber: 2

g| Total Fat: 20 g| Sodium: 113 mg| phosphorus: 227 mg| Potassium: 472 mg

5.29 Turkey Sliders with Peach Tarragon Aioli

Ingredients

- Ground turkey: 2 cups
- Parsley: 1/3 cup, chopped
- Garlic powder: 1 teaspoon
- Dijon mustard: half tablespoon
- Poultry seasoning: 1 teaspoon
- Half cup of arugula
- Six slider buns
- Red onion: 1/4 cup, diced

For Aioli

- Peaches: 2 tablespoons, pureed
- Low-fat mayonnaise: 2 tablespoons
- Tarragon: 1 teaspoon, chopped

Instructions

- Preheat grill on medium-high. In a bowl, add poultry season, red onion, mustard, turkey, garlic powder, parsley. Make it into six patties.
- Cook patties for 5 to 6 minutes on each side, until a meat thermometer, reads 165 F
- Meanwhile, make peach aioli mix all ingredients.
- Spread peach aioli on the slider, then patty and enjoy.

Nutrient per serving: Calories: 257 g| Protein: 16 g| Carbohydrates: 33 g| Fiber: 4 g| Total Fat: 11 g| sodium: 257 mg| Phosphorus: 240 mg| Potassium: 330 mg

5.30 Turkey Breast with Cranberry Orange Ginger Sauce

Ingredients

- Fresh parsley: 1 Tbsp.
- 4 lbs. of skin-on turkey breast
- Fresh thyme: 1 tsp
- Fresh rosemary: 1 tsp
- Salt: ¼ tsp
- Olive oil: ¼ cup
- Pepper: ¼ tsp
- Half tsp of lemon zest

Instructions

- Let the oven preheat to 350 F
- Mix herbs, oil, salt, and black pepper
- Loosen the turkey skin from flesh with your fingers.
- Place turkey in pan. Add 2 tbsp. Of oil mix under skin and secure with toothpicks.
- Pour the rest of the oil over the turkey breast.
- Cover it and roast for 1 to 1.5 hours.
- let the turkey rest for ten-15 minutes, pull the skin off, and discard

Nutrient per serving: Calories: 244.3 g| Protein: 32.6 g| Carbohydrates: 0.1 g| Fiber: 0.04 g| Total Fat: 11.8 g| Sodium: 108 mg| Phosphorus: 238 mg|

Potassium: 329 mg

5.31 Beef Schnitzel

Ingredients

- One lean beef schnitzel
- Olive oil: 2 tablespoon
- Breadcrumbs: ¼ cup
- One egg
- One lemon, to serve

Instructions

- Let the oven pre-heat to 400 F.

- In a big bowl, add breadcrumbs and oil, mix well until forms a crumbly mixture
- Dip beef steak in whisked egg and coat in breadcrumbs mixture.
- Place the breaded beef in the oven and cook for 20 minutes or more until fully cooked through.
- Take out from the oven and serve with the side of lemon.

Nutrition per serving: Calories 340 | Proteins 20g |Carbs 14g |Fat 10g

|Fiber 7g

5.32 Mama's Meatloaf

Ingredients

- Ground lean beef: 4 cups
- Bread crumbs: 1 cup (soft and fresh)
- Chopped mushrooms: ½ cup
- Cloves of minced garlic
- Shredded carrots: ½ cup
- Beef broth: ¼ cup
- Chopped onions: ½ cup
- Two eggs beaten
- Ketchup: 3 Tbsp.
- Worcestershire sauce: 1 Tbsp.
- Dijon mustard: 1 Tbsp.

For Glaze

- Honey: ¼ cup
- Ketchup: half cup
- Dijon mustard: 2 tsp

Instructions

- In a big bowl, add beef broth and breadcrumbs, stir well. And set it aside in a food processor, add garlic, onions, mushrooms, and carrots, and pulse on high until finely chopped

- In a separate bowl, add soaked breadcrumbs, Dijon mustard, Worcestershire sauce, eggs, lean ground beef, ketchup, and salt. With your hands, combine well and make it into a loaf.

- Let the oven preheat to 390 F.

- Put Meatloaf in the oven and let it cook for 40 minutes.

- In the meantime, add Dijon mustard, ketchup, and brown sugar in a bowl and mix. Glaze this mix over Meatloaf when five minutes are left.

- Rest the Meatloaf after for ten minutes before serving.

Nutrition per serving: Calories 330 | Proteins 19g |Carbs 16g|Fat 9.9 g |

5.33 Steak with Broccoli Bundles

Ingredients

- Olive oil spray

- Flank steak (2 pounds)- cut into 6 pieces

- Kosher salt and black pepper

- Two cloves of minced garlic

- Broccoli florets: 2 and a half cups

- Tamari sauce: half cup

- Three bell peppers: sliced thinly

- Beef broth: 1/3 cup

- 1 Tbsp. of unsalted butter

- Balsamic vinegar: 1/4 cup

Instructions

- Sprinkle salt and pepper on steak and rub.

- In a zip lock bag, add garlic and Tamari sauce, then add steak, toss well and seal the bag.

- Let it marinate for one hour to overnight.

- Equally, place bell peppers and asparagus in the center of the steak.

- Roll the steak around the vegetables and secure well with toothpicks.

- Preheat the oven.

- Spray the steak with olive oil spray. And place steaks in the oven.

- Cook for 15 minutes at 400 F or more till steaks are cooked

- Take the steak out from the oven and let it rest for five minute

- Remove steak bundles and allow them to rest for 5 minutes before serving/ slicing.

- In the meantime, add butter, balsamic vinegar, and broth over medium flame. Mix well and reduce it by half. Add salt and pepper to taste.

- Pour over steaks right before serving.

Nutrition per serving: Calories 471 | Proteins 29g |Carbs 20g |Fat 15g |

5.34 Beef Hamburger

Ingredients

- Buns:4

- Lean ground beef chuck: 4 cups

- Salt, to taste

- Slices of any cheese: 4 slices

- Black Pepper, to taste

Instructions

- Let the oven preheat to 350 F.

- In a bowl, add lean ground beef, pepper, and salt. Mix well and form patties.

- Put them in the oven in one layer only, cook for 6 minutes, flip them halfway through. One minute before you take out the patties add cheese on top.

- When cheese is melted, take out from the oven.

- Add ketchup, any dressing to your buns. Add tomatoes and lettuce and patties.

- Serve hot.

Nutrition per serving: Calories: 520kcal | Carbohydrates: 22g | Protein: 31g | Fat: 34g |

5.35 Beef Steak Kabobs with Vegetables

Ingredients

- Light sodium Soy sauce: 2 tbsp.

- Lean beef chuck ribs: 4 cups, cut into one-inch pieces

- Low-fat sour cream: 1/3 cup

- Half onion

- 8 skewers: 6 inch

- One bell peppers

Instructions

- In a mixing bowl, add soy sauce and sour cream, mix well. Add the lean beef chunks, coat well, and let it marinate for half an hour or more.

- Cut onion, bell pepper into one-inch pieces. In water, soak skewers for ten minutes.

- Add onions, bell peppers, and beef on skewers; alternatively, sprinkle with Black Pepper

- Let it cook for 10 minutes, in a preheated oven at 400F, flip halfway through.

- Serve with yogurt dipping sauce.

Nutrition per serving: Calories 268 | Proteins 20g |Carbs 15g|Fat 10g |

5.36 Beef Empanadas

Ingredients

- Square gyoza wrappers: eight pieces

- Olive oil: 1 tablespoon

- White onion: 1/4 cup, finely diced

- Mushrooms: 1/4 cup, finely diced

- Half cup lean ground beef

- Chopped garlic: 2 teaspoons

- Paprika: 1/4 teaspoon

- Ground cumin: 1/4 teaspoon

- Six green olives, diced

- Ground cinnamon: 1/8 teaspoon

- Diced tomatoes: half cup

- One egg, lightly beaten

Instructions

- In a skillet, over a medium flame, add oil, onions, and beef and cook for 3 minutes, until meat turns brown.

- Add mushrooms and cook for six minutes until it starts to brown. Then add paprika, cinnamon, olives, cumin, and garlic and cook for 3 minutes or more.

- Add in the chopped tomatoes and cook for a minute. Turn off the heat; let it cool for five minutes.

- Lay gyoza wrappers on a flat surface add one and a half tbsp. of beef filling in each wrapper. Brush edges with water or egg, fold wrappers, pinch edges.
- Put empanadas in the oven, and cook for 7 minutes at 400°F until nicely browned.
- Serve with sauce and salad greens.

Nutrition per serving: Calories 343 |Fat 19g |Protein 18g |Carbohydrate 12.9g

5.37 Rib-Eye Steak

Ingredients

- Lean rib eye steaks: 2, medium size
- Salt & freshly ground black pepper, to taste

Instructions

- Let the oven preheat at 400 F. pat dry steaks with paper towels.
- Use any spice blend or just salt and pepper on steaks.
- Generously on both sides of the steak.
- Put steaks in the oven. Cook according to the rareness you want. Or cook for 14 minutes and flip after half time.
- Take out from the oven and let it rest for about 5 minutes.
- Serve with salad.

Nutrition per serving: Calories: 470kcal | Protein: 45g | Fat: 31g | carbs: 23 g

5.38 Turkey Fajitas Platter

Ingredients

- Cooked Turkey Breast: 1/4 cup
- Six Tortilla Wraps
- One Yellow Pepper
- One Red Pepper
- Half Red Onion
- Soft Cheese: 5 Tbsp.
- Mexican Seasoning: 2 Tbsp.
- Cumin: 1 Tsp
- Kosher salt& Pepper
- Cajun Spice: 3 Tbsp.
- Fresh Coriander

Instructions

- Slice the vegetables.
- Dice up turkey breast into small bite-size pieces.
- In a bowl, add onions, turkey, soft cheese, and peppers along with seasonings. Mix it well.
- Place it in foil and the oven.
- Cook for 20 minutes at 200C.
- Serve hot.

Nutrition per serving: Calories: 379kcal | Carbohydrates: 84g | Protein: 30g | Fat: 39g |

5.39 Turkey Breast Tenderloin

Ingredients

- Turkey breast tenderloin: one-piece
- Thyme: half tsp.
- Sage: half tsp.
- Paprika: half tsp.
- Pink salt: half tsp.
- Freshly ground black pepper: half tsp.

Instructions

- Let the oven preheat to 350 F
- In a bowl, mix all the spices and herbs, rub it all over the turkey.

- Put the turkey in the oven and let it cook at 350 F for 25 minutes, flip halfway through.
- Serve with salad.

Nutrition per serving: Calories: 162kcal | Carbohydrates: 1g | Protein: 13g | Fat: 1g |

5.40 Turkey Breast with Maple Mustard Glaze

Ingredients

- Whole turkey breast: 5 pounds
- Olive oil: 2 tsp.
- Maple syrup: 1/4 cup
- Dried sage: half tsp.
- Smoked paprika: half tsp.
- Dried thyme: one tsp.
- Salt: one tsp.
- Freshly ground black pepper: half tsp.
- Dijon mustard: 2 tbsp.

Instructions

- Let the oven preheat to 350 F
- Rub the olive oil all over the turkey breast
- In a bowl, mix salt, sage, pepper, thyme, and paprika. Mix well and coat turkey in this spice rub.
- Place the turkey in an oven, cook for 25 minutes at 350°F. Flip the turkey over and cook for another 12 minutes. Flip again and cook for another ten minutes. With an instant-read thermometer, the internal temperature should reach 165°F.
- In the meantime, in a saucepan, mix mustard, maple syrup, and with one tsp. of butter.
- Brush this glaze all over the turkey when cooked.

- Cook again for five minutes. Slice and Serve with salad green.

Nutrition per serving: Cal 379 | Fat: 23 g| Carbs: 21g | Protein: 52g

5.41 Juicy Turkey Burgers with Zucchini

Ingredients

- Gluten-free breadcrumbs: 1/4 cup(seasoned)
- Grated zucchini: 1 cup
- Red onion: 1 tbsp. (grated)
- Lean ground turkey: 4 cups
- One clove of minced garlic
- 1 tsp of kosher salt and fresh pepper

Instructions

- In a bowl, add zucchini (moisture removed with a paper towel), ground turkey, garlic, salt, onion, pepper, breadcrumbs. Mix well
- With your hands, makes five patties. But not too thick.
- Let the oven preheat to 375 F
- Put in an oven in a single layer and cook for 7 minutes or more. Until cooked through and browned.
- Place in buns with ketchup and lettuce and enjoy.

Nutrition per serving: Calories: 161kcal| Carbohydrates: 4.5g| Protein: 18g|Fat: 7g|

5.42 Oven Turkey Breast

Ingredients

- Turkey breast: 4 pounds, ribs removed, bone with skin
- Olive oil: 1 tablespoon
- Salt: 2 teaspoons

- Dry turkey seasoning (without salt): half tsp.

Instructions

- Rub half tbsp. Of olive oil over turkey breast. Sprinkle salt, turkey seasoning on both sides of turkey breast with half tbsp. of olive oil.

- Let the oven preheat at 350 F. put turkey skin side down in the oven and cook for 20 minutes until the turkey's temperature reaches 160 F for half an hour to 40 minutes.

- Let it sit for ten minutes before slicing.

- Serve.

Nutrition per serving: Calories: 226kcal| Protein: 32.5g|Fat: 10g|carbs 22 g

5.43 Turkey & Noodles

Ingredients

- Dry elbow macaroni: 2 cups

- Olive oil: 1 tablespoon

- 2 pounds of lean ground turkey

- Half cup of diced green onions

- Half cup of chopped green pepper

- Italian seasoning: 1 tablespoon

- Black pepper: 1 teaspoon

- Canned tomatoes, no salt: one cup

Instructions

- Cook pasta as per instructions.

- In a pan, brown the turkey in heated olive oil.

- Add bell peppers, tomatoes, seasoning, black pepper, cooked macaroni, and onions. Mix well.

- Cover and let it simmer for five minutes. Serve right away

Nutrition per serving: 273 calories | 188 mg sodium|33 g protein| 80 mg cholesterol| 533 mg potassium|7 g total fat |22 g carbohydrates |296 mg phosphorus| 1 g saturated fat |2 g fiber| 55 mg calcium

5.44 Rotini with Mock Italian Sausage

Ingredients

- ¾ Pound of lean ground turkey

- Half cup uncooked rotini pasta

- ¾ teaspoon of Italian seasoning

- 1 cup diced onion

- Half cup of celery, chopped

- 1 clove of minced garlic

- One cup of red bell pepper, chopped

- Crushed red pepper: ¼ teaspoon

- Tomato paste, no salt added: 3 tablespoons

- Grated parmesan cheese: 2 tablespoons

- Fennel seeds: ¼ teaspoon

Instructions

- Cook pasta as per instructions. Set it aside

- Cook turkey until browned. Drain with paper towels.

- Add celery, seasonings, and onion—Cook for three minutes.

- Add tomato paste, bell pepper. Lower the heat, partially cover, and simmer for 15 minutes.

- Serve over pasta.

Nutrition per serving: 165 calories | 250 mg sodium| 13 g protein| 41 mg cholesterol | 458 mg potassium| 2 g total fat| 28 g carbohydrate |161 mg phosphorus| 1 gram saturated fat |2 g fiber| 65 mg calcium

5.45 Turkey New Orleans style

Ingredients

- Vegetable oil: 2 tablespoons
- Green peppers: ¼ cup diced
- 1-pound lean ground turkey
- Half tsp. Of cayenne pepper
- All-purpose flour: 2 tablespoons
- 1 clove of minced garlic
- Celery: ¼ cup, chopped
- Onion: ¼ cup diced
- Cooked rice: 2 cups
- Green onions: ¼ cup diced
- Chicken broth, low sodium: 1 cup

Instructions

- Let the oven preheat to 350 F
- Cook meat until browned in hot oil. Drain on a paper towel.
- Add flour and stir until light brown. Add peppers, onions, garlic, and celery. Cook till vegetables are soft.
- Add meat, rice to the pan.
- Add a little broth, so it's not too wet.
- Add into the baking dish.
- Bake for 18-20 minutes.

Nutrition per serving: 393 calories | 113 mg sodium|27 g protein| 84 mg cholesterol | 377 mg potassium|19 g total fat |28 g carbohydrate| 228 mg phosphorus|4 g saturated| 1 g fiber |43 mg calcium

5.46 Barbecue Cups

Ingredients

- One package of low-fat biscuits
- Lean ground turkey: ¾ pounds
- Onion flakes: 2 teaspoons
- Half cup of spicy barbecue sauce
- Dash of garlic powder

Instructions

- In a skillet, brown the meat.
- Add garlic powder, barbecue sauce, and onion flakes, mix it well
- Add biscuits and press in the muffin tin
- Add meat mixture in the center.
- Bake for 10-12 minutes, at 400°F.

Nutrition per serving: 134 calories | 342 mg sodium|7 g protein| 27 mg cholesterol | 151 mg potassium|5 g total fat |13 g carbohydrate| 152 mg phosphorus|1 g saturated fat| 0 g fiber| 11 mg calcium

5.47 Low Sodium Beef Stew Recipe

Ingredients

- 2 diced celery stalks
- 2 to 3 lbs. of stew meat, cut in one-inch pieces, boneless
- One diced onion
- One carrot sliced
- 2 cloves of minced garlic
- Tomato paste, no salt added: 3 tablespoons
- Frozen peas: 1 cup
- Red cooking wine: 1 cup
- One bay leaf
- Dijon mustard: 2 tablespoons, low sodium
- Beef broth, low sodium: 1 and a half cups
- Black pepper: 1 teaspoon
- Fresh parsley: 2 tablespoons, chopped

- Dried thyme: 1 teaspoon

Instructions

- Add oil to a large frying pan and bring to a simmer over medium heat. Add celery, carrots, onion, garlic, and thyme, occasionally stirring for about 10 minutes until the carrots just begin to soften.

- Add tomato paste, mustard, and wine, and stir well. Simmer for 5-10 minutes until the wine reduces by about half. Remove from heat and set aside.

- In a slow cooker, add meat, beef broth, pepper, and wine/vegetable mixture. Make sure meat is coated.

- Stir in the bay leaf, cover, and cook on high for 5-6 hours. Stir every hour, if possible.

- Add frozen peas and fresh parsley at the very end, about 10 minutes before serving.

Nutrients per serving: calories 124| total fat 1.8 g| saturated fat 0.0 g| monounsaturated fat 0.5 g| cholesterol 38 mg| calcium 7.8 mg| sodium 32 mg| phosphorus 89 mg| potassium 78 mg| | protein 12.9 g

5.48 Roast Turkey with Fresh Sage

- Olive oil: 1 teaspoon

- One fresh turkey of 12 pound

- Half diced yellow onion

- One bunch of fresh sage

- Poultry seasoning: 2 teaspoons

Instructions

- Remove turkey neck, giblets from the turkey cavity. Wash and pat dry.

- Add poultry seasoning in the cavity, add sage and onion.

- Grease the roasting pan and place turkey.

- Let the oven preheat to 350 F, bake for 2.5-3 hours, cook until juices run clear.

- Take out from the oven, cover with aluminum foil,

- Let it rest for 20 minutes, then serve.

Nutrients per serving: calories 134| total fat 2.8 g| saturated fat 0.9 g| monounsaturated fat 0.5 g| polyunsaturated fat 0.7 g| cholesterol 59 mg| calcium 16 mg| sodium 54 mg| phosphorus 186 mg| potassium 259 mg| | protein 25 g

5.49 Broccoli & Beef Stir-Fry

Ingredients

- Cooked rice: 2 cups

- 2 cloves of garlic, minced

- One cup of uncooked lean sirloin beef, cut into strips

- Olive oil: 2 tablespoons

- One and a half cups of frozen broccoli

- One small roma tomato, chopped

- Chicken broth, low-sodium: 1/4 cup

- Soy sauce, reduced-sodium: 2 tablespoons

- Cornstarch: 1 tablespoon

Instructions

- Thaw the broccoli.

- In a pan, sauté garlic for one minute, add broccoli, cook for five minutes. Take out from the pan and set it aside.

- In the same pan, add meat, cook to your desired likeness.

- In a bowl, mix soy sauce, chicken broth, and cornstarch.
- Add vegetables, tomato, and sauce to the beef. Cook and stir until sauce is thick.
- Serve with a half cup of rice.

Nutrients per serving: Calories 373| Protein 18 g| Carbohydrates 37 g| Fat 17 g| Cholesterol 42 mg| Sodium 351 mg| Potassium 555 mg| Phosphorus 255 mg| Calcium 62 mg| Fiber 5.1 g

5.50 Italian Beef with Peppers & Onions

Ingredients

- 1 tsp. of garlic powder
- Lean beef roast: 3-pound, fat trimmed
- 1 tsp. of crushed red pepper
- Black pepper: 2 teaspoons
- One sliced onion
- Oregano: 2 teaspoons
- Half cup of pepperoncini juice
- One diced green bell pepper, one red, one yellow

Instructions

- In a crockpot, add black pepper, red pepper, beef roast, garlic powder, oregano. Cook for 4-5 hours on high until soft enough.
- Take out from the pot, shred the meat, and remove the fat.
- Add shredded beef to the pot again, add onions, pepperoncini juice, and peppers.
- Cook for 50-60 minutes, on high, until vegetables are tender.

Nutrients per serving: Calories 212| Protein 25 g| Carbohydrates 3 g| Fat 11 g|

Cholesterol 84 mg| Sodium 121 mg| Potassium 280 mg| Phosphorus 196 mg| Calcium 21 mg| Fiber 0.6 g

5.51 Braised Beef Brisket

Ingredients

- Beef broth, reduced-sodium: 2 cups
- Half medium onion, chopped
- One carrot, chopped
- Fresh parsley: 1 tablespoon, chopped
- Two and a half pounds of beef brisket (trimmed fat)
- One stalk of celery, chopped
- Black pepper: 2 teaspoons
- 3 bay leaves. Crumbled
- 3 cups of water
- Two tablespoons of balsamic vinegar
- Canola oil: 2 tablespoons

Instructions

- Let the oven preheat to 350º F.
- Sprinkle the beef with black pepper.
- In a Dutch oven, brown beef for five minutes on every side in hot oil over medium heat.
- Take out the meat and add carrots, onion, and celery.
- Cook for four minutes.
- Add parsley and bay leaves to the vegetable mix, and put meat on top of the vegetables.
- Add water, broth, and balsamic vinegar.
- Let it boil.
- Cover the pot and cook in the oven for one and a half hours. Flip the meat over and cook a one and a half

hours more until beef is soft enough to shred with a fork.

- Take the meat out from the pot. Store broth for gravy

- Serve the brisket.

Nutrients per serving: Calories 230| Protein 29 g| Carbohydrates 4 g| Fat 11 g| Cholesterol 84 mg| Sodium 178 mg| Potassium 346 mg| Phosphorus 193 mg| Calcium 30 mg| Fiber 0.8 g|

Chapter 6: Kidney-Friendly Fish & Seafood Recipes

6.1 Tuna Fish Salad with Fennel & Orange Salsa

Ingredients

- Garlic-infused olive oil: 2 teaspoons
- Smoked paprika: 1 teaspoon
- Ground coriander: 1 teaspoon
- Salt: ¼ teaspoon
- Black pepper: 1/8 teaspoon
- Fresh tuna steak: 5 cups
- olive oil: 1 teaspoon
- Fennel bulb (1 bulb)
- Olive oil: 3 tablespoons
- Two oranges
- Five olives: chopped
- Parsley: 2 tablespoons
- Dried oregano: ½ teaspoon
- Cider vinegar: 2 tablespoons
- Thinly sliced scallion greens: ¼ cup
- Salt: 1/16 teaspoon
- Black pepper

Instructions

- Combine the smoked paprika, two tsp. Of garlic-infused oil, salt, coriander, and pepper into a shallow dish. Brush the tuna steak with the spice mixture on both sides and put aside.

- Break off fennel bulb stalks and throw them away. Slice pieces of fennel into 1/4 inch of the neck and put them in one layer on the baking sheet. Drizzle with two teaspoons of oil.

- Roast for about 11 to 13 minutes, till the fennel becomes medium golden brown. turn the pieces over and brown for five minutes, take out from the oven and cool it down

- Zest the orange it into a serving bowl, add 1/4 cup of orange juice. chop up another orange

- Add the oregano, juice, olives, sliced orange bits, parsley, cider vinegar, salt and peppers, scallions, two tablespoons remaining of garlic-infused liquid the orange zest.

- Coarsely chop and whisk the cooked, roasted fennel into the orange salsa.

- Preheat medium-heat a large skillet; drizzle with canola oil.

- Add the tuna steaks to the skillet and cook for five minutes until browned at the rim. Switch on the other side and cook for four minutes.

- Take the tuna off from the heat Break the tuna into pieces, following 2 or 3 minutes of rest.

- Cover 1/2 cup of Roasted Fennel Orange Salsa, then finish with 1/4 of the seared tuna strips.

Nutrition Per Serving: 351 calories| total fat 16 g | carbohydrates 14.4 g| protein 23 g | Cholesterol 4.1 mg| Sodium 142 mg| potassium 132 mg| Phosphorus 121 mg | Calcium 45 mg| Fiber 2.1 g

6.2 Baked Fish with Roasted Sweet Potatoes & Mushroom

Ingredients

- Wild Salmon: 1 and ½ cup, cut into four pieces
- sweet potatoes cubed: 2 cups, leached
- Olive oil divided: two tbsp.

- Salt: ¼ tsp.
- Herbs: 1 tsp.
- Mushrooms: 4 cups(sliced)
- Two cloves garlic: sliced
- Lemon juice: 4 tbsp.
- Ground pepper: ¼ tsp.
- Thyme

Instructions

- Let the oven heat till 425 F
- Add one tbsp. Of oil, potatoes, mushroom, pepper, and salt in a bowl.
- Transfer it to a baking dish and roast for almost forty minutes until the vegetables are soft. Stir the vegetables and add. garlic
- Place fish over it. Drizzle with one tbsp. Of oil, lemon juice. Sprinkle with herbs bake till fish is flaky for fifteen minutes.

Nutrition Per Serving: 275 calories| total fat 16.8 g | carbohydrates 15.4 g| protein 21.3 g | Cholesterol 5.3 mg| Sodium 132 mg| potassium 141 mg| Phosphorus 111 mg | Calcium 56 mg| Fiber 2.3 g

6.3 Swordfish with Olives, Capers over Polenta

Ingredients

- Chopped red peppers: 2 Cups
- Half cup of regular or coarse yellow cornmeal
- Swordfish: 4 cups, cut into four steaks
- 2 and ½ cups of water
- Extra-virgin olive oil: 1 tablespoon
- Chopped fresh basil: 3 tablespoons
- 4 medium stalks celery, chopped
- ¼ of cup green olives pitted and roughly diced
- Capers: 1 tablespoon rinsed
- A pinch of crushed red pepper
- Half teaspoon of salt, divided
- 2 cloves of pressed garlic
- For garnish Fresh basil
- Freshly ground black pepper: ⅛ teaspoon

Instructions

- Put a saucepan over medium flame and boil two cups of water with 1/4 tsp. of salt. Add the cornmeal carefully to avoid any lumps.
- Cook for three minutes, keep stirring.
- Lower the heat. Stir after every five minutes, cook for 20-25 minutes. If it becomes too hard, add a half cup of water, turn off the heat but keep it covered.
- In the meantime, in a large skillet over a medium flame, add in the oil. Add celery fry it, frequently stirring, until soft, for around five minutes.
- Then add garlic, cook for almost 30 seconds. Add in olives, bell peppers, basil, crushed red pepper, capers, freshly ground black pepper and the remaining 1/4 tsp. of Sea salt.
- Cover it lower the heat and cook for five minutes.
- Add swordfish in the sauce. Let it simmer, and Cover it cook for 10-15 minutes, till swordfish is cooked completely.

- On a serving tray, layer the cornmeal at the bottom. Add the fish over the cornmeal, cover with the sauce and, garnish with fresh basil, serve hot and enjoy

Nutrition Per Serving: 276 calories| total fat 12.1 g | carbohydrates 13.2 g| protein 22 g | Cholesterol 5.3 mg| Sodium 131 mg| potassium 124 mg| Phosphorus 104 mg | Calcium 46 mg| Fiber 2.4 g

6.4 Salmon Souvlaki Bowls

Ingredients

- 4 cups of fresh salmon sliced into four pieces
- Fresh oregano: 1 tablespoon
- Lemon juice: 6 tablespoons
- vinegar: 2 tablespoons
- Smoked paprika: 1 tablespoon or regular paprika
- Fresh dill: 1 tablespoon
- Three tablespoons of extra virgin olive oil
- 2 cloves of minced garlic minced
- Half teaspoon of salt
- One teaspoon of black pepper
- Two cucumbers cut in sliced
- Dry pearl couscous: 1 cup
- Half cup of Kalamata olives
- One-inch zucchini cut into 1/4 rounds
- Juice from one lemon
- Extra virgin olive oil: 2 tablespoons

Red peppers: 2 pieces, quartered

Instructions

- Mix balsamic vinegar, oregano, smoked paprika, black pepper, garlic, salt, olive oil, dill, and lemon juice in a big mixing bowl and mix until well combined
- Pour this marinade all over the salmon, rub gently and make sure the salmon is covered in marinade. Let it rest for 15 minutes.
- In the meantime, cook couscous to your liking.
- Mix two tablespoons of olive oil, red peppers, black pepper, salt, and zucchini in a mixing bowl. Mix well to coat the vegetables.
- Let the grill/grill pan heat up over medium flame.
- Grill the salmon on each side for about three minutes. Or cook to your liking.
- After salmon, grill zucchini, bell peppers for four minutes each side so the grill marks will appear.
- Take serving bowls, add faro or couscous on the bottom, add lemon juice to coat couscous. Then add salmon, olives, grilled veggies, cucumbers.
- Add any of your favorite sauce or Tzatziki sauce, add fresh herbs and serve.

Nutrition Per Serving: 244 calories| total fat 14 g | carbohydrates 17.1g| protein 21 g | Cholesterol 6.1 mg| Sodium 131 mg| potassium 120 mg| Phosphorus 109 mg | Calcium 48.2 mg| Fiber 2.2 g

6.5 Mediterranean Tuna- Salad

Ingredients

- One can of 5 ounces, drained chunk light tuna in water

- One and ½ tablespoons of water
- 4 Kalamata olives, pitted, diced
- Feta cheese crumbled: 2 tablespoons
- One and ½ tablespoons of tahini
- One and ½ tablespoons of lemon juice
- Parsley: 2 tablespoons
- One medium orange, sliced(peeled)

Instructions

- In a bowl, whisk together the water, tahini, and lemon juice. Add salmon, olives, parsley, and feta, toss to combine.
- Serve right away the tuna salad with the orange wedges on the side, with a cup of kale.

Nutrition Per Serving: 275 calories| total fat 11.4 g | carbohydrates 13.2 g| protein 21 g | Cholesterol 5.3 mg| Sodium 134 mg| potassium 142 mg| Phosphorus 119.9 mg | Calcium 52 mg| Fiber 2.9 g

6.6 Salmon Bowl with Faro, Green Beans, & Tahini Dressing

Ingredients

- Extra-virgin olive oil: 6 tablespoons divided
- Half of a cup cooked green beans
- Salmon: 3/4 cup
- Tahini: 2 tablespoons
- Zest and juice of one lemon
- ¼ of teaspoon garlic powder
- Half teaspoon of turmeric, divided
- Faro: ¼ cup
- Half of teaspoon cumin
- One and ½ teaspoons smoked paprika
- 2 scallions, thinly chopped

- Half teaspoon of coriander
- 4 pieces' lettuce leaves
- Fresno Chile: ¼ of a whole, thinly sliced
- Kosher salt and freshly ground black pepper

Instructions

- Mix lemon zest, the tahini, lemon juice, garlic powder, and 1⁄4 teaspoon of Turmeric and a big bowl.
- Slowly add three tablespoons of olive oil and mix until smooth and fully emulsified for the sauce. Adjust salt and pepper.
- Put a small pot over medium flame, add the faro, and one cup of water. Let it boil. Lower the heat and let it simmer for 20 -25 minutes until the faro is soft. Set it aside.
- In a bowl, add one tablespoon of olive oil, the beans, and the cumin mix well set it aside.
- With smoked paprika, 1⁄4 teaspoon of turmeric, coriander, salt, and pepper mix it and season the salmon with this pace mix.
- Heat the remaining two tablespoons of olive oil over a low flame in a medium skillet. Add in the salmon and cook for about five minutes until lightly browned on one side and opaque in the middle.
- Lay lettuce leaves at the bottom of a serving bowl. Add Faro, salmon, and green beans. Garnish with the slices of the scallions, and the diced chili add dressing on top

Nutrition Per Serving: 351 calories| total fat 18.2 g | carbohydrates 12.3 g| protein 17.1 g | Cholesterol 5.1 mg| Sodium 141 mg|

potassium 113 mg| Phosphorus 109 mg | Calcium 47.2 mg| Fiber 2.4 g

6.7 Salmon Pita Sandwich

Ingredients

- Pita bread: half (6 inches)
- Chopped fresh dill: 2 teaspoons
- Half of a teaspoon prepared horseradish
- Nonfat yogurt: 2 tablespoons(plain)
- Flaked canned sockeye salmon: 6 tbsp.(drained)
- Half of a cup watercress
- Lemon juice: 2 teaspoons

Instructions

- In a small mixing bowl, mix lemon juice, yogurt, horseradish, and dill.
- Mix well.
- Add in the salmon.
- Put the salmon salad into a pita pocket with watercress.
- Serve right away, enjoy.

Nutrition Per Serving: 239 calories| total fat 7.1 g | carbohydrates 12.3 g| protein 19.4 g | Cholesterol 5.1 mg| Sodium 132 mg| potassium 138 mg| Phosphorus 131 mg | Calcium 52 mg| Fiber 3 g

6.8 Smoked Salmon & Poached Eggs on Toast

Ingredients

With sesame seeds & soy sauce

- Lemon juice: 1/4 tsp
- Salt & pepper to taste
- Smoked salmon: 3.5 oz.
- Scallions: 1 TBSP (sliced)
- Bread toasted: 2 slices

- Two poached eggs
- Dash of soy sauce
- Microgreens is optional

Everything bagel seasoning with tomato

- Avocado: 1/2
- Bread: 2 slices
- Lemon juice: 1/4 tsp
- Smoked salmon: 3.5 oz.
- Two poached eggs
- Salt & pepper to taste
- Two thin slices of tomatoes
- Microgreens are also optional.
- Everything Bagel Seasoning: 1 tsp

Instructions

- Smash the Avocado in a dish. Add a pinch of salt and lemon juice; combine properly, and put aside.
- Poach your eggs, and toast your bread as the eggs rest in the ice water
- Place the Avocado on both slices once your bread is toasted, then add the smoked salmon to each piece.
- Place the poached eggs gently on each of the toast.
- Add a drop of Kikkoman soy sauce and some crushed pepper, scallion, and microgreen garnish.

Nutrition Per Serving: 201 calories| total fat 12.3 g | carbohydrates 6.9 g| protein 12.7 g | Cholesterol 3.1 mg| Sodium 141 mg| potassium 126 mg| Phosphorus 112 mg | Calcium 47 mg| Fiber 2.8 g

6.9 Mediterranean Couscous with Tuna & Pepperoncini

Ingredients

For Couscous

One and ¼ cups couscous

One cup of chicken broth or water

¾ teaspoon of kosher salt

For Accompaniments

- ¼ of a cup capers
- Two cans oil-packed tuna: 5-ounce each
- Half of a cup sliced pepperoncini
- ⅓ of a cup chopped fresh parsley
- Extra-virgin olive oil, for serving
- One lemon wedges
- Kosher salt and freshly ground black pepper

Instructions

- To Make the Couscous: Put a small saucepan over medium heat, add broth or water to the pan let it boil. Turn off the heat, add the couscous, and let it rest for ten minutes.
- To make the accompaniments: In the meantime, add the tuna, pepperoncini, capers, and parsley in a small bowl and mix.
- With the help of a fork, fluff the couscous, sprinkle pepper, salt, and olive oil in it, and mix well.
- On a serving plate, put couscous on the bottom, add the tuna mix on top, drizzle lemon juice and serve with lemon slices.

Nutrition Per Serving: 226 calories| total fat 4g | carbohydrates 12.3 g| protein 8.4 g | Cholesterol 4.1 mg| Sodium 131 mg| potassium 133 mg| Phosphorus 112 mg | Calcium 43 mg| Fiber 2.6 g

6.10 Salmon Cakes

Ingredients

- One tablespoon of oil
- Garlic (minced): 1/2 tsp
- Salmon: 5 oz. cooked and finely diced
- Smoked paprika: 1/4 tsp
- 3 - 4 tablespoon of flour
- Fine kosher or sea salt: 1/4 tsp
- Curry powder: 1/4 tsp (optional)
- One sprig of rosemary
- Black pepper: 1/4 tsp
- Two egg whites

Instructions

- Mashup the salmon. remove any skin, if any
- Put the salmon in a bowl, then add the mashed veggies.
- Then add one tbsp. at a time in flour. Depending on the kind of salmon you choose, you'll need just 3-4 tbsp. Then add in herbs and seasonings. Mix well.
- Finally, add in two eggs.
- Mix well that the batter gets thick enough for patties to shape. Add one tbsp. More flour if the batter is too liquid.
- Shape into small or larger balls. then turn them into patties
- Turn the skillet on to medium flame add butter
- When hot, put in at least three or four cakes at a time. Cook on either side for almost four minutes, or until the salmon is fully cooked. Canned salmon cooks early, repeat the frying process for the rest of the cakes.

- Garnish with black pepper, rosemary, chili flakes, and a sprinkle of garlic if needed, serve hot.

Nutrition Per Serving: 91 calories| total fat 4 g | carbohydrates 6 g| protein 10 g | Cholesterol 4.3 mg| Sodium 101 mg| potassium 89 mg| Phosphorus 87 mg | Calcium 33 mg| Fiber 2.8 g

6.11 Salmon Parcels with Wild Rice, Pesto, & Broccoli

Ingredients

- Salmon fillets: one cup
- rice: one cup
- Red pesto: 3 tablespoon
- One lemon: half juiced and half thinly sliced
- Purple sprouting broccoli: half cup
- Black olives chopped: 2 tablespoon
- Basil

Instructions

- Let the overheat till 200 C to gas6, a 180 C. line the baking tray with parchment paper. Separate the mixed grains and rice. Stir in the lemon juice, olives, 2 tbsp. of pesto, and half of the basil. Mix well, put in the center of the baking tray
- Place the salmon over the grains and scatter over each fillet the remaining pesto. Cover with the slices of lemon and broccoli, then cover with parchment paper on top. make it a packet around filling
- Roast for about half an hour in the oven till broccoli is soft and salmon is completely cooked
- Serve with basil on top.

Nutrition Per Serving: 361 calories| total fat 16.2 g | carbohydrates 18 g| protein 9 g |

Cholesterol 5.1 mg| Sodium 114 mg| potassium 121 mg| Phosphorus 109 mg | Calcium 56 mg| Fiber 3.2 g

6.12 Fish Taco Bowls with Chipotle Aioli over Cauliflower Rice

Ingredients

Blackened Fish

- Olive oil: 1 tablespoon
- Tilapia loins: 2 piece
- Salt: ½ tsp
- Smoked paprika: 1/2 tsp.
- Onion powder: 1/2 tsp.
- Chili powder: 1 tsp.
- Cumin: ¼ tsp
- Pepper: 1/4 teaspoon
- Garlic powder: 1/2 tsp.

Chipotle aioli

- Adobo sauce: 1 teaspoon
- Garlic powder: 1/2 tsp.
- Lime juice: ¼ tsp
- Low fat Mayonnaise: 1/4 tbsp.
- Chipotle pepper (in adoboe sauce): 1 tsp
- Soy milk: 1 tablespoon (full-fat)
- Salt: 1 tsp

Red Cabbage Slaw

Half piece of a lime juiced

Head red cabbage: 2 cups, sliced

Salt: 1 tsp

Instructions

For Fish

In a shallow bowl, mix all the spices and brush gently over the top and bottom of fish fillets.

Heat the skillet over a medium flame, add coconut oil, then add fish.

Look on either side for around four minutes, or until the fish flakes. don't let the fish overcook

Chipotle (Aioli)

- In a food processor, mix all the ingredients and pulse until creamy. Taste and mix with more salt or lime juice. if needed

Red Cabbage Slaw

- Mix all ingredients in a small bowl. mix lime juice and salt onto cabbage with your hands to tenderize before purple juices start oozing out

- Assemble your Fish Taco Bowls:

- Put coconut-lime Cauliflower rice in a bowl. Add red cabbage slaw with cauliflower rice. Cover with fish fillet, mango salsa, guacamole. while serving, add chipotle sauce.

Nutrition Per Serving: 239 calories| total fat 11 g | carbohydrates 21 g| protein 17 g | Cholesterol 5.6 mg| Sodium 121 mg| potassium 105 mg| Phosphorus 110 mg | Calcium 51 mg| Fiber 3.1 g

6.13 Fish Fajita

Ingredients

- 1 and 1/2 tsp. olive oil
- Fish: 4 cups
- One yellow, one red, one orange sliced bell peppers
- One tsp. of kosher salt
- Garlic powder: 1/2 tsp.
- Chili powder: 2 teaspoon
- Ground cumin: 1/2 teaspoon
- Lime

- Black pepper
- Cilantro
- Smoked paprika: 1/2 tsp
- Tortillas
- Onion powder: 1/2 teaspoon
- One onion sliced

Instructions

- Let the oven pre-heat to 450 F
- Add the fish, onion, olive oil, bell pepper, pepper, and salt, spices into a big bowl. mix well
- Spray oil on a baking sheet
- On that baking sheet, arrange the bell peppers, shrimp, and onions.
- Cook for about eight minutes, at 450 F. Switch the oven to broil, cook for another two minutes or until fish is completely cooked
- Squeeze lime juice over it and finish with coriander.
- Put in a warm tortilla and serve.

Nutrition Per Serving: 184 calories| total fat 9 g | carbohydrates 21 g| protein 13 g | Cholesterol 7.1 mg| Sodium 114 mg| potassium 123 mg| Phosphorus 104 mg | Calcium 45 mg| Fiber 2.8 g

6.14 Salmon with Green Bean Pilaf

Ingredients

- Olive oil: 3 tbsp.
- Pre-cooked white rice: one cup
- Wild salmon: 1 & ¼ pound (skinned and cut into four pieces)
- Green beans and cut into thirds: 12 ounces
- Low fat Mayonnaise: 2 tbsp.
- Minced garlic: one tbsp.

- Pine nuts: 2 tbsp.
- Water: 2 tbsp.
- Salt: ¾ tsp.
- Ground pepper: half tsp.
- Parsley
- Whole-grain mustard: 2 tsp.
- One lemon: zested, cut into wedges

Instructions

- Let the oven pre-heat till 425 F.
- Place parchment paper on baking sheet
- Brush the salmon with one spoonful of oil and place them on the baking sheet.
- Mash the salt and garlic together. In a small bowl, combine one teaspoon of the garlic paste with mustard, mayonnaise, 1/4 teaspoon of pepper.
- Spread the blend over the fish.
- Roast the salmon until it flakes easily —six-eight minutes per inch of thickness.
- Heat the remaining two spoons of oil over medium flame in a skillet.
- Add lemon zest, green beans, pine nuts, leftover garlic paste, and black pepper; stir for almost four minutes until the beans are soft.
- Reduce to medium heat. Add the rice and water and cook for three minutes, stirring, until hot.
- Serve with green beans and lemon and top with parsley.

Nutrition Per Serving: 242 calories| total fat 17.1 g | carbohydrates 18.1 g| protein 21.1 g | Cholesterol 6.1 mg| Sodium 125 mg| potassium 113 mg| Phosphorus 127 mg | Calcium 56 mg| Fiber 2.1 g

6.15 Fish Tacos with Broccoli Slaw & Cumin Sour Cream

Ingredients

- Eight tortillas
- Fish sticks: 2 10-oz. Packages
- Half red onion sliced
- Two limes, juiced and wedges
- Broccoli: 12 ounces
- Kosher salt: 1 tsp.
- Olive oil: 2 tablespoons
- Half cup of sour cream
- Cilantro: 1 cup
- Half tsp. of ground cumin

Instructions

- According to the direction on the package, cook the fish sticks.
- Chop broccoli' heads. Peel the stalks and cut them into matchsticks.
- In a large bowl, add the lime juice, onion, and 3⁄4 teaspoon of salt., mix and set aside around ten minutes.
- Add broccoli stalks and tops, oil, cilantro, and mix
- Mix cumin, sour cream, and salt in a small dish. Serve with fish

Nutrition Per Serving: 227 calories| total fat 14 g | carbohydrates 12.5 g| protein 20.3 g | Cholesterol 7.1 mg| Sodium 120 mg| potassium 109 mg| Phosphorus 102 mg | Calcium 6.1 mg| Fiber 3 g

6.16 Roasted Salmon with Smoky Chickpeas & Greens

Ingredients

- Wild salmon: 1 and ¼ pounds, cut in 4 pieces
- Chopped kale: 10 cups

- Olive oil: 2 tbsp.
- Salt: half tsp.
- Can of chickpeas: 15 ounces
- Garlic powder: ¼ tsp.
- Buttermilk: 1/3 cup
- Low fat Mayonnaise: ¼ cup
- Smoked paprika: one tbsp.
- Water: ¼ cup
- Ground pepper: half tsp.
- Chives: ¼ cup

Instructions

- let the oven pre-heat 'til 425 F and put the racks in the upper third portion, middle of the oven
- In a bowl, add one spoon of paprika, oil, 1/4 tsp of salt.
- Dry the chickpeas and mix with the paprika blend, put them on a baking sheet, and bake for half an hour on the upper rack.
- In the food, blender adds puree buttermilk, basil, mayonnaise,1/4 tsp of pepper, and garlic powder pulse till creamy. Set it aside.
- Heat a skillet, add one tablespoon of oil over medium flame.
- Add the kale, cook for two minutes. Add water and keep cooking, around five minutes until the kale is soft.
- Remove from flame, and add salt in the dish.
- Take out the chickpeas from the oven, transfer them to one side of the pan. Place the salmon on the other hand, and season with salt and pepper.
- Bake for 5- 8 minutes until the salmon is completely cooked.

- Top with dressing, herbs, and serve with kale and chickpeas.

Nutrition Per Serving: 247 calories| total fat 13.2 g | carbohydrates 14.2 g| protein 24 g | Cholesterol 5.3 mg| Sodium 123 mg| potassium 133 mg| Phosphorus 109 mg | Calcium 56 mg| Fiber 3.1 g

6.17 Smoked Salmon Salad with Green Dressing

Ingredients

- Smoked salmon: 180g
- Green lentils: 1/2 cup washed
- Half a cup of yogurt
- Parsley: 2 tablespoons
- Salted baby capers: 1 tablespoon
- Chives: 2 tablespoons
- Two small fennel bulbs, sliced
- Tarragon: 1 tablespoon
- Grated lemon rind: 1 teaspoon
- Half of onion, sliced
- Fresh lemon juice: 1 tablespoon
- Pinch of sugar

Instructions

- Let the lentils cook for twenty minutes or until soft, in a wide saucepan of boiling water. then drain
- In the meantime, heat a pan on high flame. Spray oil on slices of fennel. Cook per side for two minutes, or until soft.
- In a food processor, pulse the parsley, yogurt, chives, capers, tarragon, and lemon rind until creamy. season with black pepper
- In a bowl, place the sugar, onion, juice, a pinch of salt. Drain after five minutes.

- In a wide bowl, add the lentils, onion, fennel. Divide into plates. Put salmon on top. Drizzle with green dressing and fennels

Nutrition Per Serving: 310 calories| total fat 17 g | carbohydrates 12.2 g| protein 17 g | Cholesterol 5.6 mg| Sodium 141 mg| potassium 124 mg| Phosphorus 127 mg | Calcium 43 mg| Fiber 2.5 g

6.18 Greek Roasted Fish with Vegetables

Ingredients

- Four skinless salmon fillets: 5-6 ounces
- Two red, yellow, orange sweet peppers, cut into rings
- Five cloves of garlic chopped
- Sea salt: half tsp.
- Olive oil: 2 tbsp.
- Black pepper: half tsp
- Pitted halved olives: ¼ cup
- One lemon
- Parsley: 1 and ½ cups
- Finely snipped fresh oregano:1/4 cup

Instructions

- Let the oven preheat to 425 F
- Put the potatoes in a bowl. Drizzle 1 spoon of oil, sprinkle with salt (1/8 tsp.), and garlic. Mix well, shift to the baking pan, cover with foil. Roast them for half an hour
- In the meantime, thaw the salmon. Combine the sweet peppers, parsley, oregano, olives, and salt (1/8 tsp) and pepper in the same bowl. Add one tablespoon of oil, mix well.
- Wash salmon and dry it with paper towels. Sprinkle with salt (1/4 Tsp),

Black pepper, and top of it, salmon. Uncover it and roast for ten minutes or till salmon starts to flake.

- Add lemon zest and lemon juice over salmon and vegetables. Serve hot

Nutrition Per Serving: 278 calories| total fat 12 g | carbohydrates 9.2 g| protein 15.4 g | Cholesterol 7.1 mg| Sodium 131 mg| potassium 141 mg| Phosphorus 121 mg | Calcium 56 mg| Fiber 3.4 g

6.19 Garlic Roasted Salmon & Brussels Sprouts

Ingredients

- Wild salmon fillet (6 portions): 2 pounds
- Olive oil: ¼ of cup
- White wine: ¾ cup
- Oregano: 2 tbsp.
- Cloves of garlic: 14
- Salt: 1 tsp.
- Lemon
- Black pepper: ¾ tsp.

Instructions:

- Let the oven pre-heat to 450 F
- take two cloves of garlic and mink them, put them in a bowl one tbsp. Of oregano, oil, half tsp. of salt and pepper (1/4 tsp.)
- In a roasting pan, halve the remaining garlic and add with Brussels sprouts and three tbsp. Of seasoned oil.
- Roast for fifteen minutes, stirring only once
- Add the wine to the remaining oil blend.
- Take out from the oven, mix vegetables, and put salmon on top.

- Sprinkle the wine oil, and salt, pepper, and oregano. Bake for ten minutes more or till fish is cooked completely. Serve with lemon.

Nutrition Per Serving: 334 calories| total fat 15.4 g | carbohydrates 10.3 g| protein 23 g | Cholesterol 6.6 mg| Sodium 134 mg| potassium 121 mg| Phosphorus 103 mg | Calcium 45 mg| Fiber 3 g

6.20 Ginger-Tahini Oven-Baked Salmon & Vegetables

Ingredients

- Salmon: 1 and ¼ pound cut into four portions
- Olive oil: two tbsp.
- Salt: half tsp.
- Light soy sauce: 2 tbsp.
- Tahini: 3 tbsp.
- Honey
- Green beans: 1 pound
- Ginger: 1 and ½ tsp.(grated)
- Chives: 2 tbsp.
- White button mushrooms: one-pound

Instructions

- Let the oven pre-heat till 425 F.
- Add a baking sheet in the range, in the upper rack, and one six inches from the broiler
- Put a broad baking sheet rimmed into the oven, place one rack in the oven center, and another about 6 inches from the broiler.
- Combine one tablespoon of oil, and mushrooms, with salt (1/4 tsp.) in a big bowl.
- Take the baking sheet out of the oven.

- Place the mixture of vegetables in one layer on the pan; start roasting it, often stirring, around 20 minutes.
- Meanwhile, mix the remaining 1 Tbsp. of oil with green beans and salt (1/4 tsp).
- In a tiny cup, mix soya sauce, ginger, tahini, and honey.
- Take out the pan from the oven. Add mushroom and sweet potatoes on one side, and on the other side place green beans.
- Place the salmon in the center. Distribute half of the tahini sauce over the salmon. Roast, for 8 to 10 minutes more, before the salmon falls.
- Switch broiler to high, transfer the pan to the top rack, and broil for around 3 minutes until the salmon is glazed.
- In the remaining tahini oil, add vinegar and drizzle over the salmon and vegetables. If needed, garnish with the chives and eat.

Nutrition Per Serving: 334 calories| total fat 13.4 g | carbohydrates 14.5 g| protein 17 g | Cholesterol 5.6 mg| Sodium 141 mg| potassium 134 mg| Phosphorus 111 mg | Calcium 56 mg| Fiber 2.7 g

6.21 Charred Shrimp & Pesto Buddha Bowls

Ingredients

- Pesto: 1/3 cup
- Vinegar: 2 tbsp.
- Olive oil: 1 tbsp.
- Salt: half tsp.
- Ground pepper: ¼ tsp.
- Peeled & deveined large shrimp: one pound

- Arugula: 4 cups
- Cooked quinoa: 2 cups

Instructions

- In a large bowl, mix pesto, oil, vinegar, salt, and pepper. Take out four tbsp. Of mixture in another bowl.

- Place skillet over medium flame. Add shrimp, let it cook for five minutes, stirring, until only charred a little. move to a plate

- Use the vinaigrette to mix with quinoa and arugula in a bowl. Divide the mixture of the arugula into four bowls. Cover with shrimp, Add 1 tbsp. Of the pesto mixture to each bowl. And serve.

Nutrition Per Serving: 329 calories| total fat 18 g | carbohydrates 17.2 g| protein 17 g | Cholesterol 6.7 mg| Sodium 154 mg| potassium 143 mg| Phosphorus 123 mg | Calcium 45 mg| Fiber 2.1 g

6.22 Salmon with Gingery Vegetables & Turmeric

Ingredients

- Salmon fillets with skin: 4pieces, 6-ounce

- Broccoli: cut into florets along with chopped stem: 1/2 pound

- Water: 3/4 cup

- Vegetable oil: 3 tablespoons

- Cauliflower, cut into florets: 1/2 pound

- One onion sliced

- Turmeric: 1/4 teaspoon

- Salt and pepper, to taste

- Soy milk: 1/2 cup

- Chopped lime pickle: 1 tablespoon

- Minced ginger: 1and 1/2 tbsp.

Instructions

- Boil broccoli and cauliflower in a deep pan, covered, for 3 minutes in half a cup of water; move to a bowl

- Heat the three tablespoons of oil in the pan. Stir in the ginger and onion season with salt, pepper, and simmer over medium flame, stirring for around eight minutes until golden. Add the turmeric and mix until fragrant.

- Add soy milk, the pickle, and the remaining water and carry it to a simmer.

- Add the vegetables then sprinkle with salt, pepper. cover it and remove from flame

- Let the grill pan, preheat. Oil the salmon and season with salt, pepper.

- Grill, skin side down, over medium flame, for 4 minutes to crisp. Switch and grill for 2 minutes, until just cooked through. Serve the vegetables with salmon.

Nutrition Per Serving: 118 calories| total fat 6.7 g | carbohydrates 5.6 g| protein 16g | Cholesterol 8.1 mg| Sodium 123 mg| potassium 132 mg| Phosphorus 112 mg | Calcium 76 mg| Fiber 2.3 g

6.23 Simple Grilled Salmon & Vegetables

Ingredients

- Salmon fillet, cut into four portions: 1 and ¼ pounds.

- Zucchini halved lengthwise: one-piece

- Two red, orange, or yellow bell peppers: de-seeded, and halved

- One onion: cut into one wedge

- Olive oil: one tbsp.
- Salt: half tsp.
- Basil: ¼ cup
- Ground pepper: half tsp.
- Lemon into wedges

Instructions

- Let the grill pre-heat to medium-high
- Rub the onion, zucchini, and peppers with oil and salt (1/4 teaspoon).
- Sprinkle the salmon with the pepper and salt (1/4 teaspoon)
- Place the vegetables and salmon (skin side down) on the barbecue.
- Cook the vegetables, rotating once or twice, for almost five minutes per side until only soft and grill marks happen.
- Cook the salmon, without turning, for ten minutes, till it flakes.
- Cool the vegetables and Chop roughly, then put together in a dish.
- If you do not like the skin, remove it from the salmon fillets, and serve alongside the vegetables. Garnish with one tbsp. Of basil on each serving, then serve with lemon.

Nutrition Per Serving: 281 calories| total fat 12.7g | carbohydrates 10.6g|protein 20.2g | Cholesterol 7.9 mg| Sodium 154 mg| potassium 162 mg| Phosphorus 123 mg | Calcium 61 mg| Fiber 3.1 g

6.24 Broiled Salmon with Brussel sprout

Ingredients

- Steamed Brussels: 1 cup
- Fresh salmon: 4 ounces
- Light soy sauce: 2 tablespoons
- Dijon mustard: 1 and 1/2 tablespoons
- Salt & pepper, to taste

Instructions

- Let the broiler pre-heat. Cover the salmon surface with mustard and soy sauce.
- Spray the baking sheet with oil and put salmon in the baking pan, and broil for ten minutes, or until salmon completely cooked through.
- Meanwhile, steam the Brussel sprout, if not already steamed
- Serve salmon and sprinkle salt & pepper to taste.

Nutrients per serving: Calories 236|Protein 15.3 g |Carbohydrates 7.2 g| Fat 16.4 g| Cholesterol 8.9 mg| Sodium 143 mg| potassium 176 mg| Phosphorus 132 mg | Calcium 71 mg| Fiber 3 g

6.25 Zucchini Noodles with Roasted Salmon

Ingredients

- Wild Salmon: 6 ounces
- Curry paste: 1 tablespoon
- One package zucchini noodles
- Salt, pepper to taste
- Two minced cloves of garlic
- Four sliced scallions, sliced
- Half of cup of cilantro
- Two inches of ginger root(grated)
- Red pepper flakes: 1/4 teaspoon

Instructions

- Put a skillet over medium flame, and heat the coconut oil.
- Add the zoodles, curry paste, ginger and, garlic. Cook for about four minutes until the noodles are tender,

- keep stirring—season with Amino to taste.

- Put another skillet over medium flame and heat the coconut oil. Place skin-side down the fish. Season with red pepper flakes and salt.

- Turn on the broiler.

- Cook for seven minutes, then move to the broiler. Broil for five minutes or until the fish is completely cooked

- Add the noodles with scallions and cilantro, and stir to combine.

- Place on a plate, top with fish and serve.

Nutrients per serving: Calories 213|Protein 23.5 g |Carbohydrates 9.2 g| Fat 5.6 g| Cholesterol 13 mg| Sodium 132 mg| potassium 127 mg| Phosphorus 135 mg | Calcium 65 mg| Fiber 2.1 g

6.26 One-Sheet Roasted Garlic Salmon & Broccoli

Ingredients

- One head of broccoli cut into florets: 3-4 cups

- Olive oil: 2 and 1/2 tbsp.

- Salmon fillets (4 portions): 1 1/2 pounds

- Two cloves of minced garlic

- Black pepper to taste

- Lemon slices

- Sea salt: 3/4 tsp

Instructions

- Let the oven pre-heat to 450 F and line parchment paper on baking sheet

- Put the pieces of salmon on the baking sheet, with spaces in between

- Three spray one tablespoon of oil over the fish Place the minced cloves of garlic thinly over the salmon.

- Add 1/4 teaspoon salt (or to taste) and ground black pepper to sprinkle over salmon. Finally, place the cut lemon on top of the salmon. set aside

- Then, mix 1and 1/2 tablespoons of oil, half a teaspoon of salt, and ground black pepper in a medium bowl with the broccoli florets.

- Toss the florets. Arrange the broccoli around the salmon bits into the baking dish.

- Bake in the oven for almost fifteen minutes or until fish is cooked through and the broccoli florets at the ends are slightly brown.

- Sprinkle with parsley for a garnish and, if needed, layer lemon slices around. Enjoy warm.

Nutrients per serving: Calories 256|Protein 12.3 g |Carbohydrates 9.2 g| Fat 11 g| Cholesterol 12 mg| Sodium 154 mg| potassium 187 mg| Phosphorus 145 mg | Calcium 75 mg| Fiber 2.5 g

6.27 Baked Salmon & Flaxseed Crumbs(Almonds)

Ingredients

- Salmon fillet: 1 and 1/2 pounds

- Almonds: 1/4 cup

- Bread crumbs: 1/4 cup

- Scallions, green: 1/4 cup

- Salt: 1/8 teaspoon

- Flaxseeds: 2 tablespoons

- Infused with garlic, olive oil: 1 teaspoon

- Thyme leaves: 1/4 teaspoon

- Black pepper: 1/8 teaspoon
- Lemon zest

Instructions

- Let the oven pre-heat to 450 F and line foil paper on baking sheet

- Process the flaxseeds and almonds in a mixer until a consistent, sand-like texture is obtained. take out in a bowl and add the salt, bread crumbs, pepper, scallions, thyme, lemon zest

- Put the skin-side down fish onto the baking plate. Brush the fish with oil infused with garlic, sprinkle lightly with pepper, salt. Put the crumbs on the fish evenly, and press to adhere.

- Bake fish and crumbs will turn golden brown for almost 25 minutes until it flakes easily.

Nutrients per serving: Calories 293|Protein 12 g |Carbohydrates 8.8 g| Fat 10 g| Cholesterol 9.2 mg| Sodium 123 mg| potassium 222 mg| Phosphorus 132 mg | Calcium 82.3 mg| Fiber 3.3 g

6.28 Grilled Salmon with Tartar Sauce

Ingredients

- Salmon fillets: 4 pieces
- Basil: 1/4 cup
- Garlic: Four minced
- Lemon juice: 1 cup
- Curry powder: 2 teaspoons
- Thyme: 2 teaspoons
- Butter or ghee (melted ½ cup)
- Sea salt and black pepper

Ingredients (Tartar Sauce)

- Low fat Mayonnaise: 1/2 cup
- Green onion: 1 tablespoon (chopped)

- Lemon juice: 1 tablespoon.
- Fresh dill: 1/2 teaspoon
- Mustard: 1/2 teaspoon (powder)
- Paprika: 1/4 teaspoon.
- Black pepper: 1/4 teaspoon

Instructions

- Mix the marinade ingredients in a large bowl: lemon juice, basil, garlic, curry powder, ghee, basil, thyme, sea salt, and black pepper.

- Put salmon in a see-through dish, put all the marinade on the fish and cover it. Put in the refrigerator for about 28 minutes.

- In the meantime, combine all the ingredients of the tartar sauce in a small bowl: onion, mayonnaise, lemon juice, paprika, dill, ground mustard, and black pepper. You should taste it and add any more ingredients if you desire. Please keep it in the fridge until it's time to serve.

- Now the salmon has marinated, put it on the grilling pan, and cook over medium flame and Cook for about 13 minutes.

- Pour blended sauce of tartar and enjoy.

Nutrients per serving: Calories 243|Protein 11 g |Carbohydrates 11.0 g| Fat 9 g| Cholesterol 11 mg| Sodium 132 mg| potassium 213 mg| Phosphorus 127 mg | Calcium 89.2 mg| Fiber 3 g

6.29 Oven-Fried Fish

Ingredients

- One small potato: chopped, and leahced
- Salmon filets: 4 6-ounce
- (Powder) cornmeal: ¼ cup

- Half cup minced red onion
- Lime juice: 2 tablespoons
- Salt and black pepper: ¼ teaspoon each

Instructions

- let the oven pre-heat to 400 F and spray with oil generously 2. Blend salt and pepper with cornmeal.
- Dip the fish into the cornmeal blend gently. Put on the baking sheet. Put drops of olive oil at the top of the tuna, then put it in the oven.
- Bake for 20 minutes till it is cooked.
- Mix the mashed potato with the salt, red onion, and lime juice,
- Serve the fish.

Nutrients per serving: Calories 232|Protein 11 g |Carbohydrates 12 g|

Fat 6 g| Cholesterol 22 mg| Sodium 132 mg| potassium 213 mg| Phosphorus 132 mg | Calcium 78 mg| Fiber 2.3 g

6.30 Fish Tacos

Ingredients

- Cabbage: 1-1/2 cups
- Half cup red onion
- Half bunch of cilantro
- 1 garlic clove
- Two limes
- Tuna fillets: 4 cups
- Sour cream: 1/4 cup
- Half tsp. Of ground cumin
- Half tsp. Of chili powder
- Soy milk: 2 tablespoons
- Black pepper: 1/4 teaspoon
- Olive oil: 1 tablespoon

- 1/2 cup mayonnaise (low fat)- optional
- 12 flour tortillas

Instructions

- Chop up the cilantro and onion, and Shred the cabbage
- Marinate the fish in lime juice, minced garlic, black pepper, olive oil, chili powder, cumin. Mix well and chill in the fridge for half an hour.
- Make the salsa by mixing sour cream, milk, lime juice, and mayonnaise. Mix well and set it aside in the refrigerator
- Let the oven on to broil, lay the foil on the broiler pan.
- Broil the marinated fish until it turns white and flakes easily, for ten minutes.
- Take out from oven, flake fish into pieces.
- Warm up the tortillas.
- Top tortilla with fish flakes, salsa, red onion, cabbage.
- Serve right away and enjoy

Nutrients per serving: Calories 363|Protein 18 g |Carbohydrates 30 g|

Fat 19 g|Cholesterol 40 mg|Sodium 194 mg| potassium 507 mg|Phosphorus 327 mg | Calcium 138 mg|Fiber 4.3 g

6.31 Creamy fish and Broccoli Fettuccine

Ingredients

- Ground peppercorns: 3/4 teaspoon
- Half cup of fettuccine, uncooked
- One cup fresh fish
- Nondairy creamer: 1/4 cup

- Two cloves of garlic
- Broccoli florets: 1-3 cup
- Lemon juice: 1/4 cup
- Red bell pepper: 1/4 cup
- One cup of cream cheese (low fat)

Instructions

- Cook pasta to your liking without salt.
- Add the floret of broccoli in the last three minutes of pasta cooking.
- Over medium flame, in a pan, stir garlic and fish for 2 to 3 minutes. Add lemon juice, cream cheese, creamer and, ground peppercorns— Cook for two more minutes.
- Add pasta and mix with the fish mix. Add in the bell pepper.

Nutrients per serving: calories 448 |Protein 27 g| Carbohydrates 28 g| Fat 28 g| Cholesterol 203 mg| Sodium 364 mg| Potassium 369 mg| Phosphorus 315 mg| Calcium 157 mg| Fiber 2.6 g

6.32 Creamy Baked Fish

Ingredients

- All-purpose white flour: half cup
- One pound of fish (your choice)
- Salt: 1/4 teaspoon
- Pepper: 1/4 teaspoon
- Non-dairy creamer(fat-free): one cup
- Unsalted butter: 2 tablespoons
- Water: 1/4 cup
- Non-dairy creamer(regular): 1 cup

Instructions

- Let the oven preheat to 350 F
- Take an 8 by 8 baking glass dish, spray with cooking oil. Coat the dish lightly with flour.
- Place fish fillets in the dish and add pepper, salt, and flour on top.
- Pour non-dairy creamers and water on fish
- Add butter pieces on top.
- Bake for half an hour to 45 minutes or until golden brown.
- Serve with creamy sauce.

Nutrients per serving: Calories 380|Protein 23 g| Carbohydrates 46 g| Fat 11 g| Cholesterol 79 mg| Sodium 253 mg| Potassium 400 mg| Phosphorus 266 mg| Calcium 46 mg| Fiber 0.4 g

6.33 Tasty Baked Fish

Ingredients

- Olive oil: 2 tablespoons
- Half tsp. Of ground cumin
- Half tsp. Of black pepper
- One pound of any fish fillets
- Half tsp. of ground rosemary

Instructions

- Let the oven preheat to 350 F.
- Pour olive oil on fish and coat well
- Add spices over fish.
- Put in a baking dish.
- Bake for 20-25 minutes or until completely cooked through
- Serve hot

Nutrients per serving: Calories 171| Protein 20 g| Carbohydrates 0 g| Fat 10 g| Cholesterol 68 mg| Sodium 69 mg| Potassium 338 mg| Phosphorus 204 mg| Calcium 39 mg|Fiber 0.2 g

6.34 Crunchy Oven-Fried Catfish

Ingredients

- Catfish fillets: 1 pound

- One egg white
- Cornmeal: 1/4 cup
- Panko bread crumbs: 1/4 cup
- Half cup all-purpose flour
- Cajun seasoning(salt-free): 1 teaspoon

Instructions

- Let the oven preheat to 450 F.
- Spray oil on a baking tray.
- In a mixer, whisk the egg until soft peak forms.
- Add flour on a parchment paper. On another sheet of parchment, mix the Cajun seasoning, cornmeal, and panko.
- Slice the fish into four fillets.
- Coat the fillet in flour, then in egg white, then in cornmeal mix.
- Dip the fish in the flour and shake off excess.
- Place the coated fish on a baking pan.
- Spray the fish fillets with cooking spray.
- Bake for 10 to 12 minutes, turn the fish over, and bake for another five minutes.
- Serve hot

Nutrients per serving: Calories 250| Protein 22 g| Carbohydrates 19 g| Fat 10 g| Cholesterol 53 mg| Sodium 124 mg| Potassium 401 mg| Phosphorus 262 mg| Calcium 26 mg| Fiber 1.2 g

6.35 Salmon with Lemon Caper Sauce

Ingredients

- Cooked white rice: 4-1/2 cups
- Raw tuna steaks: 20 ounces
- Lemon juice: 4 tablespoons
- White wine: 1/4 cup
- Olive oil: 1 tablespoon
- All-purpose white flour: 2 teaspoons
- White pepper: 1/4 teaspoon
- Half cup of chicken broth reduced-sodium
- Unsalted butter: 2 tablespoons
- Capers: 1 teaspoon

Instructions

- In a zip lock bag, add olive oil, two tablespoons of lemon juice. Add fish in zip lock bag marinate for five minutes.
- Spray oil on a skillet over medium flame, cook the fish for three minutes.
- Flip the fish and cook for two minutes more.
- In a skillet, melt butter, add flour, and mix. Add broth cook for one minute.
- Add remaining lemon juice, pepper, wine, and capers. Continue to mix and cook for five minutes or until sauce thickens.
- Serve fish with rice and caper sauce.

Nutrients per serving: Calories 340| Protein 26 g| Carbohydrates 34 g| Fat 9 g| Cholesterol 46 mg| Sodium 118 mg| Potassium 573 mg| Phosphorus 306 mg| Calcium 79 mg| Fiber 0.6 g

6.36 Mango Ginger Mahi Mahi

Ingredients

- Mahi-mahi fillets: 1-1/2 pounds
- Sweet mango chutney: 1/2 cup
- 2 tbsp. Of vinegar
- Gingerroot: 1 tablespoon minced

- Soy sauce(reduced-sodium): 2 tablespoons

- One clove of minced garlic

- Olive oil: 2 tablespoons

- White pepper: 1 teaspoon

Instructions

- Mix all ingredients, and pour over fish.

- Chill in the fridge for 20 minutes at least

- In a pan, spray oil, and cook fish skin side down

- Cook for 4-6 minutes over medium-low heat, on each side, turn only once.

- In a pan, reduce the leftover marinade and pour over fish and Serve hot

Nutrients per serving: Calories 221 | Protein 21 g |Carbohydrates 9 g| Fat 10 g| Cholesterol 80 mg| Sodium 298 mg| Potassium 547 mg| Phosphorus 175 mg| Calcium 27 mg| Fiber 0.6 g

6.37 Grilled Salmon

Ingredients

- Salmon fillets: 1 pound

- Lemon juice: 1/4 cup

- Lemon pepper salt-free seasoning: 1 teaspoon

Instructions

- Sprinkle the salmon with seasoning. Pour lemon juice over the top. Spray with oil.

- Put on pre heated grill

- cook for 15 to 20 minutes or until cooked through.

- Serve hot.

Nutrients per serving: Calories 161| Protein 23 g| Carbohydrates 0 g| Fat 8 g| Cholesterol 63 mg| Sodium 49 mg| Potassium 556 mg| phosphorus 227 mg| Calcium 15 mg|Fiber 0 g

6.38 Grilled Blackened Tilapia

Ingredients

- Olive oil: 2 tablespoons

- Four tilapia filets

- Dried oregano: 1 teaspoon

- Half teaspoon. Of cayenne pepper

- 2 cloves of minced garlic

- Smoked paprika: 2 teaspoons

- Cumin: 3/4 teaspoon.

Instructions

- Preheat the grill on medium heat spray oil on the grill.

- Mix all the seasoning and coat the fish.

- Grill for almost three minutes on each side, or until cooked through

- Top with cilantro and serve

Nutrition per serving: Total Fat 9.3g| Cholesterol 58mg| Sodium 62.4mg| Total Carbohydrate 1.8g| Dietary Fiber 0.8g| Protein 23.7g| Iron 1.4mg| Potassium 403mg| Phosphorus 207.3mg|

6.39 Zesty Orange Tilapia

Ingredients

- Zest orange peel: 2 teaspoons

- Tilapia: 16 ounces

- Celery: ¾ cup, julien cut

- Ground black pepper: 1 teaspoon

- Half cup of sliced green onions

- Orange juice: 4 teaspoons

- Carrots: 1 cup, Julien cut

Instructions

- Let the oven preheat to 450° F.

- In a bowl, mix green onions, orange zest, carrots, celery.

- Slice the fish into four equal parts. Spray oil on four large squares of foil.

- Add ¼ of vegetables in each foil square, then add fish on top.

- Add black pepper and one tsp. of orange juice on top.

- Cover with foil and fold edges make a pouch.

- Bake for about 12 minutes or more if required.

- Serve in foil.

Nutrition Per Serving: calories 133 | Total Fat 2 g| Saturated Fat 1 g| Trans Fat 0 g| Cholesterol 57 mg| Sodium 97 mg| Carbohydrates 6 g| Protein 24 g| Phosphorus 214 mg| Potassium 543 mg| Dietary Fiber 1.7 g

Calcium 42 mg

6.40 Pesto-Crusted Catfish

Ingredients

- Pesto: 4 teaspoons

- Catfish: 2 pounds (no bones)

- Panko bread crumbs: ¾ cup

- Olive oil: 2 tablespoons

- Half cup of vegan cheese

- Seasoning Blend: (No salt added spices)

- Red pepper flakes: half teaspoon

- Garlic powder: 1 teaspoon

- Dried oregano: half teaspoon

- Black pepper: half teaspoon

- Onion powder: 1 teaspoon

Instructions

- Let the oven preheat to 400 F

- In a bowl, add all the seasoning, sprinkle over fish, both sides.

- Then spread pesto on each side of fish

- In a bowl, mix bread crumbs, cheese, oil. Coat pesto fish in crumbs mix.

- Spray oil on the baking tray. Add fish on a baking tray.

- Bake at 400° F for 20 minutes or until you want.

- Let it rest for ten minutes. Then serve

Nutrition Per Serving: Calories 312 | total Fat 16 g |Saturated Fat 3 g| Trans Fat 0 mg| Cholesterol 83 mg| Sodium 272 mg| Carbohydrates 15 g| Protein 26 g| Phosphorus 417 mg| Potassium 576 mg| Dietary Fiber 0.8 g| Calcium 80 mg

6.41 Citrus Salmon

Ingredients

- Salmon filet: 24 ounces

- Olive oil: 2 tablespoons

- Dijon mustard: 1 tablespoon

- Two garlic cloves, minced

- Dried basil leaves: 1 teaspoon

- Lemon juice: 1-1/2 tbsp.

- Unsalted butter: 1 tablespoon

- Cayenne pepper: 2 pinches

- Capers: 1 tablespoon

- Dried dill: 1 teaspoon

Instructions

- In a pan, add all the ingredients but do not add salmon. Let it boil, then

- lower the flame and cook for five minutes.
- Preheat the grill. Put the fish on a large piece of foil, skin side down.
- Fold the edges. Put the fish in foil on the grill. Add sauce over the salmon
- Cover the grill, let it cook for 12 minutes, do not flip the fish.
- Serve hot

Nutrients per serving: Calories 294| Protein 23 g| Carbohydrates 1 g| Fat 22 g| Cholesterol 68 mg| Sodium 190 mg| Potassium 439 mg| Phosphorus 280 mg | Calcium 21 mg| Fiber 0.2 g

6.42 Adobo-Marinated Tilapia Tapas

Ingredients

- Six pieces of tilapia filets
- Small wonton: 48 wrappers

Slaw Mix

- Green scallions: ¼ cup, thinly sliced
- Half cup of low-fat mayonnaise
- Fresh cabbage: 4 cups
- Lemon juice: ¼ cup
- Fresh garlic: 1 tablespoon, chopped
- Cilantro leaves: ¼ cup, roughly chopped

Adobo Sauce

- Oregano: 1 tablespoon
- Spanish paprika: 3 tablespoons
- Extra-virgin olive oil: ¼ cup
- Fresh cilantro: 3 tablespoons chopped
- Red pepper flakes: 1 teaspoon
- Half cup of red wine vinegar
- Black pepper: 1 teaspoon

Instructions

- Let the oven preheat to 400° F.
- In a bowl, mix adobo ingredients and set it aside
- Marinate the fish filets in half a cup of adobe sauce for half an hour.
- Spray oil on a baking tray and bake the fish for 15 minutes. Halfway through, flip the fish. Take out from the oven and set it aside.
- In a bowl, add claw slaw ingredients and mix well.
- Spray the oil over the muffin pan. Add one wonton wrapper in muffin cups.
- Bake for five minutes at 350 F, and then cool the crispy wontons
- Add fish in crispy wonton top with slaw mix. Top with cilantro leaves.

Nutrition Per Serving: Calories 254| Total Fat 13 g| saturated Fat 2 g| Trans Fat 0 g| Cholesterol 28 mg| Sodium 272 mg| Carbohydrates 22 g| protein 13 g | phosphorus 116 mg| Potassium 268 mg| dietary Fiber 2 g| Calcium 46 mg

6.43 Fiesta Tilapia Ceviche

Ingredients

- Chopped half cup of red bell pepper
- Fresh tilapia fillets: 1 and 1/2 pounds, cut into cubes
- Chopped red onion: 1 cup
- Chopped cilantro: 1/4 cup
- Olive oil: 2 tablespoons
- Fresh lime juice: 1-1/4 cups
- Pineapple: 1 cup
- Unsalted crackers
- Black pepper: 1/4 teaspoon

Instructions

- For three minutes, broil the fish cubes on each side

- Pour lime juice over broiled fish (cool it first for five minutes). Mix well

- Mix the oil, onion, pineapple, bell pepper, black pepper, cilantro. And pour overcooked fish.

- Let it marinate for two hours or more in the fridge

- Serve fish with unsalted crackers.

Nutrients per serving: Calories 220| Protein 19 g| Carbohydrates 20 g| Fat 7 g| Cholesterol 36 mg| sodium 168 mg| Potassium 374 mg| Phosphorus 162 mg| Calcium 43 mg| Fiber 1.3 g

6.44 Korean-Style Fried White Fish

Ingredients

- All-purpose white flour: 3 tablespoons

- Unseasoned rice vinegar: 1 tablespoon

- White fish fillets: 1 pound

- Reduced-sodium soy sauce: 1 teaspoon

- Two large egg whites whisked

- Sesame oil: 3 tablespoons

- Half tsp. of black pepper

Instructions

- In a bowl, mix soy sauce with vinegar.

- Cut the fish into one and a half-inch pieces.

- In a zip lock bag, add pepper and flour, add the fish in bag and coat well

- in a skillet heat the sesame oil, coat the flour-coated fish into eggs. Fry in hot oil until golden brown.

- Serve hot.

Nutrients per serving: Calories 273 | Protein 26 g| Carbohydrates 4 g| Fat 17 g| Cholesterol 151 mg| Sodium 134 mg| Potassium 400 mg| Phosphorus 359 mg| Calcium 42 mg| Fiber 0.1 g

6.45 Sole with Tarragon Cream Sauce

Ingredients

- Sole fillets: 1 pound

- Sliced green onions: 1/4 cup

- One clove of minced garlic

- Sliced green olives: 2 tablespoons

- Dried tarragon: 1 teaspoon

- Olive oil: 2 tablespoons

- Fresh lemon juice: 1/4 cup

- Sour cream: 1/3 cup

- Dried basil: 1/2 teaspoon

Instructions

- Sauté garlic and onion in olive oil till tender

- Add in the lemon juice, herbs, sour cream, olives.

- Mix well and heat for one minute. Turn off the heat and set it aside.

- In a microwave-proof dish, add the roll up the fish fillet, with a toothpick secure it.

- Add sauce to the fish, microwave for four minutes.

- Take out the toothpicks, serve with sauce.

Nutrients per serving: calories 216| Protein 22 g| Carbohydrates 3 g|Fat 12 g| Cholesterol 65 mg| Sodium 188 mg| Potassium 388 mg| Phosphorus 269 mg| Calcium 52 mg|Fiber 0.3 g

6.46 Eggplant Seafood Casserole

- Ingredients
- 3 eggs' white
- Eggplants: 2 medium
- One onion
- Half cup of celery
- Two garlic cloves
- Worcestershire: 1 tablespoon
- Olive oil: 1/4 cup
- One bell pepper
- Lemon juice: 1/4 cup
- Creole seasoning: 1/4 teaspoon
- Half tsp. Of tabasco
- Rice: 1/3 cup, uncooked
- Lump crab meat: 1 pound
- Unsalted butter: 2 tablespoons, melted
- Half pound boiled fish
- Half cup bread crumbs
- vegan cheese: 1/4 cup

Instructions

- Let the oven preheat to 350 F
- Chop up the celery, onion, and bell pepper.
- Dice and peel the eggplant into one-inch cubes.
- Boil eggplant for five minutes until tender, drain the water, and set it aside
- In olive oil, sauté celery, garlic, bell pepper, and onion, do not let them brown
- In a bowl, add eggplant, sautéed vegetables, Creole seasonings, lemon juice, Tabasco sauce, Worcestershire sauce, eggs, cayenne, rice, and cheese. Mix well
- Add seafood to the vegetable mix. Put in a casserole dish, oil the dish well before.
- Mix melted butter with bread crumbs and add on top of casserole.
- Bake for half an hour or until topping begins to brown.

Nutrients per serving: Calories 216 | Protein 13 g| Carbohydrates 14 g| Fat 12 g | Cholesterol 138 mg| Sodium 229 mg| Potassium 359 mg| Phosphorus 148 mg | Calcium 79 mg| Fiber 2.3 g

6.47 Honey Spice-Rubbed Salmon

Ingredients

- 16 ounces of salmon fillets
- Honey: 3 tablespoons
- Half tsp. Of black pepper
- 2 pressed cloves of garlic
- Lemon peel: 3/4 teaspoon
- Hot water: 1 teaspoon
- Arugula: 3 cups
- Olive oil: 2 tablespoons

Instructions

- In a bowl, add grated lemon peel, honey, hot water, ground pepper, garlic, and whisk well.
- With clean hands, rub the mixture over fish fillets.
- Over medium flame, heat the olive oil in a pan. Add marinated fish fillets and cook for four minutes. Turn once.
- Turn the heat to low and cook for 4-6 minutes or until fish is cooked through.

- Add half a cup of arugula to the plate. Put salmon fillet on arugula.
- Sprinkle with fresh herbs and serve.

Nutrients per serving: Calories 323 | Protein 23 g |Carbohydrates 15 g| Fat 19 g| Cholesterol 62 mg| Sodium 66 mg| Potassium 454 mg| Phosphorus 261 mg| Calcium 42 mg|Fiber 0.4 g

6.48 Cilantro-Lime swordfish

Ingredients

- Swordfish: 1 pound
- Half cup of low-fat mayonnaise
- Lime juice: 2 tablespoon
- Half cup of fresh cilantro

Instructions

- In a bowl, mix chopped cilantro, lime juice, low-fat mayonnaise, mix well.
- Take ¼ cup from the mix and leave the rest aside
- Apply the rest of the mayo mix to the fish with a brush
- In a skillet, over medium heat, spray oil
- Add fish fillets, cook for 8 minutes, turning once, or until fish is cooked to your liking.
- Serve with sauce.

Nutrients per serving: Calories 292 | Protein 20 g |Carbohydrates 1 g| Fat 23 g| Cholesterol 57 mg| Sodium 228 mg| Potassium 237 mg| Phosphorus 128 mg| Calcium 14 mg| Fiber 0 g

6.49 Grilled Mexican Swordfish Fillets

Ingredients

- Olive oil: 1 tablespoon
- Swordfish fillets: 1 and 1/2 pounds'

- Lime juice: 1/4 cup
- Fresh cilantro: 1/4 cup
- Onion: 1/4 cup
- One tablespoon honey
- Salt: 1/4 teaspoon
- One serrano chili
- One lime
- Two cloves of garlic

Instructions

- Finely dice the onion and chili (seeded).
- Place swordfish in a baking dish
- In a food blender, mix cilantro, honey, salt (1/4 tsp.), onion, garlic, oil, and lime juice. Pulse until smooth.
- Pour this mix over fish, coat the fish well, let it marinate in the fridge for half an hour.
- Let the grill preheat.
- Grill for five minutes on every side, or fish is completely cooked through.
- Serve with lime wedges and enjoy.

Nutrients per serving: Calories 198|Protein 23 g| Carbohydrates 4 g| Fat 10 g| Cholesterol 75 mg| Sodium 190 mg| Potassium 506 mg| Phosphorus 295 mg | Calcium 11 mg| Fiber 0.2 g

6.50 Lemon Pepper Salmon

- Extra virgin olive oil: 2 tablespoons
- Salmon: 2 pounds, boneless (skin on or off)
- Ten sprigs of thyme
- Chopped fresh herbs of your choice
- Kosher salt: 1 teaspoon
- Black pepper: 1/2 teaspoon

- Two medium lemons

Instructions

- Let the oven preheat to 375 F.

- Place aluminum foil over a baking tray or parchment paper

- Spray oil over the foil, place five sprigs of thyme in the middle. Add lemon slices over the thyme. Add the fish on top.

- Add zest, olive oil, salt, and pepper over fish.

- Add the remaining thyme and lemon slices and lemon juice on top of the fish.

- Pack the salmon in foil, completely closed, leave some room in the foil.

- Bake for 15-19 minutes or until salmon is cooked.

- When salmon is cooked, uncover it and let it broil for three minutes.

- Do not overcook the salmon.

- Serve with fresh lemon juice and herbs on top.

Nutrition per serving: calories 268kcal| carbohydrates: 4g|protein: 31g| fat: 14g| saturated fat: 2g| cholesterol: 83mg | potassium: 801mg| fiber: 1g|sugar: 1g| calcium: 34mg|iron: 2mg

6.51 Easy Salmon Soup

- Salmon fillet without skin: 1 lb.

- Extra virgin olive oil

- Half chopped green bell pepper

- Chicken broth(low-sodium): 5 cups

- Four cloves of minced garlic

- Four diced green onions

- 2 tbsp. Of dill chopped

- Dry oregano: 1 tsp

- One cup of potatoes(leached), thinly sliced

- One carrot cut into thinly sliced

- Ground coriander: ¾ tsp

- Salt and black pepper

- Juice and zest of one lemon

- Half tsp of ground cumin

Instructions

- In a large pot, heat two tablespoons of oil, add garlic, bell pepper, green onions, cook over medium flame. Stir often.

- Add half of the dill, and cook for 30 seconds.

- Add chicken broth, carrots, and potatoes.

- Add black pepper, spices, and salt. Let it boil, lower the heat and cook for five minutes to make sure they are tender.

- Add salt to salmon and add in the soup. Lower the heat and cook for few minutes until salmon is cooked and will flake easily.

- Add in lemon juice, zest, and dill.

- Serve hot.

Nutrients per serving: Calories 218|Protein 24 g| Carbohydrates 3.3 g| Fat 8.9 g| Cholesterol 68 mg| Sodium 181 mg| Potassium 232 mg| Phosphorus 213 mg | Calcium 9.9 mg| Fiber 8 g

Chapter 7: Kidney-Friendly Vegetables Recipes

7.1 Vegan Lettuce Wrap Recipe

Ingredients

- 2 cups of extra firm tofu
- ¼ cup of dry white rice
- Butter lettuce: 4 medium leaves
- One clove of pressed garlic
- Honey: 2 teaspoons
- 1 teaspoon of freshly grated ginger
- Cauliflower: 1 cup
- Low sodium soy sauce: 1 tablespoon
- Rice vinegar: 2 tablespoons
- Olive oil: 1 tablespoon
- Sesame oil: 1 tablespoon
- Half cup of shredded carrots

Instructions

- Let the oven Pre-heat to 400F.
- Cook the rice as you want, but do not add butter or salt.
- Cut the cauliflower in very small pieces like rice grain size.
- A small food processor mix ginger, garlic, honey, rice vinegar, soy sauce, sesame oil.
- Cut the tofu into bite-size. Spray olive oil on tofu and bake at 400F for 20 minutes' flip halfway through.
- Mix the chopped up cauliflower with freshly cooked rice.
- Toss the tofu with a sauce prepared earlier.
- Lay lettuce leaves on a flat surface, top with cauliflower/rice mix and the sauce, then tofu.

Nutrition per serving: Calories 410| Total Fat 26g| Saturated Fat 4g| Cholesterol 0mg| Sodium 187mg|Total Carbohydrate 34g| Dietary Fiber 4g| Total Sugars 9g|Protein 14g, Calcium 148mg| Iron 3mg| Potassium 441mg

7.2 Vegan Bell Pepper, Kidney Bean, & Cilantro Salad

Ingredients

- 1 tablespoon of extra virgin olive oil
- Half cup diced cilantro
- 2-3 cloves of pressed garlic
- 2 cups of red bell pepper diced
- ¼ cup of chopped macadamia nuts or walnuts
- One can chickpeas or kidney beans
- Salt, pepper to taste

Instructions

- In a big bowl, add all ingredients. Mix them well.
- Season with salt and freshly ground black pepper.
- Garnish with olive oil.

Nutrition per serving: Calories 105, Fat 9g, Sodium 8 mg, Potassium 125 mg, Carbohydrates 4g, Fiber 1g, Protein 2g, Calcium 40mg, Iron 1.4mg8%

7.3 Vegetable Paella

Ingredients

- White rice: 2 cups, uncooked
- Green beans: one and a half cups
- Olive oil: 1 tablespoon

- Green bell pepper chopped: 1 cup
- broccoli florets: 3 cups
- 1 cup of diced zucchini
- Half cup of chopped onion
- Half tsp. of salt

Instructions

- Cook rice to your preference without salt and butter.
- Add broccoli and green beans in a saucepan, add water to cover them.
- Let them boil for four minutes and drain
- In a pan, heat oil over medium flame. Sauté the broccoli, zucchini, onion, beans, and bell pepper, cook for 4-5 minutes.
- Add in the remaining ingredients. Cook for five minutes, stirring frequently.

Nutrients per serving: Calories 146, Protein 5 g, Carbohydrates 26 g, Fat 2 g, Cholesterol 0 mg, Sodium 150 mg, Potassium 305 mg, Phosphorus 89 mg, Calcium 38 mg, Fiber 1.8 g

7.4 Broccoli & Mushrooms with Sweet Potatoes

Ingredients

- Four medium-sized baked sweet potatoes
- Two tablespoons of olive oil
- 2 cups of mushrooms, sliced
- 1 head of broccoli, cut into tiny florets
- 1/3 cup broth, hot, low-sodium (veggie)
- Black pepper fresh ground, to taste
- 2/3 cup basic, low-fat yogurt

Instructions

- Make sure that the potatoes are entirely dry—dust one tablespoon of olive oil with the potatoes. Wrap Every potato in aluminum foil. Put in a slow cooker, seal, and cook for 7-8 hours at the low flame or 4-5 hours at high heat until the potatoes are tender.
- On medium flame, heat the remaining tbsp. of olive oil in a large pan. Add the mushrooms & broccoli and sauté for around ten minutes till the broccoli is tender but not soft.
- Unpack the foil from each potato. Create a slice of potatoes in the center and scrape the potato into a pan. Add broth, yogurt, and pepper. Blend to mix. Split it up back into the potato skins and stuff. Cover it with mushrooms and broccoli.

Nutrition per serving: Calories: 330, Total Fat: 7 g, Sodium: 360 mg, Total Carbs: 57 g, Dietary Fiber: 8 g, Protein: 14 g, potassium 234 mg, phosphorous 66 mg

7.5 Mediterranean Stew with Vegetables

Ingredients

- 1 sweet potato, trimmed and cut into cubes (leached)
- 1 cubed eggplant
- One big, cut into cubes zucchini
- 1 medium yellow onion, chopped
- 1 onion, sliced
- 1 carrot, finely chopped
- 2 garlic cloves, chopped up
- 1 cup of no sodium tomato sauce (homemade)

- 1/2 cup broth of vegetables, no sodium
- 1/2 teaspoon cumin ground
- 1/2 of a teaspoon of turmeric
- 1/2 teaspoon of red pepper crushed
- ¼ tsp. of the paprika

Instructions

- Add all the ingredients in a slow cooker. Mash, cover, and cook for 7-8 hours on low or 4-5 hours on high, just until the veggies are tender.
- Serve hot.

Nutrition per serving: Calories: 122| Total Fat: .5 g| Sodium: 157 mg| Total Carbs: 30 g| Dietary Fiber: 7.8 g |Protein: 3.4 g| potassium 176 mg|phosphorous 89 mg

7.6 Florentine Mushroom

Ingredients

- Half cup of whole-grain pasta
- 1/4 cup no sodium broth
- 1 cup of sliced mushrooms
- 1/4 cup of milk soybeans
- Olive oil for 1 teaspoon
- 1/2 teaspoon of Italian seasonings

Instructions

- Cook the pasta as per the direction.
- Add in the saucepan with olive oil and heat up.
- Add Italian seasonings and mushrooms. Mix well and cook for ten minutes.
- Then incorporate chicken stock and soy milk.
- Shake the combination well enough and add the cooked pasta. Cook it over low heat for 5 minutes.

Nutrition per serving: 287 calories| 12.4g protein| 20.4g carbohydrates| 4.2g fat| 9g fiber| 0mg cholesterol| potassium 123 m| phosphorus 111 mg

7.7 Bean Hummus

Ingredients

- 1 cup of soaked chickpeas
- Six Cups of Water
- 1 tbsp. of tahini paste
- Two cloves of garlic,
- Olive oil: 1/4 cup
- 1/4 Cup of Lemon Juice
- One Harissa tsp.

Instructions

- In the saucepan, add water. Add chickpeas, then close the cover.
- On the low temperature, cook the chickpeas for 40 minutes or once they're soft.
- Move the cooked chickpeas into the mixing bowl after this.
- Garnish with olive oil, lemon juice, harissa, cloves of garlic, and tahini Paste.
- Until it's smooth, mix the hummus.

Nutrition per serving: 215 calories, 7.1g protein, 21.6g carbohydrates, 12g fat, 6.1g fiber, potassium 135 mg, phosphorous 126 mg

7.8 Hassel Back Eggplant

Ingredients

- Two eggplants
- Two red peppers, sliced together
- 1 tbsp. of yogurt with low fat
- 1 tsp of powdered curry
- Olive oil for 1 teaspoon

Instructions

- Make cuts in the form of the Hassel back in the eggplants.

- Then add the curry powder on the vegetables and fill them with sliced tomatoes.

- Spray the olive oil and yogurt on the eggplants and cover them in the foil (cover each Hassel back eggplant individually).

- For 25 minutes, cook the vegetables at 375F.

Nutrition per serving: 188 calories, 7g protein, 38.1g carbohydrates, 3g fat, 21.2g fiber, Potassium 99.9 mg, phosphorous 87 mg

7.9 Roasted Cauliflower & Turmeric Curry

Ingredients

Masala

- Half cup of raw cashews

- Coriander seeds: 1 and 1/2 tablespoons

- Cardamom powder: a pinch

- Cumin seeds: 1 teaspoon

- One and 1/4-inch of cinnamon stick

- Six cloves of garlic

Curry

- Half tsp. of salt

- Turmeric powder: 1 teaspoon

- Olive oil: 2 tablespoons

- Three cloves of pressed garlic

- One cm of grated fresh ginger root

- Cauliflower florets: 2 cups

- Soy milk: 2 cups

- One chopped capsicum or bell pepper

- Red onions: 2 cups, finely chopped

- Roma tomatoes: half of a cup, finely chopped

- Half teaspoon of chili powder

- One teaspoon of Himalayan salt

- One and a 1/2 cups water

- Chopped coriander: 1 tablespoon (cilantro)

- Half teaspoon of garam masala

Instructions

Turmeric Roasted Cauliflower

- Let the oven preheat to 400 F

- In a big bowl, add the cauliflower, pinch of salt, coconut oil, and powdered turmeric, with your clean hands' mix and rub on cauliflower.

- Line a baking tray with parchment paper and pour this mixture in it and bake in the oven for half an hour. Check often to make sure cauliflower does not burn.

- Little roasted should be fine. Make sure not to overcook it.

The Curry

- In the meantime, as cauliflower is roasting.

- In a food processor bowl, add all the masala ingredients, pulse on high until completely smooth. Make sure no lumps remain.

- In a pan, over low heat, melt the coconut oil and stir in the ginger, garlic, onions and cook carefully for three minutes.

- Then add the chopped bell pepper, the tomatoes, until tomatoes are melted and falling apart.

- Add in the masala mix and stir for 2-3 minutes, do not let it burn or stick to the pan.

- When the mixture is well-combined, add in the chili powder, turmeric, and coconut milk. Add as much water as needed to get the desired consistency.

- Turn the flame down to low, let it simmer, and cook for five minutes. Adjust seasoning, and cauliflower will be ready by then, add into the pan.

- Mix well and turn off the flame. Top with cilantro and serve hot.

- It tastes well with rice or quinoa.

Nutrition per serving: Calories: 163.2, Total Fat 14.2 g, Saturated Fat 2 g, Cholesterol 0 mg, Sodium 126.7 mg, Total Carbohydrate 8.6 g, Dietary Fiber 3.5 g, Sugars 1.9 g, Protein 3 g, Potassium 187 mg, phosphorous 121 mg

7.10 One-Pot Zucchini Mushroom Pasta

Ingredients

- Two zucchinis, quartered and thinly sliced

- Grain spelt or Kamut spaghetti: 4 cups

- Two sprigs of thyme

- Walnut milk: 1/4 cup(homemade)

- Cayenne pepper and Sea salt to taste

- Cremini mushrooms: 4 cups, thinly sliced

Instructions

- In a big pot, add mushrooms, thyme, zucchini, and spaghetti with 4 and 1/2 cup of water, over medium flame. Season according to taste with cayenne pepper and sea salt.

- Let it boil, then lower the flame and let it simmer, do not cover. Let the pasta cook for ten minutes, until liquid has significantly reduced.

- Add in the milk.

- Top with cilantro and Serve hot. Enjoy.

Nutrition per serving: Calories 378.7, Total Fat 6.5g, Saturated Fat 3.4g, Trans Fat 0g, Cholesterol 17.6mg, Sodium 109.3mg, Total Carbohydrate 64.8g, Dietary Fiber 4.3g, Sugars 5.8g, Protein 15.8g, Potassium 145 mg, phosphorous 92.3 mg

7.11 Quinoa Stuffed Spaghetti Squash

Ingredients

- Two tbsp. of coconut oil

- Green peas(steamed): 1 cup

- One shallot (medium)

- One red or orange bell pepper

- Two spring of green onions, thinly sliced white part

- Cooked quinoa: 1 and 1/2 cup

- Chopped walnuts: 1/4 cup

- Two smaller or one big spaghetti squashes

- One tsp. of garlic powder

- Two tsp. of dried thyme

- Black pepper and Pink salt to taste

Instructions

- Let the oven preheat to 400 F

- Wash and pat dry the squash and half them. Take out the seeds and bake for 40 minutes. Until tender

- In a pan, add one tbsp. Of oil and add the bell pepper, shallots. Cook until tender.
- Add cooked quinoa, spices and green peas, and walnuts—season with black pepper and salt.
- Cut the squash in further half and bake for another five to 8 minutes. Take out the squash from the oven and with a fork, scratch it until resembles spaghetti.
- Serve with the vegetable mixture.

Nutrition per serving: Calories: 108kcal | Carbohydrates: 20g | Protein: 3g | Fat: 1g | Sodium: 132mg | Potassium: 251mg | Fiber: 3g | Sugar: 3g | Calcium: 29mg | Iron: 1.3mg

7.12 Kale Pesto Pasta

Ingredients

- One spiralized zucchini(zoodles)
- One bunch of kale
- Extra virgin olive oil: 1⁄4 cup
- Half cup of walnuts
- Fresh basil: 2 cups
- Fresh-squeezed: 2 limes
- Garnish with tomato, and beans
- Sea salt and pepper, to taste

Instructions

- Soak walnuts, overnight.
- Add all ingredients in a food blender.
- Pulse on high and smooth and creamy. Add this sauce over zucchini noodles
- Serve and enjoy.

Nutrition per serving: Calories: 108kcal | Carbohydrates: 10g | Protein: 3g | Fat: 0.8 g | Sodium: 102mg | Potassium: 131mg |

Fiber: 3g | Sugar: 1.9 g | Calcium: 32 mg | Iron: 1.9 mg

7.13 Quinoa Burrito Bowl

Ingredients

- Two cans of adzuki beans, black beans (15 oz. each can)
- White rice or quinoa: 1 cup
- Fresh juice from two limes
- 4 cloves of pressed garlic
- Four green thinly sliced scallions
- One teaspoon of cumin
- A handful of chopped cilantro

Instructions

- Cook the rice or quinoa. Over low flame, in the meanwhile, warm the beans.
- Add in the cumin, garlic, onions, and lime juice. Let it cook for fifteen minutes.
- When quinoa is cooked, add into two serving bowls.
- Add beans on top, and garnish with cilantro.

Nutrition per serving: Calories: 218kcal | Carbohydrates: 25g | Protein: 4 g | Fat: 0.7 g | Sodium: 192mg | Potassium: 198 mg | Fiber: 2.8g | Sugar: 1.7 g | Calcium: 27 mg | Iron: 3 mg

7.14 Raw Pad Thai Recipe

Ingredients

- A half packet of beansprouts
- Three medium zucchini
- Two spring of green onions, thinly sliced
- Shredded red cabbage: 1 cup
- Three carrots (large)

- One cup of cauliflower florets
- Olive Oil
- One bunch of cilantro, roughly chopped

Sauce

- One clove of pressed garlic
- Tahini: ¼ cup
- Tamari: ¼ cup
- One inch of grated ginger root,
- Honey: 1 tsp
- Unsalted butter: ¼ cup
- Lime or lemon juice: 2 tbsp.

Instructions

- Spiralize the carrots and zucchini into noodles.
- In a bowl, add shredded cabbage, beansprouts, coriander, spring onions, and cauliflower mix well.
- Prepare the sauce by mixing all sauce ingredients in a blender; add water if the sauce is very thick.
- Add the sauce into the bowl and coat everything well.
- Top with chopped coriander and lemon juice.

Nutrition per serving: Calories: 256 kcal | Carbohydrates: 21 g | Protein: 6 g | Fat: 2 g | Sodium: 154 mg | Potassium: 281mg | Fiber: 4 g | Sugar: 2.5g | Calcium: 21 mg | Iron: 1.2 mg| phosphorous: 121 mg

7.15 Savory Wrap

Ingredients

- ¼ chopped red onion
- One butter lettuce bunch
- One teaspoon of chopped basil
- One tomato: sliced, chopped
- loosely packed ¼ cup of spinach (leach it)
- One teaspoon of chopped cilantro
- Salt & black pepper

Instructions

- Lay lettuce leaf flat on a surface, add red onion, basil, tomato, cilantro, add spinach too, sprinkle with salt, and black pepper.
- Fold into a roll.
- Serve and enjoy.

Nutrition per serving: Calories: 99kcal | Carbohydrates: 10 g | Protein: 8g | Fat: 0.7 g | Sodium: 132mg | Potassium: 267 mg | Fiber: 6 g | Sugar: 1.2 g | Calcium: 19 mg | Iron: 1.1 mg| phosphorous 211 mg

7.16 Green Beans & Quinoa Salad

Ingredients

- Green beans: 2 cups
- Quinoa: one cup
- Chickpeas: one can drained
- Fresh parsley

Instructions

- Cook quinoa with two cups of water. Boil it and cover it, cook for 12 minutes.
- Cook until all the liquid is absorbed, fluff with a fork, and turn off the heat, set it aside.
- In a bowl, mix all ingredients with black pepper and salt.
- Serve hot with olive oil and lemon slices

Nutrition per serving: Calories: 211 kcal | Carbohydrates: 15.5 g | Protein: 5.7 g | Fat: 2 g | Sodium: 145 mg | Potassium: 213 mg |

Fiber: 4 g | Sugar: 2 g | Calcium: 11.9 mg | Iron: 2 mg| phosphorous 198 mg

7.17 Kale & Golden Beet Salad

Ingredients

Salad

- Green onions, four pieces, cut and chopped
- One bunch of kale, cut into thin strips, de-stemmed
- Carrots: 2 medium
- One yellow bell pepper
- Golden beets: 4 medium

Dressing

- Olive oil: 4 tbsp.
- Dried oregano: 2 tsp.
- Apple cider vinegar: 4 tbsp.
- Juice of a half lemon
- One-inch peeled & minced piece of ginger
- Tahini: 3 Tbs.
- Dried basil: 1 tsp.
- Three cloves of minced garlic

Instructions

Salad

- In a bowl, add green onions and chopped kale.
- Chop carrots, bell pepper, the beets and very finely in a food processor.
- Add chopped vegetables into green onion and kale.
- Mix well.

Dressing

- In a bowl, add all dressing ingredients and mix well. Or use an emulsion blender(hand-held) till smooth and creamy.
- Add sauce over the salad.
- Chill before serving and enjoy.

Nutrition per serving: Calories: 217 kcal | Carbohydrates: 9.2 g | Protein: 11g | Fat: 1.2 g | Sodium: 132 mg | Potassium: 134 mg | Fiber: 4.3 g | Sugar: 1.8 g | Calcium: 10.3 mg | Iron: 2.1 mg| phosphorous 178 mg

7.18 Apple & Almond Butter Oats

Ingredients

Green apple(grated): 1 cup

Gluten-free oats: 2 cups

Almond butter(raw): 1/3 cup

One and a ½ cups of soy milk

Half tsp of cinnamon

Instructions

- In a bowl, add milk, almond butter, add oats, and mix. Add in the grated apple.
- With plastic wrap, cover the bowl and refrigerate it overnight.
- Add coconut milk if oats become too thick.
- Top with cinnamon powder and serve

Nutrition per serving: Calories: 176 kcal | Carbohydrates: 8.9 g | Protein: 12.4 g | Fat: 1.99 g | Sodium: 121 mg | Potassium: 210 mg | Fiber: 4.3 g | Sugar: 2.7 g | Calcium: 21 mg | Iron: 1.4 mg| phosphorous 92 mg

7.19 Blueberry Pancakes

Ingredients

- Blueberries: 1/3 cup
- 1 and 1/4 cup of homemade almond milk
- Honey: 3 tbsp.

- Grapeseed oil: 2 tbsp.
- One pinch of sea salt
- 1 and 1/2 cup of spelt flour
- For serving, use extra fruit and Agave syrup

Instructions

- In a bowl, mix date sugar and flour, mix well, so no lumps remain. Add grapeseed oil, walnut milk in the flour, and date sugar mixture.
- Whisk it but do not over mix.
- Fold in the blueberries but maintain the lumps. Be careful to not over mix
- Let the griddle preheat to 350 F add a light coating with grapeseed oil.
- Add 1/4 cup of batter on the griddle in the desired shape.
- Cook until bubbles form and edges are brown
- Flip it and let it cook for 1 minute or 2.
- Top with extra fruit and agave syrup, and enjoy.

Nutrition per serving: Calories: 182 kcal | Carbohydrates: 12.4 g | Protein: 6 g | Fat: 2 g | Sodium: 121 mg | Potassium: 112 mg | Fiber: 3.2 g | Sugar: 2.1 g | Calcium: 15 mg | Iron: 1.9 mg| phosphorous 171 mg

7.20 Blueberry Delight Smoothie

Ingredients

- Flax seeds(ground): 1 tbsp.
- Blueberries: half cup
- Hemp seed powder: 1 tbsp.
- Chia seeds: 1 tbsp.
- Soy milk: one cup
- Almond butter(raw): one tbsp.-optional

- Oil: 1 tbsp.

Instructions

- Place all the ingredients in the food blender.
- Pulse on high until well combined and smooth.
- Enjoy

Nutrition per serving: Calories: 89 kcal | Carbohydrates: 7.1 g | Protein: 22 g | Fat: 1.45 g | Sodium: 106 mg | Potassium: 98 mg | Fiber: 3.9 g | Sugar: 1.2 g | Calcium: 11 mg | Iron: 2 mg| phosphorous 87 mg

7.21 Blood Orange, Carrot, & Ginger Smoothie

Ingredients

- One blood orange: peeled and diced
- Almond, coconut or cashew milk: 2 cups
- Pineapple: half cup
- One knob of one inch: minced fresh ginger
- One frozen banana
- One carrot peeled and diced (medium-sized)
- Add in half apple, de-seeded and peeled
- One scoop of vegan collagen: it is optional

Instructions

- In a food blender, add all the ingredients
- Pulse on high for almost one minute, until smooth and creamy.
- Serve with fresh basil leaves on top.
- Enjoy.

Nutrition per serving: Calories: 72 kcal | Carbohydrates: 6.5 g | Protein: 11 g | Fat: 1

g | Sodium: 104 mg | Potassium: 102 mg | Fiber: 5.6 g | Sugar: 1.4 g | Calcium: 21 mg | Iron: 2 mg| phosphorous 112 mg

7.22 Cleansing Detox Soup

Ingredients

- Vegetable broth or water: 1/4 cup
- Turmeric: 1 teaspoon
- Half of red onion, chopped
- Three stalks of chopped celery
- Three chopped medium carrots
- Two cloves of pressed garlic
- One head of small broccoli, cut into florets
- Chopped tomatoes: 1 cup
- Ginger: 1 tablespoon, peeled and freshly minced
- Cayenne pepper: 1/8 teaspoon, or to taste
- Cinnamon: 1/4 teaspoon
- Purple cabbage: 1 cup, diced
- Freshly ground black pepper, sea salt, to taste
- Water: 6 cups
- Kale: 2 cups, stem removed and torn into pieces
- Juice from half of a small lemon

Instructions

- In a big pot, over medium flame, add the vegetable broth. Once the broth is warmed, add in the garlic and onion. Cook for two minutes. Add the fresh ginger, broccoli, carrots, tomatoes, and celery.
- Cook for another three minutes. Add more water or broth if required. Add in the cayenne pepper, turmeric, cinnamon—season with pepper and salt.
- Lower the heat and let it simmer for 15 minutes. Cook until vegetables are tender.
- Add in the cabbage and kale.
- In the end, add lemon juice, let it simmer for 2-3 minutes.
- Turn off the heat
- Serve hot with fresh basil leaves.

Nutrition Per Serving: Calories 139|Fat 1g| Saturated Fat 1g|Sodium 41mg|Potassium 219mg|Carbohydrates 8g|Fiber 2g|Sugar 2g| Protein 3g|Calcium 77mg| iron 1mg| phosphorus 111 mg

7.23 Arugula & Strawberry Salad with Cayenne Lemon Vinaigrette

Ingredients

Salad

- Arugula: 2 cups,
- Walnuts (Toasted)-optional
- Diced apples: 2 tablespoons
- Three strawberries cut into slices
- Blueberries: 1/4 cup

Dressing

- Agave syrup: 1/4 teaspoon or another sweetener
- Extra virgin olive oil: 2 tablespoons
- Powder cayenne pepper: 1/8 teaspoon
- Pinch of salt
- Lemon juice: 2 teaspoon
- Freshly ground black pepper

Instructions

- In a bowl, add all the dressing ingredients, whisk to combine, and set it aside.

- In another big bowl, add all the salad ingredients, pour the dressing all over, and top with toasted walnuts.
- Serve right away and enjoy.

Nutrition Per Serving: Calories 127|Fat 0.9 g| Sodium 137 mg| Potassium 121 mg| Carbohydrates 7g|Fiber 2g|Sugar 1.4 g| Protein 4 g|Calcium 87 mg| iron 1mg| phosphorus 102 mg

7.24 Asian Cucumber Salad

Ingredients

- Grated ginger: 1 tbs.
- Key lime juice: 3 tbs.
- Half tsp. of date sugar
- Powdered, granulated seaweed: 1 tbs.
- Sea salt: 1/4 tsp
- Olive oil: 1 tbs.
- Sesame seeds: half tsp.

Instructions

- In a big bowl, add all the ingredients. Mix them well.
- Serve with your favorite dressing.

Nutrition Per Serving: Calories 121|Fat 0.8 g |Sodium 37 mg|Potassium 108 mg| Carbohydrates 5 fiber 2.3g|Sugar 1.8 g| Protein 4 g|Calcium 88 mg| iron 1.2 mg| phosphorus 89 mg

7.25 Triple Berry Smoothie

Ingredients

- One burro banana
- Strawberries: half cup
- Agave syrup, to taste
- Blueberries: half cup
- Water: one cup
- Raspberries: half cup

Instructions

- Add all ingredients in a food blender.
- Pulse it on high until smooth and creamy. Serve and enjoy.

Nutrition Per Serving: Calories 121|Fat 0.7 g| Sodium 31 mg| Potassium 102 mg| Carbohydrates 7.8g|Fiber 3 g|Sugar 1.2 g| Protein 4.4 g|Calcium 89 mg| iron 1.3 mg| phosphorus 92 mg

7.26 Mushroom Risotto

Ingredients

- Rice: 2 cups
- Olive oil: one teaspoon
- Four mushrooms
- Half onion
- Cayenne pepper, to taste
- Homemade vegetable broth: 4 cups
- Sea salt, to taste

Instructions

- In a large pot, sauté mushrooms and onions in grapeseed oil over medium heat. Cook for 5 to 7 minutes or until mushrooms are lightly browned, and liquid is evaporated, stirring occasionally.
- Stir in rice and cook an additional minute.
- Add in the vegetable broth and additional sea salt and pepper. Cover and cook on a low-heat setting for about 2 hours and 45 minutes or on a high-heat set about 1 hour 15 minutes or until rice is tender.
- Serve hot and enjoy.

Nutrition Per Serving: Calories 312|Fat 1.4 g| Sodium 89 mg| Potassium

128 mg|Carbohydrates 23 g|Fiber 2.9 g| Sugar 2 g|Protein 10 g|Calcium 87 mg| iron 1.3 mg|phosphorus 109 mg

7.27 Green Falafels

Ingredients

- Half cup of flour
- Beans, dry garbanzo (chickpeas): 2 cups
- Red bell pepper: 1/3 cup, diced
- Oregano: 1/4 teaspoon
- Fresh basil: 2/3 cup
- One large onion, diced
- Olive oil for frying
- Half cup of fresh dill
- Sea salt: one teaspoon

Instructions

- Boil the chickpeas, drain the water and wash them.
- In a food processor, add the chickpeas with the rest of the ingredients: flour, sea salt, onion, fresh herbs, red bell pepper, and oregano.
- Pulse on high until all things are finely diced and like coarse. Toss with the spoon and pulse again, taste it, and adjust the seasoning if required.
- Move this coarse meal mixture to a big mixing bowl, use your clean hands, shape them into balls or discs like structure. Place all the balls over parchment paper.
- Put in the refrigerator for one hour to chill.
- You can rather fry these falafels in one inch of oil in a deep pan. Or air fry them at 380 for ten minutes, until golden brown.
- Serve them with your favorite dipping sauce.

Nutrition Per Serving: Calories 276|Fat 1.4 g| Sodium 76 mg| Potassium

145 mg| Carbohydrates 20.3 g| Fiber 2.9 g| Sugar 1.7 g| Protein 8.9 g| Calcium 89 mg| iron 1 mg| phosphorus 87 mg

7.28 Creamy Kamut Pasta

Ingredients

Pasta

- Box of Kamut Spirals: 1 and a half cups
- Dried tarragon: 1 tablespoon
- water:6-8 cups, (to boil your pasta)
- Olive oil: 2 tablespoon
- Onion powder: 1 teaspoon (no salt)
- Sea salt: one teaspoon

Creamy Sauce

- Half medium onion: diced
- Olive oil: divided, two tablespoon
- Sea salt + plus a half teaspoon
- Water: 2 cups
- Freshly ground black pepper
- Sliced baby Bella mushrooms: 2 cups
- Chickpea flour: 1/4 cup
- Almond milk: one and a half cups
- Dried tarragon: 1 tablespoon
- Tomatoes(Roma), chopped 2-3
- Dried oregano: 1 teaspoon
- Onion powder: 2 teaspoon
- Fresh kale: 2 cups packed

- Dried basil: 1 teaspoon

Instructions

Pasta

- In a pot, add water with salt over high heat. Let it boil

- When the water has boiled, add pasta. Cook until tender to your preference.

- To enhance flavor, add seasoning while the pasta is still warm, add onion powder, sea salt, dried tarragon, and grapeseed oil.

- Taste the pasta and adjust the seasoning.

Creamy Sauce

- In a pan, add one tbsp. of grapeseed oil, over medium flame, heat for one minute

- In the hot oil, add in the sliced mushrooms and chopped onions. Stir often let it cook, until vegetables are tender for about five minutes.

- Add in the fresh ground black pepper and salt, 1/4 teaspoon of each. Add in chickpea flour and another one tbsp. of olive oil.

- Mix constantly flour with the oil and vegetables for at least one minute. Flour should not be left dry as it will help thicken the sauce.

- Then add in the can coconut milk, dried oregano, onion powder, half a teaspoon of sea salt, dried tarragon, spring water, half a teaspoon of black pepper dried basil. Mix it well. Let it simmer, uncovered for 20 minutes. Or until sauce becomes thick.

- Then add in the kale, tomatoes, and seasoned, cooked pasta. Cook until the kale is wilted for five minutes. Turn off the heat.

- With time, the sauce will become thicker from the pasta.

- Serve with fresh basil leaves and enjoy.

Nutrition Per Serving: Calories 326|Fat 3 g| Sodium 98.2 mg| Potassium 119 mg| Carbohydrates 25 g| Fiber 2.4 g| Sugar 1.5 g| Protein 22 g| Calcium 43 mg| iron 2.1 mg| phosphorus 102 mg

7.29 Vegetarian Kebabs

Ingredients

- Olive oil 1 tbsp.

- 1 dried parsley, teaspoon

- 2 spoonsful of water

- Two sweet peppers

- Two peeled red onions

- Two zucchinis shaved

Instructions

- Chop the onions and sweet peppers into medium-sized squares.

- Cut the zucchini.

- String the skewers with all the vegetables.

- Then combine the olive oil, dried parsley, wine, and balsamic vinegar in a shallow dish.

- Spray with the olive oil mixture on the vegetable skewers and switch to the hot oven 390F grill.

- Fry the kebabs on each side for three minutes just until the vegetables are light brown.

Nutrition Per serving: 88 calories|2.4g protein|13g carbohydrates|3.9g fat| 3.1g fiber| Potassium 102mg |phosphorous 87 mg

7.30 Carrot Cakes

Ingredients

- One cup of grated carrot
- Semolina 1 tablespoon
- Two egg whites
- One teaspoon of seasonings Italian
- Olive oil 1 tablespoon

Instructions

- Comb the grated carrot, semolina, egg, and Italian seasoning in a bowl and mix.
- Warm the pan with sesame oil.
- With the help of Two spoons, make the carrot cakes and place them in the skillet.
- Fry the patties on each side for four minutes.

Nutrition per serving: 70 calories|1.9g protein| 4.8g carbohydrates|4.9g fat| 0.8g fiber| Potassium 89mg|phosphorous 78 mg

7.31 Vegetables Cakes

Ingredients

- Two cups of mushroom, sliced
- Three cloves of sliced garlic
- One tbsp. of dill dry
- One beaten egg or egg alternative,
- 1/4 cup of cooked rice
- olive oil 1 tablespoon
- 1 chili powder teaspoon

Instructions

- In the mixing bowl, add the mushrooms.
- Add the chili powder, garlic, dill, egg, and rice.
- Mix for ten seconds
- Heat the sesame oil for 1 minute after that.

- Shape mushroom cakes of medium size and put them in the hot olive oil.
- Cook the mushroom cakes on a medium flame for 5 minutes per side.

Nutrition Per serving: 103 calories|3.7g protein|12g carbohydrates|4.8gfat| 0.9g fiber| 41mg calcium| Potassium 92 mg | phosphorous 76 mg

7.32 Glazed Eggplant Rings

Ingredients

- Three sliced eggplants
- One tbsp. of honey
- One minced ginger tsp
- Lemon juice 2 teaspoons
- Three tbsp. of olive oil
- 1/2 teaspoon cilantro
- Water 3 tablespoons

Instructions

- Use ground coriander to rub on the eggplants.
- And heat the olive oil for 1 minute in a pan.
- Add the diced eggplant and organize it into one layer when the oil is hot.
- Fry the vegetables on one side for 1 minute.
- Place the eggplant in a dish.
- Then fill the pan with honey, ginger, lemon juice, and water.
- Get it to a simmer and add the eggplants that have been prepared.
- Cover the vegetables well with the sweet liquid and cook for two more mints.

Nutrition per serving: 136 calories|4.3g protein|29.6g carbohydrates|2.2g fat| 15.1g fiber| Potassium 87mg |phosphorous 81 mg | sodium 109 mg

7.33 Sweet Potato Balls

Ingredients

- One cup of mashed, baked sweet potato, leached
- One tbsp. of chopped fresh cilantro
- One egg alternative
- Three tablespoons oatmeal
- One teaspoon paprika ground
- 1/2 teaspoon of turmeric
- Two spoonsful of olive oil

Instructions

- Mix the egg, ground oatmeal, paprika, sweet potato, fresh cilantro, and turmeric in the cup.
- To make the tiny balls, whisk the mixture once soft.
- Warm the saucepan with olive oil.
- Add the sweet potato balls whenever the oil is hot.
- Cook them until their golden brown.

Nutrition per serving: 133 calories|2.8g protein| 13.1g carbohydrates|8.2gfat|2.2g fiber| calcium 41mg| Potassium 86 mg| phosphorous 78 mg |sodium 103 mg

7.34 Chickpea Curry

Ingredients

- One 1/2 cup of boiled chickpeas
- One teaspoon of powdered curry
- 1/2 teaspoons of garam masala
- Kale, 1 cup
- One tsp of olive oil
- 1/4 cup of soy milk
- 1 tbsp. of tomato paste (no salt)
- Half of a cup of water

Instructions

- Warm the saucepan with oil.
- Add garam masala, curry powder, soy milk, and tomato paste.
- Stir till the batter is smooth, then take it to a boil.
- Add water, chickpeas, and kale.
- Mix and shut the lid on the meal.
- Cook it over medium flame for five minutes.

Nutrition per serving: 145 calories|8 g protein| 15.1g carbohydrates|4 gfat|3 g fiber| calcium 35 mg| Potassium 96 mg| phosphorous 81 mg |sodium 101 mg

7.35 Quinoa Bowl

Ingredients

- 1 cup of quinoa
- Two Cups of Water
- Red bell peppers: 1 cup, chopped
- 1/2 cup cooked rice
- One tbsp. of juice from a lemon
- 1/2 lemon zest teaspoon, grated
- Olive oil 1 tablespoon

Instructions

- Mix the water and quinoa, then cook for fifteen min. Then detach it from the heat and allow for ten minutes to rest.
- Move your cooked quinoa to a large bowl.
- Add the sweet pepper, sugar, lemon juice, olive oil, and lemon zest.
- Stir the mixture well in the serving bowls.

Nutrition per serving: 290 calories| 8.4g protein| 49.9g carbohydrates| 6.4gfat| 4.3g fiber| trans-fat 0mg| Potassium 88mg | phosphorous 71mg|sodium 100 mg

7.36 Vegan Meatloaf

Ingredients

- One cup cooked chickpeas
- 1 onion, diced
- 1 tbsp. flax seeds ground
- 1/2 teaspoon chili flakes
- 1 tbsp. olive oil
- 1/2 of a cup of carrot, diced
- 1/2 cup stalk of celery, chopped
- 1 tbsp. of tomato paste, no salt added

Instructions

- Warm the saucepan with olive oil.
- add the carrot, celery stalk, and onion. Cook for ten minutes or until the vegetables are tender.
- Chickpeas, ground chili flakes, flax seeds are then added.
- With the electric mixer, mix the combination until creamy.
- Later, with baking paper, cover the loaf mold and move the blended paste inside.
- Add tomato paste and scatter.
- Bake the meatloaf for twenty minutes in the oven and bake at 365 F.

Nutrition per serving: 162 calories|7.1g protein| 23.9g carbohydrates 4.7g fat|7g fiber|transfat 0mg| Potassium 88mg| phosphorous 69 mg|sodium 103 mg

7.37 Vegan Shepherd Pie

Ingredients

- 1/2 cup cooked quinoa
- 1/2 cup puree red bell pepper
- 1/2 of a cup of carrot, diced
- 1 minced shallot
- 1 tbsp. olive oil
- 1/2 cup of potato, baked, mashed
- 1 chili powder tsp
- 1/2 cup sliced mushrooms

Instructions

- In a frying pan, place the carrots, shallots, and mushrooms.
- Apply coconut oil and fry the veggies once tender but not fluffy, for ten minutes until its tender.
- Then combine the cooked vegetables with the tomato puree and chili powder.
- Move the paste and flatten even into the casserole shape.
- Cover the vegetables with mashed potatoes afterward. Contain the shepherd's pie with a baking sheet and bake 25 minutes in the preheated 375 F oven.

Nutrition per serving: 136 calories|8.2g protein| 20.1g carbohydrates|4.9gfat| 2.9g fiber| Potassium 93.2 mg |phosphorous 87mg|sodium 104 mg

7.38 Vegan Steaks

Ingredients

- 1-pound head of cauliflower
- 1 tsp turmeric
- 1/2 cayenne pepper teaspoon
- Olive oil: 2 tablespoons
- 1/2 teaspoon powdered garlic

Instructions

- Rub with cayenne pepper, ground turmeric, and garlic powder and slice the cauliflower head into the steaks.

- After which line the cookie sheet with baking paper and put the Cauliflower steaks in place.

- Spray with olive oil and cook for 25 minutes at 375F just until the veggie steaks are gentle.

Nutrition per serving: 92 calories| 2.4g protein| 6.8g carbohydrates| 7.2g fat|3.1g fiber| Potassium 85 mg |phosphorous 78 mg| sodium 93 mg

7.39 Quinoa Burger

Ingredients

- 1/3 cup cooked chickpeas

- 1/2 cup cooked quinoa

- 1 tsp of Italian seasonings

- Olive oil: 1 tsp

- 1/2 of an onion, diced

Instructions

- In a food processor, pulse the chickpeas on high, until smooth

- Then combine the quinoa, the Italian seasonings, and the grated onion with them. Till densely concentrated.

- Shape the burgers from the combination after this and position them in a lined baking tray.

- Spray olive oil on the quinoa burgers and cook them for twenty minutes at 275 F.

Nutrition per serving: 158 calories|6.4g protein| 15.2g carbohydrates|3.8g fat| 4.7g fiber| Potassium 78 mg |phosphorous 67 mg| sodium 92.3 mg

7.40 Stuffed Sweet Potatoes

Ingredients

- One sweet potato (leached)

- ¼ cup whole-grain penne pasta

- 1 tsp tomato paste

- Olive oil 1 tsp

- ¼ teaspoon minced garlic

- 1 tbsp. soy milk

Instructions

- Break the sweet potato in two and stab it 3-4 times with a fork.

- Spray the sweet potato halves with olive oil and cook in the Preheated to 375 F oven for about half an hour or when the vegetables are tender.

- In the meantime, mix up penne pasta, tomato paste, minced garlic, and soy milk.

- Whenever the sweet potatoes are baked, spoon out the vegetable meat and spice it up with a penne pasta combination.

- Cover the sweet potatoes with the pasta mix.

Nutrition per serving: 105 calories| 2.7g protein| 17.8g carbohydrates| 2.8g fat|3g fiber| Potassium 87 mg| phosphorous 66 mg |sodium 85 mg

7.41 Tofu Masala

Ingredients

- Tofu 1 cup, minced

- 1/2 cup of almond or soy milk

- 1 tsp of garam masala

- Olive oil for 1 tsp

- 1 tsp paprika ground

- 1/2 cup of red bell peppers, sliced

- 1/2 onions, sliced

Instructions

- In a frying pan, heat the olive oil.
- Add chopped onion and fry till light brown.
- Put the ground paprika, tomatoes, and garam masala in the mixture. Get it to a boil
- Add soy milk and whisk thoroughly. Let it boil for five minutes.
- And add sliced tofu and cook for three minutes with the food.
- For ten minutes, leave the cooked meal to rest.

Nutrition per serving: 155 calories|12.2g protein|20.7g carbohydrates|8.4g fat| 2.9g fiber| Potassium 78 mg|phosphorous 71 mg| sodium 94 mg

7.42 Tofu Parmigiana

Ingredients

- One cup of firm tofu, cut finely
- One olive oil tsp
- 1 tsp tomatoes sauce (no salt)
- 1/2 teaspoon Italian seasonings

Instructions

- Combine the tomato sauce and Italian seasonings in a mixing dish.
- Then add the cut tofu well with the tomato mix and leave to marinate for ten minutes.
- Heat the olive oil, too.
- Place the sliced tofu in the hot oil and roast it on each side for three minutes or until the tofu is golden brown.

Nutrition per serving: 83 calories|7g protein|1.7g carbohydrates| 6.2g fat|0.8 fiber| calcium 34 mg| Potassium 67 mg | phosphorous 56 mg|sodium 76 mg

7.43 Vegan Stroganoff

Ingredients

- Two cups of sliced mushrooms
- 1 tsp of wheat whole-grain flour
- 1 tsp olive oil
- 1 minced onion
- 1 dry tsp of thyme
- 1 clove of garlic, diced
- 1 black pepper ground tsp
- 1/2 cup of almond milk

Instructions

- Warm the saucepan with olive oil.
- add the onion and mushrooms and cook them for ten minutes. Stir the vegetables. From time to time,
- Spray them with ground black pepper, thyme, and garlic after that.
- Take the mixture to a boil and incorporate soy milk.
- Add the flour, now whisk thoroughly until it is combined.
- Heat the stroganoff mushroom until it becomes thick.

Nutrition per serving: 70 calories|2.6g protein| 6.9g carbohydrates| 4.1 fat|1.5g fiber| calcium 34 mg| Potassium 78mg | phosphorous 65 mg| sodium 87 mg

7.44 Vegan Croquettes

Ingredients

- One peeled, boiled eggplant
- Two potatoes, mashed (leached)
- Almond meal: 2 tablespoons
- 1 tsp pepper chili
- Olive oil: 1 tsp
- 1/4 teaspoon nutmeg

Instructions

- Mix the eggplant, with the mashed potato, coconut oil, chili pepper, and ground nutmeg.

- From the eggplant combination, make the croquettes.

- Warm the skillet with olive oil.

- Place the croquettes in the hot oil, then fry them on each side for two minutes until its light brown.

Nutrition per serving: 180 calories|3.6g protein| 24.3g carbohydrates| 8.8g fat|7.1g fiber| calcium 54mg| Potassium 87 mg| phosphorous 81 mg|sodium 93 mg

7.45 Stuffed Portobello

Ingredients

- Four Mushroom caps Portobello

- 1⁄2 zucchini, grated

- 1 onion, sliced

- Olive oil

- 1 tsp

- 1⁄2 teaspoon of dry parsley

- 1⁄4 teaspoon of garlic, minced

Instructions

- Combine the diced tomatoes, rubbed zucchini, dry parsley, and ground garlic in a food processor.

- And fill the mushroom caps with the blend of zucchini and move them to the baking paper tray.

- Cook the vegetables till they are cooked through or for twenty minutes.

Nutrition per serving: 84 calories|14 g protein| 10.3 g carbohydrates| 1.3 g fat| 0.9g fiber| Potassium 65 mg |phosphorous 66 mg |sodium 78 mg

7.46 Chickpeas Stir Fry

Ingredients

- One cup of garbanzo, cooked

- One zucchini, diced

- One cup of mushroom cremini, chopped

- One tablespoon olive oil

- One tsp: black pepper ground

- One tablespoon fresh, minced parsley

- 1 tsp of juice from a lemon

Instructions

- Warm the saucepan with olive oil.

- Stir in the mushrooms and cook for ten minutes.

- And add the cooked garbanzo beans and zucchini. Whisk the ingredients well enough and cook them for an extra ten minutes.

- Sprinkle the vegetables with ground black pepper and lemon juice. After this, for five minutes, cook the meal.

- Add and blend the parsley. Heat it for an extra five minutes.

Nutrition per serving: 231 calories|11.3g protein|33.9g carbohydrates| 6.6g fat| 9.6g fiber| potassium 78 mg

7.47 Chana Cha'at

Ingredients

- One cup Cooked chickpeas

- One pepper jalapeno, sliced

- 1 tsp of garlic ground

- 1 tsp extracted ginger

- Fresh cilantro 3 teaspoons, minced

- 1 tsp of masala garam

- Red bell pepper 1 cup, diced
- 1 slice of onion, minced
- Olive oil: 1 tsp
- Two Cups of Water

Instructions

- Mix the jalapeno pepper, minced garlic, ginger, and fresh cilantro.
- And heat the casserole dish with olive oil. Add in onion and roast once until light brown.
- Add the garam masala, jalapeno combination, and sliced tomatoes.
- let the mixture boil.
- Add the chickpeas and the water. Let it cook for ten minutes.

Nutrition per serving: 235 calories|10.5g protein|35.4g carbohydrates| 6.7g fat| 10g fiber| potassium 87mg

7.48 Vegan Meatballs

Ingredients

- ½ cup white beans, cooked
- ½ cup quinoa, cooked
- 1/4 cup of vegan Parmesan, grated
- 2 tbsp. of fresh cilantro, chopped
- 1 tablespoon olive oil
- ½ teaspoon chili flakes
- 1 tablespoon tomato paste
- 1 teaspoon ground black pepper

Instructions

- Put white beans, quinoa, and vegan parmesan in the blender.
- Add cilantro, chili flakes, and tomato paste and blend the mixture until smooth.

- Make the meatballs from the blended mixture and roast them in the preheated olive oil for 3 minutes per side or until they are golden brown.
- Then add tomato puree and ground black pepper. Close the lid and simmer the meatballs for 5 minutes on medium heat.

Nutrition per serving: 192 calories |12.4g protein|16.8g carbohydrates|2.5g fat| 3.2g fiber| Potassium 89 mg| phosphorous 71 mg| sodium 92 mg

7.49 Garlic Pasta

Ingredients

- One and 1/4 cup of shell pasta, cooked
- 1 cup marinara sauce with no salt
- One cup of firm tofu, crumbled
- 1 teaspoon garlic powder
- ½ cup kale, grinded
- 1 tablespoon olive oil

Instructions

- In the mixing bowl, mix up olive oil, crumbled tofu, garlic powder, and kale.
- Then fill the jumbo shells pasta with garlic mixture.
- Put the stuffed shells pasta in the casserole and top with marinara sauce.
- Cover the mold with foil and bake in the preheated to 365F oven for 15 minutes.

Nutrition per serving: 303 calories|10.5g protein| 46.4g carbohydrates| 6.4g fat|3.7g fiber| calcium 21mg | Potassium 101 mg | phosphorous 89 mg|sodium 87 mg

7.50 Smothered Brussel Sprouts

Ingredients

- One cup sprouts from Brussel, chopped
- One teaspoon of honey
- 1 white pepper teaspoon
- Low-sodium, 3 tbsp. soy sauce
- One tablespoon of olive oil,
- One tablespoon of pumpkin seeds, chopped

Instructions

- Warm the pan with olive oil.
- Add the sliced sprouts from Brussels and roast for ten minutes. Frequently, mix the vegetables.
- Add white pepper, soy sauce, and honey. Mix well and cook the vegetables for three minutes.
- Add the pumpkin seeds and blend well with them.
- Cook for an extra two minutes.

Nutrition per serving: 109 calories|5.3g protein| 7.7g carbohydrates| 7.3g fat| 1.9g fiber| calcium 62mg| Potassium 81 mg | phosphorous 76 mg| sodium 98 mg

7.51 Zucchanoush

Ingredients

- Four zucchinis, sliced
- Olive oil: Two tablespoons
- One tsp Harissa
- 1 tbsp. of tahini paste
- 1/4 teaspoon crushed garlic
- 1/2 teaspoon of dried mint

Instructions

- Let the oven preheat to 365 F
- In the baking sheet put the zucchini, spray with olive oil and bake in the oven for half an hour or until the vegetables are tender.
- Move the zucchini to the mixing bowl.
- Add tahini paste, garlic powder, nuts, harissa, and dry mint.
- Mix until combined. Serve hot.

Nutrition per serving: 123 calories| 9.2g protein| 8.1g carbohydrates| 10.1g fat| 2.6g fiber| Potassium 56 mg| phosphorous 54 mg| sodium 76 mg

Conclusion

An important part of your therapy is your diet. Your kidneys are struggling to get rid of your blood of sufficient waste materials and fluids because the body has special requirements now. Therefore, you will need to reduce fluids and adjust the consumption of those ingredients in the diet. The Dietary Guidelines emphasize that eating a variety of foods is important. This applies to patients on dialysis, too. When maintaining a renal diet, you should appreciate all items in moderation. Be reasonable: Enjoy all foods, but don't overdo it, one of the recommendations says.

But you must restrict the intake of foods containing

- High levels of sodium
- High levels of potassium
- High levels of phosphorus
- High levels of protein
- Too many fluids

Phosphorus is an important mineral mainly present in meats and dairy goods. It is used by the body to shape solid bones and teeth. The kidneys start to lose the capacity to extract excess phosphorus from the bloodstream in the early phases of chronic kidney disease. Since so much phosphorus will damage the bones, consuming fewer phosphorus makes more sense. A low-phosphorus diet is simpler if you are already on a low protein diet since foods rich in protein appear to be high in phosphorus, too.

A typical symptom of advanced kidney disease is reduced appetite. Even if you're not hungry, consuming and keeping a healthy diet is vital. You should Gain good nutrition in different ways. Normally, harm to the kidneys is permanent. You should take measures to maintain the kidneys as healthy as normal for a long period, even if the harm cannot be repaired. You can save the damage from becoming worse.

If you have diabetes, regulate your blood sugar.

- Keep your blood pressure stable.
- Follow a diet that is low-salt, low-fat.
- Exercise on certain days of the week for half an hour, at least.
- Maintaining a healthy weight.
- Must not smoke cigarettes.
- Limit alcohol consumption.
- Speak to a doctor about drugs that will support the kidneys to heal them.
- Eat more meals that are healthy or starchy.
- Prepare ahead and freeze meals so you can microwave or check for value packs that are low-salt.
- If you are hungry, Watch cooking shows to entice your cravings
- Improve the protein level by incorporating egg whites. Eat tiny amounts of protein food, such as egg salad or a frozen chicken sandwich, at a cold temperature, as well.

Get support from a renal dietitian if there is a continued loss of appetite. This could be a warning that you should start dialysis whether you are at stage 5 CHRONIC KIDNEY Disorder, and your appetite or physical well-being may not change. After some periods on dialysis, several persons find that their appetite increases.

Better self-management would then help you live a long life that is fulfilling and proceed to do the things you love. It may even help slow or avoid the progression of kidney disease, which can also prevent or postpone the kidney's collapse. Effective control of oneself begins with:

- Controlling any health conditions, you might have

- Treat kidney disorder seriously.

- Managing coronary illness

You are likely to avoid kidney failure if you detect kidney symptoms early on. You may require dialysis or a kidney transplant to live if the kidneys malfunction. Therefore, you ought to make sure that you do your utmost to start staying safe from today and start consuming kidney-friendly foods.

Vegan Meal Prep

The Kick Start Guide to Develop Vegan and Vegetarian Eating Habits for an Healthy Lifestyle - Over 115 Delicious Recipes on a Budget for Plant-Based Diet

Amanda Davis

Introduction

I want to thank you for choosing this book, *Vegan Meal Prep - Meal Prep and Recipes for Plant-based Diet: The Kick Start Guide to Develop a Healthy Lifestyle Habits.*

Veganism is steadily gaining popularity, and for the right reasons. A vegan diet is devoid of any animal-based products, including eggs and dairy. Veganism is not just a diet but also a lifestyle choice. A vegan diet can help with weight loss, reduce the risk of certain diseases, and improve your energy levels. If you want to increase your chances of sticking to this diet, concentrating on the food you consume should be your priority.

Meal prepping is essentially the practice of preparing wholesome meals, along with preparing certain components of the meals for the week ahead. In the last couple of years, this concept has steadily gained a lot of popularity. In this book, you'll find some amazing Vegan recipes that will get you started on your meal prep journey.

The recipes in the book are for breakfast, lunch, snacks, dinner, and desserts using vegan ingredients. These recipes are not only easy to follow but will help you cook delicious and nutritious meals. You no longer have to compromise on taste for the sake of nourishment. Apart from this, you will also learn the basics of vegan meal prep, the benefits of meal prepping, vegan food lists that you should have handy, and tips for getting started today.

Once you start meal prepping, you can forget about takeout and fast food! You can start saving money, eating home-cooked meals, and improving your health. By using the different recipes given in this book, you can begin prepping meals like a pro. In today's world, it is quite easy to fall into the habit of eating fast food. Regardless of whether you are trying a plant-based diet or are weakened by choice, it can become a little challenging, since finding vegan options is not always easy. Rather than depending on restaurants or food bars for your vegan meals, start meal prepping today and get access to home-cooked ready to eat.

Are you ready to learn more about all this? If yes, then let us get started immediately.

Chapter One

Going Vegan

Whenever you think of the word 'vegan', there is a good chance that you think about hippies munching on bland salads, wearing vegan leather, and being social activists who force others to give up meat. It might also remind you of the quirky yet lovable sitcom character of Phoebe Buffay! Well, veganism is so much more than the sad stereotypes society has conjured up about them. These days, veganism is steadily gaining popularity and is present everywhere. Did you know that Tesla offers cruelty-free leather in their cars? Did you know that Burger King introduced a vegan meat patty, and KFC UK came up with an original vegan chicken burger? It certainly goes to show how popular veganism has become.

The vegan diet is a plant-based diet. It is quite similar to a vegetarian diet, except that it excludes eggs as well as dairy products along with other animal-derived ingredients. Any products derived from an animal, such as meat, milk, cheese, eggs, gelatin, and honey, are not included in a vegan diet. Anything that is made out of an animal or by an animal is not vegan. A lot of vegans don't eat foods that are also produced using animal products such as some wines as well as refined white sugar.

Benefits of a Vegan Diet

In this section, let us look at the different benefits of a vegan diet.

Plenty of nutrients

If you are just getting started with a vegan diet, then it will undoubtedly be drastically different from the diet of an average American. You must ensure that your diet doesn't contain any animal-derived produce. A vegan diet consists of whole foods, vegetables, fruits, legumes, grains, nuts, and seeds. Almost all the foods contained in this diet are rich in different nutrients. Not only is the content of fiber quite high in them, but they are also rich in antioxidants, nutrients like potassium, magnesium, and vitamins A, C, and E. As long as your vegan diet isn't poorly planned, your body will get all the nourishment it requires.

Reduces the risk of certain types of cancers

According to the World Health Organization, the risk of about one-third of cancers can be reduced by following a vegan diet. The underlying factors that induce life-threatening cancers can be effectively managed through this diet. It is believed that a diet rich in fruits and legumes helps reduce the risk of colorectal cancer. Consuming plenty of soy-based products reduces the risk of breast cancer. Avoiding animal products altogether offers protection against cancer of prostate, colon, and breast.

Promotes weight loss

The consumption of plant-based foods helps speed up the process of weight loss when compared to other diets. Since the vegan diet primarily focuses on the consumption of whole foods, it helps with weight loss. All the fiber you consume tends to make you feel full for longer without being heavy on calories. Therefore, there is a natural reduction in your calorie intake. It not only helps with weight loss but also improves your overall energy levels. A vegan diet isn't usually calorie-restrictive and encourages the consumption of whole foods that will leave you feeling full. Once the calorie intake reduces, it is easy to maintain a calorie deficit. A calorie deficit is quintessential for weight loss. Also, it is a great way to tackle cravings for unhealthy foods.

Stabilizing blood sugar

A vegan diet helps reduce the risk of type II diabetes while improving the health of your kidneys. The insulin secreted by the pancreas required to balance blood sugar levels reduces whenever the blood sugar levels reduce. It, in turn, reduces the risk of diabetes. By reducing the risk of diabetes, and managing blood sugar levels, the overall function of kidneys improves.

Managing inflammation

A vegan diet can help reduce as well as manage the uncomfortable pain caused by arthritis. Inflammation is the leading cause of arthritis. A diet that's rich in processed sugars and unhealthy carbs increases the chances of inflammation. Since a vegan diet doesn't concentrate on these two types of foods, inflammation can be easily managed. Once inflammation is managed, it becomes easier to regulate pain as well.

Risk of heart diseases decreases

Consuming a diet that's rich in vegetables, legumes, fruits, and other dietary fibers help reduce the risk of several heart diseases. It also helps regulate high blood sugar. It, in turn, helps reduce the risk of several cardiovascular disorders, while improving the overall functioning of the heart. A vegan diet helps reduce the level of LDL cholesterol within the body. HDL and LDL are two cholesterol molecules present within your body. HDL stands for high-density lipoprotein, and LDL stands for low-density lipoprotein. A lipoprotein helps carry cholesterol molecules in the body. The composition of the cholesterol molecules is pretty much the same, but the functions they perform are quite different. HDL is responsible for transporting cholesterol molecules away from the body. So, a low level of LDL and a high level of HDL is directly associated with a reduction in the risk of cardiovascular disorders.

By shifting to a vegan diet, you can effectively improve your overall health and wellbeing. Not just this, you can also attain your weight loss and fitness objectives too!

Chapter Two

Meal Prep 101

What is Meal Prep?

There are plenty of creative and beautiful images of meal prep ideas on Pinterest and Instagram. Scrolling through these images can be a little intimidating. If you're thinking about cooking meals at home every week, then you need to start meal prepping. Meal prepping is not only simple but perfectly doable as well. Before we learn more about it, the first step is to understand what meal prepping means.

Meal prepping is about dedicating sufficient time to batch cook certain ingredients or prepare full meals for the week that lies ahead to make it easier to feed yourself as well as your family. It can be something as simple as preparing a sauce and chopping up a bunch of vegetables or as involved as cooking a full-fledged meal and then portioning it. If you want to get a head start on the week and reduce the time spent in the kitchen cooking, then meal prepping is quintessential.

There is no one size fits all kind of process involved in meal prepping. It differs from one person to another and from one household to another. Meal prepping does not necessarily mean preparing or prepping, cooking, and portioning every single meal you plan to consume in the following week. What might work for one person doesn't necessarily work for someone else. Also, the way you prepare meals will differ from one week to another, depending on the meals you wish to cook.

The terms meal prepping, and meal planning are often used synonymously, but they are not the same. These two techniques certainly make it easier to cook meals, but there are some differences. Meal prep is about setting a specific block of time aside to prep all the ingredients or cook meals for the week that lies ahead. On the other hand, meal planning essentially means planning the meals you wish to have. It is about answering the basic question of, "What's for dinner today?" These two tactics work hand-in-hand, and one cannot exist without the other.

Steps Involved in Meal Prep

Now that you know what meal prepping is, it is time to get started. There are three important steps involved in meal prep, and they are as follows.

Identifying your needs

Before you start prepping, you need to understand your needs and requirements. Meal prepping makes it easier to cook meals. So, what are the different things you will need to do to ensure you feel more in control of the food you eat? Think about all the pain points associated with mealtime. Do you need to cook a healthy lunch you can carry to work? Do you wish to stock up on vegan snacks? Do you want to stop spending a lot of money on breakfast?

Maybe you can start focusing by prepping ingredients required to whip up a quick breakfast in the morning. Perhaps you can start by prepping for lunch before anything else. Or maybe you want to quickly get the dinner ready and on the table within 20 minutes of reaching home. Once you identify the challenges involved, it is time to begin. Regardless of what you do, don't ever try to start prepping everything at once. Identify the biggest challenge, tackle it first, and then move onto something else. Once you get the hang of meal prepping, it becomes easier to cater to all your needs and requirements. So, start slowly and don't rush into it.

Selecting the right foods

Selecting the foods you want to prep ahead to meet your needs is the second step. It certainly sounds quite easy, doesn't it? You might want to eat healthier breakfast, a light lunch, or perhaps a quick dinner. However, where do you start? Well, this is exactly where this book comes in. It presents plenty of meal prep ideas as well as recipes you can start using.

In general, there are two options available. Whenever you think about meal prepping, you can either opt for a recipe you can make ahead and store such as a batch of chili or your favorite curry. These can be repurposed for different meals. The second option is to mix and match components such as batch cooking roasted vegetables, whole grains, or even proteins like tofu.

Creating a plan

Once you are aware of all that you wish to cook ahead, this is what you will need to do next. Start making a list of all the tasks you want to accomplish within the meal prepping time you have set aside. Make a list of items you will need to cook and think of ways in which you can multitask. Perhaps you can cook something on the stovetop while another item is baking in the oven.

When the plan is ready, it is time to create a shopping list. It becomes easier to shop when you know all the ingredients you have to purchase.

Once you have completed both these steps, it is time to start prepping. Before you start prepping, ensure that you have set sufficient time aside for meal prep. Allocate anywhere between 2 to 4 hours during the weekend to prep meals for the upcoming week. Start with a clean kitchen; gather all the dishes you will need along with the equipment and the groceries, and start cooking. Maybe you can also turn on your favorite music to lift your spirits while prepping!

When all the prep is done, you must portion and store it! Store them in the right containers, label them if you want, and keep it in the fridge or the freezer. By following these steps, meal prepping will become incredibly simple. It will no longer seem overwhelming even if you never tried it before. All the effort that you put in will certainly be worth it.

Chapter Three

Benefits of Vegan Meal Prep

Who wouldn't want to lead a healthier life and feel more energized and fit? Well, everyone would want this. However, life can get a little hectic. Setting healthy goals is quite easy, but following through and staying on track becomes a little tricky. While you are busy navigating the hectic schedule of your daily life, the thought of cooking all your meals on your own is certainly not appealing. Not to mention the difficulty in thwarting off the temptations of eating out or ordering a meal. If you are tired of eating unhealthy junk food and want to eat healthier while saving some money, then meal prepping is the answer you have been looking for. In this section, let us look at some of the benefits of meal prep.

Grocery Shopping

Once you are aware of all the different meals you will be eating in a week, it becomes easier to shop for groceries. You no longer have to wander around aimlessly looking for inspiration or ideas to decide what to eat. Use the food list discussed in this book to prepare a grocery-shopping list. You can start dividing the list into different categories like vegetables, fruits, nuts and seeds, frozen foods, fats, and dairy alternatives. It also helps ensure that you don't give in to the temptation of buying unnecessary, processed foods.

Light on the Pocket

It is not expensive to start eating healthy. In fact, you might end up saving quite a lot of money. Once you start cooking all your meals at home. The only expenses you will incur are the ones towards shopping for groceries. Once you have everything you need to cook with, cooking becomes a breeze. Also, by planning all the meals, you will know what to buy and avoid making any unnecessary trips to the grocery store. When you know there is food waiting for you, it becomes easier to stop ordering meals.

Portion Control

An important skill you will learn once you start meal prepping is portion control. With meal prep, you will be dividing the food you cook into individual portions. By storing them in different containers, the urge to reach out for more or overindulge will be reduced. If weight loss is one of your priorities, then you need to consume sufficient nutrients. Portion control will help with this. You can certainly treat yourself occasionally, but learning to become mindful of the portions you eat is quintessential.

Weight Loss

When you know what you will be eating and how much you have to eat, you will automatically become mindful of the foods you consume. Weekly meal prep makes it easier to regulate the calories you consume daily. Since most of your meals will be home-cooked, you have complete control over the quality of ingredients you use. So, it is not just the quantity, but also the quality of the food you consume that improves as well. You don't necessarily have to count calories, but by substituting unhealthy ingredients with healthier alternatives, you can improve your overall health as well.

Less Wastage

Were there instances when you probably had to throw away produce because it expired or went bad before you had a chance to eat it? Wasting food is never a good feeling. It's not just a waste of money, but it is not environmentally sustainable. When you start meal prepping, you can make the most of all the ingredients you purchase. If you plan your meals correctly, you will be able to repurpose leftovers as well.

Saves Time and Effort

It does take a little time to plan and prepare meals in advance, but it is certainly worth the while. If you can dedicate a couple of hours over the weekend or whenever you are free to do the basic meal prep, cooking during the weekdays certainly becomes easier. Think about all the time you might usually end up worrying about what you will need to eat for your next meal. Once all your meals are prepared and planned, all that you need to do is reheat them and enjoy delicious and nutritious food.

Reduces Stress

Stress hurts your overall health. It not only weakens your immune system but also affects your sleeping pattern and digestive processes. Imagine how stressful it is when you come home after a hectic day and have to start thinking about what you need to eat for dinner. All this stress will be a thing of the past with meal prep. You can relax knowing that there is food ready when you go home.

Investment in Health

One of the great things about meal prep is that you can choose what you will be eating, and do this ahead of time. All those who follow meal prepping tend to eat cleaner than those who don't. You don't have to waste time finding something vegan to eat and risk eating unhealthy options because your meal is not ready. Eating healthy and well-balanced meals will undoubtedly improve your overall health. Proper nutrition is key to leading a healthy life.

Plenty of Variety

By putting a little thought into the kind of meals you will be eating, it becomes easier to select from different categories of foods like proteins, vegetables, fruits, and so on. When you plan, you can easily include the different food groups your body requires to all your meals. Apart from this, meal prep also encourages you to get creative with the recipes you use.

Better Willpower

Once you get into the groove of healthy eating, cravings for unhealthy foods and processed sugars will reduce. As your body gets used to the diet and the concept of healthy eating, it becomes easier to stay away from foods you know you must avoid.

Keep in mind that there is no right or wrong way to go about meal prepping. You have plenty of freedom to decide what you want to do. The best way to meal prep is via trial and error. After a week or two, you will quickly realize what works best for you.

Chapter Four

Food List

Regardless of whether you have been a vegan for a while or are trying out the vegan diet, you will undoubtedly come across several people who will seem skeptical of all that you are doing. A lot of people also believe that a vegan diet is extremely restrictive and limited. Does all this sound a little familiar? Well, if you were worried about these things, you can put your fears to rest. If you take a closer look, following a plant-based diet is quite simple. There are hundreds of options available. A vegan diet includes fruits, vegetables, nuts, seeds, grains, legumes, and a variety of other ingredients. It is quite easy to cook delicious meals without using any animal-based products.

Veganism is steadily gaining popularity, and these days there are various vegan-friendly products available in the market. From vegan meats to vegan dairy products, you don't have to worry about giving up on the foods you enjoy. By merely replacing certain ingredients, you can start enjoying all sorts of foods. Also, the different recipes given in this book will undoubtedly come in handy!

Being a vegan has become quite easy and convenient these days. To give you an overview of the limitless possibilities available, here is a vegan food list you can use.

Vegetables

You are free to consume as many vegetables as you want. Most of the vegetables are low in calories and rich in dietary fiber, phytonutrients, antioxidants, minerals, and vitamins that your body needs. You can use fresh as well as frozen vegetables.

The vegetables you can include are avocados, artichokes, asparagus, bell peppers, beetroot, broccoli, cabbage, brussels sprouts, cauliflower, carrots, cherry tomatoes, celery, collard greens, eggplant, cucumber, corn, peas, green beans, olives, jalapenos, mushrooms, okra, radishes, pumpkins, potatoes, shallots, squash, fennel, onions, chilies, peppers, potatoes, sweet potatoes, rhubarb, sprouts, zucchini, turnips, yams, and parsnips. The greens you can include are kale, spinach, Swiss chard, bok choy, arugula, lettuce, mixed salad leaves, watercress, endives, and so on.

You can pretty much include any vegetables that you want, including any which haven't been mentioned in this list.

Fruits

Fruits are rich in antioxidants, minerals, enzymes, vitamins, and other phytonutrients. They pretty much includes all the good stuff that your body needs. The simple sugars present in fruits also give your body a quick boost of energy. You can use fresh, frozen, or even dried fruits.

The different fruits you can include are mango, pineapple, guava, pomegranate, kiwi, dragon fruit, apples, pears, plums, grapes, oranges, nectarines, bananas, watermelon, persimmon, mangosteen, lime, lemon, figs, apricots, prunes, peaches, honeydew melon, cantaloupe, jackfruit, lychees, cucumber, coconut, clementine, currants, durian, and grapefruit.

Berries are low in calories and rich in antioxidants and vitamins. There are various berries to choose from, like blackberries, blueberries, strawberries, goji berries, cranberries, mulberries, raspberries, and so on.

Starchy Items

Starches are rich in complex carbs that supply your body with energy while filling up your tummy. Apart from this, they contain plenty of proteins, fibers, minerals, and amino acids. Whenever you are purchasing starches, stick to whole grains instead of the processed ones.

The different whole grains, you can include are rye, buckwheat, millet, quinoa, oats, wheat, wild rice, corn, barley, amaranth, whole wheat, bulgur, farro, kamut, millet, and einkorn. Apart from whole grains, you can also consume a variety of legumes. The different legumes you can start adding to your diet are pinto beans, black-eyed peas, black beans, chickpeas, fava beans, lentils, mung beans, navy beans, white beans, red beans, split peas, snow peas, sugar snap peas, soybeans, alfalfa sprouts, cannellini beans, azuki beans, lima beans, kidney beans, and green beans.

Herbs and Spices

Herbs and spices not only help elevate the flavors of the food you consume but are also good for your health. Most of the herbs and spices tend to have anti-inflammatory properties. Regardless of whether you are using fresh or dried herbs, they are a great way to improve your overall health. While following a vegan diet, you can include all herbs and spices. For instance, you can add cilantro, bay leaf, star anise, basil, chamomile, celery, chili powder, chives, coriander, dill, garlic, ginger, lemongrass, nutmeg, nutritional yeast, onion powder, oregano, peppermint, pepper, parsley, mint, time, turmeric, saffron, rosemary, red pepper flakes, poppy seeds, and paprika.

Healthy Fats

All fats are not created equal. There are some unhealthy fats and some extremely healthy ones. Saturated fats and trans fats are undesirable and are the reasons why fats tend to get a bad rap. However, the fats present in whole plant foods are extremely good for the overall functioning of your body. They enable the proper development as well as the functioning of the nervous system, improve the absorption of nutrients, and promote the heart's health. Including a variety of healthy, plant-based fats provides Linoleic acid and alpha-linolenic acids. Consuming sufficient healthy fats ensures that there exists a balance between omega-3 fatty acids and omega-6 fatty acids in your body. However, you need to be mindful of the fat consumption.

The different sources of healthy fats include nuts, seeds, and butter made from various nuts and seeds. You can start adding chia seeds, hemp seeds, flax seeds, sesame seeds, sunflower seeds, pumpkin seeds, cashews, pistachios, almonds, Brazil nuts, chestnuts, macadamia nuts, hazelnuts, walnuts, and pine nuts to your daily diet. Other sources of healthy fats include avocados, olives, and oils made from these ingredients.

Condiments and Miscellaneous Items

The different condiments you can include are salsa, mustard, hummus, harissa, coconut milk, baked beans, applesauce, canned tomatoes, curry paste, guacamole, miso, sambal, vinegar, and tahini. Various vegan-friendly sweeteners, you can use include stevia, date syrup, coconut syrup, maple syrup, rice syrup, molasses, organic cane sugar, and agave syrup. Other miscellaneous ingredients include trail mix, coffee, cocoa, baking powder, cornstarch, tea, and potato starch.

Vegan Dairy Alternatives

These days, there are plenty of dairy alternatives available. Various plant-based dairy alternatives you can choose from include soymilk, hemp milk, flax milk, coconut milk, almond milk, rice milk, and cashew milk. Apart from this, you can also include almond yogurt, coconut yogurt, soy yogurt, and any other soy products like tofu and tempeh.

While shopping, ensure that you always read through the list of ingredients present on the product you want to purchase. Also, any product that is rich in saturated fats must be avoided. Whenever buying any processed foods, always opt for organic varieties.

Chapter Five

Meal Prep Tips

Whether you are just getting started with a vegan diet or are in it for the long haul, reducing the cooking time makes all the difference. Purchasing a ready-made meal from the veggie section of a supermarket certainly doesn't hurt once in a while, but it is always better to eat fresh and healthy meals. It is where meal prep steps in. Here are some simple tips you can start using to make vegan meal prep easy.

Frozen Foods

Frozen foods are as good as fresh produce. At times, there might not be sufficient time to wash, peel, or prep any fresh produce. So, try opting for frozen foods in such a case. They contain all the nutrients that fresh produce does. When it comes to cooking, you merely need to cook the frozen ingredients, and a meal will be ready within no time.

A Little Planning

Always plan before you start shopping for the required groceries. If you head to the grocery store without a list of ingredients you need, you will not only end up wasting your money but might also forget to pick the ingredients you want to cook with. So, spend some time and make a plan for all the meals you want to have in a week. Use the different recipes given in this book for a better idea. Combine this with the food list, and you can quickly come up with a weekly grocery list. If you like any specific recipe, you might want to cook a couple of extra portions. If that's the case, then keep all this in mind while deciding what you want to buy. Plan your meals so that certain components will overlap. For instance, if you are making a burrito bowl, you can fashion it into a salad or even a wrap for another day.

Preparing Whole Grains

Cooking grains does take some time, and after a long day, you might not want to spend hours cooking in the kitchen. So, over the weekend, you can cook whole grains such as barley, quinoa, brown rice, or even couscous and store it for later. Once you have cooked the whole grains, lentils, and legumes, you merely need to store it in the fridge. You can easily reheat them along with some veggies!

Batch Cooking

One of the main components of meal prepping is batch cooking. If you're not used to cooking big portions, then now is the time to start. For instance, you can make a big pot of chili or any soup you like and repurpose the leftovers on other days. Certain items like broths, soups, and curries are best suited for batch cooking. Apart from cooking whole grains, you can also prep roasted veggies and other legumes. Cooking an entire recipe at once is not always feasible. Therefore, try cooking portions of different recipes beforehand.

Individual Portions

Instead of baking a loaf of zucchini bread or a large casserole, start cooking recipes in individual portions. For instance, instead of a loaf tray, you can use a muffin pan! Batching cooking helps save time, but to make things easier, store the cooked food in individual serving sizes. Instead of storing curry in a huge container, store individual servings in storage bags. It certainly helps make meal prep easier.

Use a Slow Cooker

If you have a slow cooker or an instant pot, it is time to start using them frequently. If you don't, maybe you should consider investing in one. There are countless recipes you can cook using a slow cooker, and it is not just for making stews. All that you need to do is toss in the ingredients in the cooker, turn it on, and wait for it to work its magic. A slow cooker comes in handy, especially when you want to cook large portions.

Nut Butter

Start making different nut butter at home. It is quite easy to make almonds, sunflower seeds, cashews, or even peanut butter at home. You merely need to blend the nuts or seeds along with some oil, sugar, and salt. If you don't want to make it at home, you can always purchase them. Nut butter goes well with fruit, crackers, bread, carrots, and celery. Whenever hunger strikes, these nut butters will come in handy.

Using Leftovers

If you don't think you'll have time to prepare more than one meal at a time, cook multiple servings of it and then refashion it into different meals. Alternatively, you can also take elements from one meal and reuse them the next day. Leftovers from a taco can be repurposed into a pie, or leftover quinoa can be added to a salad. Leftovers certainly come in handy while prepping meals.

Fill Up on Snacks

You can have snacks for dinner as well. Whenever you are in a rush, a simple salad is a great snack. All that you need to do is merely some fruits and vegetables and top it with a simple salad dressing. Or you can even make some dips like tahini, hummus, baba ganoush, or salsa and serve it with crudités.

Right Containers

If you want to cook in batches or cook multiple portions of the same item, then you need to have the proper containers to store them. Keep in mind your favorite dishes while doing meal prep. Always opt for reusable containers instead of disposable ones. It certainly helps save time and money, not to mention that they are environment-friendly as well.

Use Canned Foods

Start using canned foods as well. A lot of people tend to look down on canned foods, but using them certainly saves time. Instead of cooking beans from scratch, opt for canned beans. The same applies to tomatoes as well. You merely need to rinse and heat the canned ingredients!

Smoothies

Whipping up smoothies is incredibly simple. You merely need to toss all the required ingredients into the blender, and that's about it. Make a batch of smoothies over the weekend and store them in individual smoothie packs. Smoothies make for a great breakfast or a healthy snack.

Safety and Storage Steps

With meal prepping, you need to ensure that you store the food safely. For instance, the food you store in the refrigerator must be consumed within 2 to 3 days. If you think you will need a while longer, then always store in the freezer. The risk of food poisoning is considerably lower when using plant foods rather than animal-based ones. It is primarily because bacteria thrive on protein-rich foods when compared to sugars and starches. However, rice and quinoa are certain exceptions to this rule. Therefore, take a little extra care while storing and reheating these foods. Before you begin, check whether the food is safe to eat or not. By simply smiling and looking at it, you'll get the idea of it.

Before you store the food in the fridge, ensure that it is at room temperature. Never leave hot food in the refrigerator. If you place warm food in the refrigerator, it increases the overall temperature present within and increases the risk of other food getting spoiled as well. If you are using any frozen foods, ensure that it is at room temperature before you consume it. So, defrosting is essential.

Chapter Six

Sticking to a Vegan Diet

Now that you're aware of all the benefits of sticking to a vegan diet, your inclination to go vegan might have grown stronger. You might even be inspired to try a diet that excludes all animal products, including eggs, as well as dairy, to improve your overall health. Or maybe you want a diet that promotes weight loss. Following a vegan diet is especially healthy because all the meals you consume from now will be full of fruits, legumes, vegetables, and whole grains. To ensure that you don't miss out on the required nutrients or end up eating only processed foods, you need to have a proper diet plan in mind. In this section, let us look at specific tips that will come in handy while following the vegan diet.

Include a Variety of Foods

If you want your body to function optimally, you need to consume all the nutrients it requires. Therefore, consuming healthy and well-balanced meals must be your priority. For instance, leafy vegetables are excellent sources of vitamins; you can get protein from beans and fiber from whole grains. You need to include different varieties of ingredients in every meal you consume, to ensure that your body gets sufficient nutrients. The simplest thing you can do is start-adding produce of different colors to reap all the benefits they offer. For instance, tomatoes contain lycopene, sweet potatoes contain vitamin K, and blueberries contain anthocyanins. Essentially, you must try to consume foods from different colors of the rainbow.

Decoding Cravings

Cravings differ from one person to another, but there are certain similarities or principles for most of the cravings. For instance, you tend to crave sugar when your body is dehydrated. You might start craving for fried foods whenever you are stressed. There are different triggers associated with cravings. Once you identify the triggers, it becomes easier to regulate cravings.

To help your body get used to the vegan diet and regulate your cravings, you need to get sufficient sleep and drink plenty of water. Learn to differentiate between real hunger and hunger caused because of dehydration or tiredness. If your usual diet was rich in meat, dairy products, or processed foods, it would take your body a while to get used to a vegan diet. You might even experience symptoms of withdrawal. So, get creative and look for vegan alternatives for the foods you love. When you don't feel like you are depriving yourself of certain foods, your willingness to stick to the diet will increase.

Select Whole Grains

Instead of different refined grains like white bread, white pasta, or any other products made of refined flour, opt for whole grains. Whole grains are rich in vitamin B, as well as iron. Apart from this, the extra fiber present in them will certainly leave you feeling full for longer while assisting in weight loss.

Load Up on Veggies

A common mistake a lot of people make while following a vegan diet is that they start thinking about all the foods they cannot eat. Instead of worrying about all this, it is better to think about all the foods you can consume. You can have a delicious meal without depending on animal-based produce. Start making vegetables the 'meat' of your meals. They are rich in different vitamins and minerals while low in calories and high in fiber.

Truth About Vegan Products

Vegan products don't need to be always healthier than regular products. For instance, vegan cookies will certainly not help you lose weight when compared with regular cookies. Likewise, any product made with vegan margarine isn't healthier for your heart than the ones made with butter. Apart from this, most of the vegan foods available in the market are rich in saturated fats like palm oil. So, make it a point to carefully go through the list of ingredients as well as the nutritional facts before you purchase any vegan food. Always opt for nutritious and whole foods. It is okay to indulge in vegan treats occasionally, but you cannot justify them as being healthy merely because they are vegan.

Plant-Based Proteins

There are various plant-based proteins available these days. Animal protein, like meat and cheese, are usually rich in unhealthy saturated fats and also bad because of all the environmental reasons. Instead, opt for vegan sources like tofu, lentils, chickpeas, beans, and edamame. If your diet is quite varied, then you don't have to worry about consciously including more sources of plant-based protein. The ideal intake of protein must be between 45 to 55 grams per day. As long as you consume the required protein, you can maintain your overall health.

Omega-3 Fatty Acids

Some nutrients are naturally present in a healthy vegan diet. For instance, EPA and DHA are two omega-3 fatty acids that are essential for maintaining the health of the eyes, brain, and heart. The primary sources of omega-3 fatty acids are fatty fish. However, by consuming plant-based foods like flaxseed, soy, walnuts, and canola oil, you can get sufficient omega-3 fatty acids. However, consult your doctor and consider taking vegan supplements for DHA and EPA.

Iron Content

Chicken and meat are amongst the best sources of iron. Iron is incredibly important because it helps the red blood cells transport oxygen in the body. Iron deficiency is a common cause of fatigue and tiredness. The best sources of iron in a vegan diet include legumes, leafy vegetables, and beans. To increase the absorption of iron, you need to consume sufficient vitamin C.

Be Mindful of Vitamin D

The best sources of vitamin D include salmon, sardines, and other fortified dairy products like yogurt and milk. However, vitamin D can also be found in fortified cereals, orange juice, soymilk, and almond milk too. Apart from this, ensure that you expose yourself to sufficient sunlight. The ideal intake of vitamin D, you must be between 600 to 1500 IU daily. Vegans might need to rely on vitamin D supplements to get their daily dose of this vitamin.

Don't Ignore Vitamin B12

Vegetarian, as well as vegan diets, are often devoid of vitamin B12. It helps convert food into energy while improving your cognitive functions. The primary sources of vitamin B12 are meat, poultry, fish, eggs, and dairy products. Since a vegan diet doesn't include any of these ingredients, it is essential that you consult a doctor about taking a supplement. You can also start adding breakfast cereals fortified with B12 to get the required dose of this vitamin.

By following the different tips discussed in this section, you can ensure that you improve your overall health while sticking to a vegan diet.

Chapter Seven

Meal Prep Mistakes to Avoid

When done right, meal prep helps save time, effort, and money while improving your overall health. Regardless of whether you have been meal prepping for a while or are just getting started with it, there is always scope for improvement. In this section, let us look at some of the most common mistakes people make while meal prepping and how to avoid them.

No Goals

Before you start meal prepping, you need to have a goal in mind. What do you plan to achieve via meal prep? Regardless of whether you want to save money and time, lose weight, or build muscle, you need to have specific goals in mind. Once you have a goal in mind, it gives you the motivation required to go through all the steps included in meal prep, like planning, shopping, and cooking.

So, take a couple of minutes and think about your goals. Maybe you can think of how you can utilize the money you save or attain your weight loss objectives. Once you make a list of these goals, stick it in a place where you can keep glancing at it regularly. Maybe you can place it on the fridge door using a magnet. So, every time you open the fridge door to grab something, you will be reminded of your goals.

Making it Complicated

Another common mistake a lot of meal preppers make is they tend to over complicate things. It is quite easy to get ambitious and think you can get a lot done. It is especially true if you have decided to spend one day a week dedicated only to cooking. However, if you start opting for recipes that require various components, you will only end up over complicating things. Chances are, you might not ever want to meal prep again. The idea of meal prep is to save time and effort. It is not about hard work, but about working smartly. You don't have to try and cook ten dishes at one go. Instead, stick to those recipes that include certain overlapping components. To get started, you can stick to one-pot recipes or even a recipe that includes various mix-ins like salads.

Reducing the Intake of Vegetables

Since you are following a vegan diet, you need to include plenty of vegetables. You cannot start skimping on vegetables. If you do this, you will be depriving your body of all the nutrients it requires. Keep in mind that vegetables need to be the star of all the meals you cook.

Quantity Matters Too

When it comes to meal prepping, you need to cook multiple portions! If the portions you cook are too less or too much, it defeats the purpose of meal prep. If you cook too little, you will soon run out of food on weekdays. If you cook too much of the same item, you will end up eating the same food every day. Neither of these is desirable. So, before you start meal prepping, plan all or at least most of your meals. Once you know the kind of meals you will be eating all week long, it indeed becomes easier to decide all the prepping that's required. So, it is a good idea to start calculating the number of meals you wish to cook as well as the serving size of every component present in each meal. It helps cut down on the time required for meal prep while making sure that every meal is planned correctly.

The Size of Containers

If you want to start meal prepping, you need to have the right boxes to store the food in. It becomes easier to regulate the portions you consume when you pick the right containers. After all, you certainly don't want to be left hungry because you picked a small container. Also, opt for reusable containers instead of disposable varieties.

Eating the Same Food

You might be quite motivated to stick to your diet, but this motivation will start dwindling. If you keep eating the same food daily it can get easily boring if you aren't careful. A little consistency is good, but excessive repetition is never desirable. You can start swapping the proteins from one source to another. If you are going to be consuming two portions of beans, maybe you can shift to chickpeas, tofu, or any other plant-based protein you want. Start adding new sources of carbs, use different herbs and spices, and don't be afraid to experiment.

Forgetting Snacks

It is good that you are prepping for all the essential meals in your day, but you must not overlook snacks. You will need a couple of snacks to get through your day. So, spend some time and think about all the snacks you can consume. Use the different snack recipes given in this book to do this. When you have a couple of snack options available readily, then the desire to mindlessly munch on junk food will reduce. The snacks don't necessarily have to be complicated. It could be something as simple as having a handful of nuts, some popcorn, or even sliced vegetables.

Not Using the Freezer

Meal prepping is wonderful, but eating the same meal seven days in a row is frustrating. Well, this is where your freezer comes in. Whenever you cook a big batch of something, freeze extra portions in different containers. Over time, you will end up with a stockpile of prepped foods that can be mixed and matched to create new meals all week long. It especially comes in handy whenever you have a busy week with little or no time left to cook.

Not Making any Sauces

The easiest way to ensure that there is some excitement to every meal you consume is by including a sauce. You can drizzle it over salads, serve it with proteins, or even turn them into soups to add a little extra flavor. To prevent things from becoming overly complicated, opt for one sauce recipe, and then make a big batch of it. If not a sauce, at least make a broth and store it. A broth can easily be turned into curries, sauces, or even soups and stews. Choose a sauce that can easily be paired with different ingredients like whole grains, proteins, and veggies.

Chapter Eight

Tips For Beginners

Tips to Get Started

Before you decide to go vegan, you need to understand your reasons for doing this. If you don't know your reasons for sticking to a diet or opting for a lifestyle, the changes you make will not last. If you are trying to go vegan because it is a fad or sounds hip, then you need to think again. When you have a solid reason in mind, it becomes easier to motivate yourself to follow a diet.

A common mistake a lot of people make whenever they go vegan is that they start skimping on carbs. Another misconception is that the lack of meat is the reason for tiredness and fatigue. However, there is no reason to trust either of these opinions because they are nothing more than misconceptions. You don't need to eat meat to feel full. When you start loading up on whole grains and other whole foods, your tummy will feel full for longer. Start adding sufficient complex carbs to your meals along with fiber-rich foods to satiate your hunger.

Contrary to popular opinion, once you decide to go vegan, there are plenty of food options available to you. Once you start going through the different recipes given in this book, the way you view vegan meals is bound to change. If you want a little extra inspiration, then you can start following different vegan accounts on various social media platforms like Instagram, Facebook, Pinterest, and so on. Start experimenting with different ingredients and spices and learn to have fun with it. Vegan meals don't have to be bland and boring; they can be exciting and mouth-wateringly delicious.

Keep in mind that shifting from an ordinary diet to a vegan diet takes time. Try to understand that you're easing into a new lifestyle and not just a diet. So, a shift like this will take time, and you need to be patient. Give your body as well as your tastes buds a while to get adjusted to the new diet.

If you are eating wholesome and healthy meals, you don't have to worry about any nutritional deficiencies. At least until you get the hang of it, it is a good idea to start tracking your nutrient intake during an initial couple of weeks. Once you are aware of all the foods that are rich in nutrients and have a sense of how much you need to eat to feel satisfied, it gets easier. A popular misconception is that vegans do not get sufficient protein. Well, the number of vegan protein sources will certainly leave you pleasantly surprised. Remember the food list previously discussed.

Vegan Mistakes to Avoid

If your usual diet was rich and processed foods, meats, and sugars, then going vegan is certainly a drastic change. Once you stop eating all animal products, you might end up sticking to easy options. You might end up eating pasta five times a week or salads every day. Well, you must avoid doing this. There needs to be plenty of variety included in your usual diet. Start using different meal prep ideas as well as recipes given in this book to add variety to your daily meals.

People might say that going vegan is expensive. Well, if you end up buying plenty of cheese and meat substitutes, it will become costly. Instead, opt for whole and natural ingredients. You don't need to depend on these meat substitutes. Also, they aren't necessarily healthy. Instead of purchasing ready-made vegan patties, you can make them at home. It is entirely up to you. If you want, you can always set a food budget and stick to it.

Don't worry that you will no longer be able to eat cookies, cakes, ice cream, or any other junk food that you love. There are vegan alternatives available for all these foods. All that you need to do is get a little creative. For instance, ice cream can be replaced with banana nice cream. Vegan cookies and cakes are quite delicious. You don't have to compromise on your taste buds for the sake of your new diet.

Your body needs protein, but you don't have to worry about it. If you are consuming wholesome meals, your body will get all the nutrients and macros it requires. Your daily intake of protein should not be higher than 10 to 20% of your total calories.

Eating vegetables is undoubtedly desirable. If you want to lose weight, then start adding non-starchy vegetables to your diet. That said, the body does need some calories to keep functioning optimally. If you start depriving your body of all the calories it requires, it cannot function as it's supposed to. Avoid severely restricting your calorie intake.

Keep an open mind and try different vegan options as much as you can. Don't restrict yourself to tried and tested recipes. Try new things, and you might start enjoying foods you never even knew existed before.

There will be times when you will slip up and accidentally consume non-vegan foods. Well, slipups are common. After all, you are human. It is okay to eat or purchase something that isn't purely vegan accidentally. However, you must not make a habit of it. After all, if you do want to stick to a new routine, you need to make a conscious effort to follow through as well.

Vegan Meal Prep on Budget

When armed with the right knowledge, a healthy diet that's full of tasty and nutritious meals can fit any budget. You don't have to burn a hole in your pocket just because you're going vegan. Use these different meal prep ideas given in this section to stick to a food budget, while staying true to your vegan lifestyle.

Perhaps the most obvious step of all is to start cooking volume meals at home. Start concentrating on whole foods. Not only are they rich in nutrients, but they are also low priced when compared to other ingredients. So, base most of your recipes around these low priced and extremely nutritious foods. Whenever possible, start purchasing in bulk. Bulk purchases are priced at a lower rate than small bags or containers. If possible, look for a wholesale food store nearby, and explore all the items on display. Different items you can purchase in bulk include whole grains, legumes, lentils, and healthy oils. However, ensure that you check the expiry date before you make any bulk purchase.

While getting started, always stick to simple recipes. Don't look for any recipes that call for multiple compliments. Start simple and slowly experiment. Simple doesn't have to be boring, and it can be quite delicious. Whenever you have any leftovers, start freezing. This stands true not just for the meals you cook, but also the ingredients you purchase. If you realize that you purchase too many vegetables, fruits, toss them in the freezer.

Start making different condiments and sauces at home instead of purchasing them. You can also make nut butter and nut flours at home. Start buying seasonal produce. Seasonal produce is not only cheaper, but it is healthier and more flavorsome as well. If possible, start visiting the local farmers market. It is a great place where you can directly buy from the farming community, and often the produce is priced at a lower rate than the local supermarkets.

Do your homework before you make any purchase. If there are a couple of grocery stores or supermarkets nearby, check for discounts and sales going on. Compare the prices; these days there are different online retailers to consider as well. Doing a little bit of research will certainly help you save money in the long run.

Ensure that you drink sufficient water. You need to drink at least eight glasses of water daily. If you don't want to get dehydrated, add fruit juices, or even a little lemon into the water you drink to enhance its flavors. Another affordable alternative you can opt for includes herbal teas!

If you have a green thumb, or you like

gardening, then start growing your food. Provided you have space available to do this. It certainly sounds like an ambitious project, but it is doable. Once you start growing your produce, you will have complete control over the end product you harvest. It certainly doesn't get any fresher than this. If not, vegetables and fruits, you can start growing herbs at home. Growing herbs is quite simple. You need a couple of planters, seeds, that's about it. You can create your kitchen garden full of herbs within no time.

Whenever you get a good deal, purchase live herbs in bulk. Fresh herbs certainly taste quite nice, but even the dried variants are equally good. Wash the herbs, dry them, and then store them! It is certainly cost-effective. By doing this, you can ensure that you have all the herbs you need all year long.

There are different ways in which you can start reducing costs, especially if you are on a tight budget. However, it doesn't mean you need to deprive yourself of flavorsome foods or compromise on your health. Fortunately, it is incredibly cheap to start cooking healthy and wholesome meals. Start being a little creative, experiment with simple recipes, and mix things up. You don't need expensive ingredients to cook mouth-watering meals. Now, all that you need to do is to get started as soon as you can!

Chapter Nine

Vegan Breakfast Recipes

Tofu Scramble with Sweet Potatoes
Serves: 3 – 4

Ingredients:

For sweet potatoes:

- ¾ pound sweet potatoes, scrubbed, chopped into ½ inch cubes
- Salt to taste
- Pepper to taste
- ½ tablespoon olive oil
- 1 teaspoon chili powder

For tofu scramble:

- 1 tablespoon olive oil
- ½ package (from a 14 ounces package) extra-firm tofu, drained, crumbled
- 1 small onion, chopped
- 1 cup chopped asparagus
- ½ teaspoon garlic powder
- 1 bell pepper, deseed if desired, finely chopped
- Salt to taste
- Pepper to taste
- ½ teaspoon ground cumin
- ½ teaspoon turmeric powder

Directions:

1. Add sweet potatoes into a bowl. Sprinkle salt, pepper and chili powder and toss well. Drizzle oil and toss well.
2. Transfer onto a lined baking sheet. Spread it evenly.
3. Bake in a preheated oven at 425° F for 30 minutes or until cooked through. Stir once halfway through baking.
4. Place a skillet over medium-high heat. Add oil. When the oil is heated, add onion, asparagus and bell pepper. Sauté for 6-7 minutes or until tender.
5. Stir in the tofu, spices, and salt. Heat thoroughly.
6. Take 3 – 4 meal prep containers and divide the scramble among them.
7. Also divide the sweet potatoes among the containers.
8. Refrigerate until use. It can last for 4 days.

Strawberry Banana Spinach Smoothie
Serves: 2

Ingredients:

For smoothie:

- 1 cup frozen, sliced bananas
- 2 cups fresh spinach
- 1 cup frozen whole strawberries
- 2 teaspoons chia seeds

Serving day ingredients (per smoothie bag):

- Unsweetened almond milk, as required
- 1 scoop vegan vanilla protein powder

Directions:

1. Divide all the ingredients for the smoothie into 2 Ziploc bags. Squeeze the bag to remove any air. Seal the bag. Label the bag with the date and name of the smoothie. Freeze until use. It can last for 3 months.
2. Serving day: Remove a bag from the freezer and thaw slightly if desired. Add all the contents of the bag into a high-speed blender.
3. Add milk and protein powder. Blend until smooth.
4. Pour into a glass and serve.

Breakfast Cookies
Serves: 12 - 15

Ingredients:

For wet ingredients:

- 1 medium overripe bananas, mashed
- 1 tablespoon maple syrup
- 1 flax egg (1 tablespoon ground flax seeds mixed with 3 tablespoons water)
- ¼ cup creamy, unsalted, peanut butter
- 1 tablespoon melted coconut oil
- ½ teaspoon pure vanilla extract

For dry ingredients:

- 1 cup gluten-free rolled oats
- ¼ teaspoon baking soda
- ¼ teaspoon baking powder

Add-ins:

- ¼ cup finely chopped walnuts
- ¼ cup raisins

Optional toppings:

> 1 tablespoon chopped walnuts
> 1 tablespoons raisins

Directions:

- Once you mix the water and ground flaxseed, set aside for 15 minutes.
- Add all the wet ingredients into a bowl and stir until well incorporated.
- Mix together all the dry ingredients in another bowl. Add the dry ingredients into the bowl of wet ingredients. Mix well into a dough.
- Divide the dough into 12 – 15 equal portions. Sprinkle optional toppings if using.
- Press them lightly into the shape of a cookie of about ½ inch thickness. Place on a baking sheet lined with parchment paper. Leave a gap between the cookies.
- Bake in a preheated oven at 350° F for 12-15 minutes or until light golden brown.
- Remove from the oven and let the cookies cool for 7 – 8 minutes on the baking sheet. Loosen the cookies with a metal spatula.
- Cool completely. Transfer into an airtight container. It can be stored at room temperature for 4 to 5 days. For longer, store the container in the refrigerator. It can last for 10 – 12 days. For even longer, transfer into freezer-safe bags. Label the bags and freeze for up to 2 months.

Carrot Cake Quinoa Breakfast Bars
Serves: 30 – 32 bars

Ingredients:

For wet ingredients:

- 2 flax eggs (2 tablespoons of ground flaxseed mixed with 6 tablespoons water)
- 1 cup mashed banana
- 2 cups cooked or canned chickpeas
- 1 cup unsweetened applesauce

For dry ingredients:

- 1 ½ cups quinoa flour
- 2 teaspoons ground cinnamon
- 1 teaspoon ground vanilla bean or 2 teaspoons pure vanilla extract
- 1/8 teaspoon salt
- 1 cup coconut sugar
- 1 teaspoon ground nutmeg
- 1 teaspoon baking soda

For add-ins:

- ½ cup hemp hearts
- ½ cup chopped walnuts
- 1 cup grated carrots

Optional toppings:

- Chopped walnuts

Directions:

1. Take a large baking dish (13 x 9 inches) and grease with some cooking spray. Place a sheet of parchment paper in it.
2. Once you mix the water and ground flaxseed, set aside for 15 minutes.
3. Add the rest of the wet ingredients into a blender and blend until smooth.
4. Add all the dry ingredients into a mixing bowl and stir.
5. Add the wet ingredients and flax eggs into the bowl of dry ingredients and mix until well incorporated.
6. Add hemp hearts, walnuts and carrots and fold gently.
7. Pour the batter into the baking dish.
8. Bake in a preheated oven at 350° F for 23 – 27 minutes. The cake is ready when a toothpick inserted in the center does not have any particles stuck on it when removed from the cake.

9. Remove the baking dish from the oven. Take out the cake from the dish after 15 – 20 minutes and place on a wire rack.
10. Let it cool to room temperature.
11. Cut into 30 – 32 equal pieces. Transfer into an airtight container. It can last for 2 – 3 days at room temperature or for 5 – 6 days in the refrigerator.

Oven Baked Beans

Serves: 4

Ingredients:

½ tablespoon olive oil
1 red onion, chopped
1 small red chili, deseeded, finely chopped
½ teaspoon smoked paprika
¼ teaspoon ground cumin
½ teaspoon chili flakes
2 – 3 sprigs fresh thyme
12 ounces tomato passata
1 tablespoon balsamic vinegar
¼ teaspoon Tabasco sauce (optional)
1 can (15 ounces) white beans like pinto beans or borlotti beans, drained, rinsed
½ teaspoon molasses
2 cloves garlic, peeled, minced
Salt to taste
Pepper to taste

Directions:

- Add onion, chili, and garlic into a baking dish. Drizzle oil over it. Add all the spices and toss well.
- Cover the baking dish with aluminum foil.
- Bake in a preheated oven at 340° F for 20 minutes.
- Remove the dish from the oven and uncover.
- Add rest of the ingredients and mix well. If you find the mixture very dry, add a little water and mix well.
- Bake for 30 – 40 minutes. Do not cover the dish while baking.

- Remove from the oven and cool completely.
- Transfer into an airtight container and refrigerate until use. It can last for 5 days. If you want to freeze it, place in freezer bags and freeze until use. It can last for 3 months.
- To serve: Thaw if frozen. Heat thoroughly in an oven or microwave.
- Serve with toasted bread if desired.

Zucchini Muffins

Serves: 9

Ingredients:

For wet ingredients:

- ¼ cup lightly packed dark brown sugar
- ¾ cup grated zucchini
- ¼ cup granulated organic sugar
- 3 tablespoons unsweetened applesauce
- 2 tablespoons canola oil
- 6 tablespoons almond milk

For dry ingredients:

1. ¼ cup almond meal
2. ¾ cup + 2 tablespoons white spelt flour
3. ½ teaspoon baking powder
4. ½ teaspoon baking soda
5. ½ teaspoon ground cinnamon
6. ¼ teaspoon salt
7. 1/8 teaspoon ground nutmeg

Directions:

1. Add all the wet ingredients into a mixing bowl and whisk well. Set aside for 5 minutes.
2. Add all the dry ingredients into another bowl and stir.
3. Add the mixture of dry ingredients into the bowl of wet ingredients and mix until well combined. Do not over mix.
4. Take 9 muffin cups and grease with olive oil. Place disposable muffin liners in it. Divide the batter into the prepared muffin cups.
5. Bake in a preheated oven at 350° F for 20 – 25 minutes or a toothpick when

inserted in the center of the muffin comes out clean. Remove the muffins from the mold and place on a wire rack. Cool completely.

6. Store in an airtight container at room temperature for up to 2 days. You can refrigerate the muffins. It can last for 4-5 days.

7. To freeze: Wrap individual muffins in plastic wrap. Place the muffins in freezer-safe bags. Freeze until use. It can last for 1 month in the freezer.

8. To serve: Thaw the muffins completely and warm for a few seconds in the microwave before serving.

Quinoa Breakfast Tacos

Serves: 8

Ingredients:

For quinoa:

- 3 cups cooked quinoa
- 2 tablespoons fresh lime juice
- ½ cup chopped cilantro
- Salt to taste
- Freshly ground pepper to taste

For butternut squash:

- 4 tablespoons coconut oil
- 1 bunch Swiss chard or kale, discard hard stems and ribs, finely chopped
- 8 cups cubed butternut squash
- Salt to taste
- Freshly ground pepper to taste
- 1 teaspoon chili powder

Serving day ingredients:

- 16 tortillas
- 8 scallions, thinly sliced
- 2 large ripe avocados, pitted, peeled, thinly sliced
- Salt to taste
- Freshly ground pepper to taste
- 2 cups shredded red cabbage

Directions:

1. To make quinoa: Add all the ingredients for quinoa into an airtight container and mix well. Close the lid and refrigerate until use.
2. To make filling: Place a large skillet over medium heat. Add oil. When the oil is heated, add squash and cook for about 8 minutes.
3. Add rest of the ingredients for the filling and cook until kale wilts. Remove from heat and cool completely. Transfer into an airtight container and refrigerate until use. The filling and quinoa can store for 4 days.
4. To serve: Remove the quinoa and filling from the refrigerator and warm it in the microwave. Heat the tortillas following the directions on the package.
5. Place the tortillas on individual serving plates. Divide the quinoa, butternut squash filling, scallions, avocados and cabbage among the tortillas. Season with salt and pepper and serve.

Blueberry Baked Oatmeal

Serves: 3 – 4

Ingredients:

1) 1/3 cup chopped pecans
2) 1 teaspoon ground cinnamon
3) 1/8 teaspoon ground nutmeg
4) 3 tablespoons maple syrup
5) 1 ½ tablespoons coconut oil, melted
6) 6 ounces blueberries, fresh or frozen, divided
7) 1 cup old fashioned oats
8) ½ teaspoon baking powder
9) ¾ cup + 2 tablespoons nondairy milk of your choice, at room temperature
10) 1 flax egg (1 tablespoon ground flax seeds mixed with 3 tablespoons water)
11) 1 teaspoon vanilla extract
12) 1 teaspoon raw sugar (optional)

Optional toppings: Use any

- Vegan vanilla yogurt
- Blueberries
- Vegan whipped cream
- Maple syrup
- Any other toppings of your choice

Directions:

1. After mixing the flaxseeds with water, set aside for 15 minutes.
2. Take a square baking dish of about 6 x 6 and grease with cooking spray. Set aside.
3. Spread pecans on a rimmed baking sheet.
4. Bake in a preheated oven at 375° F for 4 – 5 minutes or until toasted and aromatic.
5. Transfer into a mixing bowl. Also add in the oats, cinnamon, salt, baking powder and nutmeg. Stir until well incorporated.
6. Add milk, flax egg, maple syrup, vanilla, and coconut oil into a bowl and whisk

well.

7. Set aside ¼ cup of blueberries and place the rest of the berries in the prepared baking dish. Spread it evenly.
8. Spread the oat mixture over the berries. Spoon the milk mixture over the oat layer. Lightly tap the dish on your countertop.
9. Press lightly on the oats so that it is soaked in milk.
10. Sprinkle the berries (that were set aside) on top. Scatter sugar on top.
11. Bake in a preheated oven at 375° F for 30 minutes or until golden brown on top.
12. Take out the dish from the oven and let it cool to room temperature.
13. Cover the dish with foil and refrigerate until use. It can last for 4 – 5 days.
14. To serve: Cut into portions and place in a microwave-safe bowl. Heat thoroughly and serve.

Potato and Tofu Tacos
Serves: 6

Ingredients:

- 1 tablespoon vegetable oil
- ½ large bell pepper, diced
- 3 strips vegan bacon
- ½ tablespoon nutritional yeast
- Himalayan pink salt to taste
- 6 flour tortillas
- 1 medium onion, diced
- 1 cup frozen, diced potatoes
- 1 block firm tofu, drained, pressed of excess moisture, crumbled
- ½ teaspoon garlic powder
- Pepper to taste
- Salt to taste

Directions:

1. Place a large skillet over medium heat. Add ½ tablespoon of oil. When the oil is heated, add onion and bell pepper and sauté until onion turns translucent.
2. Stir in the potatoes and mix well.
3. Lower the heat to low heat and cover

with a lid. Cook until potatoes are well cooked. Stir every 5 minutes. Add salt and pepper to taste. Transfer into a bowl and let it cool.
4. Add ½ tablespoon oil into the skillet. When the oil is heated, add tofu and cook until nearly dry.
5. Stir in the vegan bacon. Cook until tofu is light brown. Add nutritional yeast and garlic powder.
6. Remove from heat. Add Himalayan pink salt and pepper and mix well.
7. Spread the tortillas on your countertop. Divide the potatoes and tofu among the tortillas. Roll and wrap in aluminum foil.
8. Place the wrapped tacos in freezer-safe bags. Freeze until use. It can last for 15 days.
9. To serve: Remove from the oven and discard the foil. Wrap the taco in paper towel and place in a microwave. Cook on high for a minute or until heated through.
10. Serve with salsa or any other dip of your choice.

Vegan Strata
Serves: 4

Ingredients:

- ½ tablespoon German mustard
- ¼ cup vegetable broth or water
- ½ cup finely chopped celery
- ½ cup finely chopped onion
- 2 ounces mushrooms, thinly sliced
- 7 ounces vegan beef crumbles
- 1 cup vegan mozzarella cheese shreds
- 1 cup chopped spinach
- 2 ½ cups diced sourdough bread

For vegan egg batter:

- ¾ cup chickpea flour
- 1 tablespoon flaxseed meal
- ½ teaspoon salt
- Pepper to taste
- A large pinch nutmeg
- 1 ½ cups unsweetened almond milk
- 1 tablespoon nutritional yeast

- ½ teaspoon turmeric powder
- ¼ teaspoon Himalayan pink salt or to taste

Serving day ingredients:

- 2 tablespoons chopped parsley
- 1 green onion, thinly sliced

Directions:

1. Spray a 6-inch freezer safe, baking dish with cooking spray.
2. Place a nonstick skillet over medium flame. Add broth. When the broth is heated, add mushrooms, celery and onion and cook until onions are pink.
3. Add vegan sausage and stir. Break it simultaneously as it cooks. Add more broth if the mixture is stuck to the bottom of the pan. Turn off the heat.
4. Add mustard and spinach and mix well.
5. To make vegan egg batter: Add all the ingredients for vegan egg batter into a bowl and whisk well.
6. Spread the sausage mixture on the bottom of the prepared baking dish.
7. Scatter bread pieces and cheese. Pour egg batter and mix the sausage mixture, bread and cheese until well coated.
8. Cover the dish with cling wrap. Chill overnight.
9. Bake in a preheated oven at 350° F for about 45 – 50 minutes or until set.
10. Let it cool to room temperature.
11. Sprinkle green onion and parsley on top and serve.

Vegan Sausage Breakfast Lasagna
Serves: 4

Ingredients:

- 4.5 ounces no-boil lasagna noodles
- 3 scallions, thinly sliced
- 4 ounces vegan mozzarella cheese shreds

For béchamel sauce:

- ¼ cup unbleached all-purpose flour
- 1 medium leek, green and white parts only

- 8 ounces frozen chopped spinach
- ½ teaspoon dried oregano
- ½ teaspoon dried sage
- 2 cloves garlic, minced
- 2 cups cashew milk or any other vegan milk of your choice
- Salt to taste
- Pepper to taste
- ½ tablespoon extra-virgin olive oil
- ¼ teaspoon ground nutmeg
- 7 ounces vegan Italian sausages, chopped

Directions:

- To make béchamel sauce: Place a skillet over medium heat. Add oil. When the oil is heated, add leeks and garlic and sauté for a minute and cook until tender.
- Stir in the sausages, salt, pepper, oregano, sage, and nutmeg.
- Stir in the flour and sauté for a couple of minutes.
- Pour cashew milk, stirring constantly. Continue stirring until thick. When the sauce begins to boil, turn off the heat.
- To assemble: Take a baking dish of about 8 inches. Spoon some of the béchamel sauce on the bottom of the baking dish. Spread a layer of noodles (about 2-3) over the sauce layer.
- Layer with half the spinach. Spread a little béchamel sauce over the spinach followed by 1/3 the cheese and 1/3 the scallions.
- Place remaining noodles over the scallions.
- Follow step 6 again.
- Spread the remaining sauce on top. Scatter remaining cheese and scallions.
- Cover the dish with plastic wrap.
- Refrigerate until use. It can last for 2-3 days.
- Remove the baking dish from the refrigerator and discard plastic wrap. Cover the dish with foil.
- Bake in a preheated oven at 350° F for about 30 minutes. Uncover and bake

until the top is golden brown.
- Remove from the oven and let it rest for 5-7 minutes.
- Serve hot, warm or cold.

Chapter Ten

Vegan Lunch Recipes

Sesame Tofu Quinoa Bowls

Serves: 2

Ingredients:

- ½ pound green beans, trimmed, halved
- 2 cups broccoli florets
- ½ block extra-firm tofu, pressed of excess moisture
- 1 cup cooked quinoa

For dressing:

- 2 tablespoons toasted sesame oil
- ½ teaspoon arrowroot or tapioca starch or cornstarch
- ¼ teaspoon ground ginger
- ¼ teaspoon garlic powder
- 1 tablespoon tamari
- Crushed red pepper flakes to taste
- Salt to taste

To garnish:

- Black sesame seeds

Directions:

- Spread the green beans on 1/3 part of a baking sheet. Spread tofu on another 1/3 portion and broccoli florets on 1/3 of the portion of the baking sheet.
- Add all the ingredients for dressing into a bowl and whisk well. Drizzle over the beans, broccoli and tofu. Mix each of them.
- Bake in a preheated oven at 375° F for about 30 minutes. Stir once halfway through baking.
- Remove from the oven and cool completely.
- Divide into 2 meal prep containers. Also divide the quinoa among the containers.
- Refrigerate until use. It can last for 3 days. Top with tamari or some hot sauce.

Portobello Fajita Meal Prep Bowls

Serves: 2

Ingredients:

For spice blend:

- ½ teaspoon garlic powder
- ½ teaspoon ground cumin
- ½ teaspoon red pepper flakes
- ½ teaspoon onion powder
- ½ teaspoon chili powder
- ½ teaspoon salt

For fajita bowls:

- 6 tablespoons quinoa
- 2 Portobello mushrooms, cut into strips
- ½ zucchini, sliced
- 1 tablespoon olive oil
- 1 bell pepper, deseed if desired, sliced
- 1 small red onion, sliced

Other ingredients:

- 2 lime wedges
- ½ cup black beans

Serving day ingredients:

- Avocado slices
- Salsa
- Vegan yogurt etc.

Directions:

1. To make spice blend: Add all the ingredients for spice blend into a bowl and stir.
2. Add half the spice blend mixture and cook the quinoa following the instructions on the package. Once cooked, set aside to cool.
3. Add all the vegetables into a baking dish. Drizzle oil over it. Sprinkle remaining spice blend mixture and toss well.
4. Bake in a preheated oven at 425° F for about 20 minutes. Stir once halfway through baking. Remove from the oven and cool completely.
5. Divide the quinoa into 2 meal prep containers. Layer with vegetables and black beans. Refrigerate until use. It can last for 5 days.
6. To serve: Heat if desired. Serve with the

suggested serving options or with any other toppings of your choice.

Miso Glazed Sweet Potato Bowls
Serves: 2

Ingredients:

- 1 medium sweet potato, peeled, cut into 2-inch cubes (about 2 cups)
- ½ teaspoon turmeric powder
- 1 tablespoon tamari
- 1 tablespoon pure maple syrup
- ½ onion, finely chopped
- ½ teaspoon garlic powder
- 4 ounces mushrooms, finely chopped
- ¾ cup uncooked farro
- 1 ½ tablespoons white miso
- ½ tablespoon rice wine vinegar
- ½ tablespoon extra-virgin olive oil
- 1 large bunch kale, discard hard stems and ribs
- Salt to taste
- Pepper to taste
- Water, as required

Serving day ingredients:

- Avocado slices
- Tahini sauce

Directions:

- Spread the sweet potatoes on a lined baking sheet.
- Bake in a preheated oven at 425° F for about 20 minutes. Stir once halfway through baking.
- Place a saucepan with 1-½ cups of water over medium heat. Bring to a boil.
- Add farro and cook until tender and dry. Add more water if it is not cooked. Stir in the turmeric. Turn off the heat and fluff with a fork. Let it cool completely.
- Place a pot over medium heat. Add oil. When the oil is heated, add onion and sauté until translucent.
- Stir in the mushrooms, salt, garlic powder and pepper and cook until slightly brown.
- Add kale and mix well. Cook until it wilts.
- Add miso, vinegar, 2 – 3 tablespoons water, tamari and maple syrup into a bowl and whisk well.
- Add the roasted sweet potatoes into the bowl of sauce mixture. Stir until well coated.
- Divide into 2 meal prep containers. Divide the farro and mushroom – kale mixture among the containers and refrigerate until use. It can last for 3 – 4 days.
- To serve: Serve warm or at room temperature with avocado and tahini sauce on top.

Tofu Burrito Bowl
Serves: 2

Ingredients:

- ½ package (from a 14 ounces package) extra-firm tofu, drained, pressed of excess moisture, chopped
- ¼ teaspoon sea salt or to taste
- ¼ teaspoon chipotle chili powder
- ¼ teaspoon paprika
- ¼ teaspoon cayenne pepper
- ¼ teaspoon chili powder
- ¼ teaspoon pepper
- 1/8 teaspoon garlic powder
- 1 tablespoon olive oil

Toppings: Use any

- Greens of your choice like kale, lettuce, spinach etc.
- Cooked or canned black beans or refried beans
- Salsa
- Guacamole
- Chopped red onion
- Any other toppings of your choice

Directions:

- Place a skillet over medium heat. Add oil. When the oil is heated, add tofu, salt and all the spices. Break the tofu simultaneously as it cooks.

- Turn off the heat and cool completely.
- Divide into meal prep containers. Refrigerate until use. It can last for 10 days.
- To serve: Heat thoroughly. Transfer into bowls. Place desired toppings and serve. If using greens, do not place in the meal prep container.

Quinoa and Seitan Fajita Bowls
Serves: 2

Ingredients:

- 1 cup cooked quinoa
- 2 cloves garlic, peeled, minced
- 6 ounces seitan, sliced
- ¼ cup sliced cherry tomatoes
- 1 tablespoon olive oil
- 1 medium bell pepper of any color, sliced
- ½ cup sliced baby Bella mushrooms
- ¼ teaspoon ground cumin
- 1/8 teaspoon red pepper flakes
- 1/8 teaspoon onion powder
- Pepper to taste
- Salt to taste
- ¼ teaspoon chili powder
- 1/8 teaspoon dried oregano
- 1 cup shredded lettuce
- 1 cup cooked or canned black beans
- 1 teaspoon lime juice or to taste + extra to serve

Directions:

- Place a pan over medium-high heat. Add oil. When the oil is heated, add garlic and cook until aromatic.
- Stir in the bell pepper, mushrooms, seitan and tomatoes.
- Add all the spices into a bowl along with oregano and salt and stir well. Add into the pan and mix well.
- Lower heat to medium heat and cook until vegetables are soft.
- Stir in the black beans and mix well.

Heat thoroughly.

- Taste and adjust seasonings if required. Turn off the heat. Cool completely.
- Add maple syrup and lime juice into the bowl of quinoa and mix well.
- Divide into 2 microwave-safe bowls. Divide the seitan mixture and place over the quinoa.
- Cover the bowls with cling wrap and refrigerate until use. It can last for 4 – 5 days.
- To serve: Warm in a microwave. Top with some lime juice and serve.

Moroccan Chickpeas
Serves: 8

Ingredients:

- 2 cans (15 ounces each) chickpeas, drained, rinsed
- 2 bell peppers, chopped
- 2 onions, chopped
- 2 cans (19 ounces each) diced tomatoes with its juices
- 4 cups cubed sweet potato (½ inch cubes)
- 3 tablespoons Moroccan spice blend
- Vegetable broth or water, if required

Serving day ingredients:

- Chopped parsley
- Lemon juice

Directions:

- Place a skillet over medium heat. Add all the ingredients into the skillet and mix well. Sprinkle some water or broth.
- Cover and cook for 30-40 minutes or until sweet potatoes are tender. Add more water or stock if the mixture is getting stuck to the bottom of the pan.
- Turn off the heat and cool completely. Transfer into an airtight container and refrigerate until use. It can last for 4 days.
- To freeze: Transfer into freezer-safe bags. Squeeze the bags to remove any air that is present. Seal and label the bags with name and date. Freeze until use. It can

last for 3 months.

- To serve: Remove from the refrigerator or freezer and thaw completely.
- Transfer into a skillet and heat thoroughly. Sprinkle some water or broth while heating.

Crispy Quinoa Patties

Serves: 10 (2 patties per serving)

Ingredients:

- 6 cloves garlic, peeled, minced
- ¼ cup chopped parsley
- Pepper to taste
- Salt to taste
- 2 teaspoons coconut oil
- 4 egg replacers
- 2/3 cup finely diced tomatoes
- 1 cup chopped onions
- 6 cup chopped spinach (bite-size pieces)
- 10 tablespoons gluten-free flour or more if required
- 3 cups cooked quinoa

For yogurt tahini sauce:

- ½ cup vegan yogurt
- ½ teaspoon garlic powder
- 2 teaspoons tahini
- Pepper to taste
- Salt to taste
- Juice of a lime
- 2 teaspoons freshly chopped parsley
- ½ teaspoon extra-virgin olive oil

Serving day ingredients:

- 3 tablespoons coconut oil or more if required

Directions:

- To make yogurt tahini sauce: Add all the ingredients for yogurt tahini sauce into a bowl and whisk well. Cover and refrigerate until use.
- To make patties: Place a pan over medium heat. Add coconut oil. When the oil is heated, add garlic and onion and cook until onion turns translucent.

- Stir in spinach, salt, and pepper and cook until spinach has wilted. Turn off the heat and let it cool for a few minutes. Transfer into a bowl.
- Add quinoa, flour, egg replacer, and tomatoes and mix well. If you find the mixture too moist, add some more flour.
- Divide the mixture into 20 equal portions and shape into patties.
- Place on a tray and refrigerate until use. It can last for 2 days. You can also freeze until firm. Once frozen, transfer into freezer-safe bags. Label the bags with name and date and freeze until use.
- To serve: Remove the patties from the refrigerator and thaw completely.
- Place a nonstick pan over medium heat. Add a little coconut oil. When the oil is heated, place 4 – 5 patties in the pan. Cook until the underside is golden brown.
- Flip sides and cook the other side until golden brown. Remove with a slotted spoon and place on a plate lined with paper towels.
- Repeat steps 8 – 9 and make the remaining patties.
- Serve with yogurt tahini sauce.

Black Bean & Plantain Arepa Sandwiches

Serves: 3

Ingredients:

For plantains:

- ½ tablespoon oil
- 1 large ripe plantains, peeled, cut into ½ inch thick slices, along the diagonal

For black beans:

- ½ can (from a 15 ounces can) black beans, with a little of its liquid
- A pinch salt

- ¼ teaspoon ground cumin

For guacamole:

- 1 ripe avocado, peeled, pitted, mashed
- Salt to taste
- 1 tablespoon chopped cilantro
- 1 – 2 tablespoons lime juice
- 2 tablespoons diced onion

Serving day ingredients:

1. 3 large arepas or corn tortillas or pita pockets
2. Thinly sliced cabbage
3. Hot sauce to taste
4. Chopped cilantro

Directions:

- Place plantains on a baking sheet lined with parchment paper. Brush oil over the plantains.
- Bake in a preheated oven at 425° F for about 20 minutes. Flip sides halfway through baking.
- Brush again with some oil. Continue baking until golden brown in color. As the plantains turn light brown, flip the banana slices a couple of times.
- Remove from the oven and let it cool completely.
- To make black beans: Add black beans, salt and cumin into a pan. Place the pan over medium heat. Heat thoroughly. Turn off the heat and let it cool.
- Transfer the banana and black beans into separate airtight containers.
- To make guacamole: Add all the ingredients for guacamole into a bowl and mix well. Cover and chill until use.
- It can last for 3 days.
- To serve: Cut the arepas into 2 halves horizontally. Place bananas, black beans, guacamole, cabbage, hot sauce and cilantro on the bottom half of the arepas. Close with the top of the arepas.
- Serve.

Moroccan Quinoa, Carrot and Chickpea Salad
Serves: 2

Ingredients:

For salad:

5. 1 cup cooked quinoa
6. ½ cup shredded carrots
7. 1 cups baby greens of your choice
8. 2 tablespoons pumpkin seeds
9. ¼ cup chopped parsley
10. 2 tablespoons sunflower seeds
11. 2 small cloves garlic, peeled, minced
12. ½ cup cooked chickpeas
13. 2 tablespoons chopped dates

For lemon ginger vinaigrette:

- 2 tablespoons olive oil
- ¼ teaspoon grated fresh ginger
- ¼ teaspoon maple syrup
- 1/8 teaspoon pepper or to taste
- Salt to taste
- ¼ teaspoon ground cinnamon
- 1/8 teaspoon cayenne pepper
- Juice of ½ lemon

Directions:

14. Divide all the ingredients for salad into 2 meal prep containers. Refrigerate until use. It can last for 3 days.
15. To make dressing: Add all the ingredients for dressing into a small jar with a lid. Fasten the lid. Shake the jar vigorously until well combined.
16. To serve: Empty the contents of the meal prep containers into 2 bowls.
17. Drizzle dressing on top. Toss well and serve.
18. Serve cold or at room temperature.

Potato Salad
Serves: 3

Ingredients:

- 1 pound baby potatoes, rinsed
- ¼ cup chopped, pickled cucumbers
- ½ cup chopped scallions

- 1 ½ cups packed, baby arugula
- 2 tablespoons whole-grain mustard
- ½ teaspoon lightly toasted caraway seeds
- Pepper to taste
- Salt to taste
- 3 teaspoons olive oil

Directions:

- Place potatoes in a pot. Pour enough water to cover the potatoes. Place the pot over medium heat. Cook until fork tender.
- Drain and place in a bowl. Let it cool completely. Add rest of the ingredients and toss well.
- Cover and refrigerate until use. It can last for 2 – 3 days.

Fennel Asparagus Salad

Serves: 2

Ingredients:

- 1 medium leek, use only the white part, cut into half-moons
- 1 medium fennel bulb, thinly sliced (about 1 cup)
- 1 ½ tablespoons olive oil
- 2 – 3 large stalks asparagus, sliced

For dressing:

1. 1 ½ tablespoons olive oil
2. ½ tablespoon minced fresh lemon thyme
3. Salt to taste
4. ½ teaspoon ground coriander
5. 1 tablespoon fresh lemon juice
6. Pepper to taste

Serving day ingredients:

- Avocado slices
- 2 tablespoons lightly toasted, chopped almonds

Directions:

- Place a pan over medium heat. Add oil. When the oil is heated, add leeks and cook until it wilts and slightly golden at a few spots.
- Add salt and stir. Turn off the heat.

- Transfer into a bowl.
- Add asparagus and fennel and toss well.
- Add all the ingredients for dressing into a bowl and whisk well. Pour over the salad. Toss well. Refrigerate until use.
- It can last for 2 – 3 days.
- To serve: Remove from the refrigerator and bring to room temperature.
- Top with avocado slices and garnish with almonds. Serve.

Kohlrabi Slaw with Cilantro, Jalapeño and Lime

Serves: 2 – 3

Ingredients:

- 3 cups sliced kohlrabi (cut into matchsticks)
- ½ teaspoon minced jalapeño or more to taste
- 1 scallion, chopped
- ¼ cup chopped cilantro
- ½ teaspoon grated orange zest
- ½ teaspoon grated lemon zest
- Juice of ½ orange
- Juice of ½ lime

For citrus dressing:

- 2 tablespoons olive oil
- 2 tablespoons fresh orange juice
- 2 tablespoons agave nectar
- ½ tablespoon rice wine vinegar
- 1 ½ tablespoons lime juice or more to taste
- Salt to taste

Directions:

- Add all the ingredients for salad into a bowl and toss well.
- Add all the ingredients for dressing into another bowl and whisk well. Pour over the salad. Toss well. Cover the bowl.
- Refrigerate until use. It can last for 2 days.

Sweet Potato, Lentil & Kale Meal Prep Salads

Serves: 2

Ingredients:

- 6 tablespoons brown lentils
- 1 teaspoon olive oil
- 1 medium red bell pepper, diced
- 2 cups cubed sweet potatoes
- 2 heaping cups chopped, curly kale
- 1 small red onion, diced
- Pepper to taste
- Salt to taste
- 1 bay leaf
- 2 tablespoons dried cranberries (optional)
- 2 tablespoons roasted pepitas (pumpkin seeds)

For curry tahini dressing:

- 3 tablespoons tahini
- ¼ teaspoon curry powder or to taste
- 1 tablespoon lemon juice
- 3 – 4 tablespoons water
- 2 small cloves garlic, peeled, minced

Directions:

1. Place sweet potatoes on a baking sheet. Drizzle oil over it. Sprinkle salt and pepper and mix well. Spread it evenly.
2. Bake in a preheated oven at 375° F for about 30 minutes or until fork tender. Stir once halfway through baking.
3. Meanwhile, add lentils into a pan. Pour enough water to cover the lentils by an inch. Add bay leaf and a bit of salt.
4. When it begins to boil, lower heat and cook until tender. Drain off the excess water.
5. To make dressing: Add all the ingredients for dressing into a bowl and whisk well.
6. Place kale in a bowl. Sprinkle some salt and lemon juice over it. Mix well using your hands, simultaneously massaging the kale leaves.
7. To assemble: Take 2 Mason's jars and add 2 tablespoons dressing in each. Divide the lentils, sweet potatoes, bell pepper, onion and kale among the jars.
8. Divide the cranberries among the jars. Fasten the lid of the jars and refrigerate

until use. It can last for 4 days.

9. To serve: Transfer the salad into a bowl. Toss well. Sprinkle pumpkin seeds on top if using and serve.

Green Pasta Salad
Serves: 2

Ingredients:

- 1 cup cooked, small, tubular pasta
- Olive oil, as required
- 1 cup shredded spinach
- ¼ cup shredded vegan parmesan cheese
- Lemon juice to taste
- 1 cup chopped green beans
- ½ jar basil and olive oil pesto
- Salt to taste
- 2 cloves garlic, peeled, sliced
- 2 tablespoons balsamic vinegar (optional)
- 2 tablespoons olive and basil oil, to drizzle (optional)

Directions:

- Drizzle a bit of olive oil over the cooked pasta and toss well.
- Place a skillet over medium heat. Add a little olive oil. When the oil is heated, add garlic and green beans and cook until slightly tender. Turn off the heat. Transfer into the bowl of pasta and toss well.
- Let it cool completely. Add rest of the ingredients and toss well. Refrigerate until use. It can last for 3 days.

Marinated Kale Salad
Serves: 4

Ingredients:

For salad:

- 2 bunches curly kale
- 5 tablespoons apple cider vinegar
- 2 tablespoons agave nectar or pure maple syrup
- 2 tablespoons natural almond butter
- 2 – 4 tablespoons tamari or soy sauce or coconut aminos

Optional toppings:

- ½ cup cherry tomatoes
- 2 tablespoons pepitas
- 1 avocado, peeled, pitted, chopped
- Any other toppings of your choice

Directions:

- Dry the kale leaves by patting with a kitchen towel.
- Tear the kale into bite size pieces and place in a large bowl.
- Add rest of the ingredients for salad into a bowl and whisk well.
- Drizzle the dressing over the kale leaves and mix it well using your hands, massaging the leaves lightly.
- Divide into 4 meal prep containers and refrigerate until use. It can last for a day.

Pea Soup

Serves: 8

Ingredients:

- 2 onions, chopped
- 2 large potatoes, peeled, cubed
- 6 cups vegetable broth or water
- 2 large cloves garlic, peeled, sliced
- 1.3 pounds peas, fresh or frozen
- 2 tablespoons vegetable oil
- A handful fresh parsley or any other herbs of your choice, chopped
- Salt to taste
- Pepper to taste

Serving day ingredients:

- ½ cup boiled peas
- Vegan yogurt or vegan cream, to drizzle
- Any other toppings of your choice
- 2 tablespoons lemon juice

Directions:

- Place a soup pot over medium heat. Add oil. When the oil is heated, add onion and garlic and sauté until pink.
- Stir in the stock, salt, pepper, parsley, potatoes and peas. When it begins to boil, lower the heat and cover with a lid. Cook until potatoes are soft. Turn off the heat.
- Blend with an immersion blender until smooth. Let it cool completely.
- Transfer into an airtight container and refrigerate until use. It can last for 4 days. You can also pour into freezer bags. Label and seal the bags and freeze until use. It can last for 2 months.
- To serve: Heat thoroughly. Add lemon juice and stir. Ladle into soup bowls. Garnish with peas, vegan yogurt and any other toppings of your choice and serve.

Cauliflower Soup

Serves: 4

Ingredients:

- 2 onions, chopped
- 1 head cauliflower, cut into florets
- 5 – 6 cups vegetable broth
- 8 cloves garlic, peeled, smashed
- 2 tablespoons chopped fresh rosemary or 2 teaspoons dried rosemary
- Salt to taste
- Pepper to taste

Directions:

- Place a soup pot over medium heat. Add oil. When the oil is heated, add onion and garlic and sauté until pink. Add a bit of salt and cook until light brown.
- Add cauliflower and rosemary and stir for a couple of minutes.
- Stir in the stock, salt and pepper. When it begins to boil, lower the heat and cover with a lid. Cook until cauliflower is soft. Turn off the heat.
- Blend with an immersion blender until smooth. Let it cool completely.
- Transfer into an airtight container and refrigerate until use. It can last for 4 days. You can also pour into freezer bags. Label and seal the bags and freeze until use. It can last for 2 months.
- To serve: Heat thoroughly. Ladle into soup bowls. Serve with toppings of your choice.

Spring Vegetables Soup

Serves: 10

Ingredients:

- 6 medium carrots, sliced
- 4 large potatoes, sliced
- 1 large onion, chopped
- 6 stalks celery, sliced
- 2 cups peas, fresh or frozen
- Salt to taste
- Pepper to taste
- 4 tablespoons sunflower oil
- 2 vegetable stock cubes

Directions:

- Place a soup pot over medium heat. Add oil. When the oil is heated, add onion, carrots, potatoes, celery and peas. Mix well. Cook for 2 – 3 minutes.
- Stir in the stock, salt and pepper. When it begins to boil, lower the heat and cover with a lid. Cook until vegetables are soft. Turn off the heat.
- Let it cool completely.
- Transfer into an airtight container and refrigerate until use. It can last for 4 days. You can also pour into freezer bags. Label and seal the bags and freeze until use. It can last for 2 months.
- To serve: Heat thoroughly. Ladle into soup bowls.

Avocado Caesar Wraps

Serves: 2

Ingredients:

- ½ avocado, peeled, pitted, sliced
- 3 tablespoons vegan Caesar dressing
- 2 tortillas
- 2 big handfuls lettuce, chopped
- ½ can (from a 15 ounces can) chickpeas, rinsed, drained
- ¼ cup chopped cherry tomatoes (optional)
- ¼ cup shredded carrots (optional)
- ½ apple, cored, chopped (optional)

Directions:

1. Add lettuce into a bowl. Pour dressing over it and stir.
2. Place tortillas on your countertop. Divide

lettuce, chickpeas, tomatoes, carrots, and apples among the tortillas.

3. Wrap like a burrito. Place in an airtight container. Refrigerate until use. It can last for a day.
4. Heat in a microwave for a few seconds if desired and serve.

Veggie Coconut Wraps

Serves: 4

Ingredients:

- 10 tablespoons hummus
- 1 medium red bell pepper, thinly sliced
- 1 large carrot, shredded
- 2 cups chopped kale
- 4 coconut wraps
- 5 – 6 tablespoons green curry paste
- ¾ cup chopped cilantro
- 1 medium avocado, peeled, pitted, sliced

Directions:

1. Place the wraps on your countertop.
2. Mix together hummus and curry paste in a bowl. Divide the mixture equally and spread on the wraps, on the area nearest to you.
3. Divide the rest of the ingredients equally and place over the wraps in layers.
4. Start rolling the wraps and place with its seam side facing down, in an airtight container.
5. Refrigerate until use. It can last for a day.

Chapter Eleven

Vegan Dinner Recipes

Butternut Squash and Lentil Curry

Serves: 4

Ingredients:

- 1 cup red lentils, rinsed
- ½ cup finely chopped onions
- 2 cups cubed butternut squash
- 1 tablespoon minced fresh ginger
- 1 large clove garlic, peeled, minced
- ½ tablespoon curry powder
- 1 teaspoon garam masala powder
- 1 teaspoon ground cumin
- 1 teaspoon ground coriander
- 1 teaspoon turmeric powder
- ½ can (from a 19 ounces can) diced tomatoes
- ½ can (from a 13.5 ounces can) coconut milk
- 1 ½ cups stock
- Salt to taste
- Lime juice to taste

Directions:

- Add all the ingredients except lime juice into a soup pot.
- Place the pot over medium heat. When it begins to boil, lower the heat and simmer until well cooked. Mash lightly if desired. Turn off the heat. Let it cool completely.
- Add lime juice and stir. Transfer into an airtight container and refrigerate until use. It can last for 4 days. To freeze: Transfer into freezer bags and freeze until use. It can last for 3 months.

Vegan Chili with Vegan Sausage

Serves: 5

Ingredients:

1. 1 tablespoon olive oil
2. ½ cup chopped red bell pepper
3. 1 cup chopped kale
4. ½ cup chopped onion
5. ½ tablespoon chopped garlic
6. ½ package (from a 12.95 ounces package) vegan sausage, chopped
7. ¼ cup white wine
8. 1 cup chopped tomato
9. Freshly ground pepper to taste
10. ½ teaspoon dried ground sage
11. 3 cups vegetable stock
12. 1 can (15 ounces) unsalted kidney beans, rinsed, drained, divided
13. 1 ½ cans (15 ounces each) cannellini beans, rinsed, drained, divided
14. ½ teaspoon salt or to taste
15. ½ teaspoon crushed red pepper

Directions

- Place a Dutch oven over medium-high heat. Add oil. When the oil is heated, add onions, garlic, sausage and bell pepper. Sauté for 3-4 minutes.
- Stir in the tomatoes, spices, wine, salt and sage. Cook until the wine reduces to half its original quantity.
- Add stock and stir. Add ½ can kidney beans and ¾ can cannellini beans into a bowl and mash with a potato masher. Add into the pot. Also add the remaining beans. Let it simmer for 5-8 minutes.
- Add kale and cook until it wilts. Add oregano and stir. Taste and adjust the seasoning if required. Turn off the heat and cool completely.
- Transfer into an airtight container and refrigerate until use. It can last for 4 days. To freeze: Transfer into freezer bags and freeze until use. It can last for 3 months.

Vegetable Chili

Serves: 8 – 10

Ingredients:

- 4 tablespoons olive oil
- 1 large red bell pepper, chopped
- 2 onions, chopped
- 2 large cloves garlic, finely chopped
- 2 small zucchinis, trimmed, diced
- 2 ears corn, use the kernels

- 2 small yellow squashes, diced
- 4 cans (10 ounces each) diced tomatoes with green chilies
- 3 cups cooked or canned kidney beans, rinsed
- 3 cups cooked or canned black beans, rinsed
- 4 tablespoons tomato paste
- 2 tablespoons chili powder
- 4 teaspoons dried oregano
- 4 teaspoons ground cumin
- Cayenne pepper to taste
- Salt to taste
- Pepper to taste

Directions:

1. Place a Dutch oven over medium-high heat. Add oil. When the oil is heated, add onions and sauté until translucent. Add garlic, spices and oregano. Sauté for few seconds until aromatic.
2. Add the vegetables and cook until tender.
3. Stir in the rest of the ingredients and bring to a boil.
4. Lower heat and cook for about 20 minutes. Taste and adjust seasonings if required. Turn off the heat and cool completely.
5. Transfer into an airtight container and refrigerate until use. It can last for 4 days. To freeze: Transfer into freezer bags and freeze until use. It can last for 3 months.

Pho Soup
Serves: 4

Ingredients:

- 2 cups very thinly sliced carrots
- 4 teaspoons minced fresh ginger
- 2 cups julienned red bell pepper
- 4 teaspoons minced garlic
- 4 cups uncooked, thin rice noodles

Serving day ingredients:

- 12 cups boiling hot vegetable stock
- 8 tablespoons soy sauce or tamari

Directions:

1. Take 4 wide-mouth Mason's jars. Divide all the ingredients into the jars, with noodles right on top.
2. Fasten the lid and refrigerate until use.
3. To serve: Add soy sauce and stock into the jars. Add some boiling water if the jar is not filled with the stock. Fasten the lid and set aside for 15 minutes.
4. Stir well. Season with salt and pepper to taste.

Baked Sheet Pan Ratatouille
Serves: 6 – 8

Ingredients:

- 6 Japanese eggplants or 2 large eggplants, cut into ½ inch thick pieces
- 4 tomatoes, cut into ¾ inch thick wedges
- 2 onions, cut into ½ inch thick slices
- 1 red bell pepper, cut into ½ inch thick strips
- 1 yellow bell pepper, cut into ½ inch thick strips
- 24 – 28 whole garlic cloves, peeled
- 4 zucchinis or summer squash, halved lengthwise, cut into ½ inch thick slices crosswise
- 1 tablespoon fresh chopped thyme
- Salt to taste
- Pepper to taste
- Olive oil, as required
- Balsamic vinegar to taste

Serving options: Use any one

- Cooked pasta
- Cooked beans or whole grains
- Cooked polenta
- Toast

Directions:

1. Line 2 large baking sheets with parchment paper.
2. Place the vegetables on the baking sheets without overlapping. Place garlic cloves at different spots on the baking sheets.
3. Trickle some oil over the vegetables. Season with salt and pepper. Sprinkle

thyme and mix using your hands.

4. Bake in a preheated oven at 400° F for about 30 minutes or until tender and slightly brown around the edges. Stir once halfway through baking.

5. Remove from the oven and transfer into an airtight container. Taste and adjust the seasoning if required. Sprinkle some vinegar and toss well.

6. Close the lid and refrigerate until use. It can last for 4 – 5 days. You can also transfer the roasted vegetables into freezer-safe bags. Freeze until use. It can last for 15 days.

7. To serve: Heat the vegetables in an oven. Serve with the suggested serving options.

Tempeh Taco Salad Bowls
Serves: 6

Ingredients:

For tempeh taco meat:

- 2 packages (8 ounces each) tempeh, crumbled
- 3 tablespoons chili powder
- ½ cup canned tomato sauce
- 2 tablespoons olive oil or avocado oil
- 5 teaspoons taco seasoning or to taste
- Salt to taste
- Pepper to taste

For bowls:

- 12 cup chopped romaine lettuce
- ½ cup chopped red onion
- 2 cups diced cherry tomatoes
- ¼ cup chopped fresh cilantro
- 1 ½ cups cooked black beans
- 2 avocados, peeled, pitted sliced
- Salt to taste

Serving day ingredients:

- 3 lime wedges
- Fresh salsa
- Tortilla chips
- Hot sauce

Directions:

- Place a large skillet over medium-high heat. Add oil. When the oil is heated, add tempeh and cook for 4 – 5 minutes.
- Add rest of the ingredients and mix well. Cook until nearly dry. Turn off the heat and let it cool.
- Add tomatoes, cilantro, onion, and salt into a bowl and toss well.
- Take 6 meal prep containers. Divide the lettuce, tomato mixture, tempeh, and black beans among the containers.
- Close the lid and refrigerate until use. It can last 4-5 days.
- Thaw completely before serving. Serve with avocado, lime wedges, salsa, hot sauce and tortilla chips.

BBQ-Flavored Seitan and Avocado Wraps
Serves: 4

Ingredients:

- 16 ounces seitan, drained, finely diced
- 4 wraps (10 – 12 inches each)
- 1 cup vegan BBQ sauce
- 4 tablespoons hemp seeds (optional)
- 1 avocado, peeled, pitted, thinly sliced
- Vegan mayonnaise or mustard (or use both), as required
- Greens of your choice
- 2 tomatoes, thinly sliced
- 1 avocado, peeled, pitted, thinly sliced

Directions:

- Place a skillet over medium heat. Add BBQ sauce and seitan and mix well. Heat thoroughly and cook until nearly dry.
- Spread the wraps on your countertop. Smear vegan mayonnaise or mustard or a little of both.
- Scatter hemp seeds if using. Spread some greens along the diameter of the wraps.
- Divide the seitan and place over the greens, along the center. Place avocados on one side and tomatoes on the other side of the seitan.
- Wrap tightly and place in an airtight container.

- It can last for a day.
- To serve: Heat in a microwave for 20 – 30 seconds and serve.

Mushroom, Spinach, and Cheddar Wraps
Serves: 2

Ingredients:

- 5 ounces white or cremini or baby mushrooms
- 2 wraps or flour tortillas (10 inches each)
- Salsa, as required (optional)
- 5 ounces fresh baby spinach
- ½ cup grated non-dairy cheddar cheese

Directions:

- Place a skillet over medium heat. Add mushrooms. Sprinkle a little water and cook until mushrooms are tender.
- Add spinach and cook until it wilts. Discard cooked water if any.
- Place wraps on your countertop. Divide equally the mixture among the wraps. Drizzle some salsa on top. Wrap and place in an airtight container with the seam side facing down.
- To serve: Heat for 20 – 30 seconds in the microwave and serve.

Teriyaki Setian with Mashed Kabocha
Serves: 2

Ingredients:

For teriyaki sauce:

- 4 tablespoons soy sauce
- 2 tablespoons orange juice
- 2 tablespoons brown sugar
- ½ teaspoon sesame oil
- ¼ teaspoon red pepper flakes or to taste
- 1 clove garlic, minced
- ½ tablespoon cornstarch
- 2 tablespoons water
- Salt to taste
- 1 teaspoon minced ginger
- 1 ½ tablespoons rice vinegar

For seitan:

- 4 ounces seitan, sliced
- ¼ pound winter squash, peeled, cubed
- ¾ cup broccoli florets
- ½ tablespoon sesame seeds
- Salt to taste

Directions:

- To make teriyaki sauce: Add all the ingredients for the sauce into a saucepan and whisk well.
- Place the saucepan over medium heat. Stir constantly until thick. Turn off the heat.
- Steam the broccoli and winter squash until tender.
- Place a nonstick pan over medium-high heat. Add seitan and cook until the underside is golden brown. Flip sides and cook the other side until brown.
- Add some of the teriyaki sauce and mix well. Turn off the heat. Cool completely.
- Place teriyaki seitan, squash and broccoli in meal prep containers. Store remaining teriyaki sauce in an airtight container. Place the containers in the refrigerator until use. It can last for 4 days.

Seitan and Mushrooms with Polenta
Serves: 4 – 5

Ingredients:

For polenta:

- 4 cups vegetable broth or water
- Salt to taste
- Pepper to taste
- 1 ½ cups instant polenta

For mushroom and seitan:

- 4 tablespoons olive oil
- 4 tablespoons flour
- ½ cup white wine
- 2 teaspoons dried parsley
- 2 packages seitan (8 ounces each), cut into strips
- 16 ounces baby Portobello mushrooms, chopped
- 2 cups vegetable broth

- 2 tablespoons chopped fresh oregano
- 1 teaspoon garlic powder
- Salt to taste
- Pepper to taste

Serving day ingredients:

- ½ - 1 cup almond milk (optional)

Directions:

1. To make polenta: Add broth or water into the saucepan. Place the saucepan over medium heat. When it begins to simmer, add polenta and cook until nearly dry. Turn off the heat.
2. To make mushroom and seitan: Place a large skillet over medium heat. Add oil. When the oil is heated, add mushrooms and cook until slightly brown.
3. Add flour and stir for a few seconds. Stir in the wine and broth.
4. Stir in the herbs, salt and spices. Cook until thick.
5. Add seitan and cook for a couple of minutes. Turn off the heat and cool completely.
6. Transfer seitan and polenta into airtight containers and refrigerate until use. It can last for 3 days.
7. To serve: Add polenta into a pan. Add milk if using or some broth and heat the polenta.
8. Heat the mushrooms and seitan mixture.
9. Divide into bowls and serve.

Vegan Tuna Lemon Pasta
Serves: 2 – 4

Ingredients:

- 4 servings cooked pasta of your choice
- 4 tablespoons olive oil
- 2 packets vegan tuna (Like Good Catch Foods Tuna)
- ½ cup chopped fresh parsley
- ½ cup cooked pasta water
- 6 large cloves garlic, pressed
- Juice of a large lemon

Directions:

1. Place a large pan over medium heat. Add oil. When the oil is heated, add garlic and cook until brown.
2. Raise the heat to high heat and add vegan tuna. Break with a fork as it cooks. Add lemon and mix well. Lower the heat and add pasta. Toss well. Add the pasta water and mix well. Turn off the heat.
3. When it cools, transfer into an airtight container. Refrigerate until use. It can last for 2 days.
4. To serve: Heat thoroughly. Add parsley and toss well. Serve.

Veggie Salad Jars
Serves: 4

Ingredients:

For salad:

- 1 tomato, chopped
- ½ courgette, sliced
- 1 medium eggplant, sliced
- 1 small cucumber, deseeded, chopped
- ○ ounces vegan feta cheese, crumbled
- ½ tablespoon olive oil
- 1.7 ounces kalamata olives
- ○ ounces canned or cooked chickpeas
- A handful of mint leaves, torn or chopped
- ½ yellow bell pepper, deseeded, chopped
- 0.8 ounce sundried tomatoes
- A handful of dill leaves, chopped
- Salt to taste
- Pepper to taste

For pickled onion dressing:

- ½ red onion, thinly sliced
- 2 tablespoons white wine vinegar
- 3 ½ tablespoons extra-virgin olive oil
- ¼ teaspoon coriander seeds
- 2 tablespoons lemon juice
- Water, as required
- Salt to taste
- Pepper to taste

Directions:

- To make pickled onion dressing: Add vinegar, onions, coriander seeds, and 3-4 tablespoons water dressing into a small pan. Place the pan over medium-low heat. Cook until the onions are translucent.
- Turn off heat and set aside to cool. Add lemon juice and oil into the pickled onion Add salt and pepper and stir.
- Brush eggplant and courgette slices with olive oil.
- Place a griddle pan over medium-high heat. When the pan begins to smoke, place eggplant and courgette slices on it.
- Cook until the underside is slightly charred. Flip sides and cook the other side until slightly charred. Remove onto a plate. Sprinkle salt and pepper and set aside.
- Divide the pickled onion into 4 mason's jars.
- Divide and layer with tomatoes, vegan feta cheese, chickpeas and olives in the jars. Press slightly with a spoon to push the salad.
- Layer with sundried tomatoes along with a little of its oil followed by the cooked vegetables. Next layer will be cucumber, followed by bell pepper, mint and dill leaves.
- Fasten the lid and refrigerate until use. It can last for 2 days.
- To serve: Empty the jars into individual serving bowls. Toss well and serve.

Smoky Tempeh Tostadas with Mango Cabbage Slaw
Serves: 6

Ingredients:

For tempeh:
- 2 packages (8 ounces each) tempeh, cut into thin pieces
- 2 teaspoons chili powder
- 1 teaspoon ground cumin
- 1 teaspoon garlic powder
- ½ teaspoon pepper
- 1 teaspoon onion powder
- Oil, as required
- ½ cup soy sauce or tamari
- Hot sauce to taste
- 1 teaspoon liquid smoke

For mango cabbage slaw:
- 3 cups shredded red cabbage
- 1 cup chopped cilantro
- 1 ½ cups diced mango
- 2 tablespoons fresh lime juice
- 2 teaspoons agave nectar
- 2 teaspoons apple cider vinegar

Serving day ingredients:
- 12 corn tortillas
- Chopped cilantro
- Chopped avocado
- Salsa

Directions:

- To make tempeh: Add soy sauce, hot sauce, liquid smoke and spices into a bowl and mix until well combined.
- Add tempeh and stir until well coated with the mixture. Let it marinate for 10 minutes.
- Place a skillet over medium heat. Add some oil. When the oil is heated, add tempeh and cook until the underside is brown. Flip sides and cook the other side until brown. Remove with a slotted spoon and place on a plate. Let it cool completely.
- To make slaw: Add all the ingredients for slaw into a bowl and toss well.
- Transfer the slaw and tempeh into meal prep containers. Refrigerate until use. It can last for 3 days.
- To serve: Place corn tortillas on a baking sheet. Bake in a preheated oven at 400° F for about 10 minutes or until golden brown.
- Heat the tempeh. Add salt to slaw and toss well.

- Divide the tempeh among the tortillas. Place slaw on top. Place the suggested toppings and serve.

Curried Cauliflower & Chickpea Burritos

Serves: 2 large or 3 medium burritos

Ingredients:

For coconut basmati rice:

- ½ cup water
- ½ cup basmati rice
- ½ cup light coconut milk
- Salt to taste

For curried cauliflower and chickpeas:

- ½ tablespoon vegetable oil
- 2 cloves garlic, peeled, minced
- ½ tablespoon garam masala
- 1 ½ cups small cauliflower florets
- ¼ cup water
- 1 tablespoon tomato paste
- Salt to taste
- Pepper to taste
- ½ onion, diced
- 1 teaspoon freshly grated ginger
- ½ teaspoon ground cumin
- ½ can (from a 14 ounces can) diced tomatoes
- ½ can (from a 14 ounces can) chickpeas, drained, rinsed
- 2 tablespoons chopped cilantro

To assemble:

- 2 large or 3 medium flour tortillas

Directions:

1. To make coconut basmati rice: Add water and coconut milk into a saucepan. Place the saucepan over high heat. When it begins to boil, add the rice and stir. Lower the heat. Cover and cook until dry. Turn off the heat. Let it rest for 5 minutes.
2. Add salt and fluff with a fork.
3. To make curried cauliflower and chickpeas: Place a skillet over medium heat. Add oil. When the oil is heated, add onion and cook until translucent. Stir in the ginger, garlic, cumin and garam masala and sauté for a few seconds until aromatic.
4. Stir in the tomatoes, cauliflower and water. Mix well. Cover with a lid. Lower the heat and simmer until cauliflower is tender.
5. Add tomato paste and chickpeas and cook uncovered until thick. Stir occasionally.
6. Turn off the heat. Add cilantro, salt and pepper and mix well.
7. Place the tortillas on your countertop. Divide the rice among the tortillas and spread on the center. Spread cauliflower and chickpeas. Over the rice. Wrap like a burrito.
8. Place in an airtight container and refrigerate until use. It can last for a day.

Buffalo Chickpea Pita Pockets with Creamy Avocado

Serves: 2

Ingredients:

- ½ can (from a 15 ounces can) chickpeas
- ½ tablespoon coconut oil
- 2 tablespoons unsweetened almond milk
- 2 pita rounds, to serve
- 1 medium cucumber, peeled, chopped
- 2 tablespoons Buffalo hot sauce
- ½ ripe avocado, peeled, pitted, chopped
- 1 tablespoon lemon juice
- A handful kale leaves, torn

Directions:

- Add chickpeas, buffalo sauce and coconut oil into a baking dish. Mix well.
- Bake in a preheated oven at 400° F for about 15 minutes. Stir a couple of times while baking. Remove from the oven and let it cool. Transfer into an airtight container. Refrigerate until use.
- Meanwhile, add avocado, almond milk, salt and lemon juice into a blender and blend until creamy.
- Pour into a bowl. Cover and chill until

use. It can last for 2 days.

- To serve: Heat chickpeas and fill the pita pockets with it. Place kale and cucumber. Spoon some avocado sauce and serve.

Baked Ziti
Serves: 8 – 10

Ingredients:

- 1 pound dried pasta
- 20 basil leaves, torn + extra to garnish
- Salt to taste
- Pepper to taste
- 2 jars (24 ounces each) marinara sauce
- 16 ounces vegan mozzarella cheese, diced
- Boiling water, as required

Directions:

- Place pasta in a large bowl. Add boiling water into the bowl such that the pasta is covered with water (about 2 inches above the pasta). Set aside for 45 minutes. Drain excess water.
- Add marinara sauce and basil leaves into a baking dish and mix well.
- Add 12 ounces mozzarella cheese and toss well. Scatter the remaining cheese on top.
- Cover the dish with foil and refrigerate until use. It can last for 2 days.
- To serve: Bake covered, in a preheated oven at 350° F for about 45 minutes. Uncover and bake for 15 minutes.
- Let it sit on the countertop for 15 minutes. Garnish with basil and serve.

Plantain Black Bean Enchilada Bake
Serves: 6

Ingredients:

For plantains:

- 1 tablespoon coconut oil, melted
- 2 large ripe plantains, peeled, cut into slices lengthwise (10 slices in all)

For black beans:

- 1 can (15 ounces) black beans, drained

- Salt to taste
- 1 teaspoon ground cumin

For cheese sauce:

- ½ cup + 2 tablespoons cashews
- ¼ teaspoon sea salt or to taste
- ¼ teaspoon ground cumin
- Warm water, to blend, as required
- 2 tablespoons nutritional yeast
- 1/8 teaspoon garlic powder
- ¼ small chipotle chili in adobo sauce or more to taste (optional)

For enchilada sauce:

- 1 cup +1 ½ tablespoons vegetable broth
- 2 cloves garlic, peeled, smashed
- ½ cup chopped onion
- 3 dried chilies, like ancho chili
- 1 dried arbol chilies
- ½ cup water
- 2 tablespoons tomato paste
- ½ teaspoon ground smoked paprika
- ½ teaspoon dried oregano
- ½ teaspoon ground cumin
- ¼ teaspoon salt

Toppings:

- Chopped cilantro
- 1 small red onion, chopped
- 1 jalapeño, chopped
- Guacamole or avocado slices

Directions:

- To make enchilada sauce: Place a skillet over medium heat. Add 1 ½ tablespoons broth, garlic, and onion and sauté until lightly brown.
- Stir in the dried chilies and sauté for a couple of minutes. Stir in water and remaining broth. When it begins to boil, lower the heat and cover with a lid. Cook for 10 – 12 minutes.
- Add tomato paste, salt, oregano, and spices and mix well. Cover and continue cooking for another 5 minutes. Turn off the heat.
- Add into a blender. Blend until smooth.

- Taste and adjust the salt if necessary.
- Use about a cup. Store leftovers in an airtight container in the refrigerator.
- Place plantain slices on a lined baking sheet. Do not overlap. Brush with oil on top. Flip sides and brush with oil on the other side as well.
- Bake in a preheated oven at 425° F for about 30 minutes or until golden brown. Flip sides halfway through baking.
- To make black beans: Add all the ingredients for black beans into a saucepan. Place the saucepan over medium heat. Mix well. Heat thoroughly. Remove from heat.
- To make cheese sauce: Add all the ingredients for cheese sauce into a blender and blend until smooth. Taste and adjust the seasonings or nutritional yeast if required.
- To assemble: Spread a little of the enchilada sauce on the bottom of a baking dish.
- Place a layer of bananas. Spread a layer of cheese sauce. Spread half the beans. Spread some good amount of enchilada sauce. Place another layer of plantain slices.
- Spread some more of the cheese sauce over the plantains. Spread the remaining beans over the plantains. Spread remaining enchilada sauce. Spread any remaining cheese sauce.
- Cover the dish with foil. Refrigerate until use. Use within 4 - 5 days. You can also freeze it for a month.
- Bake in a preheated oven at 350° F for about 30 minutes.
- Serve with suggested serving options.

Seitan Stew

Serves: 8

Ingredients:

- 6 guajillo chilies, discard stems and seeds, chopped into large pieces
- 4 dried chilies de Abrol, discard stems and seeds, chopped into large pieces
- 8 dried New Mexico chilies, discard stems and seeds, chopped into large pieces
- 8 cups vegetable broth, divided
- 4 tablespoons olive oil
- 6 cloves garlic, minced
- 4 teaspoons dried oregano
- 3 tablespoons apple cider vinegar
- 4 tablespoons masa harina
- 2 pounds seitan, chopped
- 16 ounces waxy potatoes, chopped into cubes
- Salt to taste
- 3 cups fire-roasted, canned, chopped tomatoes
- 1 onion, chopped
- 2 tablespoons ground cumin
- ½ teaspoon pepper or to taste
- 2 tablespoons soy sauce

Directions

1. Place a pan over medium heat. When the pan heats, add all the chilies and cook for a couple of minutes until slightly soft.
2. Transfer into a microwavable bowl. Add 4 cups water. Cover and cook on high for 3 minutes. Remove from the microwave and add into a blender. Also add the tomatoes and blend until smooth.
3. Place a soup pot over medium heat. Add 2 tablespoons of oil. Add onion and a bit of salt and cook until pink. Stir in the garlic and cook for a few seconds until aromatic.
4. Stir in the oregano and cumin. Cook for a few seconds stirring constantly until aromatic. Stir in the blended mixture, rest of the broth and potatoes. When it begins to boil, lower the heat and cover with a lid. Cook until potatoes are soft.
5. Meanwhile, place a pan over medium heat. Add remaining oil. When the oil is heated, add seitan and sauté for a few minutes, until light brown. Remove onto a plate and set aside.

6. Place masa harina in a bowl. Add a little of the soup and mix well. Pour it back into the pot. Also add in the vinegar, soy sauce and seitan and stir constantly until thick. Add salt and pepper to taste. Turn off the heat and cool completely.

7. Transfer into an airtight container and refrigerate until use. It can last for 4 -5 days.

8. To serve: Heat thoroughly. Ladle into soup bowls and serve.

Lentil Balls with Zesty Rice

Serves: 2

Ingredients:

For lentil balls:

- 1 can (15 ounces) brown or black lentils, drained, rinsed
- 1 ½ tablespoons chopped, dried mushrooms
- 1 ½ tablespoons tomato paste
- ¼ teaspoon pepper or to taste
- ½ cup walnut halves
- 2 teaspoons tomato paste
- ¼ cup vegan breadcrumbs
- A handful fresh parsley, chopped

For zesty rice:

- ½ cup + 1/3 cup water
- 1 tablespoon lemon juice
- 1 teaspoon grated lemon zest
- 2/3 cup uncooked basmati rice
- A handful fresh parsley, minced
- Salt to taste

For toppings:

- 1 cup chopped lettuce
- 1 small onion, thinly sliced
- ½ cup halved cherry tomatoes
- 2 lemon wedges

Directions:

1. For lentil balls: Add lentils, mushrooms, parsley, pepper, salt, tomato paste and walnuts into the food processor bowl. Pulse until chopped into smaller pieces.

Do not over process.

2. Add into a bowl. Add breadcrumbs and mix well.

3. Scoop out about 2 tablespoons of the mixture and shape into a ball. Repeat this step and make the remaining balls.

4. Place the balls on a lined baking sheet.

5. Bake in a preheated oven at 375° F for about 20 minutes. Flip sides halfway through baking.

6. Remove from the oven and cool completely.

7. To make zesty rice: Add water and rice into a saucepan. Place the saucepan over medium flame. When it begins to boil, lower the heat and cover with a lid. Cook until dry. Turn off the heat and cool completely.

8. Transfer the rice and lentil balls into meal prep containers. Refrigerate until use. It can last for 3 – 4 days.

9. To serve: Heat thoroughly the rice and lentil balls.

10. Add lettuce, onion and tomatoes into a bowl and toss well. Divide into 2 serving plates. Layer with rice. Place lentil balls on top. Serve with lemon wedges.

Butternut Squash Enchiladas

Serves: 6

Ingredients:

For enchiladas:

- 1 cup pureed, roasted butternut squash – procedure given in the directions
- 1 small jalapeño, deseeded, minced
- ½ cup thinly sliced Brussels sprouts
- ½ teaspoon chili powder
- Salt to taste
- 12 ounces mild salsa Verde
- ½ small red onion, finely chopped
- 1 – 2 cloves garlic, peeled, minced
- ½ teaspoon ground cumin
- 1/8 teaspoon cayenne pepper
- ½ can (from a 15 ounces can) black beans, drained, rinsed

- 6 corn tortillas
- ½ tablespoon extra-virgin olive oil

For cashew sour cream:

- ½ cup cashews, soaked in water for an hour
- Juice of ½ lemon
- ¼ cup water
- Salt to taste

For topping:

- A handful fresh cilantro, chopped
- 1 tablespoon pumpkin seeds

Directions:

- Place a sheet of parchment paper over a baking sheet. Take a small butternut squash. Cut into 2 halves. Discard the seeds and membrane. Brush with oil and place on the baking sheet.
- Roast in a preheated oven at 400° F for about 45 minutes.
- Remove from the oven and let it cool. Scoop out the pulp from the squash and measure out 1 cup. Add into a bowl.
- Place a skillet over medium heat. Add ½ tablespoon oil. When the oil is heated, add onion and cook until pink.
- Stir in the garlic and jalapeño and cook for a couple of minutes.
- Add Brussels sprouts, spices and salt. Sauté until slightly soft. Stir in the black beans. Turn off the heat. Let it cool completely. Transfer into the bowl of butternut squash. Mix well.
- Spread a thin layer of salsa on the bottom of a baking dish (8 x 8 inches).
- Spread the tortillas on your countertop. Place 1/3 cup of butternut squash mixture onto each tortilla, along the diameter.
- Place the rolled tortillas in the baking dish, with the seam side facing down.
- Drizzle the remaining salsa over the enchiladas. Spread the salsa evenly.
- Cover the dish and refrigerate until use. Use within a day.
- To make cashew sour cream: Add all the ingredients for cashew sour cream into a blender and blend until smooth. Pour into a bowl. Cover and chill until use.
- Remove the dish and the cashew sour cream from the refrigerator 30 minutes before baking.
- Bake in a preheated oven at 375° F for about 20 to 30 minutes.
- Remove from the oven and cool for a while. Drizzle cashew sour cream on top. Garnish with pumpkin seeds and cilantro and serve.

Chapter Twelve

Vegan Snack Recipes

Baked Samosas

Serves: 9

Ingredients:

For samosa covering:

- 9 spring roll wrappers
- Olive oil, to brush
- 2 – 3 teaspoons water

For filling:

- 1 ¼ cups chopped potatoes
- ¾ cup chopped, fresh spinach
- ½ teaspoon curry powder or to taste
- 1 onion, chopped
- Salt to taste
- 1 ½ teaspoons oil

Directions:

1. To make filling: Place potatoes in a saucepan. Pour enough water to cover the potatoes. Place the saucepan over medium heat. Cover and cook until potatoes are soft. Drain the water and set aside.
2. Place a pan over medium heat. Add oil. When the oil is heated, add onions and sauté until light brown. Add potatoes and spinach and mix well. Add salt and curry powder and mix well. Cook until spinach wilts. Turn off the heat. Let it cool completely.
3. To make samosas: Add 2 – 3 teaspoons water into a bowl. Add a little oil in another bowl.
4. Place a spring roll wrapper on your countertop. Apply a little water on one of the edges of the wrapper (the one farthest to you). Bring together this edge and its opposite edge (the one that is closest to you). Press them together to seal. So now you have a rectangle.
5. Make a cone on one of the ends of the rectangle, by folding the shorter edge.

Apply some water on the edges and press to seal, to make a cone. So one side of your cone will have extra wrapper.

6. Fill the cone with some of the potato filling. Fold in a zigzag manner until the wrapper is used. Apply some water on the edge and press to seal.
7. Repeat steps 4 – 6 and make the remaining samosas.
8. Place rack in the center of the oven. Place samosas on a baking sheet. Brush with oil.
9. Bake in a preheated oven at 350° F for about 25 - 30 minutes. Flip sides halfway through baking. It will last in the fridge for 4 days, or you can freeze them for up to one month.
10. Serve with a dip of your choice.

Cinnamon Apple Energy Bars

Serves: 20

Ingredients:

- 22 Medjool dates, pitted, soaked in water for 15 minutes, drained
- 2 teaspoons vanilla extract
- 2 teaspoons ground cinnamon
- 1 ½ cups chopped, dried apple
- 2 cups rolled oats
- 2/3 cup brown rice syrup
- ½ teaspoon salt
- ½ cup ground flaxseeds
- 3 cups puffed rice
- 1 cup cashew butter or almond butter or sunflower butter

Directions:

1. Add dates into the food processor bowl. Process until very finely chopped.
2. Transfer into a pan. Add brown rice syrup, salt, cinnamon, vanilla and cashew butter. Place the pan over medium-low heat.
3. Stir frequently until the mixture is well combined. Turn off the heat.
4. Meanwhile, add dried apple, flaxseeds, oats, and puffed rice into a large bowl

and stir.

5. Pour the date mixture and stir until well combined.

6. Place a sheet of parchment paper in a large baking pan (9 x 13 inches).

7. Transfer the mixture into the pan. Spread it evenly. Chill for 4 to 5 hours.

8. Cut into 20 equal pieces and serve. It can last one week on the countertop, or longer in the fridge.

Baked Buffalo Chickpea Bites
Serves: 6 - 8

Ingredients:

- 1 large carrot, roughly chopped
- 2 cloves garlic, peeled
- ¼ cup chopped green onions
- ¼ teaspoon salt
- ¼ teaspoon pepper
- ¼ cup rolled oats
- 7.5 ounces canned chickpeas, drained, rinsed
- 2 tablespoons hot sauce + extra to coat
- Vegan ranch dressing to serve

Vegan ranch dressing:

- ½ cup cashews, soaked in water for 5-6 hours, drained
- ½ tablespoon white vinegar
- Juice of a lemon
- ½ teaspoon garlic salt
- ¼ cup water
- ½ teaspoon onion powder
- ½ teaspoon dried dill
- ¼ teaspoon mustard powder

Directions:

1. To make vegan ranch dressing: Add all the ingredients for vegan ranch dressing into a blender and blend until smooth. Add more water or vinegar if it is too thick. Add a little at a time and blend each time.

2. Transfer into a bowl. Cover and refrigerate until use.

3. Add carrots, garlic, and oats into the food processor. Process until finely chopped. Remove and place in a bowl.

4. Add chickpeas into the food processor. Process until finely chopped. Add into the bowl of carrots. Mix well.

5. Add rest of the ingredients and mix well.

6. Place a sheet of parchment paper on a baking sheet. Spray some cooking spray on it.

7. Divide the mixture into 6 - 8 equal portions and shape into balls. Place the balls on the prepared baking sheet.

8. Place the baking sheet in the refrigerator until use. It can last for 2 – 3 days.

9. To serve: Remove the baking sheet from the refrigerator. Brush the balls lightly with hot sauce.

10. Place the baking sheet in an oven.

11. Bake in a preheated oven at 375°F for 25 - 30 minutes or until light golden brown.

12. Remove from the oven. Let it sit for about 5-6 minutes. Transfer onto a serving platter.

13. Insert toothpicks and serve with vegan ranch dressing.

Herbed Cheese Stuffed Mini Peppers
Serves: 12

Ingredients:

- 8 ounces herbed vegan cheese
- 24 ounces mini sweet peppers, halved, deseed if desired
- Balsamic reduction, to serve

Directions:

- If you do not have herbed vegan cheese, add some finely chopped herbs of your choice to crumbled vegan cheese. Mix well and use.

- Place a sheet of parchment paper on a baking sheet. Place the peppers on it, with the cut side facing up.

- Bake in a preheated oven at 400°F for 5 minutes. Remove from the oven and let it cool for 5 minutes.

- Stuff the peppers with herbed cheese. Place on a plate. Chill until use. It can last for 2 days.
- To serve: Remove from the refrigerator and bring to room temperature. Drizzle balsamic reduction on top and serve.

Baked Brussels Sprout Tater Tots

Serves: 6 (3 tater tots per serving)

Ingredients:

- 1 large russet potato, peeled
- 1 ½ tablespoons aquafaba (cooked liquid of chickpeas)
- 1 teaspoon olive oil
- ½ teaspoon salt or to taste
- 6 ounces Brussels sprouts, trimmed, shredded

Directions:

- Add potato into a saucepan. Cover with water. Place the saucepan over medium heat. Place the saucepan over medium heat.
- Let it boil until the potato it is just cooked. Do not cook until soft. Turn off the heat and drain.
- When the potato is cool enough to handle, grate using the large holes of the grater.
- Add aquafaba and salt into a bowl and whisk well using a fork. Transfer half this mixture into the bowl with the potato and mix well.
- Add Brussels sprouts into a bowl. Add remaining aquafaba and mix well. Transfer into the bowl of potatoes and mix well. Taste and adjust the salt if required.
- Divide the mixture into 18 equal portions and shape into tots. Press lightly and place on a baking sheet lined with parchment paper.
- Brush oil on the tater tots. Sprinkle some salt over it if desired.
- Bake in a preheated oven at 400°F for 20 – 25 minutes or until light brown. Flip sides halfway through baking. Remove from the oven and let it cool.
- Transfer into an airtight container and refrigerate until use. It can last for 3 days.
- To serve: Heat in an oven and serve.

Mexican Avocado Dip

Serves: 4

Ingredients:

- 2 avocados, peeled, pitted, mashed
- ½ cup medium salsa
- ½ cups nutritional yeast

To serve:

- Tortilla chips

Directions:

- Add all the ingredients into a bowl and mix well. Cover and chill until use. Use within a day.
- Serve with tortilla chips.

Beet Chips

Serves: 4

Ingredients:

- 4 medium-large sized beets, peeled, sliced, pat dried with paper towels
- Salt to taste
- 1 tablespoon grapeseed oil
- Herbs and spices of your choice

Directions:

1. Place beets in a bowl. Add rest of the ingredients except spices and toss well.
2. Spread on a lined baking sheet in a single layer.
3. Bake in a preheated oven at 325°F for 20 – 25 minutes or until crisp.
4. Remove from the oven and cool completely.
5. Transfer into an airtight container. Store at room temperature. It can last for 4 to 5 days.
6. Sprinkle some spices on top and serve.

Ginger Wasabi Roasted Almonds

Serves: 4 (¼ cup each)

Ingredients:

- 1 ½ tablespoons soy sauce
- 1 tablespoon wasabi powder
- 1 cup almonds
- 1 ½ tablespoons maple syrup or agave nectar
- 1 teaspoon ground ginger

Directions:

1. Add all the ingredients into a bowl and

mix well.

2. Transfer onto a lined baking sheet. Spread it evenly.
3. Bake in a preheated oven at 350°F for 12 – 16 minutes or until crisp. Stir a couple of times while baking. Keep a watch on it after about 10 minutes of baking.
4. Remove from the oven and cool completely. Transfer into an airtight container and store at room temperature. It can last for 4 – 5 days.

- Bake in a preheated oven at 350° F for 8 minutes. Stir a couple of times while it is baking.
- Cool completely.
- Transfer into an airtight container. Store at room temperature. It can last for 4 – 5 days.

Sun-Dried Tomato Pesto Tortilla Roll-Ups
Serves: 10

Ingredients:

- 5 tortillas (10 – 12 inches)
- 3 ounces sundried tomato pesto
- 8 ounces dairy-free cream cheese
- 5 ounces baby spinach

Directions:

- Spread the tortillas on your countertop. Divide the cream cheese equally and spread over the tortillas.
- Next spread the pesto over the tortillas. Scatter baby lettuce over the tortillas. Roll and place with its seam side facing down in an airtight container. Refrigerate until use. It can last for 2 days.
- Cut into 1-½ inch pieces. Insert toothpicks into each piece and serve.

Pistachio Granola
Serves: 10

Ingredients:

- 2 cups roasted unsalted shelled pistachios
- 4 tablespoons pure maple syrup
- ½ teaspoon ground cinnamon
- 1 cup old fashioned rolled oats
- 2 tablespoons virgin coconut oil, melted
- ¼ - ½ teaspoon fine sea salt

Directions:

- Add all the ingredients into a bowl and toss well. Transfer on to a lined baking sheet.
- Spread it evenly.

Chapter Thirteen

Vegan Dessert Recipes

Peanut Butter Banana Splits
Serves: 6

Ingredients:

- 6 bananas, sliced
- 2 tablespoons coconut oil
- 4 tablespoons peanut butter
- 1 cup chocolate chips

To serve:

- Non Dairy whipped topping
- Non Dairy frozen treats
- Maraschino cherries
- Strawberry slices

Directions:

- Add chocolate chips, coconut oil, and peanut butter into a microwave-safe bowl. Microwave on high for about a minute. Whisk well. If the mixture is not melted, place for a few more seconds. Whisk after every 5 seconds.
- Divide the banana slices into 6 glasses or bowls.
- Drizzle the chocolate sauce over the bananas. Refrigerate until use. It can last for 2 days.
- To serve: Remove the glasses from the refrigerator. Top with the suggested toppings and serve.

Salted Caramel Chocolate Cups
Serves: 6

Ingredients:

- ½ cup dark chocolate chips
- 3 tablespoons vegan caramel sauce
- 1 teaspoon coconut oil
- 1/8 teaspoon flaky sea salt

Directions:

- Place disposable cupcake liners in a 6 counts muffin pan.
- Add chocolate chips and coconut oil into a microwave-safe bowl. Microwave on

high for about 50 seconds. Whisk well. If the mixture is not melted, place for a few more seconds. Whisk after every 5 seconds.

- Divide most of the chocolate mixture among the cupcake liners. Using the back of a spoon, spread it evenly on the bottom as well as a little on the sides of the liners.
- Freeze until firm. Divide the caramel sauce among the cupcake liners. Drizzle the remaining chocolate on the caramel layer.
- Refrigerate until use. It can last for a week.

Creamy Mint Chocolate Chip Avocado Ice Cream
Serves: 7 – 8

Ingredients:

- 4 medium-large Hass avocados, peeled, pitted, chopped into chunks
- ½ cup coconut butter or coconut oil
- 2 tablespoons peppermint extract
- ½ cup chocolate chips
- 2 medium bananas, peeled, sliced
- 4 tablespoons maple syrup or coconut nectar or agave nectar
- 15-20 fresh mint leaves (optional)

Directions:

- Add all the ingredients except chocolate chips into a blender and blend until smooth.
- Pour into a freezer-safe container. Freeze for an hour.
- Remove the ice cream from the freezer and whisk well. Refreeze and beat again after 30-40 minutes.
- Repeat the previous step 2 – 3 times until well frozen without ice crystals.
- Add chocolate chips and stir when you whisk for the last time.

Apple Strudel
Serves: 8 – 10

Ingredients:

- 2 packages vegan puff pastry dough (16 x 9 inches each)
- 1 ½ teaspoons ground cinnamon
- 4 red apples, peeled, cored, cut into thin slices using a slicer
- Powdered vegan sugar, to sprinkle (optional)

Directions:

1. Sprinkle cinnamon over the apple and stir using your hands.
2. Unfold the pastry dough on your countertop. Place apple slices on one half of the dough. Fold the other half over the filling. Press the edges to seal. Place in an airtight container in the refrigerator. It can last for 2 days.
3. To serve: Bake in a preheated oven at 350° F for 15 – 20 minutes or until brown on top.
4. Serve warm or at room temperature.

Pumpkin Parfaits

Serves: 8

Ingredients:

- 4 cups vanilla soy yogurt
- ½ cup brown or raw sugar (optional)
- ½ teaspoon ground nutmeg
- 2 cups pumpkin puree
- 1 teaspoon ground cinnamon
- ¼ teaspoon ground ginger (optional)

Topping:

- 4 squares dark chocolate, melted
- 8 ginger snap cookies, broken
- Mint leaves

Directions:

1. Add pumpkin, yogurt, sugar, ginger, cinnamon, and nutmeg into a bowl and whisk until sugar dissolves completely.
2. Divide into glasses. Refrigerate until use. It can last for 3 days.
3. To serve: Top with the suggested toppings and serve.

Peanut Butter Balls

Serves: 8

Ingredients:

- 1/3 cup roasted peanuts
- 1 tablespoon cocoa powder
- 3 tablespoons rolled oats
- ½ cup pitted Medjool dates

Directions:

- Add dates into the food processor and pulse until smooth.
- Add rest of the ingredients and pulse until well combined.
- Divide the mixture into 8 equal portions and shape into balls. Place in an airtight container and refrigerate until use. It can last for a week.
- To freeze: Place in freezer-safe bags and freeze until use. It can last for 2 months.

Chocolate Fudge Cookies

Serves: 28

Ingredients:

- 2 large ripe bananas, sliced
- 1 cup peanut butter or any other nut butter of your choice
- Flaky sea salt to sprinkle
- 1 cup cocoa powder
- 1 cup + 2 tablespoons maple syrup

Directions:

- Add banana into a bowl. Using a fork, mash the bananas.
- Stir in peanut butter, maple syrup and cocoa powder. Mix until well combined.
- Place a sheet of parchment paper on 1 – 2 large baking sheets. Place tablespoonful of the mixture at different spots. You should have about 28 cookies in all.
- Bake in a preheated oven at 325° F for 15 minutes. Remove from the oven and sprinkle salt over the cookies. Let it cool to room temperature. Transfer into an airtight container. It can last for 10 – 12 days.

Apple Pie

Serves: 5

Ingredients:

For the crust:

- ½ cup + 1 tablespoon all-purpose flour
- 3 tablespoons organic vegan shortening, cut into small cubes
- 1/8 teaspoon salt
- 2 tablespoons ice water

For the filling:

- 4 cups peeled, cored, thinly sliced Granny Smith apples (about ¾ pound)
- ½ tablespoon lemon juice
- ½ tablespoon cornstarch
- ¼ cup packed light brown sugar
- ¼ teaspoon ground cinnamon

For topping:

- ¼ cup rolled oats
- 1 ½ tablespoons packed light brown sugar
- 1 tablespoon organic vegan shortening
- 2 tablespoons all-purpose flour
- ¼ teaspoon ground cinnamon

Directions:

1. To make crust: Add flour into a bowl. Add cold shortening. Cut it into the flour using a pastry cutter until crumbs are formed.
2. Add ice-cold water, a tablespoon at a time and mix until a moist dough is formed.
3. Shape into a circle of about 4-5 inches.
4. Take a sheet of plastic wrap. Sprinkle some flour on it. Place the dough in the middle of the sheet and wrap it completely. Place in the refrigerator for a maximum of 2 days.
5. Remove from the refrigerator 15 minutes before preparing.
6. To make the filling: Add apples, brown sugar, cinnamon and lemon juice into a bowl. Mix well and set aside for 15 minutes.
7. Sprinkle cornstarch and toss until well coated.
8. Place a sheet of parchment paper on your countertop. Place dough on the center of the parchment paper. Cover with another sheet of parchment paper. Roll with a rolling pin until about 6 – 7 inches in diameter. Carefully remove the top parchment paper.
9. Lift the dough along with the bottom parchment paper, carefully invert onto a 5 – 6-inch pie pan. Press the dough into the pan.
10. Carefully remove the other parchment paper.
11. Place the filling in the pie pan. Spread it all over the pan.
12. Bake in a preheated oven at 375°F for 15-20 minutes.
13. To make the topping: Add all the ingredients of the topping into a bowl. Cut it into the flour using a pastry blender or a pair of knives until smaller pieces are formed.
14. Then use your hands and mix until the mixture is crumbly. Sprinkle over the apple filling in the pie.
15. Bake for 30-40 minutes until the top is golden brown. It can last for 2 – 3 days. Place in an airtight container at room temperature.
16. Cut into wedges and serve.

Fig, Coconut, and Blackberry Ice Cream
Serves: 12 - 15

Ingredients:

- 20 fresh, ripe figs, chop each into 8 pieces
- Juice of a lemon
- Zest of a lemon, grated
- 4 teaspoons ginger, minced (optional)
- 4 cups coconut milk
- 1 1/3 cups blackberries + extra to garnish
- ¾ cup water
- 2/3 cup dried shredded coconut, unsweetened
- 1 cup agave nectar or to taste
- A few leaves lemon balm

Directions:

- Place a saucepan over medium heat. Add figs, water, lemon zest, dried coconut, and ginger. When it begins to boil, lower the heat and simmer until figs are tender.
- Add blackberries and agave nectar and cook until slightly thick.
- Turn off the heat and cool completely. Blend with an immersion blender until smooth.
- Add rest of the ingredients and blend for a few seconds until the fruits get chopped into tiny pieces. Pour into a bowl. Cover and chill for 4 – 6 hours.
- Pour into an ice cream maker and churn the ice cream following the manufacturer's instructions. Transfer into a freezer-safe container. Freeze until use.
- To serve: Remove from the freezer and place for 10 minutes on your countertop before serving. Scoop ice cream into bowls. Serve garnished with blackberries and lemon balm.

Layered Blueberry Cheesecake
Serves: 12-16

Ingredients:

For crust:

- 1 cup almond flour
- 1 cup raw pecans
- 6 dates, pitted
- 2 teaspoons ground cinnamon
- 4 tablespoons coconut oil
- ½ teaspoon kosher salt

For filling:

- 4 cups raw cashew, soaked in water for 4-8 hours
- ½ cup coconut oil, melted, cooled
- 4 tablespoons fresh lemon juice
- ½ cup freeze-dried blueberries
- ½ cup canned coconut milk, shake the can well before pouring into the cup
- 2/3 cup pure maple syrup
- 2 tablespoons vanilla extract or 1 teaspoon vanilla bean powder

For blueberry layer:

- 2 cups blueberries, fresh or frozen, thawed if frozen
- 2 tablespoons chia seeds
- 2 tablespoons fresh lemon juice

Directions:

- Grease 2 small springform pans with coconut oil. Place strips of parchment paper in it.
- Add all the ingredients of crust into the food processor and pulse until well combined and slightly sticky. Do not pulse for long.
- Divide the mixture into the prepared pans. Press it well into the bottom of the pan.
- To make filling: Add all the ingredients for filling into the food processor and pulse until smooth. Add more coconut milk if the mixture is not getting smooth while blending. Taste and adjust sweetness if desired. Set aside about 1/3 of the filling and add into a bowl. Add freeze-dried blueberries and mix well. Set aside.
- Divide the remaining 2/3 of the filling in the 2 crusts. Spread it evenly.
- Freeze for an hour.
- Divide the blueberry mixture on top of both the crusts. Place the cheesecakes in the freezer.
- To make blueberry layer: Add all the ingredients for blueberry layer into the blender and blend until smooth.
- Pour on the top of the crusts. Place the cheesecakes back in the freezer. Freeze until firm. It can last for a week.
- Serve frozen or thawed. Cut into wedges and serve.

Conclusion

I want to thank you once again for choosing this book. I hope it proved to be an enjoyable and summative read.

Perhaps the most challenging part of starting a diet or even sticking to it is committing. The vegan diet is not an exception. You might be quite motivated to stick to a plant-based diet, but then you get home after a long and tiring day, and the urge to order some takeout overcomes you. Well, this is where meal prepping steps in. Once you start making all your meals ahead of time and complete the required prep, cooking certainly becomes more accessible and easy. Meal prepping is a great way to control your cravings while sticking to a healthy diet. Apart from this, it will save you plenty of time and money.

In this book, you were given several vegan recipes to cook tasty and healthy meals without having to spend hours in the kitchen. From breakfast to desserts, there are recipes for every meal of the day within this book. Use the recipes given in this book along with a little advanced planning every week, to start cooking simple and delicious meals daily. By sticking to the diet, you can attain your weight loss objectives but also effectively improve your overall health.

All that you need to do now is to gather the required ingredients and stock up your pantry with vegan-friendly items. When everything is in place, it is time to start meal prepping!

Thank you and all the best!

References

6 Science-Based Health Benefits of Eating Vegan. (2019). Retrieved from https://www.healthline.com/nutrition/vegan-diet-benefits#section4

Benefits of Meal Prep: Top 10 Reasons Why You Should Meal Prep - Fit Fresh Blog. (2017). Retrieved from http://blog.fit-fresh.com/benefits-meal-prep-top-10-reasons-meal-prep/

Josephson, M. (2016). How to ease yourself into a vegan diet — and actually stick with it. Retrieved from https://www.google.com/amp/s/amp.insider.com/5-tips-for-becoming-vegan-and-staying-vegan-2016-6

Kot, K. (2017). The Top 10 Mistakes You'll Make When Going Vegan. Retrieved from https://thoughtcatalog.com/krista-kot/2017/04/the-top-10-mistakes-youll-make-when-going-vegan/

The Ultimate Vegan Grocery List. (2016). Retrieved from https://nutriciously.com/vegan-grocery-list/

Top 7 Meal Prep Mistakes and How to Fix Them. (2018). Retrieved from https://habit.com/blog/2018/05/03/top-meal-prep-mistakes/

Valente, L. https://eatingwell.com. Retrieved from http://www.eatingwell.com/article/279566/9-healthy-tips-to-help-you-start-eating-a-vegan-diet/

Vegan Lifestyle on a Budget » I LOVE VEGAN. Retrieved from **https://www.ilovevegan.com/resources/vegan-lifestyle-on-a-budget/**

Von Alt, S. (2018). Here Are 5 Vegan Meal Prep Tips for Beginners—and a Few Recipes to Try. Retrieved from **https://chooseveg.com/blog/vegan-meal-prep-tips-for-beginners-and-a-few-recipes-to-try/**

Meal Prep for Weight Loss

The Newest Guide to Create Your Own Healthy weekly meal plan for a progressive weight loss. Develop Your Dietetic Meal Prepping Strategies to burn fat as Fast as Possible

Amanda Davis

INTRODUCTION

Meal preppers, welcome! If you have a goal to lose weight and trim down, you've started at the right place as meal prepping can really help you to reach your goals. There's something about being organized and dedicated which makes you really want to stick to your goals and eat the foods you know will deliver you to your healthiest weight yet.

These recipes are not "diet" recipes; they are healthy, nutritious, filling, and tasty recipes. I don't believe you need to cut out food groups or deprive yourself in order to lose weight. In fact, eating properly, eating enough, and eating foods that satisfy you will result in weight loss you can maintain and sustain. So, if you're looking for a particular diet or eating style, then this might not be the book for you! But I hope it is, as I know you'll love these recipes as much as I do.

Oh, I should add a bit about me! I am not a nutritionist or dietitian. But I am someone who has successfully lost weight through sensible and healthy eating, and of course, meal prepping! I want to pass on my recipes and my knowledge of meal prepping so you too can experience the same success and health benefits.

Please consult your doctor or nutritionist for advice and guidance if you are looking to lose large amounts of weight, or if you have health issues which might be affected due to a change in diet. This book is a friendly and supportive guideline to help you lose weight in a healthy way, without extreme changes or deprivation.

Now, let's get into the ins and outs of meal prepping!

Chapter 1: What is Meal Prep?

Meal prepping is the art of preparing your meals the night (or a few nights) before eating. It usually involves preparing a few portions of each meal, packing them away in airtight containers, and storing in the fridge. Many people prep their meals these days, because it saves time, encourages healthy eating, and controls portions. Sometimes, the meal is completely prepared and cooked in its entirety before being stacked away in the fridge or freezer until it is needed. Whereas sometimes, meals are only partially prepared so they can be cooked right before eating. For example, you can prep lasagna by cooking the sauces and layering it all up before covering and storing in the fridge, raw. You would then place the lasagna into a preheated oven before eating the next night. Whatever prepping method you choose, it's a great way to manage your time and your diet!

Meal prepping is a new concept for busy cooks to help them plan the week with pre-planned meals and quick access to the ingredients. Everybody has schedule overload these days, especially if you work full-time, kids to take to school, home from school, soccer and theatre practice, after hours work obligations, meals to cook and a house to clean.

Don't you feel overwhelmed and tired already?

The basics of meal-prep works like this.

You plan the menus for the week for breakfast, lunch, and supper. Add snacks if you wish, we have plenty listed in the last chapter.

You make the list of ingredients for the week.

You buy the ingredients and the proper storage containers.

You cook everything on one afternoon, usually in two hours or less.

You refrigerate and freeze the contents, labeling each packet.

When you are ready to eat, you heat them and serve them.

You have just eliminated at least six hours of work a week, and decreased spending, and stayed on your high protein, low carb diet.

Hurray! Victory!

Benefits of Meal-Prepping

At first, meal prepping may seem like a lot of work that takes up a weekend afternoon, very precious time in my household. There are so many exciting benefits of meal-prepping I'm not quite sure where to start. Here are a few for your consideration:

Your kitchen time will be cut by as much as 75 percent, once you get the hang of it and make it a personal habit.

Your grocery bill will instantly drop. One of the reasons is because you are buying in bulk and all at one time. Another of the reasons is the impulse factor. Have you ever gone to the grocery store for just one item and came home with a trunk load of many unnecessary purchases, all because you were hungry?

Using the concepts of meal prep allows you to know what you are eating with the correct portion size. Eating out is too much a temptation to buy the wrong dinner choices, and eating leftovers so you don't have to store them is still overeating.

With the extra time you gain from eating properly and preparing your meals once a week, you can now add the exercise plan to your day that you've always wanted to start, but never had enough time.

The Helpful Equipment

Note this equipment is helpful, but not a necessity. Everything can be cooked on a stove, using a skillet, or pots and pans. Knives can be used to cut and plates can function as cutting boards. However, since the point of meal-prep is to save both time and money, these appliances pay for themselves in many ways.

A Crock-pot

This ageless appliance lets you cook and rest at the same time. Although there are only a few crock-pot recipes within these covers, these will not be the only recipes you prepare. If you use a crockpot on cooking day, you can use a larger and less expensive cut of meat. This can be a real savings.

Skillets that are oven proof and non-stick

Most likely if you cook any meals ever you have a skillet or two. In this cookbook, we strive to mess up less dishes. Some of the recipes require browning and then baking. An ovenproof skillet can do both, eliminating one more dish to wash.

At least 3 mixing bowls in large, medium and small sizes

It may be likely that you have these, but not everyone does. As you double or triple recipes when you cook, you will need more than one size and more than one in quantity.

A Blender

Some soups taste better when blended to a creamy puree. It is always easier and tastier to emulsify salad dressings, instead of whipping them by hand in a bowl. You do not have to buy an expensive model as 5 or 6 settings will be enough for the blending instructions we have included.

A Food Processor

When you are preparing multiple meals, using a food processor to chop, slice, and dice saves so much energy and time. The foods are also healthier. Did you know that purchased shredded cheese can include 10 percent wood pulp, commonly called saw dust? When you are purchasing 10 pounds of cheese, you are receiving eight pounds of cheese and two pounds of sawdust. What's more, you are eating it! Save your health by shredding your own blocks of cheese with the food processor. You can freeze it for later use and know the contents of what you are eating.

Good quality sharp knives

Sharp knives make cutting faster and help to keep you from cutting yourself by pressing too hard.

Cutting Boards

Cutting Boards come in several materials and sizes. They protect surfaces and allow the air to circulate underneath while the baked goods cool.

Keep in mind that the construction materials of a cutting board will determine its cleanliness. For example:

Bamboo cutting boards are self-healing. This allows the cuts made by knives to heal on their own. The bamboo cutting boards are very good to knives as they do not dull them quickly. Bamboo is a porous material, which allows bacteria to seep into the cuts. Even disinfecting promptly after use will never eliminate the germs that have accumulated on a wood cutting board.

Glass canning jars with lids, pint sized and quart sized

One of the lesser known secrets is that salad stored in a Ball or Mason jar with a tight sealing lid will stay fresh in the refrigerator for seven full days! This makes the dinner salad, stored in a quart jar, easy to place into serving plates. Salads stored in pint jars are perfect for toting in the thermal lunch bag for a healthy lunch. The salad dressing can be included in the jar and will still be fresh.

Foil containers

These can be expensive, but dollar stores have these priced better than grocery stores. Buy the containers that include lids, baking sizes and the individual sizes.

Plastic containers

Use the food prep containers that are custom designed for Meal-prep. These have no BPAs, are apportioned in the right serving sizes, and are inexpensive. They are dishwasher safe, freezer safe, and can be used in the microwave. Buy enough containers for all your family members to eat three meals a day for one week. You will also need zip-lock freezer bags, pint-sized and snack-sized. Using leftover whipped topping bowls or margarine containers can be less expensive, but they are not constructed to be heated in the microwave or stored for long-term in the freezer.

Chapter 2: Macronutrients and Healthy Food

The macronutrients that constitute our diet are:
The Carbohydrates: also called carbon carbohydrates, sugars or more commonly, are the primary source of energy. They also contain the fibers, which we will define a little later.
The Fat: fatty acids also called "fat" or fat are molecules that form the organic fat. They play an important role in the constitution of cell membranes, energy production, and body temperature and more generally in the metabolism of the human being.
The Proteins: they are essential molecules for the life of cells and the constitution of human tissues (muscles, hair, skin, etc.).
Macronutrients are molecules that provide energy to our body or that participate directly or indirectly in metabolism. They are called "macro" in order to differentiate them from micronutrients such as vitamins, minerals, enzymes, etc.

Carbohydrates
It is the main source of energy of the body.
As you have guessed, it's about sugars, and yes sugars, we'll always need them. Everything depends then which sugars to privilege, and there, it becomes more complicated.
In theory, these are the complex sugars to favor at the expense of simple sugars, but that does not help you much!
What are the foods based on complex sugars and those based on simple sugars?
Simple sugars have a high glycemic index (Glucose and sucrose ...) they are present in sweets, pastries, classic white sugar, in many prepared dishes, sauces (ketchup, bbq sauce, sweet and sour)
Complex sugars, meanwhile, have a low glycemic index; they are present in cereals (whole grains, attention!) and legumes.
Sugar in fruits is also an excellent source of energy, but we must not forget that fructose must first be treated in the liver before 'be used by the body, and it cannot be part of the complex sugars, it is a so-called fast sugar, but does not have a too high glycemic index, (IG: 20 against 100 for glucose), which differentiates it especially glucose classic is that the carbohydrate intake is supplemented with a contribution of fiber, minerals and vitamins.

THE PROTIDES
In common parlance we often tend to call them "proteins", but this is an abuse of language, and yes, in fact the protides is a sort of "family" grouping proteins, amino acids, and peptides.
When we talk about proteins "protiderotides" we immediately think of our muscles, and yes you know well they are made up, but we must not forget that they are also made of 70% water, moreover the water content of our body represents on average about 65% of our mass, small parenthesis
Back to our proteins, except the muscles (myosin, actin, myoglobin) , they are also present in our hair, nail our skin (keratin), but also in our red blood cells (globin).
They provide a multitude of functions within the cells:
Cell renewal
Role of protection (hair, nails, skin)
Physiological functioning (information transmission, digestion, immune defense)
Secondary energy role (after carbohydrates) and it is also our only source of nitrogen (essential for life) , and yes it is a present element to link amino acids to each other.
Proteins are of animal or vegetable origin (legumes, cereals)
Contrary to many received ideas, vegetable proteins are not of less good quality than animal proteins, on the contrary.
Indeed, animal proteins also contain so-called saturated fats (we'll talk about it later), favoring weight gain, cardiovascular risks and clot formation, on the contrary vegetable proteins are rich in fibers without any saturated fat.
LIPIDS

Despite their demonization, it is a primordial macro nutrient essential to our proper functioning.

Lipids are an important energy store, they are essential to regulate the temperature of our body, and very importantly, they are one of the major constituents of membranes   and the nervous system, indeed lipids surround and strengthen our lymph.

On the other hand, lipids are not all of the same quality!

This is where the difference, always and again, good and bad fats, so we distinguish different types of fatty acids: saturated, monounsaturated or polyunsaturated.

The saturated = to limit! They increase the cardiovascular risk as stated above (contained in fatty meats, sausages, butter or cream, vegetable fats biscuits and industrial dishes)

Mono-unsaturated = also called omega-9 contained in oilseeds (almonds, hazelnuts, walnuts ...) and avocado

Poly-unsaturated = these are omega 6 and 3, these are essential fatty acids, our body is unable to synthesize them, they contribute to the proper functioning of our cardiovascular system, some studies have demonstrated that omega-3 fatty acids promote lipolysis (provision of fat to provide energy to the body) it is not beautiful, so do not hesitate to consume virgin oils first cold pressed (olive oil, rapeseed),also in oily fish, but I cannot encourage you to consume since they too often contain heavy metals such as mercury, and especially for our biodiversity and ethics, it is better to leave them there where he is, it was the little ethical parenthesis

An individual's macros are calculated as a percentage of the total calories consumed. "So, for example, if you are an active middle-aged and 60k-weight individual who goes to the gym regularly and follow a 1600-calorie diet, you need 40% of your calories to come from carbohydrates, 30% of proteins and 30% of fats. These proportions would be normal for those who do not train for a living, or for people who are active, but not for endurance athletes. This is what those calculations would look like:

1600 x 0.40 = 640 calories from carbohydrates
1600 x 0.30 = 480 calories of protein
1600 x 0.30 = 480 calories from fat

"To convert those calories figures into grams, carbohydrates and proteins are divided by 4, because both carbohydrates and proteins provide 4 calories per gram, "and fat by 9, because fat contributes 9 calories. per gram. " This is how those calculations would work:

640/4 = 160 grams of carbohydrates
480/4 = 120 grams of protein
480/9 = 53 grams of fat

The proportion of macros will change according to your objectives. "It is important to take into account your level of activity and the type of exercises you do,

For example, if you are strength training you will need to increase your protein intake to facilitate muscle recovery and prevent injuries. While if you focus more on cardio, you will have to increase carbohydrates to prevent the wear of glycogen stores.

WHAT IS THE EASIEST WAY TO CALCULATE YOUR OWN MACROS?
When entering your data in an online macro calculator: age, height, weight, sex, activity level, target weight, frequency and intensity with which you lift weights. If It Fits Your Macros, which also asks when you want to achieve your goals, or Healthy Eater , which is simpler, but produces similar calculations.

THE BENEFITS OF COUNTING MACROS

It's about getting the right amount of each one right, so as not to fall short or exceed your body's needs. By achieving that balance, your body will function at its highest level and you will recover properly. It also activates other systems such as immune, digestive and sleep. "It's like a group of workers in which everyone does their job so that the whole body works at its maximum performance.

It is clear that this "work" depends on your level of activity and your objectives. "If you are an athlete, macros are very important. Also, if you eat adjusting to your macros, you don't have to eliminate any important food groups or deprive yourself of anything.

But if you want to lose fat, gain muscle, it is very important to consider the source and quality of the food you eat. "I have seen people who count macros stuffing themselves with donuts because 'it fits their macros', but they perform less and feel worse than if they had opted for sweet potatoes or other types of carbohydrates," he adds.

THE BAD THING ABOUT COUNTING MACROS

In an IIFYM diet, the important thing is not to deprive yourself of something, but to feed you so that your body functions in the most effective way. But counting macros can take time. Not only do you have to know the proportions, but you also have to measure food on an appropriate scale. So if you feel lazy to weigh everything you eat, counting macros is not made for you. In addition, monitoring, tracking and weighing everything you eat can create an unhealthy relationship with food. Anytime the numbers go up and you like to control your diet. But if you have suffered eating disorders in the past, counting macros is probably not a good idea. Like any other diet, counting macros is not a panacea. It can help you make the body function very effectively, and even serve you to reach certain goals, but remember that the most important thing is the quality of what you eat. As an athlete, you know that diet is only part of the equation, so the best is what best suits your lifestyle and, therefore, you manage to maintain in the long term.

Chapter 3: Success in Meal Prepping

Utilize the freezer

Frozen prepped meals are a lifesaver during busy and chaotic times. A good way to utilize the freezer is to double the recipe for a particular meal and put half of the servings in the fridge for the consequent days, and put the other half in the freezer for later down the track. You'll be very pleased you did so, especially during times when your meal-prep game schedule is slipping!

Keep your macros in mind: proteins, carbs, fats

You don't want to sit down to your prepped lunch only to find that it's too filling or not filling enough due to unbalanced macros. Remember to include a portion of protein, some good fats, and some healthy wholegrain carbs for optimum energy and satiety. Most of the recipes in this book have a great balance of macros, but you can adjust them to suit your needs and preferences.

Stock-up on flavor-packing non-perishables

Herbs, spices, vinegars, oils, and natural flavorings can turn any simple dish into a tasty masterpiece, with very little added calories. What's more, they last a very long time in the pantry so you don't need to worry about using them up before their best-before date. Splash out on a big haul of natural, flavor-giving ingredients to pack into your meal-prep box. This means that you can use simple base ingredients, and adjust the flavors with the addition of healthy and low-cal seasonings.

Invest in storage equipment

This is an important one. To successfully prep, you need containers to store your meals in. High-quality plastic or glass containers with airtight lids are ideal, especially if you can find a set which includes different sizes. Small, single-serve containers are really handy for breakfasts such as oats and chia pudding, and snacks such as fruit and nut mix. Pyrex bowls which have airtight lids are ideal for large salads and soups. Have a shop around and find yourself a few value packs, and allocate a special box, drawer, or cupboard, especially for your meal-prep containers.

Get creative with color

During my own meal prepping journey I found that using bright and varied colors really helped me to get excited about making, and eating my prepped meals. A pile of red cabbage with bright red bell peppers and some vibrant green cilantro – beautiful! Rich yellow corn kernels, inky black beans, glossy red chili, and pale green avocado, it looks as amazing as it tastes. If you're like me, then you'll get a kick out of putting together beautiful and fresh-looking meals to fill your containers. Fresh fruits, veggies, herbs, and rich spices are the best sources of edible color.

Predict your cravings and prep accordingly

If you don't feel like eating a particular meal, then don't prep it. Don't think that you must eat a certain type of dish simply because it seems like the healthiest option. You can make any dish healthy! Even if it's traditionally a junk food. For example, you will find recipes for burgers and rich pastas in this book, but they are nutritious versions which fit in with your weight loss plans. If you've got a craving for sweeter dishes, then try a yummy oatmeal with dates for breakfast! If you feel like something a bit heavier for dinner (tiredness, hormones, and overindulgence can make us crave comfort foods) then choose a recipe for dinner with sweet potatoes and beans to fill you up. The bottom line? Prep foods you want to eat that particular week! This way, you'll avoid seeking other foods or snacks to satisfy you in between meals.

Make a plan and stick to it

This is where you need to be a bit strict and structured. Decide on a day to complete your prepping, set the time aside, and stick to it. Get your shopping done on the same day so your produce and meats are fresh, then set aside a couple of hours to prep, prep, prep! If you end up missing a prep day and you don't have the time to make up for it, you might find you slip back into day-to-day meals and the unhealthy choices and unbalanced portion sizes may creep back. Once the routine has been established it will be so easy!

Make it fun

Cooking should be as fun as eating, in my opinion! And the same goes for prepping. If you enjoy yourself, you'll get into a positive mindset about meal prepping, and a positive mindset about food will follow on. There are many ways to make meal-prep sessions fun! Play music, have a glass of wine, watch your favorite TV show, anything that relaxes you and puts you at ease as you work. Weight loss needn't be a drag, it can actually be an enjoyable and nourishing experience if you make the process work in a way that you enjoy

Chapter 4: Diet Meal Planning

By planning your meals in advance, you're able to buy in bulk which will save you money. You can usually store a meal for at least two weeks in the freezer too. It can help you save money at lunchtime too when you have prepped leftovers.

Weight Loss

The ketogenic diet already helps you to lose weight but planning your meals in advance will help you to save a little more cash too. With meal planning, you know exactly how much you're going to eat at a time, which can help to keep you from overeating.

A meal routine will also make it easier to know how many net carbs you're putting in your body each day. You can even label the meals with the amount of net carbs in each one.

Easy Grocery Shopping

It's easy to go grocery shopping when you know exactly what you'll be eating and when. Make a list, and just get everything off it. If you are prepping your snacks too, you don't even have to deviate off the list for everything you need. Just divide your shopping list into different categories like fruits, protein, frozen food, etc., and it'll be easier than ever to avoid aisles where you'd spend too much money or end up straying from the ketogenic diet.

Less Waste

Most of the time, you can just eat out of the dish that you've stored your food in. this helps you to cut down on paper plates, plastic utensils, and will keep you from wasting your food if you've prepped in advance. You unitize all the ingredients that you bought during the week, and it helps you to plan accordingly.

Time Saver

This is the main reason that people decide to start meal prepping. It's hard to find time to cook three meals a day, but that's exactly what the ketogenic diet requires. By saving time when cooking, you're less likely to eat junk food or fast food too.

Stress Reduction

Stress can affect your digestive system, disrupt your sleep and even cause your immune system to suffer. It can be hard to come home from a long day of work and then pan for dinner. With meal prep, you have a dedicated day to get the dinners ready, which allows you to relax most of the time.

How to Start Prepping Today

Let's

look at everything you need to start meal prepping today. There are certain ingredients you'll need as well as equipment to get started with.

Meal Prepping Equipment

You'll find essential equipment and what it's used for below.

- Cutting Board: You should try to get boards made from solid materials because they're corrosion resistant and non-porous which makes them easier to clean than wood or bamboo boards. Try plastic, glass, or even marble cutting boards for easier clean up.

- Measuring Cups: It's important that you measure out your spices and condiments accurately.

- Measuring Spoons: Even when you're prepping in bulk, you may still only need a small amount of some spices.

- Glass Bows: Glass bowls are considered easier, but nonmetallic containers will also be needed for storing meat and marinades.

- Packaging Materials: Your non-metallic containers and glass bowls will be important for this as well, but you may also want bento boxes that are freezer safe or even Tupperware. Make sure that you have freezer safe containers too.

- Paper Towels & Kitchen Towels: These will be required for draining meat.

- Knives: Your knives should be sharp to slice meat accordingly. Remember to cut away from your body, and you should wash your knives while cutting different food types

- Kitchen Scale: A kitchen scale can make some recipes much easier, allowing for much more accurate measurements.

- Internal Thermometer: You'll need to check the internal temperature of many meats, especially if you're making snacks like jerky.

- Baking Sheet: This will be needed for many recipes, especially sheet cakes, cookies, or even jerky.

- Colander: You'll have to drain some vegetables and rices.

- Skillets & Pans: It's going to be easier to cook if you have the right sized pan or skillet for what you're doing. You'll need baking dishes too!

- Stocking Your Kitchen

- While it's impossible to give you a list of each ingredient you'll ever use, there are some basics that you'll want to keep on hand. Before you start prepping for the week, make a comprehensive shopping list according to your meal plan.

- Cupboard Ingredients: Sea Salt, Black Pepper, Tomato Sauce, Tomato Paste, Crushed Tomatoes, Garlic Powder, Onion Powder, Ground Spices, Powdered Sweeteners, Liquid Sweeteners, Canned Vegetables, Almond Flour, Coconut Oil, Coconut Milk, Desiccated Coconut, Nuts & Seeds, Olive Oil, Balsamic Vinegar, White Wine Vinegar.

- Vegetables: Avocado, Onions, Fresh Garlic, Zucchini.

- Fridge: A Pound of Butter, Cream, Yogurt, Eggs, Baby Carrots, Cherry Tomatoes.

Simple Steps for Meal Prep

For whatever day you get started, you're going to want to streamline the process as much as possible. To do that, just follow the simple steps below to help you get started.

Step 1: Make a Shopping List

You'll want to make a shopping list the day before for best results. In the beginning of your 21-day plan, you'll need to make it for a few short days, but at the end, your shopping list will be for a week at a time. Expect to dedicate most of the day to meal prep but remember that it will make life easier.

Step 2: Go Shopping

You'll want to go in and get out when it comes to the grocery store so that you aren't tempted by unhealthy snacks that will pull you out of ketosis. If you have mostly vegetables, try going to the local farmers market where there's less temptation too. A butcher's shop for your meat can also help.

Step 3: Start with a Clean Area

It's going to be easier to start cooking if you clean your area beforehand, and make sure that you have your containers clean too. It's important to make sure you have everything on hand, and it'll help to make it all go by a little quicker.

Step 4: Start Cooking!

Now the only thing left is to start cooking, but make sure that you let your food completely cool before packing it up. If you don't let your food cool, then you can ruin the texture and it may

become soggy upon reheating.

Ketogenic diet is not one of those fad diets that you have probably used before, this diet is completely different because it does not put you in a "fast" or "calorie deprivation" mode, rather it works by simply switching your body's mechanism from the usual high carb reliant to a fat-burning mode – this mode makes it easier for your body to build more muscles and cut down fat deposit.

Contrary to the beliefs in some quarters that Low carb Ketogenic diet will cause high fat deposits in the body, due to the presence of low carbs and high protein and fat contents, the reverse is completely the case. The "Low carb" rule here does not mean you have to consume excess saturated fats that cause high cholesterol, it simply allows you to lower your carb supplies enough, and increase other components marginally. The main benefit of Ketogenic diet is that it forces the body to rely on stored fat and fat from diet, as the primary source of energy. Ketogenic diet helps build more lean muscles while losing fat. The main reason for this is that individuals placed on Ketogenic diets have been found to force their bodies to use up more water, and secondly, the lowered Insulin hormones will force the kidneys to remove excess Sodium and the combined effect of these is that there is a speedy loss of weight within the shortest possible period of time.

Another benefit of Ketogenic diet is that, it targets fat deposit in the most difficult parts of the body, most especially the abdominal region, thighs and the upper chest areas. Starving yourself may not help cut fat in the most difficult regions, even when you lose fat in such areas, they may return quickly, but this is not the case with Ketogenic diets. Losing weight around your mid-section and around vital organs is necessary in order to avoid serious fat-related diseases. Ketogenic diets increases the amount of HDL cholesterols while reducing LDL cholesterol levels. Choosing the right type of unsaturated fats in your Ketogenic diet will help increase good cholesterols (HDL cholesterols), and these are healthy for the heart and general wellbeing. Ketogenic diets also help regulate blood sugar levels while reducing the risks of insulin intolerance. When carbs are broken down, they release sugar into the blood quickly and this increases blood sugar rapidly, a condition that triggers more supply of Insulin hormones, but when Ketogenic diets replace high carb diets, less sugar are released slowly into the body, a situation that can stabilize the secretion of Insulin hormones.

Chapter 5: Shopping List

When shopping applies: Well-planned is usually already won. Anyone who thinks before, what he wants to cook buys more targeted and provides more variety. Generally good: Buy fresh and seasonal goods as much as possible. It tastes better and is often cheaper.

FRUIT AND VEGETABLES

Season: Buy seasonally. Tomatoes, radishes or strawberries have a long journey in the winter and come mostly from the greenhouse. This is at the expense of taste and vitamin content.

Fresh or frozen: Let withered spinach or yellowish broccoli lie down. When in doubt, frozen vegetables are better. It is processed harvest fresh, the vitamin content is higher and the taste better than long-stored goods. Sometimes the handle to preserve is worthwhile. Example tomatoes: Here come fully ripe fruit in the can.

Mature or immature: Ripe fruits give on finger pressure usually slightly and smell good. Some fruits and vegetables can also be bought immature. Apples, bananas, kiwis or avocados ripen at home.

Appearance: The appearance is often secondary: the shinier the apple, the more likely it has been treated with pesticides. You should also ignore size and commercial classes: Especially small fruits are often big in taste.

Packaged fruit: Should you weigh. For cardboard trays, check that the soil is moist. Then down is slush.

Street stalls. Small greengrocers often offer particularly appetizing greens. But you should intensively brush it at home. Car exhaust and abraded brake pads are deposited.

FISH

Storage: If possible, fresh fish should be on ice and covered with it. Also packaged smoked fish must be sufficiently cooled. As a precaution, do not buy goods that have almost reached the end of their shelf life.

Appearance and smell: Moist, bright red gills, shiny skin, clear mucus and clear eyes characterize fresh fish. If the fish smells severe, do without it.

Fish sticks: Are a viable alternative for anyone who likes neither the sight nor the taste of raw fish. They contain all essential ingredients. But: A stick is 35 percent breadcrumbs, which fat and energy levels grow enormously. Who wants to reduce the fat content, can bake the fish fingers in the oven.

Shellfish: Filtering with food also pollutants from the water. If possible, avoid mussels from near-industrial regions. Mussel meat spoils even easier than fish. Open mussels have to close on pressure themselves. Otherwise they should be sorted out.

Surimi: Is not an exquisite delicacy, but a crustacean or crabmeat from fish leftovers. It can also contain dyes and is flavored with sugar, salt and spices. Allergy sufferers should carefully examine the list of ingredients.

Sustainable fishing: The oceans are overfished. About half of the food fish comes from farms today (aquaculture). If you have wild fish, pay attention to the MSC seal or else opt for organic aquaculture.

MEAT

Appearance: Good meat should not be absolutely lean. A light marbling not only serves better cooking, but also the taste. Fresh meat should not be too light, too shiny, dry or too moist.

Self-service: Take a good look at meat: the blood on the bone must be fresh and bright red.

Cool. Meat spoils quickly at room temperature. That means go home quickly and put it in the refrigerator or prepare it.

Whitewashing: Sometimes the rosy fresh offer from the meat counter on the way home gets a pale, unappealing color. This may be due to the lighting in the counter. Anyone who believes that they have been "duped" should change the butcher.

CHEESE

Arrangement: Cheese should be arranged by kinship, ie hard and white and white mold with white cheese. Molds can migrate, and taste notes can influence them.

Aroma: Buy cheese in one piece. Pre-cut, it dries out and quickly loses its aroma. Press soft cheese lightly. Young cheese is firm, more mature gives way

Blueberry Scones
- Preparation time: 10 minutes
- Cooking time: 15 minutes
- Servings: 12

Ingredients:
- Baking powder -2 tsp.
- Vanilla -2 tsp.
- Stevia -.5 c.
- Raspberries -.75 c.
- Almond flour -1.5 c.
- Beaten eggs -3

Directions:
- Allow the oven to heat up to 375 degrees and add some parchment paper to a baking sheet.
- Take out a bowl and beat together the almond flour, eggs, baking powder, vanilla, and stevia. Fold the raspberries in.
- Scoop this batter onto the baking sheet. Add to the oven. After 15 minutes, take the scones out and let them cool down before serving.
- Nutrition Value:
- Calories: 133
- Fats: 8g
- Carbs: 4g
- Protein: 2g

Cinnamon Porridge
- Preparation time: 5 minutes
- Cooking time: 5 minutes
- Servings: 4
- **Ingredients:**
- Cinnamon -1 tsp.
- Stevia -1.5 tsp.
- Butter -1 Tbsp.
- Flaxseed meal -2 Tbsp.
- Oat bran -2 Tbsp.
- Shredded coconut -.5 c.
- Heavy cream -1 c.
- Water -2 c.

Directions:

- Combine all of your ingredients into a pot and mix around.
- Place it on a low flame and bring to a boil. Stir it well when it is boiling and then remove from the heat.
- Divide into four servings and set aside for a bit to thicken.
- Nutrition Value:
- Calories: 171
- Fats: 16g
- Carbs: 6g
- Protein: 2g

Scotch Eggs
- Preparation time: 15 minutes
- Cooking time: 25 minutes
- Servings: 6

Ingredients:
- Pepper -.5 tsp.
- Salt -.33 tp.
- Garlic powder -1.5 tsp.
- Breakfast sausage -1.5 c.
- Peeled hard-boiled eggs

Directions:
- Allow the oven to heat up to 400 degrees. Add the sausage to a bowl and add the garlic, pepper, and salt.
- Divide this into 6 equal parts and add to some baking paper. Flatten them out and then place the hard boiled eggs on top. Wrap the sausage around the egg.
- Arrange onto a baking sheet and place into the oven. After 25 minutes, take these out and allow to cool down.
- Nutrition Value:
- Calories: 258
- Fats: 21g
- Carbs: 1g
- Protein: 17g

Breakfast Tacos
- Preparation time: 10 minutes
- Cooking time: 5 minutes
- Servings: 2

Ingredients:
- Pepper

- Salt
- Tabasco sauce
- Cilantro sprigs -4
- Butter -1 Tbsp.
- Sliced avocado -.5
- Eggs -4
- Low carb tortillas -2

Directions:
- Whisk the eggs until they are smooth. Take out a skillet and heat up the butter on it.
- Add the prepared eggs and spread it out. cook until done and then move to a bowl. Warm up the tortillas and then put on a platter.
- Spread mayo over one side of the tortillas. Divide up the egg on the tortilla and top with the avocado and cilantro. Add the pepper, salt, and pepper sauce.
- Roll up the tortillas and then serve or store.
- Nutrition Value:
- Calories: 289
- Fats: 27g
- Carbs: 6g
- Protein: 7g

Vanilla Smoothie
- Preparation time: 2 minutes
- Cooking time: 0
- Servings: 1

Ingredients:
- Whipped cream
- Liquid stevia -3 drops
- Vanilla -.5 tsp.
- Ice cubes -4
- Water -.25 c.
- Mascarpone cheese -.5 c.
- Egg yolks -2

Directions:
- Take out your blender and add in all the ingredients.
- Place the lid on top and blend. When the ingredients are well mixed, pour into a glass and serve.

- Nutrition Value:
- Calories: 650
- Fats: 64g
- Carbs: 4g
- Protein: 12g

Blackberry Egg Bake
- Preparation time: 10 minutes
- Cooking time: 15 minutes
- Servings: 4

Ingredients:
- Chopped rosemary -1 tsp.
- Orange zest -.5 tsp.
- Salt
- Vanilla -.25 tsp.
- Grated ginger -1 tsp.
- Coconut flour -3 Tbsp.
- Butter -1 Tbsp.
- Egg -5
- Blackberries -.5 c.

Directions:
- Allow the oven to heat up to 350 degrees. Take out a blender and add all the ingredients inside to blend well.
- Pour this into each muffin cup and then add the blackberries on top. Place into the oven to bake.
- After 15 minutes, take the dish out and store!
- Nutrition Value:
- Calories: 144
- Fats: 10g
- Carbs: 2g
- Protein: 8.5g

Coconut Pancakes
- Preparation time: 10 minutes
- Cooking time: 5 minutes
- Servings: 2

Ingredients:
- Maple syrup -4 Tbsp.
- Shredded coconut -.25 c.
- Salt
- Erythritol -.5 Tbsp.
- Cinnamon -1 tsp.
- Almond flour -1 Tbsp.

- Cream cheese -2 oz.
- Eggs -2

Directions:
- Beat the eggs together before adding in the almond flour and cream cheese.
- Now add in the rest of the ingredients and stir until well combined.
- Take out a frying pan and fry the pancakes on both sides. Add to a plate and sprinkle some coconut on top.
- Nutrition Value:
- Calories: 575
- Fats: 51g
- Carbs: 3.5g
- Protein: 19g

Chocolate Chip Waffles
- Preparation time: 8 minutes
- Cooking time: 10 minutes
- Servings: 2

Ingredients:
- Maple syrup -.5 c.
- Cacao nibs -50g
- Salt
- Butter -2 Tbsp.
- Separated eggs -2
- Protein powder -2 scoops

Directions:
- Take out a bowl and beat the egg whites until soft peaks form. In a second bowl mix the butter, protein powder, and egg yolks.
- Now fold the egg whites into this mixture and add the cacao nibs and salt.
- Pour the mixture into a waffle maker and let it cook until golden brown on both sides. Serve with maple syrup.
- Nutrition Value:
- Calories: 400
- Fats: 26g
- Carbs: 4.5g
- Protein: 34g

Chocolate and Peanut Butter Muffins
- Preparation time: 20 minutes
- Cooking time: 20 minutes

- Servings: 6

Ingredients:
- Eggs -2
- Almond milk -.33 c.
- Peanut butter -.33 c.
- Salt
- Baking powder -1 tsp.
- Erythritol -.5 c.
- Almond flour -1 c.

Directions:
- Bring out a bowl and mix the salt, baking powder, erythritol, and almond flour together. Add the eggs, almond milk, and peanut butter next.
- Finally, mix in the cacao nibs before pouring this into a muffin tin.
- Allow the oven to heat up to 350 degrees. Place the muffin tray into the oven to bake.
- After 25 minutes, the muffins are done and you can store.
- Nutrition Value:
- Calories: 265
- Fats: 20.5g
- Carbs: 2g
- Protein: 7.5g

Blender pancakes
- Preparation time: 5 minutes:
- Cooking time: 5 minutes
- Servings: 1

Ingredients:
- Salt
- Cinnamon
- Protein powder -1 scoop
- Eggs -2
- Cream cheese -2 oz.

Directions:
- Add the salt, cinnamon, protein powder, eggs, and cream cheese to a blender and combine well.
- Take out a skillet and fry the batter on both sides until done. Serve warm.
- Nutrition Value:
- Calories: 450

- Fat: 29g
- Carbs: 4g
- Protein: 41g

Butter Coffee
- Preparation time: 5 minutes
- Cooking time
- Servings: 1

Ingredients:
- Coconut oil -1 Tbsp.
- Butter -1 Tbsp.
- Coffee -2 Tbsp.
- Water -1 c.

Directions:
- Bring out a pan and boil the water inside. When the water is boiling, add in the coffee, coconut oil, and butter.
- Once these are all melted and hot, pour into a cup through a strainer and enjoy.
- Nutrition Value:
- Calories: 230
- Fat: 25g
- Carbs: 0g
- Protein: 0g

Mocha Chia Pudding
- Preparation time: 5 minutes
- Cooking time: 10 minutes
- Servings: 2

Ingredients:
- Cacao nibs -2 Tbsp.
- Swerve -1 Tbsp.
- Vanilla -1 Tbsp.
- Coconut cream -.33 g
- Chia seeds -55g
- Water -2 c.
- Herbal coffee -2 Tbsp.

Directions:
- Brew the herbal coffee with some hot water until the liquid is reduced in half. Strain the coffee before mixing in with the vanilla, swerve, and coconut cream.
- Add in the chia seeds and cacao nibs net. Pour into some cups and place in the fridge for 30 minutes before serving.
- Nutrition Value:

- Calories: 257
- Fat: 20.25g
- Carbs: 2.25g
- Protein: 7g

Keto Green Eggs
- Preparation time: 5 minutes
- Cooking time: 12 minutes
- Servings:2

Ingredients:
- Ground cayenne -.25 tsp.
- Ground cumin -.25 tsp.
- Eggs -4
- Chopped parsley -.5 c.
- Chopped cilantro -.5 c.
- Thyme leaves -1 tsp.
- Garlic cloves -2
- Coconut oil -1 Tbsp.
- Butter -2 Tbsp.

Directions:
- Melt the butter and coconut oil in a skillet before adding the garlic and frying. Add in the thyme, parsley and cilantro and cook another 3 minutes.
- At this time, add in the eggs and season. Cover with a lid and let this cook for another 5 minutes before serving.
- Nutrition Value:
- Calories: 311
- Fat: 27.5g
- Carbs: 4g
- Protein: 12.8g

Cheddar Souffles
- Preparation time: 15 minutes
- Cooking time: 25 minutes
- Servings: 8

Ingredients:
- Cheddar cheese -2 c.
- Heavy cream -.75 c.
- Cayenne pepper -.25 tsp.
- Xanthan gum -.5 tsp.
- Pepper -.5 tsp.
- Ground mustard -1 tsp.
- Salt -1 tsp.
- Almond flour -.5 c.

- Salt -1 pinch
- Cream of tartar -.25 tsp.
- Eggs -6
- Chopped chives -.25 c.

Directions:

- Allow the oven to heat up to 350 degrees. Take out a bowl and mix all the ingredients besides the eggs and cream of tartar together.
- Separate the egg whites and yolks and add the yolks in with the first mixture. Beat the egg whites and cream of tartar until you get stiff peaks to form.
- Take this mixture and add into the other mixture. When done, pour into the ramekins and place in the oven.
- After 25 minutes, these are done and you can serve or store.
- Nutrition Value:
- Calories: 288
- Fat: 21g
- Carbs: 3g
- Protein: 14g

Ricotta Pie

- Preparation time: 10 minutes
- Cooking time: 30 minutes
- Servings: 6

Ingredients:

- Mozzarella -1 c.
- Eggs -3
- Ricotta cheese -2 c.
- Swiss chard -8 c.
- Garlic clove -1
- Chopped onion -.5 c.
- Olive oil -1 Tbsp.
- Mild sausage -1 lb.
- Pepper
- Salt
- Nutmeg
- Parmesan -.25 c.

Directions:

- Heat up the garlic, onion, and oil on a pan. When those are warm, add in the swiss chard and fry to make the leaves wilt.
- Add in the nutmeg and set it aside. In a new bowl, beat the eggs before adding in the cheeses. Now add in the prepared swiss chard mixture.
- Roll out the sausage and press it into a pie tart. Pour the filing inside. Allow the oven to heat to 350 degrees.
- Place the pie inside and let it bake. After 30 minutes, it is done and you can store or serve.
- Nutrition Value:
- Calories: 344
- Fat: 27g
- Carbs: 4g
- Protein: 23g

Vegetarian Red Coconut Curry

- Servings: 2
- Preparation time: 35 mins
- Ingredients
- ¾ cup spinach
- ¼ medium onion, chopped
- 1 teaspoon ginger, minced
- 1 cup broccoli florets
- 4 tablespoons coconut oil
- 1 teaspoon garlic, minced
- 2 teaspoons coconut aminos
- 1 tablespoon red curry paste
- 2 teaspoons soy sauce
- ½ cup coconut cream

Directions

- Heat 2 tablespoons of coconut oil in a pan and add garlic and onions.
- Sauté for about 3 minutes and add broccoli.
- Sauté for about 3 minutes and move vegetables to the side of the pan.
- Add curry paste and cook for about 1 minute.
- Mix well and add spinach, cooking for about 3 minutes.
- Add coconut cream, remaining coconut oil, ginger, soy sauce and coconut aminos.
- Allow it to simmer for about 10 minutes

and dish out to serve.

- Nutrition Value:Calories: 439 Carbs: 12g Fats: 44g Proteins: 3.6g Sodium: 728mg Sugar: 3.5g

Zucchini Noodles with Avocado Sauce

- Servings: 2
- Preparation time: 10 mins
- Ingredients
- 1¼ cup basil
- 4 tablespoons pine nuts
- 1 zucchini, spiralized
- 1/3 cup water
- 2 tablespoons lemon juice
- 2 cherry tomatoes, sliced
- 1 avocado

Directions

- Put all the ingredients except the cherry tomatoes and zucchini in a blender and blend until smooth.
- Mix together the blended sauce and zucchini noodles and cherry tomatoes in a serving bowl and serve.
- Nutrition Value:Calories: 366 Carbs: 19.7g Fats: 32g Proteins: 7.1g Sodium: 27mg Sugar: 6.4g

Tomato Basil and Mozzarella Galette

- Servings: 2
- Preparation time: 35 mins
- Ingredients
- 1 large egg
- 1 teaspoon garlic powder
- ¾ cup almond flour
- 2 tablespoons mozzarella liquid
- ¼ cup Parmesan cheese, shredded
- 3 leaves fresh basil
- 2 plum tomatoes
- 1½ tablespoons pesto
- 1/3-ounce Mozzarella cheese
- Directions
- Preheat oven to 365 degrees F and line a cookie sheet with parchment paper.
- Mix together the garlic powder, almond flour and mozzarella liquid in a bowl.
- Add Parmesan cheese and egg and mix to

form a dough.

- Form balls out of this dough mixture and transfer on the cookie sheet.
- Press the dough balls with a fork and spread pesto over the centre of the crust evenly.
- Layer mozzarella, tomatoes and basil leaves, and fold the edges of the crust up and over the filling.
- Transfer in the oven and bake for about 20 minutes.
- Dish out to serve.
- Nutrition Value:Calories: 396 Carbs: 17.6g Fats: 29.2g Proteins: 17.5g Sodium: 199mg Sugar: 6.2g

Cheesy Spaghetti Squash with Pesto

- Servings: 2
- Preparation time: 25 mins
- Ingredients
- ½ tablespoon olive oil
- ¼ cup whole milk ricotta cheese
- 1/8 cup basil pesto
- 1 cup cooked spaghetti squash, drained
- Salt and black pepper, to taste
- 2 oz fresh mozzarella cheese, cubed

Directions

- Preheat the oven to 375 degrees F and grease a casserole dish.
- Mix together squash and olive oil in a medium-sized bowl and season with salt and black pepper.
- Put the squash in the casserole dish and top with ricotta and mozzarella cheese.
- Bake for about 10 minutes and remove from the oven.
- Drizzle the pesto over the top and serve hot.
- Nutrition Value:Calories: 169 Carbs: 6.2g Fats: 11.3g Proteins: 11.9g Sodium: 217mg Sugar: 0.1g

Vegan Sesame Tofu and Eggplant

- Servings: 2
- Preparation time: 30 mins
- Ingredients

- ½ cup cilantro, chopped
- 2 tablespoons toasted sesame oil
- ½ teaspoon crushed red pepper flakes
- ½ eggplant, julienned
- ½ pound block firm tofu, pressed
- 1½ tablespoons rice vinegar
- 1 clove garlic, finely minced
- 1 teaspoon Swerve
- ½ tablespoon olive oil
- 1/8 cup sesame seeds
- Salt and black pepper, to taste
- 1/8 cup soy sauce

Directions
- Preheat the oven to 200 degrees F.
- Mix together cilantro, eggplant, rice vinegar, half of toasted sesame oil, garlic, red pepper flakes and Swerve in a bowl.
- Heat olive oil in a skillet and add the marinated eggplant.
- Sauté for about 4 minutes and transfer the eggplant noodles to an oven safe dish.
- Cover with a foil and place into the oven to keep warm.
- Spread the sesame seeds on a plate and press both sides of each piece of tofu into the seeds.
- Add remaining sesame oil and tofu to the skillet and fry for about 5 minutes.
- Pour soy sauce into the pan and cook until the tofu slices are browned.
- Remove the eggplant noodles from the oven and top with tofu to serve.
- Nutrition Value:Calories: 333 Carbs: 13.9g Fats: 26.6g Proteins: 13.3g Sodium: 918mg Sugar: 4.5g

Cheesy Spinach Puffs
- Servings: 2
- Preparation time: 25 mins
- Ingredients
- ½ cup almond flour
- 1 large egg
- ¼ cup feta cheese, crumbled
- ½ teaspoon kosher salt
- ½ teaspoon garlic powder

- 1½ tablespoons heavy whipping cream

Directions
- Preheat the oven to 350 degrees F and grease a cookie sheet.
- Put all the ingredients in a blender and pulse until smooth.
- Allow to cool down and form 1-inch balls from this mixture.
- Arrange on a cookie sheet and transfer into the oven.
- Bake for about 12 minutes and dish out to serve.
- Nutrition Value:Calories: 294 Carbs: 7.8g Fats: 24g Proteins: 12.2g Sodium: 840mg Sugar: 1.1g

Lobster Salad
- Servings: 2
- Preparation time: 15 mins
- Ingredients
- ¼ yellow onion, chopped
- ¼ yellow bell pepper, seeded and chopped
- ¾ pound cooked lobster meat, shredded
- 1 celery stalk, chopped
- Black pepper, to taste
- ¼ cup avocado mayonnaise

Directions
- Mix together all the ingredients in a bowl and stir until well combined.
- Refrigerate for about 3 hours and serve chilled.
- Put the salad into a container for meal prepping and refrigerate for about 2 days.
- Nutrition Value:Calories: 336 Carbohydrates: 2g Protein: 27.2g Fat: 25.2g   Sugar: 1.2g Sodium: 926mg

Beef Sausage Pancakes
- Servings: 2
- Preparation time: 30 mins
- Ingredients
- 4 gluten-free Italian beef sausages, sliced
- 1 tablespoon olive oil
- 1/3 large red bell peppers, seeded and sliced thinly
- 1/3 cup spinach

- ¾ teaspoon garlic powder
- 1/3 large green bell peppers, seeded and sliced thinly
- ¾ cup heavy whipped cream
- Salt and black pepper, to taste

Directions
- Mix together all the ingredients in a bowl except whipped cream and keep aside.
- Put butter and half of the mixture in a skillet and cook for about 6 minutes on both sides.
- Repeat with the remaining mixture and dish out.
- Beat whipped cream in another bowl until smooth.
- Serve the beef sausage pancakes with whipped cream.
- For meal prepping, it is compulsory to gently slice the sausages before mixing with other ingredients.
- Nutrition Value:Calories: 415 Carbohydrates: 7g Protein: 29.5g Fat: 31.6g Sugar: 4.3g Sodium: 1040mg

Holiday Chicken Salad
- Servings: 2
- Preparation time: 25 mins
- Ingredients
- 1 celery stalk, chopped
- 1½ cups cooked grass-fed chicken, chopped
- ¼ cup fresh cranberries
- ¼ cup sour cream
- ½ apple, chopped
- ¼ yellow onion, chopped
- 1/8 cup almonds, toasted and chopped
- 2-ounce feta cheese, crumbled
- ¼ cup avocado mayonnaise
- Salt and black pepper, to taste

Directions
- Stir together all the ingredients in a bowl except almonds and cheese.
- Top with almonds and cheese to serve.
- Meal Prep Tip: Don't add almonds and cheese in the salad if you want to store the

salad. Cover with a plastic wrap and refrigerate to serve.
- Nutrition Value:Calories: 336 Carbohydrates: 8.8g Protein: 24.5g Fat: 23.2g Sugar: 5.4g Sodium: 383mg

Luncheon Fancy Salad
- Servings: 2
- Preparation time: 40 mins
- Ingredients
- 6-ounce cooked salmon, chopped
- 1 tablespoon fresh dill, chopped
- Salt and black pepper, to taste
- 4 hard-boiled grass-fed eggs, peeled and cubed
- 2 celery stalks, chopped
- ½ yellow onion, chopped
- ¾ cup avocado mayonnaise

Directions
- Put all the ingredients in a bowl and mix until well combined.
- Cover with a plastic wrap and refrigerate for about 3 hours to serve.
- For meal prepping, put the salad in a container and refrigerate for up to 3 days.
- Nutrition Value:Calories: 303 Carbohydrates: 1.7g Protein: 10.3g Fat: 30g Sugar: 1g Sodium: 314mg

Italian Platter
- Servings: 2
- Preparation time: 45 mins
- Ingredients
- 1 garlic clove, minced
- 5-ounce fresh button mushrooms, sliced
- 1/8 cup unsalted butter
- ¼ teaspoon dried thyme
- 1/3 cup heavy whipping cream
- Salt and black pepper, to taste
- 2 -6-ounce grass-fed New York strip steaks

Directions
- Preheat the grill to medium heat and grease it.
- Season the steaks with salt and black pepper, and transfer to the grill.

- Grill steaks for about 10 minutes on each side and dish out in a platter.
- Put butter, mushrooms, salt and black pepper in a pan and cook for about 10 minutes.
- Add thyme and garlic and thyme and sauté for about 1 minute.
- Stir in the cream and let it simmer for about 5 minutes.
- Top the steaks with mushroom sauce and serve hot immediately.
- Meal Prep Tip: You can store the mushroom sauce in refrigerator for about 2 days. Season the steaks carefully with salt and black pepper to avoid low or high quantities.
- Nutrition Value:Calories: 332 Carbohydrates: 3.2g Protein: 41.8g Fat: 20.5g Sugar: 1.3g Sodium: 181mg

Meat Loaf

- Servings: 12
- Preparation time: 1 hour 15 mins
- Ingredients
- 1 garlic clove, minced
- ½ teaspoon dried thyme, crushed
- ½ pound grass-fed lean ground beef
- 1 organic egg, beaten
- Salt and black pepper, to taste
- ¼ cup onions, chopped
- 1/8 cup sugar-free ketchup
- 2 cups mozzarella cheese, freshly grated
- ¼ cup green bell pepper, seeded and chopped
- ½ cup cheddar cheese, grated
- 1 cup fresh spinach, chopped

Directions
- Preheat the oven to 350 degrees F and grease a baking dish.
- Put all the ingredients in a bowl except spinach and cheese and mix well.
- Arrange the meat over a wax paper and top with spinach and cheese.
- Roll the paper around the mixture to form a meatloaf.

- Remove the wax paper and transfer the meat loaf in the baking dish.
- Put it in the oven and bake for about 1 hour.
- Dish out and serve hot.
- Meal Prep Tip: Let the meat loafs cool for about 10 minutes to bring them to room temperature before serving.
- Nutrition Value:Calories: 439 Carbohydrates: 8g Protein: 40.8g Fat: 26g Sugar: 1.6g Sodium: 587mg

Grilled Steak

Servings: 2
- Preparation time: 15 mins
- Ingredients
- ¼ cup unsalted butter
- 2 garlic cloves, minced
- ¾ pound beef top sirloin steaks
- ¾ teaspoon dried rosemary, crushed
- 2 oz. parmesan cheese, shredded
- Salt and black pepper, to taste

Directions
- Preheat the grill and grease it.
- Season the sirloin steaks with salt and black pepper.
- Transfer the steaks on the grill and cook for about 5 minutes on each side.
- Dish out the steaks in plates and keep aside.
- Meanwhile, put butter and garlic in a pan and heat until melted.
- Pour it on the steaks and serve hot.
- Divide the steaks in 2 containers and refrigerate for about 3 days for meal prepping purpose. Reheat in microwave before serving.

Nutrition Value:Calories:
- 83 Carbohydrates: 1.5g   Protein:
- 41.4g Fat: 23.6g Sugar: 0g Sodium: 352mg

Roasted Veggie Salad

Total time: 30 minutes

Ingredients

- 2 cups cubed butternut squash (I keep the skin on but you can remove it if you wish)
- 2 cups cubed sweet potato
- 2 carrots, chopped into chunks
- 2 large Portobello mushrooms, thickly sliced
- 2 large zucchinis, cut into chunks
- 1 head of broccoli, cut into florets
- 2 tbsp. sunflower seeds
- 2 tbsp. pumpkin seeds
- 3 tbsp. olive oil (I've added the oil in here because it's quite a lot and it adjusts the calorie count)
- Salt and pepper, to taste

Directions

- Preheat the oven to 356 degrees Fahrenheit and prepare a tray by lining it with baking paper.
- Place all ingredients onto the tray and add a sprinkle of salt and pepper.
- Combine the ingredients together with your hands, making sure everything gets coated in olive oil.
- Place into the oven and bake for approximately 30 minutes or until the veggies are soft and the seeds are toasted.
- Divide into your 4 containers, cover and place into the fridge until needed.

Pita Pockets with Lamb and Salad

Total time: 20 minutes

Ingredients

- 12 oz. lamb steaks, cut into cubes
- 1 tsp. ground cumin
- Salt and pepper, to taste
- 4 whole-meal pita breads
- 2 cups salad greens (mixed kale, lettuce and arugula is ideal)
- 4 tbsp. plain yogurt
- 1 lemon, cut into quarters

Directions

- Drizzle some olive oil into a fry pan and place over a medium heat.
- Add the lamb, cumin, salt and pepper and stir to combine, sauté for about 7 minutes or until the lamb cubes are cooked but still a little pink.
- Make a slit in each pita bread and fill each one with mixed salad greens, lamb, and a drizzle of yogurt.
- Place the filled pitas into your 4 containers and place a lemon quarter in each one so you can squeeze it over the pita when you're ready to eat!
- Cover the containers and store in the fridge until needed.

Sticky Chicken and Broccoli Prep Bowls

Total time: 30 minutes

Ingredients

- 2 tbsp. honey
- 2 tsp. soy sauce (tamari is best)
- 4 boneless, skinless chicken thighs
- 1 head of broccoli, cut into florets
- 1 tsp. sesame oil

Directions

- Drizzle some olive oil into a frying pan and place over a medium heat.
- Add the honey and soy sauce, place the chicken thighs into the pan and stir to coat in soy and honey, sauté for approximately 15 minutes or until the chicken is almost cooked.
- Add the broccoli to the pan, increase the heat to high, splash a few teaspoons of water into the pan and immediate place a lid onto the pan – this will steam the broccoli.
- Once the water has evaporated, remove the lid and check that the chicken has cooked through and the broccoli is cooked yet crunchy.
- Drizzle the sesame oil over the broccoli before dividing the chicken and broccoli

- between your 4 containers.
- Cover and store in the fridge until needed!

Quinoa and Fresh Greens Salad
Total time: 25 minutes
Ingredients
- 1 cup dry quinoa
- 1 ½ cups (12floz) salt-reduced chicken broth/stock
- 3 cups shredded lettuce (use any, I use iceberg)
- 2 cups baby spinach leaves
- 2 green bell peppers, core and seeds removed, sliced
- 3 oz. feta cheese, cut into small chunks
- Salt and pepper, to taste

Directions
- Thoroughly rinse the quinoa in a sieve to remove the bitter outer layer.
- Bring the chicken broth to the boil in a small pot and add the quinoa, stir to combine then turn the heat down to a simmer, cover, and cook for 12-15 minutes or until the liquid has disappeared and the quinoa is soft.
- Divide the cooked quinoa between your 4 containers, then divide the lettuce, spinach, bell peppers and feta between the containers and place on top of the quinoa.
- Sprinkle with salt and pepper and a drizzle of olive oil to finish.
- Cover and place into the fridge until needed!

Homemade Hummus, Tomato, and Ham Rice Wafer Stacks
Total time: 20 minutes
Ingredients
- 1 can of chickpeas, drained
- 1 tbsp. tahini
- 1 garlic clove
- 4 tbsp. olive oil
- 1 lemon
- Salt and pepper, to taste

- 12 rice wafers
- 2 large tomatoes, sliced
- 4 large slices of deli ham

Directions
- Make the hummus by placing the chickpeas, tahini, garlic clove, olive oil, juice of one lemon, salt and pepper into a blender or food processor and blending until smooth.
- Wrap your rice wafers in plastic wrap to keep them fresh and place them into the pantry.
- Place a good drop of hummus into one corner of your airtight containers, then divide the tomato and ham between the containers too.
- Place the lid onto your containers and place them into the fridge until needed.
- When it's time to pack your lunch into your work bag, simply place a container of toppings into your bag and grab a packet of wrapped rice wafers too.
- Assemble just before eating for a fresh and crunchy lunch!

Grilled Salmon and Seasonal Greens
Total time: 30 minutes
Ingredients
- 4 small-medium salmon filets
- Salt and pepper, to taste
- Olive oil
- 1 head of broccoli, cut into florets
- 2 large zucchinis, chopped into chunks
- 1 tsp. sesame oil

Directions
- Preheat the oven to 356 degrees Fahrenheit and line a baking tray with baking paper, place the salmon filets onto the tray and sprinkle with salt, pepper and a little olive oil.
- Place into the oven and bake for approximately 12 minutes or until cooked to your liking.
- As the salmon cooks, prepare the greens by placing a pot of water over a high heat

and bringing to the boil, place a steaming basket or double boiler over the pot and place the greens inside, place the lid onto the basket.

- Steam the veggies for a few minutes until just cooked, sprinkle with the sesame oil and some salt and pepper.
- Place a salmon filet into each container and divide the veggies between each container.
- Place the lid onto each container and place into the fridge to store before serving.
- Eat hot or cold!

Chicken, strawberry, and black rice salad

Total time: 40 minutes
Ingredients
- 2 cups dry black rice
- 1 large chicken breast
- Olive oil
- Salt and pepper, to taste
- 1 cup strawberries, stalks removed, sliced
- 1 lemon

Directions
- Preheat the oven to 356 degrees Fahrenheit and line a baking tray with baking paper.
- Place the rice into a pot and add 4 cups of water and a pinch of salt, bring to the boil then reduce to a simmer, cover and let simmer until the water has disappeared and the rice is cooked.
- While the rice is cooking, cook the chicken by placing it onto the lined baking tray, drizzling with olive oil, and sprinkling with salt and pepper, bake in the preheated oven for approximately 20 minutes or until cooked through.
- Shred the cooked chicken breast and add to the pot with the cooked black rice.
- Place the strawberries into the pot and squeeze in the juice of one lemon.
- Season with salt and pepper before

stirring to combine.
- Divide between your 4 containers, cover and store in the fridge until needed!

Cauliflower Rice and Chili Chicken
Total time: 30 minutes
Ingredients
- 1 head of cauliflower, core removed, florets cut into chunks
- Salt and pepper, to taste
- 4 boneless, skinless chicken thighs
- 2 tbsp. olive oil
- 1 fresh red chili, finely chopped
- 1 garlic clove, crushed
- 1 lemon, cut into quarters

Directions
- Preheat the oven to 356 degrees Fahrenheit and line a baking tray with baking paper.
- Place the cauliflower into a food processor and blend until it resembles the size and consistency of rice.
- Place the cauliflower into a bowl and sprinkle with salt and pepper, place in the microwave and cook on HIGH for 1 minute increments until cooked through.
- Place the chicken thighs onto the lined baking tray and sprinkle the olive oil, chili, garlic, salt and pepper on top rub to combine and make sure the chicken is well-coated.
- Place the chicken into the preheated oven and bake for approximately 20 minutes or until the chicken is cooked through.
- Divide the cauliflower rice between the 4 containers and place a chicken thigh into each container on top of the "rice".
- Place a lemon quarter into each container, cover and place into the fridge until needed!

Loaded Broccoli Salad with Toasted Seeds
Total time: 20 minutes
Ingredients
- Olive oil

- 1 large head of broccoli, stalk removed, cut into florets
- ¼ red onion, finely chopped
- 2 tbsp. pumpkin seeds
- 2 tbsp. sunflower seeds
- 3 tbsp. grated Parmesan cheese
- Salt and pepper, to taste

Directions
- Drizzle some olive oil into a frying pan and place over a medium heat.
- Add the broccoli and sauté for a few minutes.
- Pour a few tablespoons of water into the pan and immediately place a lid on top to trap the steam, this will steam the broccoli.
- Once the water has evaporated and the broccoli is cooked but still has a "bite", add the red onion, pumpkin seeds and sunflower seeds, continue cooking for about 1 minute until the seeds are gently toasted.
- Divide the broccoli mixture between your 4 containers and sprinkle the Parmesan over each one.
- Finish with a sprinkle of salt and pepper and a little drizzle of olive oil.
- Cover and place into the fridge until needed!

White Bean and Tomato Salad with Balsamic Dressing

Total time: 10 minutes
Ingredients
- 2 cans white beans, drained
- 3 ripe tomatoes, cut into chunks
- Small handful of fresh basil, roughly chopped
- 2 tbsp. balsamic vinegar mixed with 2 tablespoons of olive oil
- Salt and pepper, to taste

Directions
- Place the beans, tomatoes, basil, balsamic, olive oil, salt and pepper into a small bowl and mix to combine.

- Divide into your 4 containers, cover and place into the fridge to store until needed.
- Eat cold!

One-Tray Chicken Thigh and Root Veggie Baked "Bowls"

Total time: 35 minutes
Ingredients
- 4 boneless, skinless chicken thighs
- 2 carrots, cut into small chunks
- 2 parsnips, peeled and cut into chunks
- 2 raw beets, cut into chunks
- 1 large red onion, cut into wedges
- 1 tsp. mixed dried herbs
- Olive oil
- Salt and pepper, to taste
- 1 lemon, cut into quarters

Directions
- Preheat the oven to 356 degrees Fahrenheit and line a baking tray with baking paper.
- Place the chicken thighs, carrots, parsnips, beets, onion, herbs and a drizzle of olive oil onto the tray, add a pinch of salt and pepper and combine all of the ingredients with your hands.
- Place the tray into the oven and bake for approximately 30 minutes or until the chicken is cooked through and the veggies are soft.
- Divide the chicken and veggies between the 4 containers and place a lemon quarter into each container.
- Place into the fridge to store until needed!

Cold Soba Noodle Salad with Cashews, Carrot and Tofu

Total time: 20 minutes
Ingredients
- 14 oz. dry soba noodles
- 2 tbsp. sesame oil
- 2 tbsp. soy sauce
- 1 tbsp. honey
- 9 oz. firm tofu, sliced
- 1/3 cup raw cashew nuts
- 2 carrots, peeled and chopped into small

pieces

Directions

- Place a pot of water over a high heat, bring to the boil and add the soba noodles, cook until soft.
- While the noodles are cooking, drizzle the sesame oil, soy sauce and honey into a small non-stick fry pan and place over a medium heat.
- Place the tofu slices into the hot pan and cook for a couple of minutes on each side until golden.
- Drain the noodles and place into a bowl.
- Add the cashews, carrots, and cooked tofu with any oil/soy sauce left over in the fry pan.
- Stir to combine.
- Divide into your 4 containers, cover and place into the fridge to store until needed!
- Best eaten cold!

Basil, Tomato and Haloumi Salad with Cos and Cucumber

Total time: 20 minutes

Ingredients

- 7 oz. halloumi cheese, sliced into 12 slices
- 2 cos or Romaine lettuces, roughly chopped
- 1 cup chopped cucumber
- 3 large tomatoes, sliced
- Large handful of fresh basil, roughly chopped
- 2 tbsp. apple cider vinegar mixed with 2 tbsp. olive oil

Directions

- Heat a non-stick frying pan over a high heat.
- Add the halloumi slices to the pan and cook on both sides until golden.
- Divide the lettuce, cucumber, tomatoes, basil, and halloumi between the 4 containers.
- Sprinkle with salt and pepper and the oil/ vinegar mixture, gently toss to combine and coat with dressing.

- Cover and place into the fridge to store until needed.

Prepped Topping Packs for Rice Wafers

Total time: 10 minutes

Ingredients

- 1 cup cottage cheese
- 4 tbsp. chopped chives
- 1 fresh tomato, sliced
- 4 slices of deli ham or turkey
- 4 tbsp. peanut butter
- 1 banana, cut into 4 chunks
- (plus 4 rice wafers per lunch serving)

Directions

- Place the cottage cheese, chives, tomato, ham or turkey, peanut butter, and banana into a container with separated compartments.
- Cover and place into the fridge to store until needed.
- Wrap the rice wafers in sealable bags or plastic wrap, or keep them in an airtight container at work to pull out whenever you need them!

Minced Lamb Meat Balls with Yogurt and Cucumber Dip

Total time: 25 minutes

Ingredients:

- 17.5 oz. minced lamb
- ½ red onion, finely chopped
- 1 egg
- ½ cup almond flour
- Salt and pepper, to taste
- Olive oil
- ½ cup plain Greek yogurt
- ¾ cup finely chopped cucumber

Directions

- Place the minced lamb, red onion, egg, almond flour, salt and pepper into a bowl and stir to combine.
- Drizzle some olive oil into a non-stick fry pan and place over a medium heat.
- Roll the lamb mixture into 16 balls and place them in 2 batches into the hot pan,

cook for about 7 minutes, turning a few times until golden and cooked through.

- Stir together the yogurt and cucumber in a small bowl.
- Place 4 lamb balls into each container and place a drop of yogurt mixture over top.
- Cover and place into the fridge to store until needed.
- Eat cold or hot! (Place the yogurt on the side if you want to eat the lamb balls hot, so then you don't have to heat the yogurt as well).

Smoked Salmon and Avocado Wholegrain Wraps

Total time: 20 minutes

Ingredients

- 4 wholegrain wraps
- 2 cups lettuce, roughly sliced
- 2 avocadoes, flesh sliced
- 3 oz. smoked salmon
- Olive oil
- 1 tbsp. balsamic vinegar mixed with 1 tablespoon of olive oil

Directions

- Place your wraps onto a large board or clean bench.
- Place a pile of lettuce onto each one, then add ½ an avocado (sliced) on top, place the salmon on top of the avocado and drizzle with olive oil and vinegar.
- Carefully wrap your wraps into tight parcels, place into your containers and store in the fridge until needed.

Cold Tuna and Pasta Salad

Total time: 30 minutes

Ingredients

- 1 ½ cups whole-meal penne pasta (or any other shapes you have handy!)
- 2 cans tuna (the single-serve cans) drained
- 2 carrots, peeled and cut into small pieces
- ¾ cup corn kernels
- 1 avocado, flesh cut into chunks
- 1 red bell pepper, core and seeds removed, flesh cut into small pieces

- Salt and pepper, to taste

Directions

- Bring a pot of water to boil and add pinch of salt and the dry pasta, cook until the pasta is al dente (some pastas differ so use the instructions on your packet).
- Drain the pasta and leave to cool slightly before adding the tuna, carrots, corn, avocado, bell pepper, salt, pepper and a drizzle of olive oil.
- Divide the pasta salad between your 4 containers, cover and place into the fridge to store until needed.
- Serve cold!

Tuna, Corn, and Cheese Hot Sandwiches (for cheat days and cravings)

Total time: 15 minutes

Ingredients

- 4 slices of cheddar cheese
- 8 slices of wholegrain bread
- 1 cup corn kernels, fresh or canned
- 2 small cans of tuna (single-serve cans, half a can per sandwich)
- Salt and pepper, to taste

Directions

- Place a slice of cheese onto 4 of your bread slices, top with corn kernels and tuna, sprinkle with salt and pepper then place the other slice of bread on top of each sandwich.
- Wrap in plastic wrap to keep the sandwiches together and place into your airtight containers.
- Store in the fridge until need, and place into a hot sandwich press to toast before eating!

Stuffed Sweet Potatoes

Total time: 20 minutes

Ingredients

- 4 sweet potatoes, pricked all over with a fork
- 1 scallion, finely chopped
- Small handful of parsley, finely chopped

- 1 cup cottage cheese
- 1 cup baby spinach leaves
- Salt and pepper, to taste

Directions

- Place the sweet potatoes into the microwave and cook on HIGH for 1 minute increments until soft all the way through.
- Cut the sweet potatoes in half and remove the flesh and place it into a small bowl.
- Add the scallions, parsley, cottage cheese, spinach, salt and pepper, stir to combine.
- Re-fill the sweet potato skins with the filling and place 2 halves into each of your 4 containers.
- Place into the fridge to store until needed!

Grilled Chicken with Sweet Potatoes and Asparagus

Total time: 35 minutes

Ingredients

- 4 small chicken breasts
- 1 large sweet potato, cut into chunks
- 16 spears of asparagus, tough ends removed
- 2 tbsp. olive oil
- 1 tsp. dried rosemary
- Salt and pepper, to taste

Directions

- Preheat the oven to 356 degrees Fahrenheit and prepare a tray by lining it with baking paper.
- Place the chicken, sweet potato, asparagus, olive oil, rosemary, salt and pepper onto the tray and combine with your hands until everything is coated in oil and seasoning.
- Place into the oven and bake for approximately 30 minutes or until the chicken is cooked through and the sweet potatoes are soft.
- Divide between your 4 containers, cover, and place into the fridge until needed.
- Eat hot or cold!

Brown Rice and Tuna Bowls

Total time: 25 minutes

Ingredients

- 2 cups dry brown rice
- 4 small cans of unflavored tuna (the single-serve cans)
- 1 carrot, peeled and chopped into small pieces
- 1 red bell pepper, core and seeds removed, cut into small pieces
- 1 cup chopped cucumber
- 1 tbsp. balsamic vinegar

Directions

- Place the brown rice into a pot and add 3 ½ cups of water and a pinch of salt, bring to the boil then reduce to a simmer, leave covered until the water has disappeared and the rice is soft (but still with a bite!).
- Divide the cooked rice between your 4 containers and add the contents of one tuna can into each, divide the carrot, bell pepper, cucumber and balsamic vinegar between the 4 containers and stir to combine with the rice.
- Cover and place into the fridge to store until needed!

Rainbow Chicken Salad

Total time: 30 minutes

Ingredients

- 2 chicken breasts
- Olive oil
- Salt and pepper, to taste
- ½ head of red cabbage, thinly sliced
- 2 carrots, grated
- 1 cup cubed cucumber
- 2 yellow bell peppers, core and seeds removed, thinly sliced
- ½ head iceberg lettuce, roughly chopped
- 2 tomatoes, chopped into chunks
- 2 tbsp. balsamic vinegar mixed with 2 tbsp. olive oil

Directions

- Preheat the oven to 356 degrees Fahrenheit and line a baking tray with baking paper.
- Place the chicken breasts onto the tray and rub with olive oil, salt and pepper, place into the oven and bake for approximately 25 minutes or until cooked all the way through.
- Slice the cooked chicken breasts into thin slices.
- Place the cabbage, carrot, cucumber, bell peppers, lettuce, tomatoes, balsamic vinegar, olive oil and chicken into a large bowl and gently toss to combine and coat in oil and vinegar.
- Divide the salad between your 6 containers, cover and place into the fridge to store until needed!
- Eat within 3 nights of cooking (3 dinners for 2 people).

Veggie Stacks with Feta and Mint

Total time: 25 minutes

Ingredients

- 8 large Portobello mushrooms
- 2 large zucchinis, sliced lengthways
- 1 large eggplant, sliced into 8 slices
- 2 large tomatoes, sliced
- 2 tbsp. olive oil
- 2 garlic cloves, crushed
- Salt and pepper, to taste
- 3.5 oz. feta cheese
- Small handful fresh mint leaves

Directions

- Preheat the oven to 356 degrees Fahrenheit and line a baking tray with baking paper.
- Lay the mushrooms, zucchini slices, eggplant slices, and tomato slices onto the tray and drizzle over the olive oil, garlic, salt and pepper.
- Place the tray into the oven and bake for approximately 20 minutes until tender and golden.
- Create your stacks by layering in this order: mushrooms, feta, zucchini slices, feta, eggplant slices, mint, tomato slices, feta, mint.
- Place a skewer through the middle of each stack to keep them together if you like!
- Pack away into your containers, cover and place into the fridge until needed.

Mexican-Inspired Shepherd's Pie

Total time: 45 minutes

Ingredients

- Olive oil
- 1 onion, finely chopped
- 17 oz. minced beef
- 2 cans (14 oz.) black beans, drained
- 1 tsp. chili powder
- 1 tsp. coriander
- 1 can (14 oz.) chopped tomatoes
- 2 large sweet potatoes, chopped into chunks
- Salt and pepper, to taste
- Large handful cilantro, roughly chopped

Directions

- Preheat to oven to 356 degrees Fahrenheit.
- Drizzle some olive oil into a large pot and place over a medium heat.

- Place the onions into the pot and sauté until soft.
- Add the minced beef and sauté until browned.
- Add the black beans, chili powder, coriander and canned tomatoes, stir to combine.
- Leave to simmer for about 10 minutes as you prepare the sweet potatoes.
- Prick the sweet potatoes all over and place into the microwave, cook on HIGH for 1 minute increments until soft all the way through.
- Cut the sweet potatoes into chunks and place into a bowl, mash with a potato masher or fork, add a pinch of salt and pepper and stir through.
- Pour the mince and bean mixture into a large baking dish and spread the mashed sweet potatoes over top.
- Sprinkle the coriander over the top of the sweet potatoes.
- Place into the oven and bake for approximately 30 minutes until golden.
- Leave to cool before cutting into 8 pieces, stacking into your airtight container/and store in the fridge or freezer until needed.

Swiss Chard and Ricotta Crust-Less Pie
Total time: 30 minutes
Ingredients
- Butter or cooking oil spray
- 5 eggs
- 9 oz. ricotta cheese
- 4 cups shredded Swiss chard
- 1 onion, finely chopped
- ½ cup grated cheddar cheese
- Handful of fresh parsley, finely chopped
- ½tsp baking powder
- Salt and pepper, to taste
Directions
- Preheat the oven to 356 degrees

Fahrenheit and grease a baking dish with butter or cooking oil spray.
- Place all ingredients, plus a pinch of salt and pepper into a bowl and whisk until fully combined.
- Pour into your prepared baking dish and place into the oven.
- Bake for approximately 25 minutes or until just set and beginning to turn golden on top.
- Slice into 6 pieces, pack into your chosen containers cover and store in the fridge or freezer until needed!
- A small drop of tomato relish goes really well on the side of this crust-less pie.

Steak and Zoodle Salad
Total time: 25 minutes
Ingredients
- 3 large zucchinis, cut into noodles with a spiralizer
- Saltand pepper, to taste
- Olive oil
- 2 sirloin steaks (or 1 really large one, use your judgment to figure out how much steak you'd like for each serving)
- Juice of one lemon mixed with 2 tbsp. olive oil
- 2 tbsp. sesame seeds
Directions
- Place the zucchini noodles into a microwave-safe bowl and cook in the microwave for 1 minute. Don't overcook them, as you don't want them to be slushy or mushy! Sprinkle with salt and pepper and set aside.
- Heat a small amount of olive oil in a non-stick frying pan and place over a high heat.
- Place your steak onto the hot frying pan and cook to your liking, place onto a board to rest. You can season the steak with salt and pepper at this stage.
- Keep the pan on the heat and add the sesame seeds to the pan and toast them in

the leftover steak juices until golden and fragrant.

- Thinly slice your steak and add to the bowl of zoodles, add the sesame seeds and the olive oil and lemon dressing, stir to combine.
- Pack away into your container/s, cover and place into the fridge to store until needed!
- I love to eat this salad cold, right out of the fridge.

Breaded Fish for the Freezer

Total time: 15 minutes
Ingredients

- 2 eggs, lightly beaten
- 1 cup breadcrumbs mixed with a pinch of salt and pepper
- 4 large white fish filets, cut into 3 pieces each

Directions

- Prepare by setting the working space with your beaten egg in a small bowl, and your breadcrumbs mixed with salt and pepper spread onto a plate, have your fish pieces next to them on a plate, ready to be dipped.
- Have a tray lined with baking paper ready too, so you can put the coated fish on it to freeze.
- Dip the fish pieces into the beaten eggs and transfer them straight into the breadcrumbs, turning to coat thoroughly on all sides.
- Place the coated fish onto your lined tray, cover with plastic wrap and place into the freezer until almost frozen.
- Place the almost-frozen fish pieces into your small container lined with baking paper, place another layer of paper between each layer of fish so they don't stick together.
- Place straight into the oven from the freezer when you want to eat them! Don't thaw them out first.

Green Bean, Potato, and Pea Curry

Total time: 30 minutes
Ingredients

- Olive oil
- 4 garlic cloves, finely chopped
- 1 onion, finely chopped
- 4 tbsp. store-bought green curry paste
- 5 large potatoes, cut into cubes or chunks
- 2 cups frozen green beans
- 2 cups frozen peas
- 1 cup (8fl oz.) chicken or vegetable broth
- 3 cups (24fl oz.) coconut milk
- Salt, to taste

Directions

- Drizzle some olive oil into a large pot or pan and place over a medium heat.
- Add the garlic, onions and curry paste, stir to combine and leave to sauté for a couple of minutes until the curry paste is fragrant.
- Add the potatoes, beans, peas, broth and coconut milk to the pot and stir to combine, add a pinch of salt to season.
- Allow the curry to boil for approximately 20 minutes or until the potatoes are soft but not mushy.
- Leave to cool before dividing between your 6 containers, covering and placing into the fridge or freezer.

Coconut-Poached Fish with Peanuts and Asian Greens

Total time: 25 minutes
Ingredients

- 1 ½ cups (12fl oz.) coconut milk
- 1 tsp. soy sauce
- 1 tsp. fish sauce
- 1 tsp. chili flakes
- 4 white fish filets
- 2 bunches of bok choi, base removed, leaves washed
- ½ cup roasted, salted peanuts
- 1 tsp. sesame oil

Directions

- Add the coconut milk, soy sauce, fish sauce, chili flakes and fish filets into a deep fry pan or pot and place over a medium heat.
- Bring to a gentle boil and leave to simmer for about 10 minutes or until the fish is just cooked.
- Add the bok choi to the pot and place the lid onto the pot, leave for 1 minute to gently steam the bok choi.
- Divide the fish, bok choi, and coconut milk between your 4 containers and sprinkle the peanuts and sesame oil over the top, cover and place into the fridge or freezer to store until needed.
- If you like, a sprinkle of fresh chili and cilantro is a gorgeous addition before eating.

Marinated Steak Freezer Packets

Total time: 15 minutes

Ingredients

- 4 beef steaks, cut into slices
- 2 tbsp. olive oil
- 2 tbsp. soy sauce
- 1 tbsp. honey
- Salt and pepper, to taste

Directions

- Place the steak strips, olive oil, soy sauce, honey, and a pinch of salt and pepper into a bowl and stir to combine, making sure each piece of beef is coated in oil, honey and sauce.
- Divide the marinated steak between your 8 freezer-safe, sealable bags and stack into the freezer to store until needed.
- To cook, leave to thaw in the bag before emptying into a hot frying pan to sauté with veggies, rice, egg or whatever you fancy!

Marinated Pork Packets

Total time: 30 minutes

Ingredients

- 4 pork steaks, cut into slices
- 2 tbsp. olive oil
- Juice of 1 lemon
- 1 small sprig of fresh rosemary, roughly chopped
- 1 tsp. dried mixed herbs (use fresh herbs if you have them, but don't worry if you don't, dried herbs are fine)
- 4 garlic cloves, crushed

Directions

- Place all ingredients into a bowl and stir to combine, making sure the pork is thoroughly coated in oil, lemon juice, garlic and herbs.
- Divide between your 8 freezer-safe bags, seal and stack into the freezer to store until needed.
- Leave to thaw before cooking in a hot frying pan.

Prepped Pasta Sauce: Tomato

Total time: 30 minutes

Ingredients

- Olive oil
- 6 garlic cloves, finely chopped
- 2 onions, finely chopped
- 3 cans (14 oz.) chopped tomatoes
- 2 tbsp. balsamic vinegar
- 1 tsp. honey
- 1 tsp. mixed dried herbs
- Salt and pepper, to taste

Directions

- Drizzle the olive oil into a frying pan and place over a medium heat.
- Add the garlic and onions to the pan and sauté until soft.
- Add the tomatoes, balsamic vinegar, honey, herbs, and a pinch of salt and pepper, stir to combine.
- Cover the pot and leave to simmer on a low heat for 20 minutes.
- Leave the sauce to cool slightly before dividing between your 4 containers, cover, and pack into the freezer to store until needed!
- You could also use this sauce for zucchini

noodles and meatballs!

Healthy Lamb Curry with Couscous
Total time: 30 minutes
Ingredients
- Olive oil
- 2 onions roughly chopped
- 1 tsp. ground turmeric
- 1 tsp. chili powder
- 1 tsp. dried cumin
- 1 tsp. dried coriander
- ½ tsp. cinnamon
- 20 oz. lamb steak (leg steak works great), cut into cubes
- 2 cups (16fl oz.) lamb stock
- 2 cans (14 oz.) chopped tomatoes
- Salt and pepper, to taste
- 2 cups dried couscous

Directions
- Drizzle some olive oil into a large frying pan or pot and place over a medium heat.
- Add the onions, turmeric, chili powder, cumin, coriander and cinnamon and heat until the onions are soft.
- Add the lamb cubes and stir to coat in spices and onions, sauté for a couple of minutes to brown the meat.
- Add the lamb stock, tomatoes, salt and pepper, stir to combine.
- Place the lid onto the pot or pan and allow it to simmer over a low heat for about 25 minutes until the lamb is cooked and the curry sauce is rich and beginning to thicken.
- While the curry cooks, prepare the couscous: place the dried couscous into a bowl and pour 2 and a half cups of boiling water over, cover the bowl and leave for about 5 minutes until the couscous is soft.
- Uncover the couscous and add a pinch of salt and pepper, use a fork to fluff the couscous and then divide it between your 6 containers.
- Divide the lamb curry between the containers and spoon it on top of the

couscous, cover and place into the fridge or freezer to store until needed!

Salmon with Mango and Lentils
Total time: 20 minutes
Ingredients
- Olive oil
- 2 large salmon steaks, cut in half to make 4 even pieces
- 1 tbsp. soy sauce
- 1 tsp. sweet chili sauce
- 2 cups cooked brown lentils (I used canned ones, so much easier!)
- 1 ripe mango, skin removed, flesh cut into small chunks
- 4 fresh mint leaves, finely chopped

Directions
- Drizzle some olive oil into a non-stick fry pan and place over a medium heat.
- Add the salmon pieces to the hot pan skin-side down and cook for 2 minutes on each side or until just cooked through.
- Pour the soy sauce and chili sauce over the salmon.
- Divide the lentils between your 4 containers, add the mango to each container, then place a piece of salmon on top, finish by sprinkling each pieces of salmon with the fresh mint.
- Cover the containers and place into the fridge or freezer until needed!

Freezer Chicken Soup
Total time: 30 minutes
Ingredients
- 5 boneless chicken thighs, cut into small pieces
- 1 onion, finely chopped
- 4 cups (32fl oz.) chicken broth
- 2 cups (16fl oz.) water
- 1 can (14 oz.) corn kernels, drained
- 2 scallions, finely sliced
- Salt and pepper, to taste

Directions
- Place all ingredients into a pot and add a pinch of salt and pepper, place over a

medium heat and cover.

- Leave to simmer for approximately 30 minutes until the chicken is cooked through.
- Leave to cool slightly before dividing into your 6 containers, cover and stack into the freezer to store until needed.
- Leave the frozen containers on the bench to thaw before thoroughly reheating, or simply place the frozen soup in a pot over a high heat to speed the process up!

Prepped Pasta Sauce: Pesto

Total time: 10 minutes

Ingredients

- 2 cups fresh basil leaves
- 3.5 oz. parmesan cheese, broken into small chunks
- 1/3 cup olive oil
- 3 garlic cloves, roughly chopped
- ½ cup pine nuts, (they are very expensive so just use cashew nuts for a cheaper option!)
- Salt and pepper, to taste

Directions

- Place all ingredients into a blender or small food processor and add a pinch of salt and pepper.
- Blend until smooth but still with a few small pieces of nuts remaining.
- Pour into your jar or container and store in the fridge until needed!
- You can also use this as a salad dressing for potato salads or chicken salads.

Prepped Pasta Sauce: Creamy Mushroom

Total time: 20 minutes

Ingredients

- 2 tbsp. olive oil
- 5 cups chopped mushrooms, (use a range of different kinds of mushrooms if you like! I use white button mushrooms and Portobello mushrooms)
- 8 garlic cloves, finely chopped
- 1 sprig of fresh rosemary, finely chopped

- 3fl oz. white wine
- ½ cup (4fl oz.) sour cream
- ½ cup (4fl oz.) plain yogurt

Directions

- Drizzle the olive oil into a frying pan and place over a medium heat.
- Add the mushrooms, garlic and rosemary or mixed herbs, sauté for a few minutes until the mushrooms have begun to shrink and become colored.
- Add the wine and simmer until the alcohol evaporates.
- Add the sour cream and yoghurt and stir to combine.
- Turn off the heat and leave the sauce to cool slightly before dividing into your 4 containers, cover and place into the freezer to store until needed!

Taco Freezer Packets

Total time: 30 minutes

Ingredients

- 3 large chicken breasts, cut into small slices
- 3 red bell peppers, core and seeds removed, thinly sliced
- 2 red onions, red onions, thinly sliced
- 2 cans (14 oz.) chopped tomatoes
- 6 garlic cloves, finely chopped
- 2 tsp. paprika
- 1 tsp. ground cumin
- 1 tsp. ground coriander
- 1 tsp. chili powder
- 2 tbsp. olive oil

Directions

- Place all ingredients into a large bowl and stir to combine, making sure every piece of chicken and vegetables is coated in olive oil and spices.
- Divide the mixture between your 8 freezer-safe sealable bags, seal and stack into the fridge to store until needed.
- Leave to thaw before sautéing in a hot frying pan until cooked all the way through and the onions and bell peppers

are slightly charred.

Breaded Chicken Freezer Packets

Total time: 15 minutes
Ingredients
- 2 eggs, lightly beaten
- 2 cups breadcrumbs mixed with a pinch of salt and pepper
- 4 large chicken breasts, each cut into 6 pieces

Directions
- Prepare your work space by placing the beaten egg in a small bowl next to a plate of breadcrumbs, salt and pepper.
- Line a baking tray with baking paper and keep nearby so you can place your breaded chicken onto it.
- Take your chicken pieces and dip them into the egg, then straight into the breadcrumbs, turning a few times to thoroughly coat in breadcrumbs.
- Place the breaded chicken pieces onto your lined tray and place in the freezer.
- Once frozen, divide the chicken pieces between your 8 freezer bags and stack into the freezer to store until needed!
- To cook, simply preheat your oven to 356 degrees Fahrenheit, place the chicken pieces onto a lined baking tray and bake for about 25 minutes or until cooked through, no need to thaw first.

Stir-Fried Brown Rice with Chicken and Veggie Jewels

Total time: 30 minutes
Ingredients
- 2 large chicken breasts
- Olive oil
- Salt and pepper
- 1 tsp. chili flakes
- 1 ½ cups dry brown rice
- 1 garlic clove, crushed
- 2 red bell peppers, core and seeds removed, cut into small pieces
- 2 scallions, finely chopped
- 8 spears of asparagus, cut into small pieces (the same size as the bell pepper pieces)
- 2 carrots, peeled and cut into pieces to match the asparagus and bell pepper pieces
- 2 tbsp. olive oil mixed with 1 tbsp. soy sauce

Directions
- Preheat the oven to 356 degrees Fahrenheit and line a baking tray with baking paper.
- Place the chicken breasts on the tray and drizzle with olive oil, salt, pepper and chili flakes, place into the oven for approximately 20 minutes or until the chicken is cooked through.
- Leave the chicken to rest for a few minutes before cutting into small pieces.
- Cook the rice while the chicken is cooking: place the brown rice into a pot and add 2 cups of water, place over a high heat and bring to the boil, reduce to a simmer and cook with the lid on until the water has disappeared and the rice is cooked.
- Add the garlic, peppers, scallions, asparagus and carrot to the pot of rice and add the olive oil and soy sauce mixture, turn the heat up to high and keep stirring as the veggies cook in the rice – you can use a wok or fry pan for this step, but I just use the pot the rice cooked in to save myself another dish to wash up! It works perfectly well.
- Add the chopped cooked chicken to the pot, stir through and leave to cool before dishing into your containers, cover and store in the fridge or freezer until needed!

Prepped Quinoa Sushi Rolls

Total time: 25 minutes
Ingredients
- 1 cup quinoa
- 1 ½ cups water

- 14 oz. firm tofu, cut into strips
- 2 tbsp. soy sauce
- 1 tsp. sesame oil
- 1 tbsp. honey
- 6 nori sheets (sushi seaweed)
- 2 tbsp. sesame seeds, lightly toasted in a dry fry pan
- 1 red bell pepper, core and seeds removed, sliced
- 1 carrot, peeled and sliced into thin strips

Directions
- Thoroughly rinse the quinoa in a sieve to remove the bitter outer layer.
- Bring the water to the boil in a small pot and add the quinoa, stir to combine then turn the heat down to a simmer, cover, and cook for 12-15 minutes or until the liquid has disappeared and the quinoa is soft.
- While the quinoa is cooking, prepare the tofu: place the soy sauce, sesame oil, honey and tofu into a small fry pan over a medium heat, cook for a few minutes until golden and cooked through, set aside.
- Lay the nori sheets onto a large board, have your tofu, cooked quinoa, toasted sesame seeds and sliced veggies close by.
- Spread a thin layer of quinoa onto each nori sheet, leaving an inch-wide gap at the top of each sheet.
- Lay the tofu, carrot and bell peppers in a line in the center of the nori sheet (horizontally).
- Sprinkle the sesame seeds on top of the tofu and veggies on each nori sheet.
- Tightly roll the sushi and seal the ends with warm water.
- Don't slice yet, wait until you're ready to eat to slice just before eating.
- Pack the sushi rolls into your container and store in the fridge until needed!

Lamb and Red Onion Skewers

Total time: 25 minutes
Ingredients
- 4 lamb leg steaks, cut into cubes
- 2 red onions, cut into 6 wedges each
- 2 tbsp. olive oil
- Salt and pepper, to taste
- 8 skewers

Directions
- Preheat the oven to 400 degrees Fahrenheit and line a baking tray with baking paper.
- Load the skewers by alternating lamb and onion until full (but leave an inch on either side of the skewers so you can pick them up easily).
- Rub the onion and lamb with olive oil and sprinkle with salt and pepper and place on the tray.
- Place the tray into the oven and bake for approximately 20 minutes, turning once, until the onions are cooked and beginning to turn golden, and the lamb is cooked but still pink inside.
- Leave the skewers to cool slightly before packing away into a large container, covering and storing in the fridge until needed.

Veggie Burgers Patties

Total time: 25 minutes
Ingredients
- 5 Portobello mushrooms, cut into small pieces
- 1 cup corn kernels
- 1 cup chickpeas, drained and rinsed
- 2 eggs, lightly beaten
- 1 cup almond flour
- Large handful of fresh parsley, finely chopped
- 1 tsp. ground cumin
- 1 tsp. ground coriander
- 1 tsp. chili powder
- Salt and pepper, to taste

Directions
- Preheat the oven to 356 degrees Fahrenheit and line a baking tray with baking paper.
- Place all ingredients into a large bowl and

- add a pinch of salt and pepper.
- Vigorously stir until thoroughly combined.
- Shape the mixture into 8 large patties.
- Place the patties onto the baking tray and place into the oven.
- Bake for about 7 minutes on each side (just take the tray out of the oven and turn the patties over after 7 minutes then put them back in for another 7) or until cooked through and golden on the outside.
- Stack into an airtight container and store in the fridge until needed.

Freezer Soup (Pumpkin and Coconut)
Total time: 45 minutes
Ingredients
- 6 cups cubed pumpkin (skin removed, about 1 medium-sized pumpkin)
- 1 onion, finely chopped
- 2 carrots, cut into chunks
- 3 cups (24fl oz.) chicken stock
- Salt and pepper, to taste
- 1 cup (8fl oz.) coconut milk
Directions
- Place the pumpkin, onion, carrots, stock, salt and pepper into a pot and bring to the boil, reduce to a simmer and simmer covered for about 25 minutes or until the veggies are soft.
- Using a hand-held stick blender, blend until smooth.
- Stir the coconut milk into the soup, taste, and add more salt and pepper if needed.
- Allow it to cool slightly before pouring into your 6 containers, covering, then packing away into the freezer!
- Remember to label the containers with masking tape and a sharpie so you can keep track of when the soup was made.
- Simply take out of the freezer the morning of the day you want to have the soup for dinner, and leave to thaw on the kitchen bench.
- Throw it into a pot or place into the microwave in a bowl to heat.

Spicy Lentil Stew with Sweet Potato Mash and Cilantro
Total time: 40 minutes
Ingredients
- Olive oil
- 1 onion, finely chopped
- 1 tsp. cumin
- 1 tsp. chili powder
- 1 tsp. ground coriander
- 1 can (14 oz.) chopped tomatoes
- 2 cans (14 oz.) brown lentils, drained
- Salt and pepper, to taste
- 1 cup (8fl oz.) chicken stock
- 2 large sweet potatoes, cut into cubes
- Large handful of cilantro, roughly chopped
Directions
- Drizzle some olive oil into a pot and place over a medium heat.
- Add the onion, cumin, chili, ground coriander, tomatoes, lentils, salt and pepper, stir to combine.
- Add chicken stock to the pot.
- Allow it to simmer for about 20 minutes until thick and rich.
- As the lentil stew simmers, cook the sweet potatoes by pricking all over with a fork and cooking in the microwave on HIGH for 1 minute increments until soft all the way through.
- Cut the cooked sweet potatoes into chunks and place into a bowl (I keep the skin on, it has nutrients!), add some salt and pepper and mash with a fork.
- Divide the sweet potato mash between your 6 containers then divide the lentil stew between the containers and spoon on top of the sweet potatoes.
- Sprinkle with fresh cilantro, cover and place into the fridge or freezer (or both, freeze 3, fridge 3!) until needed.

Chapter 9: Dessert Meal Plan

Fruit Kebab
Total time: 30 minutes
Ingredients
- 3 apples
- ¼ cup orange juice
- 1 ½ lb. watermelon
- ¾ cup blueberries

Directions
- Use a star-shaped cookie cutter to cut out stars from the apple and watermelon.
- Soak the apple stars in orange juice.
- Thread the apple stars, watermelon stars and blueberries into skewers.
- Refrigerate for 30 minutes before serving.

Roasted Mangoes
Total time: 15 minutes
Ingredients
- 2 mangoes, peeled and sliced into cubes
- 2 tablespoons coconut flakes
- 2 teaspoons crystallized ginger, chopped
- 2 teaspoons orange zest

Directions
- Preheat your oven to 350 degrees F.
- Put the mango cubes in custard cups.
- Top with the ginger and orange zest.
- Bake in the oven for 10 minutes.

Figs with Yogurt
Total time: 8 hours 5 minutes
Ingredients
- 8 oz. low fat yogurt
- ½ teaspoon vanilla
- 2 figs, sliced
- 1 tablespoon walnuts, toasted and chopped
- Lemon zest

Directions
- Refrigerate yogurt in a bowl for 8 hours.
- After 8 hours, take it out of the refrigerator and stir in yogurt and vanilla.
- Stir in the figs.
- Sprinkle walnuts and lemon zest on top before serving.

Strawberry & Watermelon Pops
Total time: 6 hours 10 minutes
Ingredients
- ¾ cup strawberries, sliced
- 2 cups watermelon, cubed
- ¼ cup lime juice
- 2 tablespoons brown sugar
- ⅛ teaspoon salt

Directions
- Put the strawberries inside popsicle molds.
- In a blender, pulse the rest of the ingredients until well mixed.
- Pour the puree into a sieve before pouring into the molds.
- Freeze for 6 hours.

Cinnamon Almond Balls
Total time: 15 minutes
Ingredients
- 1 tsp cinnamon
- 3 tbsp erythritol
- 1 ¼ cup almond flour
- 1 cup peanut butter
- Pinch of salt

Directions:
- Add all ingredients into the mixing bowl and mix well.
- Cover and place bowl in fridge for 30 minutes.
- Make small bite size ball from mixture and serve.

Choco Frosty
Total time: 10 minutes
Ingredients
- 1 tsp vanilla
- 8 drops liquid stevia
- 2 tbsp unsweetened cocoa powder
- 1 tbsp almond butter
- 1 cup heavy cream

Directions:
- Add all ingredients into the mixing bowl and beat with immersion blender until soft peaks form.
- Place in refrigerator for 30 minutes.

- Add frosty mixture into the piping bag and pipe in serving glasses.
- Serve and enjoy.

Moist Avocado Brownies

Total time: 45 minutes

Ingredients

- 2 avocados, mashed
- 2 eggs
- 1 tsp baking powder
- 2 tbsp swerve
- 1/3 cup chocolate chips, melted
- 4 tbsp coconut oil, melted
- 2/3 cup unsweetened cocoa powder

Directions:

- Preheat the oven to 325 F.
- In a mixing bowl, mix together all dry ingredients.
- In another bowl, mix together avocado and eggs until well combined.
- Slowly add dry mixture to the wet along with melted chocolate and coconut oil. Mix well.
- Pour batter in greased baking pan and bake for 30-35 minutes.
- Slice and serve.

Mix Berry Sorbet

Total time: 0 minutes

Ingredients

- ½ cup raspberries, frozen
- ½ cup blackberries, frozen
- 1 tsp liquid stevia
- 6 tbsp water

Directions:

- Add all ingredients into the blender and blend until smooth.
- Pour blended mixture into the container and place in refrigerator until harden.
- Serve chilled and enjoy.

Chia Almond Pudding

Total time: 10 minutes

Ingredients

- 2 tbsp almonds, toasted and crushed
- 1/3 cup chia seeds

- ½ tsp vanilla
- 4 tbsp erythritol
- ¼ cup unsweetened cocoa powder
- 2 cups unsweetened almond milk

Directions:

- Add almond milk, vanilla, sweetener, and cocoa powder into the blender and blend until well combined.
- Pour blended mixture into the bowl.
- Add chia seeds and whisk for 1-2 minutes.
- Pour pudding mixture into the serving bowls and place in fridge for 1-2 hours.
- Top with crushed almonds and serve.

Choco Peanut Cookies

Total time: 20 minutes

Ingredients

- 1 cup peanut butter
- 1 tsp baking soda
- 2 tsp vanilla
- 1 tbsp butter, melted
- 2 eggs
- 2 tbsp unsweetened cocoa powder
- 2/3 cup erythritol
- 1 1/3 cups almond flour

Directions:

- Preheat the oven to 350 F.
- Add all ingredients into the mixing bowl and stir to combine.
- Make 2-inch balls from mixture and place on greased baking tray and gently press down each ball with fork.
- Bake in oven for 8-10 minutes.
- Serve and enjoy.

Chocolate Macaroon

Total time: 30 minutes

Ingredients

- 1 tsp vanilla
- ¼ cup coconut oil
- 2 eggs
- 1/3 cup unsweetened coconut, shredded
- 1/3 cup erythritol
- ½ tsp baking powder
- ¼ cup unsweetened cocoa powder

- 3 tbsp coconut flour
- 1 cup almond flour
- Pinch of salt

Directions:
- Add all ingredients into the mixing bowl and mix until well combined.
- Make small balls from mixture and place on greased baking tray.
- Bake at 350 F for 15-20 minutes.
- Serve and enjoy.

Mocha Ice-Cream

Total time: 20 minutes

Ingredients
- ¼ tsp xanthan gum
- 1 tbsp instant coffee
- 2 tbsp unsweetened cocoa powder
- 15 drops liquid stevia
- 2 tbsp erythritol
- ¼ cup heavy cream
- 1 cup unsweetened coconut milk

Directions:
- Add all ingredients except xanthan gum into the blender and blend until smooth.
- Add xanthan gum and blend until mixture is slightly thickened.
- Pour mixture into the ice cream maker and churn according to machine instructions.
- Serve chilled and enjoy.

Fruit Salad

Total time: 10 minutes

Ingredients
- 1 tsp erythritol
- 1 tsp lemon juice
- 1 sage leaf, chopped
- 1 tbsp blueberries
- ¼ cup strawberries, sliced
- ½ cup raspberries
- ½ cup blackberries

Directions:
- Add all ingredients into the bowl and toss well.
- Serve and enjoy.

Blackberry Pops

Total time: 20 minutes

Ingredients
- 1 tsp liquid stevia
- ½ cup water
- 1 fresh sage leaf
- 1 cup blackberries

Directions:
- Add all ingredients into the blender and blend until smooth.
- Pour blended mixture into the ice pop molds and place in refrigerator for overnight.
- Serve and enjoy.

Peanut Butter Banana Splits

Total time: 10 minutes

Ingredients:
- 6 bananas, sliced
- 2 tablespoons coconut oil
- 4 tablespoons peanut butter
- 1 cup chocolate chips

To serve:
- Non Dairy whipped topping
- Non Dairy frozen treats
- Maraschino cherries
- Strawberry slices

Directions:
- Add chocolate chips, coconut oil, and peanut butter into a microwave-safe bowl. Microwave on high for about a minute. Whisk well. If the mixture is not melted, place for a few more seconds. Whisk after every 5 seconds.
- Divide the banana slices into 6 glasses or bowls.
- Drizzle the chocolate sauce over the bananas. Refrigerate until use. It can last for 2 days.
- To serve: Remove the glasses from the refrigerator. Top with the suggested toppings and serve.

Apple Strudel

Total time: 20 minutes

Ingredients:

- 2 packages vegan puff pastry dough (16 x 9 inches each)
- 1 ½ teaspoons ground cinnamon
- 4 red apples, peeled, cored, cut into thin slices using a slicer
- Powdered vegan sugar, to sprinkle (optional)

Directions:

- Sprinkle cinnamon over the apple and stir using your hands.
- Unfold the pastry dough on your countertop. Place apple slices on one half of the dough. Fold the other half over the filling. Press the edges to seal. Place in an airtight container in the refrigerator. It can last for 2 days.
- To serve: Bake in a preheated oven at 350° F for 15 – 20 minutes or until brown on top.
- Serve warm or at room temperature.

Pumpkin Parfaits

Total time: 10 minutes
Ingredients:

- 4 cups vanilla soy yogurt
- ½ cup brown or raw sugar (optional)
- ½ teaspoon ground nutmeg
- 2 cups pumpkin puree
- 1 teaspoon ground cinnamon
- ¼ teaspoon ground ginger (optional)

Topping:

- 4 squares dark chocolate, melted
- 8 ginger snap cookies, broken
- Mint leaves

Directions:

- Add pumpkin, yogurt, sugar, ginger, cinnamon, and nutmeg into a bowl and whisk until sugar dissolves completely.
- Divide into glasses. Refrigerate until use. It can last for 3 days.
- To serve: Top with the suggested toppings and serve.

Peanut Butter Balls

Total time: 10 minutes
Ingredients:

- 1/3 cup roasted peanuts
- 1 tablespoon cocoa powder
- 3 tablespoons rolled oats
- ½ cup pitted Medjool dates

Directions:

- Add dates into the food processor and pulse until smooth.
- Add rest of the ingredients and pulse until well combined.
- Divide the mixture into 8 equal portions and shape into balls. Place in an airtight container and refrigerate until use. It can last for a week.
- To freeze: Place in freezer-safe bags and freeze until use. It can last for 2 months.

Fig, Coconut, and Blackberry Ice Cream

Total time: 6 hours 20 minutes
Ingredients:

- 20 fresh, ripe figs, chop each into 8 pieces
- Juice of a lemon
- Zest of a lemon, grated
- 4 teaspoons ginger, minced (optional)
- 4 cups coconut milk
- 1 1/3 cups blackberries + extra to garnish
- ¾ cup water
- 2/3 cup dried shredded coconut, unsweetened
- 1 cup agave nectar or to taste
- A few leaves lemon balm

Directions:

- Place a saucepan over medium heat. Add figs, water, lemon zest, dried coconut, and ginger. When it begins to boil, lower the heat and simmer until figs are tender.
- Add blackberries and agave nectar and cook until slightly thick.
- Turn off the heat and cool completely. Blend with an immersion blender until smooth.
- Add rest of the ingredients and blend for a few seconds until the fruits get chopped into tiny pieces. Pour into a bowl. Cover

and chill for 4 – 6 hours.

- Pour into an ice cream maker and churn the ice cream following the manufacturer's instructions. Transfer into a freezer-safe container. Freeze until use.
- To serve: Remove from the freezer and place for 10 minutes on your countertop before serving. Scoop ice cream into bowls. Serve garnished with blackberries and lemon balm.

Layered Blueberry Cheesecake

Total time: 1 hour 10 minutes
Ingredients:
- For crust:
- 1 cup almond flour
- 1 cup raw pecans
- 6 dates, pitted
- 2 teaspoons ground cinnamon
- 4 tablespoons coconut oil
- ½ teaspoon kosher salt
- For filling:
- 4 cups raw cashew, soaked in water for 4-8 hours
- ½ cup coconut oil, melted, cooled
- 4 tablespoons fresh lemon juice
- ½ cup freeze-dried blueberries
- ½ cup canned coconut milk, shake the can well before pouring into the cup
- 2/3 cup pure maple syrup
- 2 tablespoons vanilla extract or 1 teaspoon vanilla bean powder
- For blueberry layer:
- 2 cups blueberries, fresh or frozen, thawed if frozen
- 2 tablespoons chia seeds
- 2 tablespoons fresh lemon juice

Directions:
- Grease 2 small springform pans with coconut oil. Place strips of parchment paper in it.
- Add all the ingredients of crust into the food processor and pulse until well combined and slightly sticky. Do not pulse for long.

- Divide the mixture into the prepared pans. Press it well into the bottom of the pan.
- To make filling: Add all the ingredients for filling into the food processor and pulse until smooth. Add more coconut milk if the mixture is not getting smooth while blending. Taste and adjust sweetness if desired. Set aside about 1/3 of the filling and add into a bowl. Add freeze-dried blueberries and mix well. Set aside.
- Divide the remaining 2/3 of the filling in the 2 crusts. Spread it evenly.
- Freeze for an hour.
- Divide the blueberry mixture on top of both the crusts. Place the cheesecakes in the freezer.
- To make blueberry layer: Add all the ingredients for blueberry layer into the blender and blend until smooth.
- Pour on the top of the crusts. Place the cheesecakes back in the freezer. Freeze until firm. It can last for a week.
- Serve frozen or thawed. Cut into wedges and serve.

Chocolate Fudge Cookies

Total time: 30 minutes
Ingredients:
- 2 large ripe bananas, sliced
- 1 cup peanut butter or any other nut butter of your choice
- Flaky sea salt to sprinkle
- 1 cup cocoa powder
- 1 cup + 2 tablespoons maple syrup

Directions:
- Add banana into a bowl. Using a fork, mash the bananas.
- Stir in peanut butter, maple syrup and cocoa powder. Mix until well combined.
- Place a sheet of parchment paper on 1 – 2 large baking sheets. Place tablespoonful of the mixture at different spots. You should have about 28 cookies in all.

- Bake in a preheated oven at 325° F for 15 minutes. Remove from the oven and sprinkle salt over the cookies. Let it cool to room temperature. Transfer into an airtight container. It can last for 10 – 12 days.

Apple Pie

Total time: 90 minutes

Ingredients:

For the crust:
- ½ cup + 1 tablespoon all-purpose flour
- 3 tablespoons organic vegan shortening, cut into small cubes
- 1/8 teaspoon salt
- 2 tablespoons ice water
- For the filling:
- ¼ teaspoon ground cinnamon
- ½ tablespoon lemon juice
- ½ tablespoon cornstarch
- ¼ cup packed light brown sugar
- For topping:
- ¼ cup rolled oats
- 1 ½ tablespoons packed light brown sugar
- 1 tablespoon organic vegan shortening
- 2 tablespoons all-purpose flour
- ¼ teaspoon ground cinnamon

Directions:
- To make crust: Add flour into a bowl. Add cold shortening. Cut it into the flour using a pastry cutter until crumbs are formed.
- Add ice-cold water, a tablespoon at a time and mix until a moist dough is formed.
- Shape into a circle of about 4-5 inches.
- Take a sheet of plastic wrap. Sprinkle some flour on it. Place the dough in the middle of the sheet and wrap it completely. Place in the refrigerator for a maximum of 2 days.
- Remove from the refrigerator 15 minutes before preparing.
- To make the filling: Add apples, brown sugar, cinnamon and lemon juice into a bowl. Mix well and set aside for 15 minutes.
- Sprinkle cornstarch and toss until well coated.
- Place a sheet of parchment paper on your countertop. Place dough on the center of the parchment paper. Cover with another sheet of parchment paper. Roll with a rolling pin until about 6 – 7 inches in diameter. Carefully remove the top parchment paper.
- Lift the dough along with the bottom parchment paper, carefully invert onto a 5 – 6-inch pie pan. Press the dough into the pan.
- Carefully remove the other parchment paper.
- Place the filling in the pie pan. Spread it all over the pan.
- Bake in a preheated oven at 375°F for 15-20 minutes.
- To make the topping: Add all the ingredients of the topping into a bowl. Cut it into the flour using a pastry blender or a pair of knives until smaller pieces are formed.
- Then use your hands and mix until the mixture is crumbly. Sprinkle over the apple filling in the pie.
- Bake for 30-40 minutes until the top is golden brown. It can last for 2 – 3 days. Place in an airtight container at room temperature.
- Cut into wedges and serve.

Salted Caramel Chocolate Cups

Total time: 10 minutes

Ingredients:
- ½ cup dark chocolate chips
- 3 tablespoons vegan caramel sauce
- 1 teaspoon coconut oil
- 1/8 teaspoon flaky sea salt

Directions:
- Place disposable cupcake liners in a 6 counts muffin pan.
- Add chocolate chips and coconut oil into

a microwave-safe bowl. Microwave on high for about 50 seconds. Whisk well. If the mixture is not melted, place for a few more seconds. Whisk after every 5 seconds.
- Divide most of the chocolate mixture among the cupcake liners. Using the back of a spoon, spread it evenly on the bottom as well as a little on the sides of the liners.
- Freeze until firm. Divide the caramel sauce among the cupcake liners. Drizzle the remaining chocolate on the caramel layer.
- Refrigerate until use. It can last for a week.

Creamy Mint Chocolate Chip Avocado Ice Cream

Total time: 50 minutes
Ingredients:
- 4 medium-large Hass avocados, peeled, pitted, chopped into chunks
- ½ cup coconut butter or coconut oil
- 2 tablespoons peppermint extract
- ½ cup chocolate chips
- 2 medium bananas, peeled, sliced
- 4 tablespoons maple syrup or coconut nectar or agave nectar
- 15-20 fresh mint leaves (optional)

Directions:
- Add all the ingredients except chocolate chips into a blender and blend until smooth.
- Pour into a freezer-safe container. Freeze for an hour.
- Remove the ice cream from the freezer and whisk well. Refreeze and beat again after 30-40 minutes.
- Repeat the previous step 2 – 3 times until well frozen without ice crystals.
- Add chocolate chips and stir when you whisk for the last time.

Quick Mug Brownie

Total time: 6 minutes
Ingredients

- 2 eggs
- 1 tbsp heavy cream
- 1 scoop protein powder
- 1 tbsp erythritol
- ¼ tsp vanilla

Directions:
- Add all ingredients into the mug and mix well.
- Place mug in microwave and microwave for 1 minute.
- Serve and enjoy.

Protein Peanut Butter Ice Cream

Total time: 10 minutes
Ingredients
- 5 drops liquid stevia
- 2 tbsp heavy cream
- 2 tbsp peanut butter
- 2 tbsp protein powder
- ¾ cup cottage cheese

Directions:
- Add all ingredients into the blender and blend until smooth.
- Pour blended mixture into the container and place in refrigerator for 30 minutes.
- Serve chilled and enjoy.

Chia Raspberry Pudding

Total time: 10 minutes
Ingredients
- ¼ tsp vanilla
- ¾ cup unsweetened almond milk
- 1 tbsp erythritol
- 2 tbsp proteins collagen peptides
- ¼ cup chia seeds
- ½ cup raspberries, mashed

Directions:
- Add all ingredients into the bowl and stir until well combined.
- Place in refrigerator for overnight.
- Serve chilled and enjoy.

Chocolate Chia Pudding

Total time: 30 minutes
Ingredients
- ½ cup chia seeds

- ½ tsp vanilla
- 1/3 cup unsweetened cocoa powder
- 1 ½ cups unsweetened coconut milk

Directions:
- Add all ingredients into the mixing bowl and whisk well.
- Place bowl in refrigerator for overnight.
- Serve chilled and enjoy.

Cheesecake Fat Bombs

Total time: 20 minutes

Ingredients
- 8 oz cream cheese
- 1 ½ tsp vanilla
- 2 tbsp erythritol
- 4 oz coconut oil
- 4 oz heavy cream

Directions:
- Add all ingredients into the mixing bowl and beat using immersion blender until creamy.
- Pour batter into the mini cupcake liner and place in refrigerator until set.
- Serve and enjoy.

Matcha Ice Cream

Total time: 1030 minutes

Ingredients
- ½ tsp vanilla
- 2 tbsp swerve
- 1 tsp matcha powder
- 1 cup heavy whipping cream

Directions:
- Add all ingredients into the glass jar.
- Seal jar with lid and shake for 4-5 minutes until mixture double.
- Place in refrigerator for 3-4 hours.
- Serve chilled and enjoy.

Grilled Peaches

Total time: 8 minutes

Ingredients
- 1 cup balsamic vinegar
- ⅛ teaspoon ground cinnamon
- 1 tablespoon honey
- 3 peaches, pitted and sliced in half

- 2 teaspoons olive oil
- 6 gingersnaps, crushed

Directions
- Pour the vinegar into a saucepan.
- Bring it to a boil.
- Lower heat and simmer for 10 minutes.
- Remove from the stove.
- Stir in cinnamon and honey.
- Coat the peaches with oil.
- Grill peaches for 2 to 3 minutes.
- Drizzle each one with syrup.
- Top with the gingersnaps.

Fruit Salad

Total time: 5 minutes

Ingredients
- 8 oz. light cream cheese
- 6 oz. Greek yogurt
- 1 tablespoon honey
- 1 teaspoon orange zest
- 1 teaspoon lemon zest
- 1 orange, sliced into sections
- 3 kiwi fruit, peeled and sliced
- 1 mango, cubed
- 1 cup blueberries

Directions
- Beat cream cheese using an electric mixer.
- Add yogurt and honey.
- Beat until smooth.
- Stir in the orange and lemon zest.
- Toss the fruits to mix.
- Divide in glass jars.
- Top with the cream cheese mixture.

Choco Banana Bites

Total time: 2 hours 10 minutes

Ingredients
- 2 bananas, sliced into rounds
- ¼ cup dark chocolate cubes

Directions
- Melt chocolate in the microwave or in a saucepan over medium heat.
- Coat each banana slice with melted chocolate.
- Place on a metal pan.
- Freeze for 2 hours.

Blueberries with Yogurt

Total time: 5 minutes

Ingredients

- 1 cup nonfat Greek yogurt
- ¼ cup blueberries
- ¼ cup almonds

Directions

- Add yogurt and blueberries in a food processor.
- Pulse until smooth.
- Top with almonds before serving.

Chocolate & Raspberry Ice Cream

Total time: 12 hours 20 minutes

Ingredients

- ¼ cup almond milk
- 2 egg yolks
- 2 tablespoons cornstarch
- ¼ cup honey
- ¼ teaspoon almond extract
- ⅛ teaspoon salt
- 1 cup fresh raspberries
- 2 oz. dark chocolate, chopped
- ¼ cup almonds, slivered and toasted

Directions

- Mix almond milk, egg yolks, cornstarch and honey in a bowl.
- Pour into a saucepan over medium heat.
- Cook for 8 minutes.
- Strain through a sieve.
- Stir in salt and almond extract.
- Chill for 8 hours.
- Put into an ice cream maker.
- Follow manufacturer's directions.
- Stir in the rest of the ingredients.
- Freeze for 4 hours.

Mocha Pops

Total time: 4 minutes

Ingredients

- 3 cups brewed coffee
- ½ cup low calorie chocolate flavored syrup
- ¾ cup low fat half and half

Directions

- Mix the ingredients in a bowl.
- Pour into popsicle molds.
- Freeze for 4 hours.

Crab Dip
- Preparation time: 10 minutes
- Cooking time: 30 minutes
- Servings: 8

Ingredients:
- bacon strips, sliced
- ounces crab meat
- ½ cup mayonnaise
- ½ cup sour cream
- ounces cream cheese
- poblano pepper, chopped
- tablespoons lemon juice
- Salt and black pepper to the taste
- garlic cloves, minced
- green onions, minced
- ½ cup parmesan cheese+ ½ cup parmesan cheese, grated
- Salt and black pepper to the taste

Directions:
- Heat up a pan over medium high heat, add bacon, cook until it's crispy, transfer to paper towels, chop and leave aside to cool down.
- In a bowl, mix sour cream with cream cheese and mayo and stir well.
- Add ½ cup parmesan, poblano peppers, bacon, green onion, garlic and lemon juice and stir again.
- Add crab meat, salt and pepper and stir gently.
- Pour this into a heat proof baking dish, spread the rest of the parmesan, introduce in the oven and bake at 350 degrees F for 20 minutes.
- Serve your dip warm with cucumber stick.
- Enjoy!
- Nutrition Value: calories 200, fat 7, fiber 2, carbs 4, protein 6

Simple Spinach Balls
- Preparation time: 10 minutes
- Cooking time: 12 minutes
- Servings: 30

Ingredients:
- tablespoons melted ghee
- eggs
- 1 cup almond flour
- 16 ounces spinach
- 1/3 cup feta cheese, crumbled
- ¼ teaspoon nutmeg, ground
- 1/3 cup parmesan, grated
- Salt and black pepper to the taste
- 1 tablespoon onion powder
- tablespoons whipping cream
- 1 teaspoon garlic powder

Directions:
- In your blender, mix spinach with ghee, eggs, almond flour, feta cheese, parmesan, nutmeg, whipping cream, salt, pepper, onion and garlic pepper and blend very well.
- Transfer to a bowl and keep in the freezer for 10 minutes
- Shape 30 spinach balls, arrange on a lined baking sheet, introduce in the oven at 350 degrees F and bake for 12 minutes.
- Leave spinach balls to cool down and serve as a party appetizer.
- Enjoy!
- Nutrition Value: calories 60, fat 5, fiber 1, carbs 0.7, protein 2

Garlic Spinach Dip
- Preparation time: 10 minutes
- Cooking time: 35 minutes
- Servings: 6

Ingredients:
- bacon slices
- ounces spinach
- ½ cup sour cream
- ounces cream cheese, soft
- 1 and ½ tablespoons parsley, chopped
- ounces parmesan, grated
- 1 tablespoon lemon juice
- Salt and black pepper to the taste
- 1 tablespoon garlic, minced

Directions:
- Heat up a pan over medium heat, add

bacon, cook until it's crispy, transfer to paper towels, drain grease, crumble and leave aside in a bowl.

- Heat up the same pan with the bacon grease over medium heat, add spinach, stir, cook for 2 minutes and transfer to a bowl.
- In another bowl, mix cream cheese with garlic, salt, pepper, sour cream and parsley and stir well.
- Add bacon and stir again.
- Add lemon juice and spinach and stir everything.
- Add parmesan and stir again.
- Divide this into ramekins, introduce in the oven at 350 degrees f and bake for 25 minutes.
- Turn oven to broil and broil for 4 minutes more.
- Serve with crackers.
- Enjoy!
- Nutrition Value: calories 345, fat 12, fiber 3, carbs 6, protein 11

Mushrooms Appetizer

- Preparation time: 10 minutes
- Cooking time: 20 minutes
- Servings: 5

Ingredients:

- ¼ cup mayo
- 1 teaspoon garlic powder
- 1 small yellow onion, chopped
- 24 ounces white mushroom caps
- Salt and black pepper to the taste
- 1 teaspoon curry powder
- ounces cream cheese, soft
- ¼ cup sour cream
- ½ cup Mexican cheese, shredded
- 1 cup shrimp, cooked, peeled, deveined and chopped

Directions:

- In a bowl, mix mayo with garlic powder, onion, curry powder, cream cheese, sour cream, Mexican cheese, shrimp, salt and pepper to the taste and whisk well.

- Stuff mushrooms with this mix, place on a baking sheet and cook in the oven at 350 degrees F for 20 minutes.
- Arrange on a platter and serve.
- Enjoy!
- Nutrition Value: calories 244, fat 20, fiber 3, carbs 7, protein 14

Simple Bread Sticks

- Preparation time: 10 minutes
- Cooking time: 15 minutes
- Servings: 24

Ingredients:

- tablespoons cream cheese, soft
- 1 tablespoon psyllium powder
- ¾ cup almond flour
- cups mozzarella cheese, melted for 30 seconds in the microwave
- 1 teaspoon baking powder
- 1 egg
- tablespoons Italian seasoning
- Salt and black pepper to the taste
- ounces cheddar cheese, grated
- 1 teaspoon onion powder

Directions:

- In a bowl, mix psyllium powder with almond flour, baking powder, salt and pepper and whisk.
- Add cream cheese, melted mozzarella and egg and stir using your hands until you obtain a dough.
- Spread this on a baking sheet and cut into 24 sticks.
- Sprinkle onion powder and Italian seasoning over them.
- Top with cheddar cheese, introduce in the oven at 350 degrees F and bake for 15 minutes.
- Serve them as a keto snack!
- Enjoy!
- Nutrition Value: calories 245, fat 12, fiber 5, carbs 3, protein 14

Italian Meatballs

- Preparation time: 10 minutes
- Cooking time: 6 minutes

- Servings: 16

Ingredients:
- 1 egg
- Salt and black pepper to the taste
- ¼ cup almond flour
- 1 pound turkey meat, ground
- ½ teaspoon garlic powder
- tablespoons sun dried tomatoes, chopped
- ½ cup mozzarella cheese, shredded
- tablespoons olive oil
- tablespoon basil, chopped

Directions:
- In a bowl, mix turkey with salt, pepper, egg, almond flour, garlic powder, sun dried tomatoes, mozzarella and basil and stir well.
- Shape 12 meatballs, heat up a pan with the oil over medium high heat, drop meatballs and cook them for 2 minutes on each side.
- Arrange on a platter and serve.
- Enjoy!
- Nutrition Value: calories 80, fat 6, fiber 3, carbs 5, protein 7

Parmesan Wings
- Preparation time: 10 minutes
- Cooking time: 24 minutes
- Servings: 6

Ingredients:
- pound chicken wings, cut in halves
- Salt and black pepper to the taste
- ½ teaspoon Italian seasoning
- tablespoons ghee
- ½ cup parmesan cheese, grated
- A pinch of red pepper flakes, crushed
- 1 teaspoon garlic powder
- 1 egg

Directions:
- Arrange chicken wings on a lined baking sheet, introduce in the oven at 425 degrees F and bake for 17 minutes.
- Meanwhile, in your blender, mix ghee with cheese, egg, salt, pepper, pepper flakes, garlic powder and Italian

seasoning and blend very well.
- Take chicken wings out of the oven, flip them, turn oven to broil and broil them for 5 minutes more.
- Take chicken pieces out of the oven again, pour sauce over them, toss to coat well and broil for 1 minute more.
- Serve them as a quick keto appetizer.
- Enjoy!
- Nutrition Value: calories 134, fat 8, fiber 1, carbs 0.5, protein 14

Cheese Sticks
- Preparation time: 1 hour and 10 minutes
- Cooking time: 20 minutes
- Servings: 16

Ingredients:
- eggs, whisked
- Salt and black pepper to the taste
- mozzarella cheese strings, cut in halves
- 1 cup parmesan, grated
- 1 tablespoon Italian seasoning
- ½ cup olive oil
- 1 garlic clove, minced

Directions:
- In a bowl, mix parmesan with salt, pepper, Italian seasoning and garlic and stir well.
- Put whisked eggs in another bowl.
- Dip mozzarella sticks in egg mixture, then in cheese mix.
- Dip them again in egg and in the parmesan mix and keep them in the freezer for 1 hour.
- Heat up a pan with the oil over medium high heat, add cheese sticks, fry them until they are golden on one side, flip and cook them the same way on the other side.
- Arrange them on a platter and serve.
- Enjoy!
- Nutrition Value: calories 140, fat 5, fiber 1, carbs 3, protein 4

Tasty Broccoli Sticks
- Preparation time: 10 minutes
- Cooking time: 20 minutes
- Servings: 20

Ingredients:

- 1 egg
- cups broccoli florets
- 1/3 cup cheddar cheese, grated
- ¼ cup yellow onion, chopped
- 1/3 cup panko breadcrumbs
- 1/3 cup Italian breadcrumbs
- tablespoons parsley, chopped
- A drizzle of olive oil
- Salt and black pepper to the taste

Directions:

- Heat up a pot with water over medium heat, add broccoli, steam for 1 minute, drain, chop and put into a bowl.
- Add egg, cheddar cheese, panko and Italian breadcrumbs, salt, pepper and parsley and stir everything well.
- Shape sticks out of this mix using your hands and place them on a baking sheet which you've greased with some olive oil.
- Introduce in the oven at 400 degrees F and bake for 20 minutes.
- Arrange on a platter and serve.
- Enjoy!
- Nutrition Value: calories 100, fat 4, fiber 2, carbs 7, protein 7

Bacon Delight

- Preparation time: 15 minutes
- Cooking time: 1 hour and 20 minutes
- Servings: 16

Ingredients:

- ½ teaspoon cinnamon, ground
- tablespoons erythritol
- 16 bacon slices
- 1 tablespoon coconut oil
- ounces dark chocolate
- 1 teaspoon maple extract

Directions:

- In a bowl, mix cinnamon with erythritol and stir.
- Arrange bacon slices on a lined baking sheet and sprinkle cinnamon mix over them.
- Flip bacon slices and sprinkle cinnamon

mix over them again.

- Introduce in the oven at 275 degrees F and bake for 1 hour.
- Heat up a pot with the oil over medium heat, add chocolate and stir until it melts.
- Add maple extract, stir, take off heat and leave aside to cool down a bit.
- Take bacon strips out of the oven, leave them to cool down, dip each in chocolate mix, place them on a parchment paper and leave them to cool down completely.
- Serve cold.
- Enjoy!
- Nutrition Value: calories 150, fat 4, fiber 0.4, carbs 1.1, protein 3

Taco Cups

- Preparation time: 10 minutes
- Cooking time: 40 minutes
- Servings: 30

Ingredients:

- 1 pound beef, ground
- cups cheddar cheese, shredded
- ¼ cup water
- Salt and black pepper to the taste
- tablespoons cumin
- tablespoons chili powder
- Pico de gallo for serving

Directions:

- Divide spoonfuls of parmesan on a lined baking sheet, introduce in the oven at 350 degrees F and bake for 7 minutes.
- Leave cheese to cool down for 1 minute, transfer them to mini cupcake molds and shape them into cups.
- Meanwhile, heat up a pan over medium high heat, add beef, stir and cook until it browns.
- Add the water, salt, pepper, cumin and chili powder, stir and cook for 5 minutes more.
- Divide into cheese cups, top with pico de gallo, transfer them all to a platter and serve.
- Enjoy!

- Nutrition Value: calories 140, fat 6, fiber 0, carbs 6, protein 15

Tasty Chicken Egg Rolls

- Preparation time: 2 hours and 10 minutes
- Cooking time: 15 minutes
- Servings: 12

Ingredients:

- ounces blue cheese
- cups chicken, cooked and finely chopped
- Salt and black pepper to the taste
- green onions, chopped
- celery stalks, finely chopped
- ½ cup tomato sauce
- ½ teaspoon erythritol
- egg roll wrappers
- Vegetable oil

Directions:

- In a bowl, mix chicken meat with blue cheese, salt, pepper, green onions, celery, tomato sauce and sweetener, stir well and keep in the fridge for 2 hours.
- Place egg wrappers on a working surface, divide chicken mix on them, roll and seal edges.
- Heat up a pan with vegetable oil over medium high heat, add egg rolls, cook until they are golden, flip and cook on the other side as well.
- Arrange on a platter and serve them.
- Enjoy!
- Nutrition Value: calories 220, fat 7, fiber 2, carbs 6, protein 10

Halloumi Cheese Fries

- Preparation time: 10 minutes
- Cooking time: 5 minutes
- Servings: 4

Ingredients:

- 1 cup marinara sauce
- ounces halloumi cheese, pat dried and sliced into fries
- ounces tallow

Directions:

- Heat up a pan with the tallow over medium high heat.

- Add halloumi pieces, cover, cook for 2 minutes on each side and transfer to paper towels.
- Drain excess grease, transfer them to a bowl and serve with marinara sauce on the side.
- Enjoy!
- Nutrition Value: calories 200, fat 16, fiber 1, carbs 1, protein 13

Jalapeno Crisps

- Preparation time: 10 minutes
- Cooking time: 25 minutes
- Servings: 20

Ingredients:

- tablespoons olive oil
- jalapenos, sliced
- ounces parmesan cheese, grated
- ½ teaspoon onion powder
- Salt and black pepper to the taste
- Tabasco sauce for serving

Directions:

- In a bowl, mix jalapeno slices with salt, pepper, oil and onion powder, toss to coat and spread on a lined baking sheet.
- Introduce in the oven at 450 degrees F and bake for 15 minutes.
- Take jalapeno slices out of the oven, leave them to cool down.
- In a bowl, mix pepper slices with the cheese and press well.
- Arrange all slices on a another lined baking sheet, introduce in the oven again and bake for 10 minutes more.
- Leave jalapenos to cool down, arrange on a plate and serve with Tabasco sauce on the side.
- Enjoy!
- Nutrition Value: calories 50, fat 3, fiber 0.1, carbs 0.3, protein 2

Delicious Cucumber Cups

- Preparation time: 10 minutes
- Cooking time: 0 minutes
- Servings: 24

Ingredients:

- cucumbers, peeled, cut in ¾ inch slices and some of the seeds scooped out
- ½ cup sour cream
- Salt and white pepper to the taste
- ounces smoked salmon, flaked
- 1/3 cup cilantro, chopped
- teaspoons lime juice
- 1 tablespoon lime zest
- A pinch of cayenne pepper

Directions:
- In a bowl mix salmon with salt, pepper, cayenne, sour cream, lime juice and zest and cilantro and stir well.
- Fill each cucumber cup with this salmon mix, arrange on a platter and serve as a keto appetizer.
- Enjoy!
- Nutrition Value: calories 30, fat 11, fiber 1, carbs 1, protein 2

Caviar Salad
- Preparation time: 6 minutes
- Cooking time: 0 minutes
- Servings: 16

Ingredients:
- eggs, hard boiled, peeled and mashed with a fork
- ounces black caviar
- ounces red caviar
- Salt and black pepper to the taste
- 1 yellow onion, finely chopped
- ¾ cup mayonnaise
- Some toast baguette slices for serving

Directions:
- In a bowl, mix mashed eggs with mayo, salt, pepper and onion and stir well.
- Spread eggs salad on toasted baguette slices, and top each with caviar.
- Enjoy!
- Nutrition Value: calories 122, fat 8, fiber 1, carbs 4, protein 7

Marinated Kebabs
- Preparation time: 20 minutes
- Cooking time: 10 minutes
- Servings: 6

Ingredients:
- 1 red bell pepper, cut in chunks
- 1 green bell pepper, cut into chunks
- 1 orange bell pepper, cut into chunks
- pounds sirloin steak, cut into medium cubes
- garlic cloves, minced
- 1 red onion, cut into chunks
- Salt and black pepper to the taste
- tablespoons Dijon mustard
- and ½ tablespoons Worcestershire sauce
- ¼ cup tamari sauce
- ¼ cup lemon juice
- ½ cup olive oil

Directions:
- In a bowl, mix Worcestershire sauce with salt, pepper, garlic, mustard, tamari, lemon juice and oil and whisk very well.
- Add beef, bell peppers and onion chunks to this mix, toss to coat and leave aside for a few minutes.
- Arrange bell pepper, meat cubes and onion chunks on skewers alternating colors, place them on your preheated grill over medium high heat, cook for 5 minutes on each side, transfer to a platter and serve as a summer keto appetizer.
- Enjoy!
- Nutrition Value: calories 246, fat 12, fiber 1, carbs 4, protein 26

Simple Zucchini Rolls
- Preparation time: 10 minutes
- Cooking time: 5 minutes
- Servings: 24

Ingredients:
- tablespoons olive oil
- zucchinis, thinly sliced
- 24 basil leaves
- tablespoons mint, chopped
- 1 and 1/3 cup ricotta cheese
- Salt and black pepper to the taste
- ¼ cup basil, chopped
- Tomato sauce for serving

Directions:

- Brush zucchini slices with the olive oil, season with salt and pepper on both sides, place them on preheated grill over medium heat, cook them for 2 minutes, flip and cook for another 2 minutes.
- Place zucchini slices on a plate and leave aside for now.
- In a bowl, mix ricotta with chopped basil, mint, salt and pepper and stir well.
- Spread this over zucchini slices, divide whole basil leaves as well, roll and serve as an appetizer with some tomato sauce on the side.
- Enjoy!
- Nutrition Value: calories 40, fat 3, fiber 0.3, carbs 1, protein 2

Simple Green Crackers

- Preparation time: 10 minutes
- Cooking time: 24 hours
- Servings: 6

Ingredients:
- cups flax seed, ground
- cups flax seed, soaked overnight and drained
- bunches kale, chopped
- 1 bunch basil, chopped
- ½ bunch celery, chopped
- garlic cloves, minced
- 1/3 cup olive oil

Directions:
- In your food processor mix ground flaxseed with celery, kale, basil and garlic and blend well.
- Add oil and soaked flaxseed and blend again.
- Spread this into a tray, cut into medium crackers, introduce in your dehydrator and dry for 24 hours at 115 degrees F, turning them halfway.
- Arrange them on a platter and serve.
- Enjoy!
- Nutrition Value: calories 100, fat 1, fiber 2, carbs 1, protein 4

Cheese And Pesto Terrine

- Preparation time: 30 minutes
- Cooking time: 0 minutes
- Servings: 10

Ingredients:
- ½ cup heavy cream
- ounces goat cheese, crumbled
- tablespoons basil pesto
- Salt and black pepper to the taste
- sun dried tomatoes, chopped
- ¼ cup pine nuts, toasted and chopped
- 1 tablespoons pine nuts, toasted and chopped

Directions:
- In a bowl, mix goat cheese with the heavy cream, salt and pepper and stir using your mixer.
- Spoon half of this mix into a lined bowl and spread.
- Add pesto on top and also spread.
- Add another layer of cheese, then add sun dried tomatoes and ¼ cup pine nuts.
- Spread one last layer of cheese and top with 1 tablespoon pine nuts.
- Keep in the fridge for a while, turn upside down on a plate and serve.
- Enjoy!
- Nutrition Value: calories 240, fat 12, fiber 3, carbs 5, protein 12

Avocado Salsa

- Preparation time: 10 minutes
- Cooking time: 0 minutes
- Servings: 4

Ingredients:
- 1 small red onion, chopped
- avocados, pitted, peeled and chopped
- jalapeno pepper, chopped
- Salt and black pepper to the taste
- tablespoons cumin powder
- tablespoons lime juice
- ½ tomato, chopped

Directions:
- In a bowl, mix onion with avocados, peppers, salt, black pepper, cumin, lime juice and tomato pieces and stir well.

- Transfer this to a bowl and serve with toasted baguette slices as a keto appetizer.
- Enjoy!
- Nutrition Value: calories 120, fat 2, fiber 2, carbs 0.4, protein 4

Tasty Egg Chips

- Preparation time: 5 minutes
- Cooking time: 10 minutes
- Servings: 2

Ingredients:

- ½ tablespoon water
- tablespoons parmesan, shredded
- eggs whites
- Salt and black pepper to the taste

Directions:

- In a bowl, mix egg whites with salt, pepper and water and whisk well.
- Spoon this into a muffin pan, sprinkle cheese on top, introduce in the oven at 400 degrees F and bake for 15 minutes.
- Transfer egg white chips to a platter and serve with a keto dip on the side.
- Enjoy!
- Nutrition Value: calories 120, fat 2, fiber 1, carbs 2, protein 7

Chili Lime Chips

- Preparation time: 10 minutes
- Cooking time: 20 minutes
- Servings: 4

Ingredients:

- 1 cup almond flour
- Salt and black pepper to the taste
- 1 and ½ teaspoons lime zest
- 1 teaspoon lime juice
- 1 egg

Directions:

- In a bowl, mix almond flour with lime zest, lime juice and salt and stir.
- Add egg and whisk well again.
- Divide this into 4 parts, roll each into a ball and then spread well using a rolling pin.
- Cut each into 6 triangles, place them all on a lined baking sheet, introduce in the

oven at 350 degrees F and bake for 20 minutes.
- Enjoy!
- Nutrition Value: calories 90, fat 1, fiber 1, carbs 0.6, protein 3

Artichoke Dip

- Preparation time: 10 minutes
- Cooking time: 15 minutes
- Servings: 16

Ingredients:

- ¼ cup sour cream
- ¼ cup heavy cream
- ¼ cup mayonnaise
- ¼ cup shallot, chopped
- 1 tablespoon olive oil
- garlic cloves, minced
- ounces cream cheese
- ½ cup parmesan cheese, grated
- 1 cup mozzarella cheese, shredded
- ounces feta cheese, crumbled
- 1 tablespoon balsamic vinegar
- 28 ounces canned artichoke hearts, chopped
- Salt and black pepper to the taste
- ounces spinach, chopped

Directions:

- Heat up a pan with the oil over medium heat, add shallot and garlic, stir and cook for 3 minutes.
- Add heavy cream and cream cheese and stir.
- Also add sour cream, parmesan, mayo, feta cheese and mozzarella cheese, stir and reduce heat.
- Add artichoke, spinach, salt, pepper and vinegar, stir well, take off heat and transfer to a bowl.
- Serve as a tasty keto dip.
- Enjoy!
- Nutrition Value: calories 144, fat 12, fiber 2, carbs 5, protein 5

Baked Parsley Cheese Fingers

- Preparation Time: 15 minutes
- Servings: 2-4

Ingredients

- 1 cup pork rinds, crushed
- 1 egg
- 1 tbsp dried parsley
- 1 lb cheddar cheese, cut into sticks
- Directions
- Preheat oven to 350 F and line a baking sheet with parchment paper. Combine pork rinds and parsley in a bowl to be evenly mixed. Beat the egg in another bowl.
- Coat the cheese sticks in the egg and then generously dredge in pork rind mixture. Arrange on the baking sheet. Bake for 4 to 5 minutes, take out after, let cool for 2 minutes, and serve with marinara sauce.
- Nutrition Value:
- Calories: 213, Fat: 19.5g, Net Carbs: 1.5g, Protein: 8.7g

CONCLUSION

Once you get the hang of meal prepping you will never want to go back! Having packets of fresh, healthy food packed away in the fridge and freezer, ready to be eaten is a satisfying and gratifying feeling. If these recipes do not quite fit in with your particular weight-loss diet, then simply modify them until the macronutrients are where you want them to be! Less carbs? No worries. More protein? Easy. Just download a calorie-counting app, load the recipes in, and shuffle things around to reach your desired numbers.

Always remember to prep meals that you **want to eat!** In my opinion, the best foods are healthy **and** delicious, and once you hit that sweet-spot you can lose weight without even noticing that you've changed your diet! You'll be so satisfied and full from your yummy, nutrient-filled foods that you won't get that horrible sense of deprivation and craving which comes with many strict diets.

Make a day of it and go shopping for containers, oils, spices, non-perishables, masking tape and sharpies for labeling, a diary to plan your meals and prep days, and put it all in a pretty and space-saving box. Make your prep-sessions fun and relaxing, as they should be! You deserve to enjoy your life, your diet, and your kitchen.

Good luck and have fun!

The Wholesome Optavia Diet Cookbook

The 83-Day Anti-Obesity Challenge For a Progressive Weight Loss

—

3 Exclusive Meal Plans to Burn Fat

—

250 Lean & Green Recipes on a budget

Dedication:

This book is dedicated to all those people who strive to find a new way to lose weight and stay fit to improve their health

ABIGAIL SMITH

Introduction

With advancements in science and technology, machines have taken over humans' role while humans are left with their brains only. No doubt, the inventions in science have made humans' lives very easy but have made him inactive. On the other hand, competition has grown to a greater extend, pushing us into a hectic work schedule. In addition to that, the food industry, with its flourishment, has started offering various junk food, daily eating of them is hazardous to health. All of these factors have contributed to elevating the severity of obesity in our societies. As a result, nowadays, people are becoming more and more concerned about their weight because obesity can call other fatal diseases such as heart attack, hypertension, joint pains, and much more. So if you are looking for a diet plan that can help you lose weight to regain your true shape and size to enhance your beauty, then it's a good time for you to read this book till the end. The meal replacement company named Medifast, founded in 1980 by William Vitale, has revised its product called "take shape for life" in 2017 and called it "Optavia," a low carbs diet with high protein intake and moderate fat consumption. Various diet plans accompany the Optavia diet program, each with a discrete target audience from various groups ranging from individuals wanting to lose less than 15 kg to those who want to lose more than 40 kg, from young overweight masses to senior citizens, from healthy to diabetic patients, from those who want to lose weight to those who want to maintain weight. Thus, it guides not only weight loss but also shepherds on managing and retaining your weight.

If we talk about the meal options that it offers, it has its standing among other weight-loss diet plans by providing a combination of home-cooked and prepacked food. One of its target customers are those who don't go for a diet plan though they need that, but the hassle of thinking and searching what to eat when it's time for a meal and how to cook low carb food is frustrating and time-consuming. Optavia offers users a coach to discuss their weight issues,o help them formulating a whole diet plan with weight loss goals and schedule meal plans for their customers. Users, if want, can have ready-made at their doorsteps right on time.

The first program offered by Optavia is 5 and 1 diet schedule in which the client has to eat five fuelings and one lean and green meal per day with eating intervals of two or three hours. The second program is the 4-2-1 plan asking users to take four servings for the fueling category, two from lean and green, and one from healthy fat. The first two programs are aimed to lose weight while the third program, the 3-3 plan, allows clients to maintain their desired weight. Optavia fueling is prudently designed with the right balance of nutrients from all three groups: fats, proteins, and carbohydrates, including bars, shakes, biscuits, puddings, brownies, and much more: various fueling options are also given in this book with simple and easy recipes for your assistance. Fueling is formulated to give you a fulfillment feeling to easily restrict yourself from calories to achieve your weight loss target set by you. Simultaneously, lean and green sanctioned almost seven ounces of protein, three servings of vegetables included in the non-starchy group, and two healthy fat servings.

In the upcoming sections, details about Optaiva diet plan, its advantages and health concerns, types of food that are allowed, how Optavia is more beneficial as compared to other related diets, several meal plans offered by it followed by quick and easy to made recipes from all categories of meals (lean and green, fuelings and snacks) are discussed.

Part 1: Introduction to Optavia

Chapter 1: Optavia Diet Program

What is a diet called Optavia?

The ease of nutritional supplement diets that bring the guesswork out of reducing weight has long attracted consumers. The Optavia Diet is a famous meal replacement plan.

The Optavia Diet seeks to help people lose weight by eating small quantities of calories during the day by incorporating "fueling" (Bars, shakes, and other ready-made foods), six times small-meals-per-day ideology. A meal replacement strategy is the Optavia diet. Followers eat a minimum amount of fuel every day (plus one home-cooked meal), resulting in a drop in calories and weight loss. Optavia is a weight reduction or maintenance plan that recommends a combination of purchased, refined foods called "fuels" and "lean and green" homemade meals. No carbs or calories are counting; instead, as part of six meals every day, adherents add water to processed food or unwrap a cookie.

Furthermore, the strategy suggests doing about 30 minutes of normal moderate-intensity exercise. Medifast, a nutritional supplement firm, owns the Optavia diet. Low-calorie, reduced carb plans that incorporate processed foods with home-cooked meals to support weight loss are both the primary diet (also labeled Medifast) and Optavia. The Optavia diet, however, requires one-on-one coaching, unlike Medifast.

They all include branded items called Optavia Fuelings and home-cooked entrées recognized as Lean and Green meals, although you can choose from many choices. Optavia Fuelings include some low carbohydrates products but rich in probiotic culture and protein that contain helpful bacteria that can enhance your gut's health, such as soups, pasta, bars, cereals, cookies, shakes, and puddings contain certain foods. While they may appear to be very high in carbohydrates, they are built to be lower in carbohydrates and sugar than conventional forms with the same foods. The firm utilizes sugar substitutes, and limited portion sizes to do this. Also, several fuels are packaged with soy protein isolate and powdered whey protein.

The company has a line of pre-made low-carbohydrate meals labeled Tastes of Home that are supplements of Lean and Green meals for anyone not interested in cooking.

History

As the term itself hasn't been around for long, the Optavia Diet could sound unfamiliar. You're probably have learned of the diet advertised as Optavia in July 2017 under its original title, Take Shape for Life. Take Shape for Life started as a subsidiary of the weight-reducing product of the firm. Medifast was established in 1980 by Dr. William Vitale, a medical doctor.

The goal of taking Shape for Life was to deliver Medifast's goods in an electronic platform better suited to the digital era when it was launched in 2002. The Optavia Diet isn't targeted for a particular group but aims to cater to individuals who want to avoid "overanalyzing" an eating plan.

Five out of the six small meals a day are pre-packaged and pre-planned with Optavia's famous '5 & 1' plan, removing the need for any major adjustments when it's time to eat. Users consume five of the "fuelings" of Optavia and one low-calorie "lean and green" home-cooked meal per day on this schedule. Optavia seems to be a favorite of individuals with a busy life, but the plan's reduced-calorie technique is meant for anybody who wants to lose weight.

Optavia includes lifestyle schedules for weight maintenance and weight reduction targets. The plans of Optavia, the "3 & 3" and "4 & 2 & 1", combine "actual" meals with substitutes for meals. These plans are better for people who want to steadily lose weight or maintain their weight. Both "fueling" and "lean and green" home-cooked meals are kept inside strict calorie ranges on all Optavia plans.

The basic concept behind the Optavia diet

The tagline of Optavia is "Lifelong Transition, One Healthy Practice at a Time." The primary emphasis of the Optavia diet is a diet focused on several mini-meals (called "fuels") consumed during the day, complemented by a homemade meal (termed "lean and green").

The program is designed around six optimal health "main building blocks":

Weight Management

Alimentation and hydration

Motion

Sleeping

Spirit

The environs

The argument goes that you are less likely to wander into unhealthy eating regions if you have a diet to execute and recommended mini-meals to consume. And weight loss is almost guaranteed when you only consume the small number of calories that the diet offers, even as small as 1,100 calories a day. The home cooking

becomes a routine every night by preparing your own "lean and green" meal, making the switch from the diet back to "normal" healthy eating easier.

Optavia also provides an aspect of social support that separates it from several other diets that substitute meals. As emotional support is a significant factor in the success of weight loss, those who participate in their programs have access to a mentor, usually someone who has completed the program successfully. This mentor will answer all the questions for your weight loss program, offer education, and act as a cheerleader.

How is Optavia expected to assist with weight loss?

To encourage weight loss, Optavia depends on intensively limiting calories. Most "fuels" contain about 100-110 calories each, which means you can eat about 1,000 calories a day on this diet. The U.S. Owing to the dramatic strategy of Optavia, in its Best Easy Weight-Loss Diets ranking, News and world study published ranked it # 2. The Optavia Diet offers consumers, like many other meal replacement diets, its variety of advertised items that take over many meals during the day.

The "5 & 1" plan is the most successful and is intended for drastic weight loss. Users consume five of the "fuelings" of Optavia and one low-calorie "lean and green" home-cooked meal per day on this schedule. The other plans of Optavia, the "3 & 3" and "4 & 2 & 1", combine "actual" meals with substitutes for meals.

Advantages of the Optavia Diet

If you'd like a diet plan that is simple and easy to follow, which will help with weight loss easily, and provides developed-in social support, Optavia 's program may be a good match for you.

Give convenience for packaged goods

The shakes, soups, and other meal replacement items from Optavia are delivered straight to your door, a degree of convenience not offered by many other diets. Whereas for "lean and green" meals, you will have to shop with your ingredients, the home delivery choice for the "fuels" of Optavia saves time and energy. They're simple to process and make great fetch-and-go meals once the items arrive.

Accomplishes Quick Weight Loss

To maintain their weight, most healthy individuals need about 1600 to 3000 calories a day. For most people, reducing the number of calories to as minimal as 800 guarantees weight reduction. The 5 & 1 plan of Optavia is intended for accelerated weight loss, allowing it a solid choice for rapidly shed pounds for those with a health purpose.

Removes Guesswork

Some people learn that the most difficult part of dieting is the psychological effort needed to find out what to eat every day or even every meal. Optavia mitigates the tension of meal preparation and "choice fatigue" by providing "fueling" and "lean and green" meal guidelines to users with pretty obvious-cut approved foods.

Social Service Offers

For every weight loss strategy, social reinforcement is a critical determinant of success. The coaching service and community calls from Optavia provide built-in motivation and user support.

Easiness and potential efficacy of meal substitutions

The Optavia Diet focuses on meal alternatives, catering to all those who deal with meal and cooking preparation. While there is no significant research directly aiming only at Optavia Diet, there has been researched exploring the feasibility of using substitutes for Medifast meals. The Medifast and Optavia plans have, according to the company, the same macronutrient compositions, and the items are interchangeable; the only distinction is between the particular products provided by each of them. Over this, Optavia relates to the Medifast research to support the program's efficacy, and some studies show promising outcomes compared to merely decreasing consumption using other approaches while implementing the Medifast pre-packaged food plan.

One 2010 study indicated that compared to those who consumed a reduced-calorie diet, including foods of choice, those adopting the Medifast 5 & 1 program had substantially higher weight and fat loss at one year. Similarly, when a study of charts was conducted in 2015 for individuals pursuing the 4 & 2 & 1 plan at Medifast centers, the total weight loss was 24 lbs. at three months and 42 lbs. at six months, lean mass loss was held to a minimal, and both heart rate and blood pressure decreased. Individuals that then adopted the maintenance strategy have seen less than a 2% improvement in weight recovery.

Available for particular circumstances and ages Variations

The Optavia Diet is intended for healthy people with weight to lose more than 15lbs, but they often have programs customized to work with people with certain health or lifestyle requirements. Optavia provides recommendations for those over 65 and sedentary, very healthy people, people who have less weight to lose, people who want to add more carbs into their diet, new mothers, and strategies for anyone with gout, and it suggests that it should be followed under the guidance of a doctor by those with diabetes. Also, it provides a teen program for those between 13 and 18 years of age, rendering it among one of the few such commercial diets available for teenagers.

Intake of Nutrients

The Optavia diet brings it closer to fulfilling certain nutrient recommendations than most other programs commercially available, thanks to the fortification of minerals, vitamins, and other nutrients. The nutrient profile of Optavia indicates that fiber and calcium requirements can be completely met, both chronically ill-utilized by the American population. Furthermore, Optavia defines its products as "clean," and they seem to identify them as having no artificial colors, flavorings, or sweeteners.

Is the diet for Optavia healthy?

A protein-rich diet is the Optavia diet, including protein making up 10-35 percent of the daily value calories.

For all items, Optavia offers nutrition statistics, and the 5 & 1 program is marketed as having at least 72 g of protein, 80 to 100 g of carbs, and less than 30 percent of daily fat calories. The daily nutrient averages indicated a macronutrient breakdown on the 5 & 1 program of 40 percent carbohydrates, 40 percent protein, and 20 percent fat dependent on a daily nutritional breakdown that Optavia supplied to U.S. News & Report on the Planet. "The material of the program also states that almost all fueling have added minerals and vitamins and contain" high-quality protein that preserves lean muscle mass, "as well as a patented probiotic named GanedenBC30 to" make it easier for a healthy digestive tract.

Chapter 2: Optavia vs. other low-carb diets

why is the optavia diet so innovative from the other diet?

Regardless of advancements in the medical field, obesity is still posing a serious threat to the health of people worldwide, with its mortality rate of 3 million deaths in a year. Obesity, resulting from an inactive lifestyle and unhealthy eating habits, is a major concern in the medical world because it can lead to many serious diseases such as diabetes, cardiac diseases, and hypertension.

Thus, scientists and dietitians are continuously trying to develop weight reduction programs with scientifically and carefully designed meal plans that will assist the targets with their weight loss. Below are some of today's most popular diets plans to help reduce obesity and weight management, followed by the advantages of Optavia over other similar diet plans.

Ketogenic diet

Keto diet is a low carbohydrate diet comprising 35% of proteins, 60% of fats, and 5% carbohydrates. When on a keto diet, you are allowed to take in 2000 kcal in a day, out of which carbohydrates make 50 grams. Thus, the ketogenic diet is a low carb and high-fat diet plan. In this diet, dietitians decrease carbohydrate intake, which reduces glucose production by the body; thus, your body shifts to ketogenesis mode for continuous energy supply. In the ketogenesis process, fats are broken down, thus reducing weight by metabolizing stored fats.

The ketogenic diet's main theory is the drastic reduction of glucose, the primary energy source for the body's cells. Thus to meet the energy demands of cells, the body shifts its energy production mechanism from endogenesis to ketogenesis in which energy is extracted from the stored fats through the production of ketones bodies by the liver. Continuous energy supply should be given to the brain for its proper functioning. Thus, when the body is deprived of carbohydrates (main energy source), it starts breaking down fats as the main fuel source for energy production. Thus, utilizing stored fats as energy fuel by reducing carbohydrate intake leads to weight reduction. The ketogenic diet was very popular because of its outcomes, but it faces some serious drawbacks. Firstly, the user must be very careful in monitoring the diet to not rise the ketone bodies to harmful levels, leading to ketoacidosis, severely affecting the brain activity.

Secondly, as the liver becomes very active when the body is on ketogenesis, it can develop keto stones, affecting liver function and anatomy. Furthermore, carbohydrates are also the source of some essential nutrients; reducing carbohydrates also causes nutrient deficiency, which leads to many other serious diseases. In addition to these, constipation, headache, fatigue, and digestive system issues are also the outcomes of being on a keto diet. The digestive issues arise because fibers in food keep GIT healthy, but the keto diet restricts its amount, thus not letting the body to have enough fibers to keep GIT healthy.

Intermittent fasting

Intermittent fasting is not as such a diet plan rather an eating pattern that runs between the cycles of eating and fasting because no specification regarding the food items is given, but only the times of eating are guided. Since the stone age, it has its routes because man struggles for food as hunting and natural edibles are the only food source. And to get those, he has to go from here and there and fasts during that time.

This weight reduction program's main objective is to allow the body to use stored fat by not providing it with new carbohydrates, proteins, and fats when you are not eating means you are in a fasting state. Your body is always in one state among the two; feeding state and fasting state. The feeding state activates the moment to start eating food and lasts 10-12 hours until it digests all the food. During this state, the body does not feel needed to burn stored fat for energy production because it is always getting fresh fuel supplies. Normally, we eat three times a day. Before our body is finished up digesting previous food, we again fill our stomach with the next fresh meal. Our body digests it, uses it, and stores the leftover as fat instead of decreasing weight, putting extra fat load.

Next comes the fasting state; when we don't eat for a longer period, glucose level drops, and the body does a metabolism switching from glucose to fat for energy production. This diet plan is when the body has to burn stored fat to produce energy, reducing fat load, and decreasing weight. There are different eating times recommended, but all have the same basic objective of shifting body glucose to fat metabolism for producing energy.

Intermittent fasting has several benefits, weight loss, and cardiac health but followed by some concerns too. Fasting for a longer time makes you tired and unproductive because you are not getting an efficient energy source. It's human nature that it wants to get rewarded when odes something good or after a long work period; thus, man considers fasting hard work to control himself from eating. He wants to reward himself, and this reward is eating a lot of calories. As there are not specific edibles recommended, so user eats what he wanted to eat after hours of fasting without being conscious of the number of calories he is taking in.

DASH Diet

Dietary Approaches to Stop hypertension is the full abbreviation of diet. As the name suggests, it is initially not designed to lose weight rather reduce hypertension/ blood pressure by restricting sodium and red meat intake with increased vegetables and fruits and lean meat.

Later, dietitians discovered that it is also a good diet plan for lower weight besides decreasing blood pressure. Vegetables, whole grains, fruits, lean meats, and edibles rich in nutrients such as potassium and calcium are recommended in this diet program because they help the body reduce hypertension and be good eating plans/habits.

DASH is effective in lowering blood pressure, but it is not designed as a weight-loss program; thus, if someone wishes to reduce weight quickly, DASH is not a good option. Furthermore, it is hard to follow due to its strict meal surveillance and even doesn't have much variety in foods to wat.

Atkins diet

It is also a low carb diet plan with lots of proteins and fats intake as a ketogenic diet. These low-carb diets usually work on the principle that reduced carbohydrates and rich intake of fats and proteins give you fulfillment feeling, reduces your appetite, thus restricting you to eat many calories in the form of carbohydrates and body will meet up is energy demands by burning stored fats which reduces the body mass.

Atkins diet program runs in phases, moving from one phase to next with a steady increase of calories and fat and proteins keeping your calorie intake and utilization in check. Dietitians work with their customers to change their eating patterns and habits from unhealthy and unchecked to healthy and monitored to reduce weight and live healthy lives.

But despite the encouraging outcomes of weight loss, it is not free from pitfalls. The sudden decrease in carbs intake can cause nutrient deficiency resulting in other health issues. Reduction in carbohydrates can lead to ketoacidosis due to the unavailability of a sufficient amount of carbohydrates to generate energy; the body shifts towards ketogenesis. The liver starts breaking down stored food and produces ketone bodies, becoming the source of ketoacidosis and liver dysfunctionality.

Optavia Diet Plan

Nowadays, the most trendy diet, an improved version of the Medifast diet program, is Optavia. Optavia is a low carbohydrate diet, not that low as in ketogenic diet or other related diets, and high in proteins with a moderate amount of fats. Unlike low carbs diet plans such as ketogenic diet, the optavia program doesn't shift your body to ketogenesis but allows the body to use stored fat at a steady rate by providing a decrease amount of carbs. This program offers various diet plans according to your requirements. For instance, it's one of three programs for those who want to reduce weight in a short period, while the second attracts those looking for a flexible diet plan because of health, age or lifestyle and the third one is targets weight retentions, ones who want to maintain their current weight. The high protein content gives user fulfillment feeling, which reduces their carb intake and helps you reduce weight. It restricts your carbs up to 100 calories a day for the first six weeks, but when you start achieving your weight loss goals, more edibles are allowed to give you variety on your dining table at mealtimes. This diet asks you to take 6 to 7 meals per day after every 2 to 3 hours to don't feel hungry and tired, which hinders your daily routine. The most prominent benefit that optavia provides is offering you prepacked food at your doorstep if you don't like standing in the kitchen cooking. It also saves you from the hassle of spending hours

thinking about what to eat and what not to eat by providing you with the whole meal schedule for the full month. Furthermore, you can also get guidance from a trained coach and can also discuss your concerns.

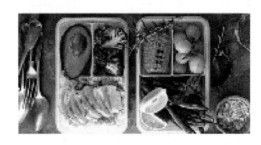

Chapter 3: How to follow the optavia program?

How do you follow the Optavia Diet?

The everyday experience on Optavia implicates eating multiple small meal replacements after every two to three hours. These fuelings consist of options of low-carbs pre-packaged stuff like bars, brownies, shakes, soups, and other snack-like meals ordered directly from the company.

Optavia offers various programs that must contain fueling whose numbers depend on which program you are following. Fueling makes up 3 to 5 daily meals out of six recommended meals and is scientifically designed to provide a balanced amount of nutrients; thus, users are free to pick any fueling at any time for any mealtime.

Once in a day, users usually have to make dinner by themselves labeled lean and green. Items included in lean and green are recommended, and the whole list is given on websites to help customers decide and choose with ease. According to the nutritional guide plan, a lean protein of about 50 to 6 oz., non-starchy items, and healthy fats make three and two servings.

Three basic diet plans offered by Optavia are there for users to choose that best suits and fulfill their requirements. For losing weight, the user has to select from 5-1 and 4-2-1 diet plan in which they will eat five fuelings and one lean and green in the first plan and four fuelings, two servings of protein from lean and green category with one serving of healthy fats in the second plan. You should not stop here, proceed further, and stay healthy with the same weight. Optavia is again there for its users to help maintain their current weight and formulate a 3-3 plan in which three servings from a balanced meal and three servings of fueling are advised.

All three diet plans are easy to follow because Optavia designs a detailed meal plan for your whole day and offers a guiding coach with whom users can consult their concerns. Furthermore, while keeping users' hectic routine and lifestyle, Optavia also offers to deliver pre-prepared food at your doorstep right on time, thus keeping you free from the hassle of choosing and how to choose how to cook.

For the counseling of the customers, the Optavia plan can be jaw downed into phases. Firstly, with the coach's help and advice, you will decide which plan you will follow. The meals you are eating in the Optavia plan are low in carbohydrates, not more than 100 carbohydrates in a day, and eating time is scheduled after every two to three hours

Another ease that Optavia provides is that it offers a flexible meal plan to accommodate a wide range of customers such as customers with type 2 and 1 diabetes, those who don't want much reduction in their weight, and, more importantly, senior citizens (people above 65 years of age). 4-2-1 plan is specifically formulated to cater to such customers because it is much more flexible than other plans offered by Optavia.

The maintenance stage begins with a six-week transition time, where you progressively surge your regular caloric intake. After you've shifted, you'll have 3 Fueling and three lean & green meals every day. After selecting the diet plan, the coach will help you set your goals related to the weight loss plan and teach you about the program and its nutritional values, supporting you in getting habituated. Furthermore, the following section will clear your concerns about who to follow this diet and what to do in it, and who is easy to follow.

Starting Phase

The coach mostly recommends following a 5-1 program in which eight hundred to thousand calories are allowed, helping you lose around 5.4 kilograms of your weight in twelve weeks. To loss 12 lb. in 12 weeks, this program asks you to take one serving from lean and green and five servings from fueling in a day in such a way that you are eating after every two to three hours on daily bases with thirty minutes of normal exercise four times a week. Just keep in mind while eating that you have to take in just 100 grams of carbohydrates only in one day. Meals on the Optavia diet are low in carbohydrate and high in proteins with 145 to 200 g of prepacked protein, vegetables which are non-starchy and healthy fats in addition to one snack such as a half cup of low-carb gelatin, half an ounce of nuts, celery sticks. Furthermore, a complete guide plan is also offered through which you can easily choose a meal from any dining-out place without much worries about weight because this guide will keep adherent with your diel plan. In general, alcohol is strongly discouraging in Optavia diet plans because of its high carbohydrate content.

Maintenance phase

After the initial phase comes the most important part of the Optavia program that is to maintain your weight, most people start a diet and follow a particular plan, but once they have achieved the weight loss goals, they don't know what to do next, and within weeks, they are back to their previous weight. But the Optavia plan is a full-fledged program that guides and supports losing weight and will also help maintain it.

When you are up on your required weight goal, Optavia gives a transition chapter of six weeks. In the transition phase, you must steadily increase your calories and intake up to 1550 calories a day. Foods that were not allowed in the initial phase because of their calorie counts that exceed their threshold are permitted in the maintenance phase as they are now within the range of required calorie counts.

Followed by a transition phase of six weeks, the program asks you to shift to a 3-3 meal plan in which you have a meal consisting of three serving of fueling and three serving from the lean and green group to provide you with the number of calories that you can easily burn in during your daily work out.

Part 2: Meal plans offered by Optavia

Chapter 1: what type of food you can eat on the Optavia diet?

Foods to Include and Foods to avoid

Eating arrangements on the Optavia Diet differ somewhat based on how long you are following the weight loss program and on the desired amount of weight you ought to lose, but both programs consist of two major parts: Optavia meal labeled as lean and green Fueling.

Fueling our Optavia's pre-portioned prepared meals formulated to have been "nutritionally compatible meal substitutes that are low in fat and controlled carbs and choices vary from bars and shakes to more nutritious meals like cheese and spinach pesto Mac.

Lean and Green portions of the meal are cooked on your own and concentrate on lean protein, reduced carbohydrates, veggies, and healthy fats. Plans differ depending on the amount of lean and green, and Fueling recommended daily steadily rising carbs and calories. Mostly on Optavia 5&1 Package, the only foods permitted are a single lean and green portion for a meal along with the Optavia Fueling. These meals usually consist of low carbohydrates, healthy fats, and lean proteins, suggesting two fatty fish meals once a week. Some low carb spices and drinks are also permitted in limited quantities.

Since meal replacements make up most of your daily meals on Optavia, many of your food choices are more or less made for you. However, certain foods are emphasized, while others are discouraged.

Amenable Foods

The lean and green portions of the meal contain; healthy fats, vegetables, and proteins. In the Optavia meal list, separate options are given under leanest, leaner and lean meat and proteins extracted from plants. The amount of lean decides the number of proteins to include.

The number of vegetables permitted in the Optavia diet can be selected from higher carbohydrates, moderate carbohydrates, and lower carbohydrates, ranging from lettuce to spaghetti. In addition to that, healthy fat is included to enhance the flavor, such as salad dressing or olive oil.

In the Optavia diet strategy, three main meal courses are offered depending upon what you want to do with your weight; either you want to lose weight or maintain your current weight. The basic concept of these diet plans is described here but discussed in detail in the coming sections.

The first two diet schemes cater to your wish to lose weight by offering a whole set of multiple meals per day: in the 5 and 1 program, you are allowed to have one cooked lean and green portion with five fuelings in a day, making a total of six meals per day while on the other hand 4, and 2 and 1 programs permit you to have four fuelings, two cooked lean and green and one snack in a day. At the same time, the third meal plan teaches you how to maintain your current weight and is named as 3 and 3 plans. As per diet instructions, three home-cooked balanced meals are endorsed per day.

Regular exercise with caution is recommended, but if there is already some sort of work out intervals in your lifestyle, it is suggested to reduce it at the start and restart after a provisional period. Here is the amount of calories allowed in each meal plan.

800 to 1000 calories are allowed in 5-1 plan, 1100 to 1300 calories in 4-2-1, and 1500 to 1800 calories are permitted in a 3-3 diet plan.

Even though no such food is rigorously forbidden when you are on an Optavia diet plan, sweets and other such edibles are discouraged. Furthermore, there is a whole list of food items that are strongly suggested and healthy fats. A list of certified food items in the everyday meal plan of lean and green is given below in different categories.

- Eggs: egg whites, beaten eggs, and whole eggs
- Soy product: tofu
- Meat: pork tenderloin, chicken, lean beef, ground and game meat, pork chops, turkey.
- Healthy fats: avocado, salad dressings which are low in carbohydrates, low-fat margarine and butter, pistachios, walnuts, olive, almonds
- Oils: olive oil, canola oil, walnut oil, flaxseed oil
- Vegetables: bell pepper, eggplant, jicama, collard greens, celery, mushrooms, cauliflower, spaghetti squash, zucchini, spinach, broccoli, cucumbers, cabbage, and all other vegetables having low carbohydrates
- Seafood: shrimps, tuna, trout, scallops, halibut, crab, salmon, lobster, trout
- Snacks: mints, gum, popsicles, gelatin, and all sugar-free snacks
- Condiments: ketchup half tsp, BBQ sauce, dried herbs, pepper, lemon and lime juice, mustard, salsa, spices, soy sauce, cocktail sauce, calorie-free sweeteners
- Beverages: coffee, sugar-free milk, tea, water

Suggestions for food items that are allowed and not allowed can also be divided according to the following list to help customers choose their meal wisely. There is no specific list of edibles that users should adhere to, but recommended items are given supporting users to lose weight in addition to providing necessary nutrients, are summarized as follows

- Optavia fuelings
- Healthy fats: Lean meats contain almost 7 oz of cooked lean protein. According to the amount of protein a meal provides, lean, leaner, and leanest categories are made to help customers select items as per requirement.
- Low-fat dairy,
- Fresh fruit with reduce carbs
- Low carb/fat whole grains
- According to carbohydrates consumed after eating, greens and other non-starchy vegetables are classified as low, medium, and high carbohydrates veggies.

Note: Once using an Optavia meal replacement strategy, have lost the desired weight, then users can shift to the next stage, which is the weight-maintaining stage. In the weight-maintaining phase, customers can incorporate low-fat products prohibited in the previous phase, such as fresh fruit, whole grains, some drinks, etc.

Besides providing pre-packaged meals at your doorstep, this diet plan also encourages you to practice preparing your meal at home to be cautious about how much calories you are taking in. Thus, the Optavia diel plan does not demand to follow any specific recipe for cooking your lean and green meal at home, but it highly recommends cooking methods such as baking, broiling, grilling, and poaching.

Non- Amenable Foods

- Some fuels obstruct your way to weight loss and are not either nutritious.
- Sugary beverages
- Indulgent desserts
- Alcohol
- High-calorie additions

- Fried foods: Fish, chicken, vegetables, meats
- Refined grains, such as pasta, biscuits, cakes, crackers, white bread, and white rice
- Alcohol
- Butter
- Coconut oil
- Milk
- Cheese
- Soda, fruit juice, and other sugar-sweetened beverages
- Undermentioned edibles are prohibited at the start of the diet plans (5-1 plan); nevertheless, after six weeks of transition, it is reintroduced in the meal plan list. Furthermore, these items are permitted when on a 3-3 diet plan.
- Starchy vegetables: corn, potatoes (sweet)
- Fruit: fresh fruits
- Legumes: soybeans, lentils, peas, beans
- Whole grains: brown rice, wheat pasta, high fiber cereal
- Low fat or fat-free dairy: cheese, milk, yogurt
- As per expectations, high calories food is not allowed in the Optavia program. While some foods are not permitted at the start, but later, you can reintroduce them in your diet schedule when you start meeting weight loss targets, such as fresh fruits, low-fat dairy products, and starchy vegetables.
- Mentioned below are some of the food items with the number of calories they provide

Food	Calories
Decadent double chocolate brownie	110 kcal
Indonesian cinnamon and hot honey cereal	110 kcal
Creamy vanilla shake	110 kcal
Spinach pesto mac and cheese	110 kcal
Chia bliss smoothie	110 kcal
Campfire S' more crisp bar	110 kcal
Wild rice and chicken-flavored soup	100 kcal
Cranberry honey granola bar	110 kcal
Sharp cheddar and sour cream popcorn	70 kcal
Buttermilk cheddar herb biscuit	110 kcal
Golden chocolate chip pancakes	110 kcal
Spiced gingerbread	110 kcal

Chewy chocolate chip cookie	110 kcal
Sour cream and chives mashed potatoes	110 kcal
Silky peanut butter shake	110 kcal
Smashed potatoes, sour cream, and chive	110 kcal
Soup wild rice and chicken flavor	100 kcal
Poppers jalapeno cheddar	110 kcal
Pancakes	90 kcal
Oatmeal orchard apple and cinnamon-spiced	110 kcal
Redberry crunchy cereal	100 kcal
Mocha blast shake	110 kcal
Caramel macchiato shake	100 kcal
Rustic tomato herb penne	110 kcal
Yogurt berry blast	90 kcal
Cinnamon sugar sticks	110 kcal
Home-style chicken and vegetable noodle soup	100 kcal
Chocolate fudge pudding	110 kcal
Olive oil and sea salt popcorn	70 kcal
Sweet blueberry biscuit	110 kcal
Golden pancakes	90 kcal
Frosted cookie dough bar	110 kcal
Beef and garden vegetable soup	100 kcal
Sticks honey mustard and onion	110 kcal

Smashed potatoes, roasted garlic creamy	110 kcal
Smoky BBQ crunchers	100 kcal
Puffed ranch snacks	50 kcal
Popcorn, olive oil, and sea salt	70 kcal
Parmesan garlic poppers	110 kcal

Chapter 2: Optavia 5 & 1 diet plan

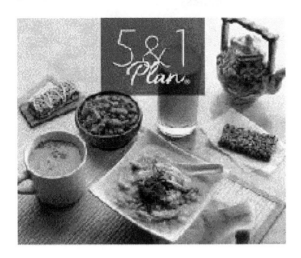

The Optimal Weight 5 & 1 Plan

5 & 1 meal plan is among the three meal programs that Optavia offers. In this plan, users have to eat six times a day after every two to three hours consisting of five meals for fueling category and one cooked either pre-packaged ordered meal or home-cooked meal but controlled carbs intake. Besides weight loss, another objective of the Optavia diel plan is to develop healthy eating habits to reduce weight and maintain it. 5 & 1 diet plan is simple and easy to follow, quick action, and in-cooperating good healthy eating habits in you.

Five among six meals recommended in this plan are fueling, having enormous scientifically deigned nutritional rich and convenient edible comprising hot beverages, soups, biscuits, brownies, shakes, puddings, and much more. Every item included in Optavia fueling is very carefully designed based on its scientific rationale having the right and required balance of fats, carbs, and proteins, helping to stimulate a fat-burning state that is moderate but proficient. Fueling is aimed to be low in carbohydrates but rich in protein so that one should retain his/her lean muscle mass.

As mentioned earlier, Optavia is a low carb diet plan to help reduce your weight by pushing the body to burn stored fats; thus, it is not recommended for pregnant women to follow Optavia or any low carb diet. Pregnancy is a crucial time for women and her baby; risk can't be taken in this regard as, during pregnancy, it is not only you but also another small individual who depends on you for their nourishment. If you are following any diet lose program, the body's calorie depends are hardly fulfill, and you are feeding two individuals. The lack of required amount of calories pose serious health issues to the users and puts the fetus at risk.

What do you need to know about Lean & Green Meal?

In lean-green meal, non-starchy vegetables make three portions that fill the green section of lean and green while one cooked protein about 7 oz. Makes a lean portion of lean and green. Furthermore, it also includes healthy fats making two servings. Stated below are the lean, green meal's nutritional parameters followed by some lean, green, and healthy fats food options for you to choose from.

Nutritional Parameters of Lean and Green

Calories ranging from 300 to 400 kcal

Fat in between 10 - 20g

Protein more than 25g

Carbohydrates less than 20g

Meal: Lean & Green

The "Lean"

- Pick broiled, baked, poached, or grilled but not fries

- Once a week, have two portions of omega-three rich fish (herring, salmon, trout, tuna) in a meal
- Can select meat-free meal such as tempeh or tofu

The proteins make the lean portion, classified into a lean, leaner, and leanest group depending on the number of proteins the food items included in these categories provides.

Nutritional Value of Lean

Calories in the range of 180 to 300 kcal

Protein greater and equals to 25g

Carbohydrates less than 15g

LEANEST: Pick a cooked portion of 7 ounces comprising 4 grams of healthy fat.

Choices from Meat

- Shellfish: shrimp, crab, lobster, scallops
- Fish: tilapia, haddock, cod, catfish, mahi-mahi, flounder, tuna
- Meat: elk., buffalo, deer, buffalo, turkey

Choices from Meatless

- 1.5 cups making 12 ounces' cottage cheese
- 5 ounces' seitan
- 2 cups of egg whites or 14 egg whites
- 12 ounces' fat-free yogurt

LEANER: Select, cooked meal making 6 ounces' containing almost 9 grams of healthy fat.

Choices from Meat

Chicken: skinless white meat, breast piece

Fish: trout, swordfish, halibut

Turkey has 95% – 97% lean

Choices from Meatless

Two eggs and four egg whites

1.5 cups, which makes almost 12 ounces of cottage cheese

12 ounces' yogurt (low fat almost less than 15 grams)

LEAN: Go for 5 ounces cooked meal, including 20 grams of healthy fat.

Choices from Meat

Turkey (ground)

Fish: mackerel, tuna, salmon, catfish, herring

Lamb

Pork tenderloin or chop

Chicken

Beef: roast, steak, ground

Choices from Meatless

5 ounces' tempeh

15 ounces' tofu

1 cup shredded (4 ounces') low-fat cheese

Three eggs (whole) twice a week

1 cup (8 ounces') ricotta cheese

Healthy Fats

Your meal should have a minimum of 2 portions of healthy fats, including fats 5 g and carbs not more than 5 g because fats assist your body in taking in some essential vitamins such as D, K, A, and E and facilitating your gallbladder to stay healthy and work appropriately.

1 tsp of any kind of oil

2 tbsp. low fat/carb salad dressing

1.5 ounces' avocado

1 tbsp of reduced carbs salad dressing

half tbsp margarine, butter, mayonnaise

5 to 10 olives (black/green)

⅓ ounces' nuts (almonds, pistachios, peanuts)

1 tbsp seeds (chia, sesame, pumpkin seeds, flax)

The "Green"

The green in lean and green means the non-starchy green vegetables grouped in low, medium, and high carbs according to the carbs offered by food items in each group, making three servings of your daily meal schedule.

Each serving consists of half cup of vegetables with up to 25 calories and not more than 5 grams of carbs.

Level with HIGH CARBS Level

Half cup of any non-starchy veggies such as turnips, leeks, mustard, cabbage, kabocha squash, summer squash, palm, green/wax beans, chayote squash, kohlrabi, broccoli, okra, tomatoes, all bell pepper, spaghetti, scallions

Level with MEDIUM CARBS

Half cup of summer squash, eggplant, cabbage, spinach, a fennel bulb, cauliflower, asparagus, mushrooms, kale

Level with LOW CARBS

One cup of lettuce, fresh or raw spinach, watercress, fresh or raw collards, green mustard, raw bok choy endive, spring mix, and a half cup of raw Swiss chard, turnip, celery, radish, cucumber, cooked bok choy, mushrooms, jalapeno, alfalfa, escarole, mung bean

Additional items for Optimal Weight 5 & 1

You are free to add a daily basis, a non-compulsory snack in your 5 and 1 diet program.

Puffed Snacks

Popcorn

One carb-free Popsicle (fruity flavor)

A half-ounce of nuts such as seven walnuts (half), 20 kernels of pistachios, ten almonds

Half cup of sugar-free gelatin

Three pieces of gum or mints (sugar-free)

Three stalks of celery

Two dill pickles

Food with home-cooked food flavor

A complete set of nutritious and delightful meals with the required amount of green veggies, lean protein, and healthy fat tastes like home-cooked yet ready in one minute is available at the doorstep when you have a hectic schedule and too tired to cook your dinner.

Proper and purposeful liquid intake is as important and crucial as to eat healthy food to transform your life by losing the desired weight.

Here are some of the products offered by the Optavia program to fulfill your proper and purposeful hydration supplies.

The first one is to **start strong,** which comprises Vitamin C equivalent to six oranges to keep your immune system strong and healthy.

Second is **B active** good source of vitamin B assisting the body in producing cellular energy**.**

Third and the last one is **replenishment** through which one can regain his/her electrolytes that as lost during our day-to-day activities.

Seasoning Options

The flavor of your meal can be enhanced, condiments can be in-cooperated, but carbs present will also be counted restricted to one gram per serving allowed a day thrice.

Examples:

Half tsp of dried spices and herbs, cocktail sauce, catsup, pepper, BBQ sauce, Worcestershire sauce

One-fourth tsp of salt

One tbsp. of chopped onion, soy sauce, salsa, reduced-fat milk, fat-free soy milk, yellow mustard

Two tsp. of lemon juice or lime juice

Two tbsp. of flavored syrup (sugar-free)

One packet of calorie-free sweetener

One cup of cashew or vanilla milk (sugar-free and refrigerated)

Chapter 3: Optavia 4 & 2 & 1 diet plan

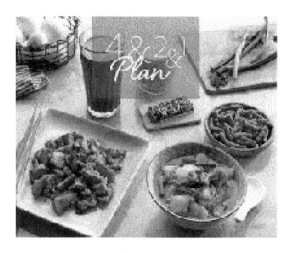

4 & 2 & 1 Meal Plan for Optimal Weight

The 4-2-1 diet plan is best suited to those users who want a quick reduction in weight and desire somewhat flexible meal plans to attain it. The group of people that can follow the 4-2-1 diet plan includes

Patients with type 1 and 2 diabetes

Age above 65 years

Desire to have a variable meal program

Work out more than 45 mins per day

This second meal plan offered by Optavia is simple, quick, and easy to follow, with a wide range of meals that you can take or add to your diet plan. It allows having a meal seven times per day after every two or three times a day with four meals from fueling, two meals from the lean and green section, and one from snacks portion, thus fulfilling your desire to have different things on your dining table after every few hours.

Food scientists have formulated the fueling items with the same nutritious worth with nutritionists and dietitians' help. It has the required amount of fat, carbs, and proteins to attain healthy weight if you follow the 4-2-1 diet plan. The fueling included in the Optavia diet is free of artificial flavors, colors, and sweeteners; they contain cultures from the probiotic category, helping our digestive system stay healthy, which keeps us healthy with an optimal diet. This plan will help you choose healthy meals for everyone around and make you aware of the nutritional value of the food you are eating, and eventually, you will get to know how to cook lean and green meals.

Snacks

Following items can be the part of diet plan as snacks

olive oil Popcorn (salty)

Puffed Snacks (salty /sweet)

Cream or Cheddar Starchy Popcorn

Puffed Snacks (ranch)

A snack meal might include

One-third cup of cooked pasta

One-third cup of cooked brown rice

Half cup of cooked lentils or beans

Two slices of bread low-calorie (one slice contains almost around 40 calories

Three fourth cup of whole-grain cereal making almost 3 grams

Half cup of peas or corns

One-fourth part of potato baked making almost 3 ounces

Half cup of cooked cereal

One cup of squash

Dairy

Three fourth cup of low-fat yogurt (6 ounces')

1 cup of milk reduced fat

Half cup of fat-free condensed milk

Fruit

A fruit serving includes:

17 grains of grapes

One cup of melon sliced

Half grapefruit

Half banana

¾ cup berries

Citrus fruits about 4 ounces' (canned or frozen)

Chapter 4: Optavia 3 & 3 diet plan

Optavia diet place 3 and 3

3 & 3 program is the last stage of the Optavia program, which starts when you have attained the desired weight loss, and now you have to maintain this weight. For this, you need not follow the previous diet plan rather than add low carbohydrates edibles that were not permissible in the 5-1 or 4-2-1 meal plan. You just have to have three fueling with three servings of a healthy balanced meal per day. Thus to stick to your desired weight, you have to plan your meals sensibly; balance your calorie intake with the calories utilization.

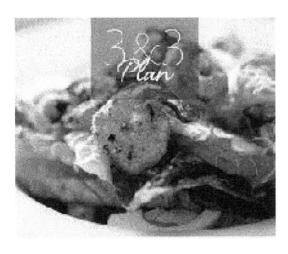

The 3 and 3 plan is simple and convenient to follow with these easy steps. Firstly, estimate how many calories you can burn daily according to your work routine. The 3-3 diet plan can also be called assessing total energy expenditure (TEE). According to your TEE design, your meals contain the number of calories that you can easily burn in a day. Optavia also assists its users in choosing meals with calories ranging from 12oo to 25oo. Scientists and dietitians have carefully designed these daily meal plans for Optavia customers. In addition to that, in 3 and 3, you can add variety to your meals by adding items from different food groups such as healthy fats, vegetables, fruits, proteins, and starchy edibles.

Tip: Steady increase in your workout is also a part of sustaining a healthy weight.

Mentioned below are one complete sample meal plan details for one a day when you aimed to have to take 12oo, 13oo, 1400, 1500, 1600, 1700, 1800, 1900, 2000, 2100, 2200, 2300, 2400 and 2500 calories a day.

As a sample meal plan when taking **1200 calories** per day

Breakfast

1 starch serving - three fourth cup of cooked cereal (sugar free)

1 dairy serving – one cup of skimmed milk

Nibble

1 Fueling serving – Yogurt bar strawberry flavor

Lunch

1 dairy serving – three fourth cup of yogurt (low fat)

1 vegetable serving – half cup of cauliflower (ready to eat)

1 protein serving – three ounces of chicken (grilled or baked)

Evening

1 fueling serving – smoothie (banana and/or strawberry flavor)

Dinner

1 fruit serving – one apple

1 protein serving - three ounces of baked tuna

2 vegetables servings – one cup of chopped mushrooms, tomatoes and/or cucumbers with two cups of spinach (raw)

1 fat serving – two tablespoons of salad dressing (low fat)

Midnight

1 serving as desired

As a sample meal plan when taking **1300 calories** per day

Breakfast

1 starch serving - three fourth cup of cooked cereal (sugar free)

1 dairy serving – one cup of low fat milk

Nibble

1 Fueling serving – Yogurt bar fruity flavor

Lunch

1 dairy serving – three fourth cup of yogurt (low fat)

1 vegetable serving – half cup of broccoli (ready to eat)

1 protein serving – three ounces of chicken (grilled or baked)

Evening

1 fueling serving – smoothie (banana and/or strawberry flavor)

Dinner

1 fruit serving – one apple

1 protein serving - three ounces of baked tuna

2 vegetables servings – one cup of chopped mushrooms, tomatoes and/or pepper with two cups of spinach (raw)

1 fat serving – two tablespoons of salad dressing (low fat)

Mid-Evening

1 fueling – Biscuits (blueberry flavor)

Midnight

1 serving as desired

As a sample meal plan when taking **1400 calories** per day

Breakfast

1 starch serving - three fourth cup of cooked cereal (sugar free)

1 dairy serving – one cup of skimmed milk

1 fruit serving – 1 ¼ cup strawberries

Nibble

1 Fueling serving – Yogurt bar strawberry flavor

Lunch

1 dairy serving – three fourth cup of yogurt (low fat)

1 vegetable serving – half cup of broccoli (ready to eat)

1 protein serving – three ounces of chicken (grilled or baked)

Evening

1 fueling serving – smoothie (banana and/or strawberry flavor)

Dinner

1 fruit serving – one apple

1 protein serving - three ounces of baked tuna

2 vegetables servings – one cup of chopped mushrooms, tomatoes and/or peppers with two cups of spinach (raw)

2 fat serving – eight black olives and two tablespoons of salad dressing (low fat)

Midevening

1 fueling – Biscuits (blueberry flavor)

Midnight

1 serving as desired

As a sample meal plan when taking **1500** calories per day

Breakfast

1 starch serving - three fourth cup of cooked cereal (sugar free)

1 dairy serving – one cup of skimmed milk

1 fruit serving – 1 ¼ cup strawberries

Nibble

1 Fueling serving – Yogurt bar strawberry flavor

Lunch

1 dairy serving – three fourth cup of yogurt (low fat)

1 dairy serving – three fourth cup of yogurt (low fat)

1 vegetable serving – half cup of broccoli (ready to eat)

1 starch serving – whole-grain bread (one slice)

1 protein serving – three ounces of chicken (grilled or baked)

Evening

1 fueling serving – smoothie (banana and/or strawberry flavor)

Dinner

1 fruit serving – one apple

1 protein serving - three ounces of baked tuna

2 vegetables servings – one cup of chopped mushrooms, tomatoes and/or cucumbers with two cups of spinach (raw)

2 fat servings – eight black olives and two tablespoons of salad dressing (low fat)

Mid evening

1 fueling serving – Biscuits (any fruity flavor)

Midnight

1 serving as desired

As a sample meal plan when taking **1600** calories per day

Breakfast

1 fruit flavor – 1 ¼ cup strawberries

1 starch serving - three fourth cup of cooked cereal (sugar free)

1 dairy serving – one cup of skimmed milk

Nibble

1 Fueling serving – Yogurt bar strawberry flavor

Lunch

1 starch serving – whole grain bread (one slice)

1 dairy serving – three fourth cup of yogurt (low fat)

1 vegetable serving – half cup of broccoli (ready to eat)

1 protein serving – four ounces of chicken (grilled or baked)

Evening

1 fueling serving – smoothie (banana and/or strawberry flavor)

Dinner

1 fruit serving – one apple

1 protein serving - four ounces of baked tuna

2 vegetables servings – one cup of chopped mushrooms, tomatoes and/or cucumbers with two cups of spinach (raw)

2 fat servings – 8 black olives and two tablespoons of salad dressing (low fat)

Midevening

1 fueling serving – cream shake and cookies

Midnight

1 serving as desired

As a sample meal plan when taking **1700** calories per day

Breakfast

1 starch serving - three fourth cup of cooked cereal (sugar free)

1 fruit serving – 1 ¼ cup of strawberries

1 dairy serving – one cup of skimmed milk

Nibble

1 Fueling serving – Yogurt bar strawberry flavor

Lunch

1 dairy serving – three fourth cup of yogurt (low fat)

1 starch serving – whole grain bread (one slice)

1 vegetable serving – half cup of broccoli (ready to eat)

1 protein serving – four ounces of chicken (grilled or baked)

Evening

1 fueling serving – smoothie (banana and/or strawberry flavor)

Dinner

1 fruit serving – one apple

1 dairy serving – one cup skimmed milk

1 protein serving - four ounces of baked tuna

2 vegetables servings – one cup of chopped mushrooms, tomatoes and/or cucumbers with two cups of spinach (raw)

2 fat serving – eight black olives and two tablespoons of salad dressing (low fat)

Midevening

1 fueling serving – cream shake and cookies

Midnight

1 serving as desired

As a sample meal plan when taking **1800** calories per day

Breakfast

1 starch serving - three fourth cup of cooked cereal (sugar free)

1 fruit serving – 1 ¼ cup of strawberries

1 dairy serving – one cup of skimmed milk

Nibble

1 Fueling serving – Yogurt bar strawberry flavor

Lunch

1 dairy serving – three fourth cup of yogurt (low fat)

1 starch serving – whole grain bread (one slice)

1 vegetable serving – half cup of broccoli (ready to eat)

1 protein serving – four ounces of chicken (grilled or baked)

Evening

1 fueling serving – smoothie (banana and/or strawberry flavor)

Dinner

1 fruit serving – one apple

1 dairy serving – one cup skimmed milk

1 protein serving - four ounces of baked tuna

2 vegetables servings – one cup of chopped mushrooms, tomatoes and/or cucumbers with two cups of spinach (raw)

2 fat serving – eight black olives and two tablespoons of salad dressing (low fat)

Midevening

1 fueling serving – cream shake and cookies

Midnight

1 serving as desired

As a sample meal plan when taking **1900** calories per day

Breakfast

1 starch serving - three fourth cup of cooked cereal (sugar free)

1 fruit serving – 1 ¼ cup of strawberries

1 dairy serving – one cup of skimmed milk

Nibble

1 Fueling serving – Yogurt bar strawberry flavor

Lunch

1 dairy serving – three fourth cup of yogurt (low fat)

1 serving of healthy fat – 1 tsp of olive oil

1 starch serving – whole grain bread (one slice)

1 vegetable serving – half cup of broccoli (ready to eat)

1 fruit serving – half cup of chopped pears (canned)

1 protein serving – five ounces of chicken (grilled or baked)

Evening

1 fueling serving – smoothie (banana and/or strawberry flavor)

Dinner

1 fruit serving – one apple

1 dairy serving – one cup skimmed milk

1 protein serving - five ounces of baked tuna

2 vegetables servings – one cup of chopped mushrooms, tomatoes and/or cucumbers with two cups of spinach (raw)

2 fat serving – eight black olives and two tablespoons of salad dressing (low fat)

Midevening

1 fueling serving – cream shake and cookies

Midnight

1 serving as desired

As a sample meal plan when taking **2000** calories per day

Breakfast

1 starch serving - three fourth cup of cooked cereal (sugar free)

1 fruit serving – 1 ¼ cup of strawberries

1 dairy serving – one cup of skimmed milk

Nibble

1 Fueling serving – Yogurt bar strawberry flavor

Lunch

1 dairy serving – three fourth cup of yogurt (low fat)

1 fat serving – 1 teaspoon of olive oil

1 starch serving – whole grain bread (one slice)

2 vegetable serving – One cup of broccoli and cauliflower (ready to eat)

1 fruit serving – half cup of chopped pears (canned)

1 protein serving – five ounces of chicken (grilled or baked)

Evening

1 fueling serving – smoothie (banana and/or strawberry flavor)

Dinner

1 fruit serving – one apple

1 dairy serving – one cup skimmed milk

1 protein serving - five ounces of baked tuna

1 starch serving – half cup potato (baked)

2 vegetables servings – one cup of chopped mushrooms, tomatoes and/or cucumbers with two cups of spinach (raw)

2 fat serving – eight black olives and two tablespoons of salad dressing (low fat)

Midevening

1 fueling serving – cream shake and cookies

Midnight

1 serving as desired

As a sample meal plan when taking **2100** calories per day

Breakfast

1 starch serving - three fourth cup of cooked cereal (sugar free)

1 fruit serving – 1 ¼ cup of strawberries

1 dairy serving – one cup of skimmed milk

Nibble

1 Fueling serving – Yogurt bar strawberry flavor

Lunch

1 dairy serving – three fourth cup of yogurt (low fat)

1 fat serving – 1 teaspoon of olive oil

1 starch serving – whole grain bread (one slice)

2 vegetable serving – One cup of broccoli and cauliflower (ready to eat)

1 fruit serving – half cup of chopped pears (canned)

1 protein serving – six ounces of chicken (grilled or baked)

Evening

1 fueling serving – smoothie (banana and/or strawberry flavor)

Dinner

1 fruit serving – one apple

1 dairy serving – one cup skimmed milk

1 protein serving - six ounces of baked tuna

1 starch serving – half cup potato (baked)

2 vegetables servings – one cup of chopped mushrooms, tomatoes and/or cucumbers with two cups of spinach (raw)

2 fat serving – eight black olives and two tablespoons of salad dressing (low fat)

Midevening

1 fueling serving – cream shake and cookies

Midnight

1 serving as desired

As a sample meal plan when taking **2200** calories per day

Breakfast

1 starch serving - three fourth cup of cooked cereal (sugar free)

1 fruit serving – 1 ¼ cup of strawberries

1 dairy serving – one cup of skimmed milk

Nibble

1 Fueling serving – Yogurt bar strawberry flavor

Lunch

1 dairy serving – three fourth cup of yogurt (low fat)

1 fat serving – 1 teaspoon of olive oil

1 starch serving – whole grain bread (one slice)

2 vegetables serving – One cup of broccoli and cauliflower (ready to eat)

1 fruit serving – half cup of chopped pears (canned)

1 protein serving – six ounces of chicken (grilled or baked)

Evening

1 fueling serving – smoothie (banana and/or strawberry flavor)

Dinner

1 fruit serving – one apple

1 dairy serving – one cup skimmed milk

1 protein serving - six ounces of baked tuna

1 starch serving – half cup potato (baked)

2 vegetables servings – one cup of chopped mushrooms, tomatoes and/or cucumbers with two cups of spinach (raw)

3 fat serving – eight black olives, 1 teaspoon of fat free margarine and two tablespoons of salad dressing (low fat)

Midevening

1 fueling serving – cream shake and cookies

Midnight

1 serving as desired

As a sample meal plan when taking **2300** calories per day

Breakfast

1 starch serving - three fourth cup of cooked cereal (sugar free)

1 fruit serving – 1 ¼ cup of strawberries

1 dairy serving – one cup of skimmed milk

Nibble

1 Fueling serving – Yogurt bar strawberry flavor

Lunch

1 dairy serving – three fourth cup of yogurt (low fat)

1 fat serving – 1 teaspoon of olive oil

1 starch serving – whole grain bread (one slice)

2 vegetables serving – One cup of broccoli and cauliflower (ready to eat)

2 fruit serving – one cup of chopped pears (canned)

1 protein serving – seven ounces of chicken (grilled or baked)

Evening

1 fueling serving – smoothie (banana and/or strawberry flavor)

Dinner

1 fruit serving – one apple

1 dairy serving – one cup skimmed milk

1 protein serving - seven ounces of baked tuna

1 starch serving – half cup potato (baked)

2 vegetables servings – one cup of chopped mushrooms, tomatoes and/or cucumbers with two cups of spinach (raw)

3 fat serving – eight black olives, 1 teaspoon of fat free margarine and two tablespoons of salad dressing (low fat)

Midevening

1 fueling serving – cream shake and cookies

Midnight

1 serving as desired

As a sample meal plan when taking **2400** calories per day

Breakfast

1 starch serving - three fourth cup of cooked cereal (sugar free)

1 fruit serving – 1 ¼ cup of strawberries

2 dairy serving – three fourth cup of yogurt (low fat) and one cup of skimmed milk

Nibble

1 Fueling serving – Yogurt bar strawberry flavor

Lunch

1 dairy serving – three fourth cup of yogurt (low fat)

1 fat serving – 1 teaspoon of olive oil

1 starch serving – whole grain bread (one slice)

2 vegetables serving – One cup of broccoli and cauliflower (ready to eat)

2 fruit serving – one cup of chopped pears (canned)

1 protein serving – seven ounces of chicken (grilled or baked)

Evening

1 fueling serving – smoothie (banana and/or strawberry flavor)

Dinner

1 fruit serving – one apple

1 dairy serving – one cup skimmed milk

1 protein serving - seven ounces of baked tuna

1 starch serving – half cup potato (baked)

2 vegetables servings – one cup of chopped mushrooms, tomatoes and/or cucumbers with two cups of spinach (raw)

3 fat serving – eight black olives, 1 teaspoon of fat free margarine and two tablespoons of salad dressing (low fat)

Midevening

1 fueling serving – cream shake and cookies

Midnight

1 serving as desired

As a sample meal plan when taking **2500** calories per day

Breakfast

1 fat serving – six almonds

1 starch serving - three fourth cup of cooked cereal (sugar free)

1 fruit serving – 1 ¼ cup of strawberries

2 dairy serving – three fourth of yogurt (low fat) and one cup of skimmed milk

Nibble

1 Fueling serving – Yogurt bar strawberry flavor

Lunch

1 dairy serving – three fourth cup of yogurt (low fat)

1 fat serving – 1 teaspoon of olive oil

1 starch serving – whole grain bread (one slice)

2 vegetables serving – One cup of broccoli and cauliflower (ready to eat)

2 fruit serving – One cup of chopped pears (canned)

1 protein serving – six ounces of chicken (grilled or baked)

Evening

1 fueling serving – smoothie (banana and/or strawberry flavor)

Dinner

1 fruit serving – one apple

1 dairy serving – one cup skimmed milk

1 protein serving - six ounces of baked tuna

2 starch serving – one third of brown rice (cooked) and half cup potato (baked)

2 vegetables servings – one cup of chopped mushrooms, tomatoes and/or cucumbers with two cups of spinach (raw)

3 fat serving – eight black olives, 1 teaspoon of fat free margarine and two tablespoons of salad dressing (low fat)

Midevening

1 fueling serving – cream shake and cookies

Midnight

1 serving as desired

Part 3: Recipes

Chapter 1: Recipes for lean and green meal

Lean and Green Recipes

Things you can cook at home with extremely easy and staying within your budget.

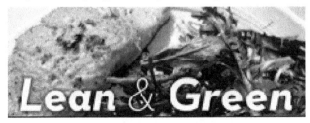

Tarragon chicken with asparagus, lemon, and leeks

Preparation Time: 15 minutes Cook Time: 20 minutes Total Time: 35 minutes Serving: 4

Ingredients

1.5 lb. trimmed asparagus

Two lemons

1.5 lb. boneless chicken breast

1/4 cup olive oil

1 oz. pkg of chopped tarragon leaves

Five chopped garlic cloves

½ tsp black pepper

2 tsp. salt

Two leeks sliced

Instructions

Combine oil, salt, lemon juice and zest, garlic, and pepper. Whisk to dissolve the salt.

Mix half tarragon.

In a bowl, add asparagus and marinade and toss. Add leeks and chicken and mix well.

Spread the mixture over a pan lined sheet, squeeze lemon over the mixture, slice it, and place it at the top.

Place the pan in a preheated oven at 450 degrees for 20 minutes.

Toss the mixture and serve after drizzling tarragon.

Nutrition

326 kcal calories, 35 grams' protein; 103 milligrams cholesterol; 18 grams' fat; 7.5 grams' carbohydrates.

Lemon Herb Chicken

Preparation time: 5 minutes Cook Time: 20 minutes Total Time: 25 Minutes Serving: 2

Ingredients

Two boneless chicken breast

1 tbsp olive oil

One lemon

Salt to taste

One pinch of oregano

Pepper to taste

Two sprigs of parsley

Instructions

Squeeze juice from the half lemon on chicken and sprinkle salt. Set aside.

Heat oil in a pan over a low flame and sauté chicken.

Squeeze juice from the second of lemon and add oregano and pepper.

Cook chicken from both sides for 10 minutes each

Garnish with parsley and serve.

Nutrition

212 kcal calories, 29 grams' protein; 68 milligrams cholesterol; 9 grams' fat; 8 grams' carbohydrates.

Italian Chicken

Preparation Time: 5 minutes Cook Time: 60 minutes Total Time: 65 minutes Serving: 6

Ingredients

Six chicken breast

16 oz. Italian salad dressing

Instructions

In a bowl, put the chicken and pour dressing, and coat well.

Put in refrigerator for an hour, at least.

Put the chicken in a greased pan without marinade and bake in preheat oven at 350 degrees for one hour and serve hot.

Nutrition

344 kcal calories, 25 grams' protein; 68 milligrams cholesterol; 11 grams' fat; 7.7 grams' carbohydrates.

Asian Orange Chicken

Preparation Time: 40 minutes Cook Time: 40 minutes Total Time: 80 minutes Serving: 4

Ingredients

For Sauce

½ tsp chopped ginger

1.5 cups water

¼ cup lemon juice

1 cup of sugar

1/3 cup vinegar

1 tbsp grated zest of orange

½ tsp chopped garlic

2 tbsp. water

2 tbsp. chopped onion

2 tbsp. orange juice

¼ tsp red pepper flakes

2.5 cup soy sauce

3 tbsp. cornstarch

For Chicken

Two chicken breast boneless

3 tbsp. olive oil

¼ tsp salt

1 cup flour

¼ tsp pepper

Instructions

In a saucepan, add lemon and orange juice, soy sauce, and one and a half cup of water, heat the mixture.

Mix zest, ginger, onion, sugar, garlic, and flakes. Let the mixture boil.

Turn off the flame and let it cool.

Place chicken and one cup of sauce and mix well in a large bowl and place the bowl in refrigerate for two hours.

After two hours, take out the chicken pieces in another bowl and combine pepper, flour, salt, and toss to coat chicken well.

Over medium flame, heat oil in a skillet and cook chicken from both sides until turned brown.

Take out the chicken pieces on the plate and clean the skillet.

In the same skillet, pour remaining sauce and boil on high flame.

Add in water and starch and mix.

At low heat, place chicken pieces and simmer for five minutes.

Nutrition

445 kcal calories, 18 grams' protein; 34.2 milligrams cholesterol; 11 grams' fat; 69 grams' carbohydrates.

Rosemary Chicken

Preparation Time: 5 minutes Cook Time: 35 minutes Total Time: 40 minutes Serving: 5

Ingredients

1 tbsp olive oil

1.25 lb. chicken breasts boneless

pepper to taste

2 tsp. chopped rosemary leaves

3 tbsp. melted butter

1.25 tsp. chopped garlic

1 tbsp minced fresh parsley

2 tbsp. lemon juice

lemon slices for garnishing

1/4 cup chicken broth

salt to taste

Rosemary sprigs for garnishing

Instructions

Drizzle salt and pepper on chicken and rub on both sides.

Cook chicken pieces in heated oil in a skillet on a medium flame for three minutes.

When chicken turns brown, place it on a baking pan greased with oil.

Combine butter, chicken broth, rosemary, and lemon juice and pour the mixture over chicken.

Bake in a preheated oven at 400 degrees for 25 minutes.

Spread sauce over the chicken and drizzle parsley.

Garnish with rosemary sprigs and lemon slices and serve.

Nutrition

271 kcal calories, 30 grams' protein; 113 milligrams cholesterol; 15 grams' fat; 40 grams' carbohydrates.

Slow Cooker Cilantro Lime Chicken

Preparation Time: 10 minutes Cook Time: 240 minutes Total Time: 255 minutes Serving: 6

Ingredients

16 oz. salsa jar

1 tbsp lime juice

3 lb. chicken breast boneless

1.25 oz. taco seasoning

3 tbsp. chopped cilantro

Instructions

Combine taco seasoning, cilantro, salsa, lemon juice, chicken in a slow cooker and toss to coat.

Close the cooker and set the cooker on high for four hours.

Using forks, shred chicken, and serve.

Nutrition

272 kcal calories, 45 grams' protein; 117 milligrams cholesterol; 4.7 grams' fat; 9.3 grams' carbohydrates.

Spinach Mushroom Stuffed Chicken Breast

Preparation Time: 10 minutes Cook Time: 15 minutes Total Time: 25 minutes Serving: 3

Ingredients

Three boneless chicken breasts

2 tbsp. Olive Oil

200 g sliced mushrooms

Two chopped garlic cloves

3/4 cup grated mozzarella cheese

1/2 tsp Italian Seasoning

2 cups chopped spinach leaves

Salt to taste

1 tsp Butter

Pepper to taste

Instructions

In a pan, stir fry garlic and mushrooms and add salt and Italian seasoning.

Cook for 3 minutes and set aside.

Make pockets in chicken for stuffing.

Drizzle pepper and salt over chicken.

Fill the chicken with mushrooms, spinach leaves, and cheese.

Close the opening and use a toothpick to secure it.

In a pan, heat butter and oil and cook chicken breasts from both sides for 7 minutes from each side at the medium flame or until chicken is done.

Nutrition

461 kcal calories, 57 grams' protein; 167 milligrams cholesterol; 23 grams' fat; 5 grams' carbohydrates.

Chicken with Sun-Dried Tomato Cream Sauce

Preparation Time: 5 minutes Cook Time: 45 minutes Total Time: 50 minutes Serving: 4

Ingredients

Eight thighs

Kosher salt to taste

Three chopped garlic cloves

1/4 tsp red pepper flakes

1/2 cup heavy cream

1/4 tsp dried basil

1/4 cup grated Parmesan

Pepper to taste

1/4 tsp dried thyme

1 cup chicken broth

1/4 tsp dried oregano

3 tbsp. butter

1/4 cup basil leaves

1/3 cup dried tomatoes in olive oil

Instructions

Drizzle pepper and salt over chicken.

Over medium flame, heat 2 tbsp butter and chicken in it from both sides for 3 minutes from each side and remove from flame and set aside.

In the same skillet, heat 1 tbsp of butter and stir flakes and garlic for 2 minutes.

Add broth, sun-dried tomatoes, cream, thyme, basil, parmesan, and oregano.

Let the mixture boil and simmer for 5 minutes on low flame.

Add chicken and mix. Turn off the flame.

Place the mixture in a preheated oven at 400 degrees for 30 minutes.

Sprinkle basil and serve.

Nutrition

277 kcal calories, 16 grams' protein; 95 milligrams cholesterol; 22 grams' fat; 2.6 grams' carbohydrates.

Honey Teriyaki Chicken Strips

Preparation Time: 15 minutes Cook Time: 45 minutes Total Time: 60 minutes Serving: 2

Ingredients

Two chicken breasts boneless sliced

4 tbsp. butter

Eight fluid oz. honey teriyaki marinade

Instructions

Mix all the ingredients with chicken and marinate for 30 minutes in the refrigerator.

Over medium flame, melt butter and cook it for 25 minutes.

Nutrition

365 kcal calories, 34 grams' protein; 106 milligrams cholesterol; 15 grams' fat; 22 grams' carbohydrates.

Asian Chicken Tenders with Zesty Lemon Sauce

Preparation Time: 15 minutes Cook Time: 35 minutes Total Time: 50 minutes Serving: 12

Ingredients

Three chicken breasts boneless

2 tbsp. soy sauce

1 tbsp honey

½ tsp powdered ginger

¼ tsp powdered garlic

1 cup crispy bread crumbs

½ cup sweet-and-sour sauce

½ tsp lemon peel grated

Instructions

Cut chicken pieces into slices.

In a bowl, mix chicken slices with honey, garlic and ginger powder, and soy sauce. Set aside for 20 minutes.

Coat chicken with bread crumbs and place in baking pan greases with oil.

Bake chicken in a preheated oven at 400 degrees. For 5 minutes from each side until turned brown.

Mix lemon peel and sauce and serve with chicken.

Nutrition

100 kcal calories, 9 grams' protein; 25 milligrams cholesterol; 2.5 grams' fat; 11 grams' carbohydrates.

Shredded Chicken with Chinese Cauliflower Salad

Preparation Time: 20 minutes Cook Time: 20 minutes Total Time: 40 minutes Serving: 4

Ingredients

Salad

Chicken broth 2 cup

Chinese cooking wine 3 tbsp

Ginger 4 slices

Four chicken tenderloin

Chinese cauliflower 1

Avocado oil ½ tbsp

Garlic 1 clove

Water ¾ cup

One handful of purple coral lettuce

Chopped ½ cup chives

Salad Dressing

Grated 1 ½ ginger

Rice wine vinegar 4 tbsp

Plum sauce 2 tbsp

Olive oil 1 tbsp

Instructions

The Salad

Boil 2 cups of chicken broth in a shallow saucepan over medium to high flame. To the broth, add three tablespoons of Chinese cooking wine and four slices of ginger. Attach the chicken tenderloin strips until it begins to boil and simmer for 10 minutes.

To cool, remove the chicken and put it aside. Shred the chicken by using the fingertips to rip the meat away. Just set aside.

Split into tiny florets with the Chinese cauliflower.

Add 1/2 tbsp of avocado oil into a wok over medium to high flame. Add one chopped garlic clove once it is warmed. 45 seconds to fry.

In the wok, introduce the Chinese cauliflower accompanied by a 1/4 cup of water. For 2 minutes, stir fry. Connect another 1/4 cup of water and fry for an extra 2 minutes. Add another 1/4 cup and fry for another 2 minutes if any water starts to dry up. When finished, use a pair of tongs to cut the finished Chinese cauliflower. As we do not want the garlic or the sauce for the salad, do not spoon it out or spell it out.

Thinly sliced a bunch of purplish reef lettuce.

Split the chives to a length of around 3 cm to produce 1/2 cup.

Dressing with Salad

Peel and grate the ginger enough to produce 1 1/2 tsp.

Add the plum sauce, rice wine vinegar, olive oil, and grated ginger to a small mixing bowl until well mixed.

Assembly

Apply both salad ingredients to a big mixing cup.

Pour on the salad with the dressing and toss until well mixed.

Place the mixed salad in a heap on a wide serving tray.

Immediately serve.

Notes

For this dish, you can use any cut of chicken. Tenderloin strips have been selected because they are leaner and are simpler to shred. The breast is quick to shred as well.

If you are unable to get Chinese cauliflower, it is nice to use standard cauliflower. If you like, you may also use broccoli or broccoli.

If you're shopping for chives in the Asian grocery store, make sure you don't purchase the garlic chives by accident because when consumed fresh, it is too powerful a taste.

If you don't have a wok, they'll do a huge fry pan. However, make sure it has a bit of depth since it will make the stir-frying less messy.

In any Asian grocer, you can find Chinese cooking wine quickly.

Nutrition

144 kcal calories, 13 grams' carbohydrates, 14 grams' protein, 4 grams' fat, 32 milligrams cholesterol.

Tarragon Scallops on Asparagus Spears

Preparation time: 5 minutes Cook time: 20 minutes' Total time: 25 minutes Servings: 4

Ingredients

Fresh or frozen sea scallops one ¼ lb.

Water 1 cup

Asparagus spears, trimmed 1-pound

Lemons 2 medium

Ground pepper ½ tsp

Salt ¼ tsp

Extra virgin olive oil 1 tbsp

Vegetable oil spread 3 tbsp

chopped fresh tarragon 1 tbsp

Instructions

If frozen, thaw the scallops, set aside. Bring water to a boil over medium-high heat in a broad nonstick skillet, introduce the asparagus, return to a boil, minimize heat, cover the pot 3 to 5 minutes, or until soft-crisp. Drain well, put on a serving plate, and gently cover to stay warm.

Break the wedges out of one of the lemons. Finely shred one peel of a teaspoon of the remaining lemon. Squeeze out two teaspoons of lemon juice.

With paper towels, pat scallops off. Sprinkle pepper and salt on the scallops.

Wipe dry in the skillet. Over medium pressure, pressure the liquid. Cook the scallops for 3 minutes, change and cook two more minutes or until golden brown and only opaque in the middle, operating in two batches. Atop the asparagus, position the cooked scallops, and keep warm.

Apply the combination of vegetable oil, lemon peel, one tablespoon of lemon juice, and tarragon to the skillet. Cook for 1 minute to thicken somewhat. If needed, apply the remaining lemon juice. Squeak over the scallops. Serve with wedges of lemon.

Nutrition

253 kcal calories; 27 grams' protein, 13.8 grams' carbohydrates, 11.9 grams' fat; 46.8-milligrams cholesterol

Ginger Turmeric Cauliflower Rice

Preparation Time: 15 minutes Cook Time:10 minutes Total Time: 25 minutes Serving: 6

Ingredients

Cauliflower 1 head

Olive oil 3 tbsp

Onion diced one medium

Garlic, minced five cloves

Freshly grated ginger 1 1/2 tbsp

Ground turmeric 2 tsp

Salt 1 1/4 tsp

Ground pepper 1 tsp

Instructions

Cut the cauliflower's head into four quadrants and then carve off the center of the central stalk. Split the florets into smaller parts or dice them and put them in the food processor tank.

Pulse before the cauliflower's florets is broken up into small pieces equivalent to rice in scale. You will need to replicate this step more than once, depending on your food processor's size, before all the cauliflower is harvested.

Heat 2 teaspoons of olive oil over medium heat in a large skillet. Add the onion, garlic, and grated ginger and roast for 5-6 minutes or until the onion are crispy, stirring periodically. Remove everything to a plate until finished and set the skillet back on the burner.

Set back over medium pressure, heat the remaining 1 tbsp of olive oil in the skillet. To the skillet, add bits of cauliflower and stir. To mix uniformly, apply salt, turmeric, and pepper and stir. Cover and simmer for 5 minutes, stirring regularly, until the bits of cauliflower have been tender and softened slightly.

Add the sautéed onion/garlic/ginger with the cauliflower rice to the skillet and whisk to mix uniformly. To reheat the onion mixture, you can want to hold the skillet over medium heat for a couple of minutes. Serve with parsley, green onions, or a garnish of your choice herbs.

Nutrition

96 kcal calories: 8 grams' carbohydrates: 2 grams' proteins: 7 grams' fat: 0 milligrams cholesterol.

Low Carb Shakshuka

Preparation Time:10 minutes Cook Time:40 minutes Total Time:50 minutes Serving: 4

Ingredients

2 tbsp olive oil

4 tsp crushed garlic

One diced red pepper without seeds

One finely chopped onion

2 tsp Turmeric

1 tsp ground coriander

1 tsp ground cumin

5 tsp ground cinnamon

3 tbsp harissa homemade

pepper to taste

Two chopped tomatoes

14 oz. diced tomatoes

Eight eggs

200 g diced feta cheese

salt to taste

fresh coriander to garnish

Instructions

Cook the garlic and onions in the EVOO in a large frying pan/ovenproof skillet until soft and opaque. Connect the spices and red pepper and proceed to cook until tender.

Incorporate the new and tinned tomatoes and begin cooking for another 20 minutes at a simmer.

Remove the pan, turn off the heat, and apply the sauce with the sliced feta.

Using the back of a spoon, build the appropriate number of shallow 'nests' in your sauce.

Crack each egg one at a time in a small bowl and slip the egg into the nests you already made, seasoning each with pepper and salt.

On a very low heat environment, return the pan to the stovetop and allow the eggs to poach for about 5-8 minutes or until cooked. To help with the cooking of the egg tops, cover them with a close-fitting lid or foil. Notice that you can cook the eggs in the oven for around 10-12 minutes at 160 C/320 F or until the eggs are fried if you have an ovenproof plate.

Spray the dish with minced coriander to eat.

Nutrition

390 kcal calories, 12 grams' carbohydrates, 20 grams' protein, 28 grams' fat, 0 milligrams cholesterol.

Niçoise Salad

Preparation Time: 15 minutes Cook Time:30 minutes Total Time: 45 minutes Serving: 5 -6 people

Ingredients

mixed potatoes ½ lb.

Three eggs

French green beans 1 cup

cherry tomatoes 1 ½ cup

cooked fresh tuna 1 ½ cup

pitted Niçoise olives 1/2 cup

mixed greens 3 cups

Dressing

minced one garlic clove

red wine vinegar 2 tbsp

balsamic vinegar 2 tbsp

Dijon mustard 1 tbsp

olive oil ¼ cup

One mashed anchovy fillet

Sugar 1 -2 tsp

salt and fresh ground black pepper to taste

chopped fresh parsley 2 tsp

Instructions

The way to prepare tuna

When using new tuna, over medium-high pressure, heat the skillet. Season the tuna with pepper and salt. If needed, use some salad dressing on the tuna. Using olive oil to rub.

Put the tuna in the skillet and sear on each side for around 3 minutes; cook until the tuna is cooked through, as in the image for medium-rare.

The Vegetables Preparation

Cook the scrubbed potatoes in a saucepan of water over high heat until soft, around 10 minutes. Drain and put in cold water in a tub, then drain again. 1/4-inch-thick, sliced into slices. Only put back.

Place the eggs and cold water in a saucepan. Carry to a boil over medium-high pressure, then simmer for 17 minutes or so. Drain, put the cold water in a bowl, and let it cool. Stir, peel and break into pieces.

Blanch the green beans by putting them for 2 or 3 minutes in hot water. Remove, then put for around 5 minutes in ice-cold water. Drain then and put aside.

Halve the cherry tomatoes and put them aside.

Drain the tuna from a can and position it in a little bowl if you use canned tuna. For the olives, repeat this process.

Arrange a salad plate of mixed vegetables, olives, French beans, hard-boiled eggs, potato quarters, onions, and tuna. Garnish with, if needed, fresh herbs.

Dressing Now

In a blender or screw-top pot, combine the red wine, garlic, balsamic vinegar, olive oil, Dijon mustard, anchovy fillet, salt, and pepper and shake or pulse until well mixed. You should do this in a bowl and mix before all the components are thoroughly mixed. Serve with salad dressing and garnish with new parsley.

Nutrition

238 kcal calories: 11 grams' carbohydrates: 15 grams' proteins: 15 grams' fat: 115 mg cholesterol.

Garden Chicken Cacciatore

Preparation Time: 15 minutes Cook Time: 510 minutes' Total time: 525 minutes Servings: 12

Ingredients

skinless chicken thighs (about 3 pounds) 12

green peppers chopped two mediums

diced tomatoes with basil, oregano, and garlic, one can (14-1/2 ounces)

tomato paste one can (6 ounces)

One medium onion, sliced

reduced-sodium chicken broth 1/2 cup

dry red wine 1/4 cup

minced three garlic cloves

salt 3/4 tsp

pepper 1/8 tsp

cornstarch 2 tbsp

cold water 2 tbsp

Instructions

Position 4- or 5-qt of chicken. With a slow cooker, mix the green peppers, onions, tomato paste, salt, broth, garlic, wine, and pepper in a medium bowl, spill over the chicken. Cook, wrapped, for 8-10 hours or until the chicken is soft.

Combine cornstarch and water in a small bowl until smooth; steadily stir in a slow cooker. Cook, wrapped, for 30 minutes or until thickened in the sauce.

Nutrition

207 kcal calories, 9 grams' fat, 76 milligrams cholesterol, 8 grams' carbohydrate, 23 grams' protein.

The best chicken crust low-carb pizza

Preparation Time:10 minutes Cook Time: 25 minutes Total Time: 35 minutes Serving: 5

Ingredients

Crust

chicken breast one 1/4lb raw

grated parmesan 1/2 cup

dried oregano one teaspoon

dried rosemary one teaspoon

pinch of pepper

sage one teaspoon

Topping

reduced-calorie pizza sauce 3 tbsp

grated parmesan 1/4 cup

chopped basil 1/4 cup

reduced-fat shredded mozzarella 1/2 cup

bell pepper chopped 1/2 green

Garnish

Red pepper flakes

Dried chives

Instructions

Get the oven adjusted to 450F/232C.

Add a food processor or high-powered blender to the ingredients for the crust. Mix the pulses before they are blended and minced.

Line a baking sheet and add the pizza crust with parchment paper. Mash it flat, less than 1/4-inch wide, to create a thin circle or a broad rectangle. Bake in the oven for 14 minutes, or until the chicken is cooked through and the sides are browned.

In the order mentioned, add the ingredients for the topping and feel free to incorporate your low-calorie ingredients.

Bake in the oven for about 6 minutes until the butter melts, browned, and bubbled.

Remove, garnish, slice, and eat from the oven! Like conventional pizza, enabling the pizza to cool slightly would make it much smoother to treat and keep.

Nutrition

246 kcal calories, 38 grams' protein, 9 grams' fat, 3 grams' carbohydrates, 0 milligrams cholesterol

Loaded Pizza Cauliflower

Preparation Time: 20 minutes Cook Time: 40 minutes Total Time: 60 minutes Serving: 4

Ingredients

Oven Roasted Cauliflower 1 batch

canned diced tomatoes drained 1 cup

slice mushrooms, drained 4-ounce can

red onions 1/4 cup diced

sliced black olives drained 1 - 4-ounce can

green pepper 1/2 cup diced

shredded mozzarella cheese 1 1/3 cups

mini pepperonis 1/2 cup

Instructions

The oven should be preheated to 425 degrees, according to recipe instructions, roast cauliflower.

In a cup, mix the olives, strawberries, onions, mushrooms, and green peppers. Divide the mixture equally into two cups, such that the latter divided into the pans is smoother.

Place half the florets equally in 2-6-inch cast iron pans until the cauliflower is finished frying. Between the two pots, split one bowl of vegetables.

Using 1/3 cup mozzarella cheese or a few mini pepperonis to top each skillet. Beginning with the remaining cauliflower, replicate the layers again.

Sprinkle the cheddar cheese and some dried oregano for each skillet.

For 5-7 minutes, bake. Immediately serve.

Nutrition

156 kcal calories, 9 grams' fat, 28 milligrams cholesterol, 9 grams' carbohydrates, 10 grams' proteins

Cauliflower "fried rice."

Preparation Time: 20 minutes Cook Time:10 minutes Total Time:30 minutes Servings: 4

Ingredients

One med head, about 24 oz. cauliflower, rinsed

sesame oil 1 tbsp

whites two egg

egg one large

pinch of salt

cooking spray

diced fine 1/2 small onion

frozen peas and carrots 1/2 cup

Two garlic cloves, minced

diced, whites and greens separated five scallions,

soy sauce, or more to taste 3 tbsp

Instructions

Remove the core and allow the cauliflower to dry.

Coarsely cut into florets, then in a food processor, position half of the cauliflower and pulse until the cauliflower is tiny and has the rice or couscous texture-do, not over process, or it may become mushy. Place aside with the remaining cauliflower and repeat.

In a shallow cup, mix the egg and egg whites and whisk with a fork.

Over medium pressure, pressure a broad saucepan or wok and spray with oil.

Add eggs and cook until set, rotating a few times; set aside.

Add the scallion whites, onions, peas and carrots and garlic, sesame oil for 3 to 4 minutes, or until tender. Increase the heat to medium-high.

With soy sauce, apply the cauliflower' rice' to the plate. Comb, cover, and cook for around 5 to 6 minutes, stirring regularly until the cauliflower's exterior is slightly crispy, but the inside is soft.

Then extract the egg from the heat and blend in the scallion greens.

Nutrition

108 kcal calories, 14 grams' carbohydrates, 9 grams' protein, 3 g fat, 47 milligrams cholesterol

Cauliflower Breadsticks

Preparation Time: 7 minutes Cook Time: 30 minutes Total Time: 37 minutes Serving: 12

Ingredients

cauliflower (7″ – 8″ wide and 3–3.5 lbs.) 1 large head

egg whites 1/4 cup or two large eggs

Mozzarella cheese shredded 1/2 cup + 3/4 cup (for topping)

Italian seasoning 1 tsp

black pepper 1/4 tsp

Marinara sauce for dipping

Pinch of salt

Cooking spray

Instructions

Preheat the oven to 375 ° F. Rinse the cauliflower, cut the outer leaves, and use a paring knife to divide them into florets. In a food processor, place cauliflower florets and process until "rice" is textured. A few coarse chunks are okay.

Put in an ovenproof baking dish and bake for 20 mins. Take the roasted cauliflower from the oven and put it in a tea/linen towel-lined dish. Let the cauliflower cool down a little for around 15 minutes before it is healthy to handle.

Fold the towel at the ends and squeeze the liquid as hard as you can out of the "ball" of cauliflower. Be careful and continue this before hardly any liquid falls out several times. I had 1 cup of liquid squeezed out.

Raise the T-oven to 450 degrees F. Move the cauliflower and egg whites, 1/2 cup of cheese, black pepper, herb seasoning, a touch of salt, and combine to a mixing bowl.

Move the cauliflower mixture lined with unsalted parchment paper to the baking sheet. Flatten a rectangle with your palms, around 9 "x 7" in dimension and 1/4 "wide.

Bake, extract from the oven and cover with the remaining 3/4 cup of cheese for 18 minutes. Bake and broil for about 5 minutes before the cheese becomes golden brown. Break into 12 breadsticks and, if wanted, eat warm with warm marinara sauce. Hey. P.S. Do not cover it with cheese for a lighter version.

Nutrition

51 kcal calories, 6.5 milligrams cholesterol, 4.8 grams' carbohydrates, 4.6 grams' proteins, 0.2 grams' fats.

Spring Chicken Salad with Lemon Dill Vinaigrette

Preparation Time: 15 minutes Cooking time: 0 minutes Total Time:15 minutes Serving: 2

Ingredients

trimmed and sliced in half 12 asparagus spears

baby greens 2 cups

strawberries trimmed and sliced in half 1 cup

peas 1/2 cup

radicchio sliced 1/2 cup

package Lilydale Oven Roasted Carved Chicken Breast 1 200-gram

Lemon Dill Vinaigrette

olive oil extra virgin 2 tbsp

lemon juice 1/2

Dijon mustard 2 tbsp

Honey 2 tsp

fresh dill chopped 3 tbsp

salt 1/4 tsp

freshly ground black pepper 1/4 tsp

Instructions

Cook the asparagus in a pot of boiling water for around 4 minutes, depending on the asparagus's size and thickness, until tender-crisp.

Take the asparagus from the pot, immerse it in ice water, rinse it, and cool it.

Toss the greens, tomatoes, radicchio, peas, and cooled asparagus together.

Cover with Roasted Cut Chicken Breast.

Lemon Dill Vinaigrette

Add all the vinaigrette ingredients to a container with a cap and shake until mixed.

Over the salad, add the vinaigrette and toss gently to cover.

Nutrition

245 kcal calories, 26 grams' carbohydrates, 6 grams' protein, 15 grams' fat, 1-milligram cholesterol.

Roasted Radishes and Carrots with a Lemon Butter Dill Sauce

Preparation Time: 10 minutes Cook Time: 20 minutes Total Time: 30 minutes Servings: 6

Ingredient

radishes trimmed and cut in half 1-pound

baby carrots 1-pound

olive oil 2 Tbsp

salt to taste

pepper to taste

Lemon Butter Dill Sauce

butter 1 Tbsp

lemon juice 1 Tbsp

fresh dill chopped 1 tsp

Instructions

1. Preheat the oven to 400 ° F.

2. Toss the olive oil with the carrots and radishes.

3. On a baking sheet spread the vegetables out in a thin layer.

4. Use salt and black pepper to sprinkle.

5. Cook for around 20 minutes until it's soft with a fork.

6. Create the lemon butter dill sauce as the vegetable roast.

7. In a little pot or the oven, heat the butter.

8. Stir in the dill and lemon juice.

9. Drizzle and eat the sauce over the vegetables.

Nutrition

97 kcal calories, 9 grams' carbohydrates, 1-gram protein, 6 grams' fat, 5-milligram cholesterol.

Zucchini pad Thai noodles "zoodles."

Preparation time: 5 minutes Cooking time: 15 minutes Total Time: 20 minutes Servings: 2

Ingredients

Zucchini Noodle Pad Thai

zucchinis two medium

olive oil (30ml), 2 Tbsp

peeled and deveined shrimp (225g) 1/2 pound

garlic, minced three cloves

red bell pepper, 1/2

onions sliced three green

egg one large

bean sprouts (480ml), 2 cups

roasted peanuts (80ml) 1/3 cup

Sauce

rice vinegar (30ml), 2 Tbsp

fish sauce (30ml), 2 Tbsp

ketchup (45ml), 3 Tbsp

packed brown sugar (5ml), 1 tsp

cayenne pepper or one small red chili sliced 1/2 tsp

chili garlic sauce, 1 tsp

Instructions

Create the sauce: Mix all the ingredients (vinegar, ketchup, fish sauce, cayenne pepper, brown sugar, garlic sauce) in a small cup, and set aside.

Using a vegetable spiralizer method to slice the zucchini into noodles or long pasta.

On medium-high fire, fire a wide skillet. Apply one tablespoon of olive oil. Then add the zucchini noodles and cook the zucchini noodles for 2-3 minutes or until soft. Don't have the pasta overcooked. With a tender bite, the zucchini noodles should be mildly crunchy.

To encourage as much moisture to be released as possible, let the noodles rest for around 3 minutes. Remove the noodles and clear the excess water from the tub.

To extract the excess water, gently clean the same pan, and reheat the pan over low, high heat. The residual cooking oil and garlic are applied. Cook the garlic for around 30 seconds until it is smooth and translucent. Add the seafood shrimp and cook for around 3 minutes, until the shrimp is soft and fried.

Add the green onions and bell peppers. Cook until tender or for around 1-2 minutes. Attach the egg and mix in the vegetables before the egg is ready to fry.

Back in the same pan, add the zucchini noodles, then add the sauce. Cook for another 1 minute or until the zucchini noodles are fully heated. Stir in the bean sprouts then.

Serve with roasted peanuts, cilantro, and lime wedges for the warm zucchini pad Thai noodles.

Nutrition

545 kcal Calories, 30 grams' carbohydrates, 41 grams' protein, 31 grams' fat, 379 milligrams cholesterol.

Clean Vegan Pad Thai

Preparation time: 5 minutes Cook time: 25 minutes Total Time: 30 minutes Serving: 2

Ingredients

natural peanut butter 2 tbsp

rice vinegar 2 tbsp

tomato paste 2 tsp

low-sodium soy sauce or tamari sauce, 2 tsp

Chili flakes

zucchinis end trimmed, two media

bell peppers and carrots, 1 cup mixed

snap peas 1 cup

scallions, sliced, two smalls

shelled edamame 1 cup

Instructions

In a small bowl, stir together tomato paste, rice vinegar, soy sauce, peanut butter, and chili flakes to taste until smooth.

Spiralizer the zucchini or peel the julienne peeler, potato peeler, or mandolin into ribbons. Placed the zucchini noodles in the sauce in a wide tub. (If you can boil the zucchini in peanut sauce for at least 20 minutes, this recipe tastes much better.) Substitute the remaining vegetables and toss to blend.

If wanted, serve topped with avocado, peanuts, coriander, and lime wedges.

Nutrition

305 kcal calories, 12 grams' fat, 34 grams' carbohydrates, 17 grams' proteins, 0-milligram cholesterol.

Caprese chicken

Preparation Time: 5 minutes Cook Time: 40 minutes Total Time: 45 minutes Serving: 3

Ingredients

chicken breasts boneless and skinless 1 ½ lbs.

salt ½ tsp

pepper ¼ tsp

Italian seasoning 1 tbsp

olive oil 2 tbsp

cherry tomatoes halved 2 cups

mozzarella cheese shredded 1 cup

fresh basil chiffonade 2-3 tbsp

Instructions

Preheat up to 400F in your oven.

Season your chicken breasts generously with salt, pepper, and all sides with Italian seasoning. To coat the bottom of a 9 to 13-inch baking dish, drizzle the olive oil. Chicken and cherry tomatoes are added. Disperse the tomatoes around the chicken equally.

Bake for 30 minutes or until the breasts, in the thickest region, reach an internal temperature of 165F. Remove the baking sheet out of the oven and cover each chicken breast with around 1/3 cup of the mozzarella. Place the dish back in the oven and bake for a further 10 minutes.

Sprinkle over the chicken with the basil.

Nutrition

263 kcal calories, 6 grams' carbohydrates, 33 grams' protein, 11 grams' fat, 101 milligrams cholesterol.

Turkey Stracciatella Soup

Preparation time: 15 minutes Cooking time: 15 minutes' Total time: 30 minutes Servings: 4

Ingredients

cooked pasta Two cups

chicken stock 2 quarts

leftover cooked turkey, 1-pound

eggs three whole

salt ½ tsp

freshly grated Parmesan cheese, divided, ¼ cup

freshly Italian flat-leaf parsley, chopped, 2 tbsp

Instructions

Cook the pasta for ten minutes in boiling water, wash but do not clean.

Three tablespoons of cold stock are extracted and placed in a medium bowl. Bring the remaining stock to a boil in a medium pot and minimize it to 11/2 quarts.

When supplies are declining and pasta is frying, shred turkey into bite-sized shreds with your fingertips.

Add the eggs, salt, and half the Parmesan together with the minced parsley into the bowl with cool stock. Shake by hand with a whip for three minutes or use an electronic mixer.

If the stock has been limited, incorporate a little egg mixture when you whip the stock. What you want is to separate the chickens.

Add the cooked pasta and the cooked turkey, and boil for five minutes and simmer.

Serve with the remaining Parmesan cheese and parsley, sliced.

Nutrition:

543 kcal calories, 29 grams' protein, 30 grams' carbohydrates, 12 grams' fat, 0 milligrams cholesterol

Slow Cooker Southwestern Pulled Chicken Sandwiches

Preparation time: 15 minutes Cook time: 245 minutes' Total time: 260 minutes Serving: 4

Ingredients

10oz. chopped tomatoes

1.5 lb. chicken breasts boneless

1/3 cup chopped white onion

Four garlic cloves

10 oz. chopped green chilies

3 tbsp honey

4 tbsp Worcestershire sauce

1 tsp powdered coriander

1 tsp powdered cumin

1.5 tsp chili powder

½ tsp salt

1 tbsp cilantro leaves

¼ tsp black pepper

2 tbsp lime juice

Ten sandwich buns cut in half

Instructions

Together with the garlic, onion, honey, coriander, Worcestershire sauce, cumin, salt, ground black pepper & chili powder, Put the sliced tomatoes in a blender. Pulse till smooth.

Place the chicken in the crockpot on low heat. Put the Ro-Tel combination on the chicken, cover it, & cook for four hrs.

Turn the crockpot off and cut the chicken. Chop the chicken into bits using two forks.

To a bowl, place the chicken. On the chicken, squeeze your lime juice & put the crushed leaves of cilantro.

Add around one cup of leftover sauce to your chicken. Mix it to combine.

Serve your chicken with additional sauce on the sandwich buns.

Nutrition

1120 kcal calories: 156 grams' protein, 497 milligrams cholesterol, 19 grams' fat, 76 grams' carbohydrates.

Ten minutes' tacos

Preparations time: 10 minutes Cook time: 0-minute Total time: 10 minutes Serving: 8

Ingredients:

For the tacos

1 tbsp olive oil

½ large onion, diced

1 ½ tsp chili powder

½ tsp ground cumin

¼ tsp kosher salt, plus more as needed

1 (15-ounce) black beans

1/4 c water

Eight corn tortillas

For serving

One bag cabbage slaw/shredded cabbage

One med avocado, sliced

Salsa

Lime wedges

Instructions:

Heat oil on med-high heat in a large saucepan till it shimmers. Place the onion & fry for around 2 mins, often stirring, till tender. Mix in the powder of chili, cumin & 1/4 tsp of salt. Add the beans & water.

To sustain a simmer, cover the skillet & lower the heat. Cook for five min, then uncover & partly mash the beans with the fork's back, preserve about half of them. If there is any leftover water in the bowl, boil the combination uncovered for around thirty seconds till it has evaporated. When required, taste as well as adjust the seasoning.

Warm the tortillas meanwhile. Place them on a plate that is suitable for microwaves and cover them with such a damp towel. Microwave it for 30 secs till hot

With the black bean combination, fill the tortillas & season with slaw/cabbage, salsa & avocado. Serve it with wedges of lime.

Nutrition

325 kcal calories, 11 grams' protein; 0 milligrams cholesterol; 12.6 grams' fat; 46 grams' carbohydrates.

Rosemary garlic beef stew in a Slow cooker

Preparations time: 30 minutes Cook time: 240 Total time: 270 minutes Servings: 1

Ingredients

Four carrots

1/2 bunch celery

½ tbsp brown sugar

One onion

2 lbs. red potatoes

4 tbsp olive oil

Salt to taste

Four chopped garlic cloves

1 tbsp soy sauce

1.5 lb. beef stew meat

Black pepper to taste

½ tbsp dried rosemary

1/4 cup all-purpose flour

2 cup beef broth

2 tbsp. Dijon mustard

1 tbsp Worcestershire sauce

½ tsp dried thyme

Instructions

Chop the onion & chop the carrots & celery. Clean the potatoes properly, & break them into 1-inch cubes. In a big crockpot, add the carrots, onion, celery, & potatoes together.

In a wide bowl, place the stew meat & sprinkle pepper & salt. Put the flour & toss meat till it is coated. Place aside the floured beef.

Heat olive oil on med heat in a big heavy pan. Sauté the garlic for around a min in hot oil, till it is tender & fragrant. Add to the pan the floured meat and all the flour from its bottom of the dish. To make it brown on one side, let the beef cook without mixing for a couple of mins. Stir & repeat till the whole beef is browned. Put the browned beef in the crockpot & stir to mix with the vegetables.

Place the pan back on the burner & lower the heat. Fill the skillet with the Dijon, beef broth, soy sauce, Worcestershire sauce, brown sugar, thyme & rosemary. Stir to mix the components, and from the bottom of the pan, dissolve the browned pieces. When it is dissolved in the crockpot from the pan's bottom, add the sauce over the ingredients. The sauce is not going to cover the crock pot's contents, but it's all right. There would be more moisture produced when it cooks.

Put the cover on the crockpot & cook for 4 hrs, on high heat. Remove the cover after 4 hrs. & stir the stew, splitting the beef into smaller parts. Taste the stew &, if required, adjust the salt. Serve warm as is or over a plate of pasta/rice.

Nutrition

228 kcal calories: 17.32 grams' protein, 0 milligrams cholesterol, 7 grams' fat, 23.66 grams' carbohydrates.

Strawberry-lemonade marinated chicken

Preparation Time: 5 minutes Cook time: 10 minutes' Total time: 15 minutes Serving: 2

Ingredients

½ cup lemon juice

1 tsp pepper

1 tsp chopped basil

1 tsp lemon zest

¼ c strawberries

½ tsp salt

¼ tbsp oil

Four chicken breasts

Instructions

In a blender, mix the first seven ingredients & process till smooth.

Remove fat all from chicken, pour marinade on chicken, refrigerate for 2-4 hrs.

With cooking spray, coat the grill & preheat for five min (for the indoor grill).

Cook the chicken for 5-7 mins.

Nutrition

296.5 kcal calories: 30.5 grams' protein, 92.8 milligrams cholesterol, 14 grams' fat; 4.3 grams' carbohydrates.

1.31. Strawberry Vinaigrette

Preparation Time: 10 minutes Cook time: 0 minutes Total Time: 10 minutes Servings: 9

Ingredients

8 oz. strawberries

2 tbsp honey

2 tbsp apple cider vinegar

2 tbsp olive oil

¼ tsp salt

¼ tsp black pepper

Instructions

In a processor, add the honey, strawberries, olive oil, apple cider vinegar, salt, & black pepper, mix till smooth.

Nutrition

50 kcal calories, 0.1 grams' protein; 0 milligrams cholesterol; 3 grams' fat; 6.2 grams' carbohydrates.

Mardi Gras Jambalaya

Preparation Time: 15 minutes Cook Time: 20 minutes Total Time: 35 minutes Servings: 6

Ingredients

2 tbsp oil

8 oz. shrimp

8 oz. boneless chicken breasts

4 oz. andouille sausage

Two chopped celery

Two chopped red and green bell peppers

One chopped garlic clove

Two cups of water

oz. pkg Red Beans & Rice

Instructions

Heat 1 tbsp oil on med heat in a big pan. If needed, season the shrimp with pepper & salt. Cook shrimp till its color changes to pink, remove & reserve for around one min a side (shrimp won't be completely cooked).

If needed, season the chicken with pepper & salt, then cook chicken on both sides in the same pan for around five min, extract & reserve.

Put the leftover tbsp oil in the pan & fry the sausage, often stirring for around 4 minutes till browned, for around four mins.

Stir the celery into the pan & cook for around three minutes, till translucent. Place the peppers in the pan & cook for around two min, till slightly tender. Stir in the garlic and cook for around thirty secs till it's fragrant.

Place water to the pan & Knorr Cajun Sides, Rice, Red Beans mix to combine. Carry to a simmer, cover, slowly lower the heat & boil for five min. Stir in the reserved shrimp & chicken, then simmer for 3-4 mins or till the rice is soft. Let sit for two mins. Now serve.

Nutrition

274 kcal calories, 18.5 grams' protein; 87 milligrams cholesterol; 11.5 grams' fat; 22.2 grams' carbohydrates.

Asian Chicken Salad Wraps

Preparations Time: 20 Cook time: 0 minutes Total Time: 20 minutes Servings: 6

Ingredients

3 cup cooked chicken breasts-shredded

Four chopped green onions

1 cup shredded cabbage

1/2 cup shredded carrot

Dressing

3 tbsp seasoned rice vinegar

3 tbsp canola oil

2 tbsp honey

1 tbsp water

One chopped garlic clove

¾ tsp minced gingerroot

¼ tsp pepper

1 cup cilantro leaves

Six lettuce leaves

Six whole-wheat tortillas

Instructions

Combine the green onions, chicken, carrot & cabbage in a large dish. For the dressing, mix the oil, vinegar, water, garlic, honey, pepper & ginger in a small blender. Process it till blended. Add coriander, cover & process till diced. Pour over the mixture of chicken; toss to cover.

Put each tortilla with a lettuce leaf; finish with the chicken combination. Tightly roll-up.

Nutrition

370 kcal calories, 26 grams' protein; 60 milligrams cholesterol; 13 grams' fat; 14 grams' carbohydrates.

Buttery Garlic Green Beans

Preparation Time: 10 minutes Cook Time: 10 minutes Total Time: 20 minutes Servings: 4

Ingredients

1 lb. green beans

3 tbsp butter

Three chopped garlic cloves

Lemon pepper to taste

Salt

Instructions

In a big pan, put the green beans & fill with water; carry to a simmer. Lower the heat to med-low & boil for around five min before the beans begin to soften. Drain the water. Put the butter to the green beans; mix & cook for 2 - 3 mins till the butter is melted.

Cook & mix garlic only with green beans for 3-4 mins, till garlic is soft & fragrant. Garnish with lemon pepper & salt.

Nutrition

116 kcal Calories, 23 grams' protein; 23 milligrams cholesterol; 8.8 grams' fat; 8.9 grams Carbohydrates.

Mexican Shrimp Cocktail Recipe

Preparation Time: 10 Minutes Cook Time: 5 Minutes Total time: 15 minutes Servings: 10

Ingredients

3 lb. shrimp

1 tsp olive oil

¾ cup ketchup

1/4 cup lime juice

1/4 cup beer

1 tbsp Worcestershire sauce

1 tbsp prepared horseradish

1 tbsp hot sauce

Pepper to taste

2 tbsp simple syrup

1 tbsp Tajin seasoning

Salt to taste

Instructions

Oven preheated to 230 C. With a clean towel, pat a shrimp to dry & put them on a wide-rimmed cookie sheet. Drizzle the oil on the shrimp and top it with pepper & salt. To coat, toss the shrimp & spread them out in a single layer on the cookie sheet. Cook for five min in the oven till its color changes to pink. Do not leave any longer than required for the shrimp in the oven; otherwise, they can become tough and rubbery.

Meanwhile, combine the lime juice, ketchup, beer, horseradish, hot sauce & Worcestershire in a big bowl. To mix, stir well.

Remove the shrimp from the oven & allow them to cool.

On two tiny plates, pour the basic syrup as well as the Tajin seasoning. Dip the rims often four to six-ounce serving cups in the basic syrup and the Tajin seasoning rims.

Toss them into the cocktail sauce when the shrimps are cold. Spoon your shrimp into the cups once they are coated. Chill before it's fit for serving.

Nutrition

173 kcal calories, 28 grams' protein; 343 milligrams cholesterol; 2 grams' fat; 8 grams' carbohydrates.

Pasta with Zucchini and Mushrooms

Preparation Time: 15 Minutes Cook Time: 10 Minutes Total Time: 25 Minutes Servings: 6

Ingredients

1 lb. thin spaghetti

Two shredded zucchinis

8 oz. chopped mushrooms

1/2 c extra-virgin olive oil

Eight chopped garlic cloves

Salt to taste

Black pepper to taste

1/4 tsp red pepper flakes

1/2 cup grated Parmesan cheese

Instructions

Set the water in a big pot to simmer. Cook pasta till al dente, approx. Eight minutes, as per the instructions.

Heat a big nonstick skillet on med-high heat whereas the pasta is cooking. Place oil of olive to the skillet; after this, put the garlic. Add the zucchini as the garlic begins to sizzle within the oil. Sprinkle with salt red pepper flakes to taste; sauté for three minutes.

Place the mushrooms, then sauté for another four minutes.

Add drained pasta (hot) to the skillet. Add the zucchini & mushroom combination to the spaghetti.

To combine, put the Parmesan & mix. Serve it warm.

Nutrition

501 kcal calories, 15 grams' protein; 7 milligrams cholesterol; 22 grams' fat; 62 grams' carbohydrates.

Baby Bok Choy Salad with Sesame Dressing Recipe

Preparations Time: 5 minutes Cook Time: 25 minutes Total Time: 30 minutes Servings: 8

Ingredients

Sesame dressing

1/4 cup brown sugar

1/4 cup olive oil

2 tbsp red wine vinegar

2 tbsp sesame seeds (toasted)

1 tbsp soy sauce

Salad

2 tbsp olive oil

One pkg ramen noodles

1/4 cup sliced almonds

One bunch baby boy choy sliced

Five chopped scallions

Instructions

To make the dressing:

Combine the olive oil, brown sugar, sesame seeds, vinegar, & soy sauce in a tiny jar/bowl with a tight-fitting cover. Let the flavors mix at room temp as the rest of the salad is being prepared.

To make the salad:

In a wide saucepan, heat the olive oil till it shimmers, on med heat. Lower the heat. Add the ramen noodles & almonds; sauté for around ten min till toasted, stirring regularly to prevent scorching.

Combine the baby bok choy, the scallions, and the crunchy mix in a wide bowl. Sprinkle salad dressing on the top & toss till evenly mixed. At room temperature, serve.

Notes

You can buy toasted sesame seeds/toast standard sesame seed by yourself.

For toasting sesame seeds

Warm the sesame seeds in a med pan on med heat till they are golden brown & fragrant, often stirring, for around 3 to 5 mins.

Take it from heat & move it to a plate instantly to cool fully. Place in an airtight jar in the pantry for six months or up to one year in a freezer.

To make ahead:

Mix the sesame dressing and store it in the fridge.

Scallions & Baby bok choy can be minced & kept separately in the fridge within the containers.

The crunchy combination can be toasted in advance, cooled, and kept at room temp.

Nutrition

222 kcal calories, 3 grams' protein; 0 milligrams cholesterol; 17 grams' fat; 16 grams' carbohydrates.

Salmon

Preparation Time: 5 minutes Cook Time: 10 minutes' Total time: 15 minutes Serving: 4

Ingredients

4 * 6 oz. salmon fillets

1/2 tsp. salt

1/2 tsp. pepper

1 tbsp. olive oil

Instructions

Oven preheated to 230 ° C.

Drizzle with pepper & salt on each side of the salmon.

Over med-high heat, preheat a wide oven-safe pan

Put the oil once the pan is fine and warm.

Once the oil is hot, Place the salmon & cook undisturbed till just browned, 3-4 mins.

Flip the salmon & put the pan in the oven for 3-4 mins, till the salmon is scarcely opaque fully.

Remove the pan (be alert, it will be really hot) from the oven. Move the salmon to the plates and leave to rest before serving for around 5 mins.

Nutrition

404 kcal calories, 65.5 grams' protein; 167.4 milligrams cholesterol; 16 grams' fat; 0.2 grams' carbohydrates.

Easy Cole Slaw (Coleslaw)

Preparation Time: 5 minutes Cook time: 0 minutes Total Time: 5 minutes Servings: 8

Ingredients

14 oz. coleslaw combined with red cabbage and carrots

½ cup mayonnaise

2 tbsp white sugar

½ tbsp lemon juice

1 tbsp white vinegar

¼ tsp kosher salt

½ tsp black pepper

Instructions

In a big mixing bowl, combine the butter, mayonnaise, white vinegar, lemon juice, pepper & salt, then whisk together till thoroughly mixed.

Put it in the coleslaw milk & mix well.

Before you eat, refrigerate for at least two hrs.

Nutrition

120 kcal calories, 7 grams' protein; 5 milligrams cholesterol; 10 grams' fat; 6 grams' carbohydrates.

Chicken curry

Preparation time: 30 minutes Cooking time: 30 minutes' Total time: 60 minutes Serving: 4

Ingredients

1 tsp ground ginger

Three garlic cloves

2 tbsp vegetable oil

200 g chopped tomatoes

2 tbsp curry powder

Salt to taste

14oz chicken thigh boneless

Six spring onions

100ml yogurt

Pepper to taste

Instructions

Cut the spring onions finely, reserving a few of the green cut pieces for garnish. Peel the garlic and cut it. Over med pressure, heat the oil in a wide saucepan & cook the garlic & spring onions for a few mins. Cook for 3 to 4 mins & add the curry powder, ground ginger & tomatoes. Add water splash if the pan becomes dry to guarantee that the spices do not burn.

Place the chicken, then cook for five mins. Making sure that the whole chicken is coated on the sides and is turning brown.

Add water 250 ml & carry it to a simmer. Lower the heat and cook for 10 to 15 mins, or till the chicken is fully cooked & there is no sign of pink color juices in the center of the pieces.

Prepare the rice, whereas the chicken is frying. To take out some cloudy starch, put the rice into a skillet & rinse it under a cold tap. Drain out the cloudy water. To cook the rice, add clean drinking water. Then carry it to a simmer and lower the heat. Cover it & cook nicely for ten min. Take it from the heat & wait for around ten mins with the cover on to allow the rice to be cooked fully. It is necessary to hold the lid on, so hardly any of the vapor escapes.

Remove the curry from the heat, add the yogurt and sprinkle with salt. With the rice, serve the curry & sprinkle with a yogurt drizzle.

Nutrition

232 kcal calories, 25 grams' protein; 0 milligrams cholesterol; 11 grams' fat; 6.5 grams' carbohydrates.

Roasted cauliflower hummus

Preparation Time: 10 minutes Cook time: 20 minutes Total Time: 30 minutes Serving: 4

Ingredients

1/4 tsp salt

One garlic clove

One large head cauliflower

3 tbsp olive oil

1/4 cup tahini

juice from 1 lemon

pinch of ground coriander

2 tbsp water

pepper to taste

Olive oil for garnishing

chopped parsley for garnishing

1/4 tsp ground cumin

sunflower seeds for garnishing

Instructions

Oven preheated to 200 C.

Take the cauliflower head from the florets and put florets on a cookie tray. Add 1 tbsp of olive oil & toss to mix. In the oven, put the cookie tray and bake for twenty mins.

Move the cauliflower to the food processor. Put the leftover two tbsp of olive oil, lemon juice, water, garlic cloves, cumin, salt, coriander & tahini. To taste, add pepper. Mix on high till creamy & smooth.

Move it to a bowl & season with seeds of a sunflower & minced parsley.

Nutrition

235.5 kcal calories, 6.7 grams' protein; 0 milligrams cholesterol; 18.8 grams' fat; 14.7 grams' carbohydrates.

1.42. Stuffed Portobello Mushrooms

Preparation Time: 15 minutes Cook Time: 30 minutes Total Time: 40 minutes Servings: 4

Ingredients

1 tbsp olive oil

Four Portobello mushrooms

Two chicken breasts

1/2 chopped red pepper

1/2 chopped red onion

One egg

1/4 cup breadcrumbs

Two chopped garlic cloves

1/2 tsp each salt & pepper

1/4 c chopped parsley

1 cup cheddar cheese (shredded)

Instructions

Oven preheated to 200 C. On chicken, put 1/2 tablespoon of olive oil & season with pepper & salt. Bake for fifteen mins, till the chicken, is barely done. Then leave to cool and shred or chop into tiny bits.

When chicken is baking in the oven, scrape out & de-stem the Portobello's, reserving within the mushroom gills & disposing of stems.

In a big bowl, place the mushroom gills & toss in the cooked chicken, red onion, parsley, red pepper, bread crumbs, egg, garlic, pepper & salt, and half of the cheese. Changing the temperature of the oven to 175 C.

Add topping to mushroom caps and then top with the leftover cheese. Bake for 18 to 20 mins in the oven till the mushroom caps are fully cooked, and the cheese melts. Serve it.

Nutrition

313 kcal calories, 35 grams' protein; 142 milligrams cholesterol; 35 grams' fat; 10 grams' carbohydrates.

Bruschetta Stuffed Balsamic Chicken

Preparation Time: 10 minutes Cook Time: 50 minutes Total Time: 60 minutes Serving: 5

Ingredients

Two chopped tomatoes

1/3 cup basil

1 cup shredded mozzarella cheese

6 * 4 oz. chicken breasts boneless

Salt to taste

Pepper to taste

2 tbsp extra virgin olive oil

1/4 cup balsamic vinegar

1/3 cup chicken broth

Three chopped garlic cloves

1 tsp Italian seasoning

Instructions

Oven preheated to 175 C.

Combine the peppers, 1/2 cup of cheese & basil in a mixing bowl; whisk until mixed & set aside.

Pound every chicken breast to a thickness of 1/4-inch, taking caution not to split or rip through.

Season the chicken with pepper & salt.

Spoon the tomato combination previously prepared on every breast of chicken.

Roll the chicken breasts up, wrap them firmly, and use toothpicks to protect the ends.

Heat additional virgin olive oil in a cooktop on an oven-safe big pan.

Add the ready chicken breasts to the hot oil & cook for around six mins on med-high heat or slightly browned on each side.

Meanwhile, make the sauce of Balsamic.

Mix the balsamic sauce, garlic, chicken broth, & Italian seasoning in a med bowl; whisk till completely mixed.

Take the chicken from the heat.

Spoon it on the chicken if you have any leftover tomato paste.

Pour ready balsamic vinegar on chicken.

Move to oven & cook for twenty min; Take it from the oven, turn the chicken over, & put it back to the oven for Fifteen further mins.

Sprinkle with the rest of the cheese of mozzarella and proceed to cook for another five min.

Take off the heat & leave it for some mins.

Serve with a fresh salad, potatoes, pasta, or veggies.

Nutrition

239 kcal calories, 29 grams' protein; 0 milligrams cholesterol; 10 grams' fat; 4 grams' carbohydrates.

Fresh tomato bruschetta

Preparation Time: 10 minutes Cook Time: 10 minutes Total Time: 20 minutes Servings: 4

Ingredients

For the fresh tomato topping

1 lb. ripe tomatoes

Salt to taste

2 tbsp chopped basil

1 tbsp olive oil

2 tsp lemon juice

Pepper to taste

For the bruschetta

Eight slices bread

3 tbsp olive oil

1 tbsp butter

One garlic clove halves

Instructions

Cut the tomatoes and put them in a food processor to prepare the tomato paste.

Put the lemon juice, olive oil & basil, after this sprinkle to taste & combine well. Let wait for 10 to 20 mins to allow the tomatoes to produce some juice.

To prepare the bruschetta, add the olive oil & butter together in a big skillet.

Additionally, brush the bread with oil & barbecue it in a grill pan.

Fry the bread slices till the two sides are golden brown.

Take it out of the pan & rub it with the garlic.

With the tomato paste, fill up the toasted bread & serve.

Nutrition

154 kcal calories, 4 grams' protein; 0 milligrams cholesterol; 7 grams' fat; 20 grams' carbohydrates.

Skillet Chipotle Shrimp

Preparation Time: 5 minutes Cook Time: 20 minutes Total Time: 25 minutes Serving: 4

Ingredients

14.5 oz. Tomatoes

Kosher salt

Four chipotle chilies in adobo sauce

Black pepper

¼ cup olive oil

1.5 lb. shrimp

¼ cup lime juice

½ chopped yellow onion

Four chopped garlic cloves

½ tsp dried oregano

¼ cup white wine

½ cup chopped cilantro

For serving

Eight corn tortillas

Four avocado slices

1 cup sour cream

Four lime wedges

Instructions

Oven preheated to 100 ° C. Stack your tortillas, cover them in foil. After this, put them in the oven to warm up.

Put the chilies, tomatoes & 3⁄4 tsp of flake salt in a blender. Blend one min. In this recipe, only half of the sauce would be used. For later usage, the leftover sauce should be frozen.)

Heat 2 tbsp oil on med-high heat in a 12-inch nonstick pan only till it starts to smoke. Place half of the shrimp & cook for 1 min, rotating around periodically. Move to a bowl with the cooked shrimp & repeat with the left shrimp. Put the fried shrimp in the bowl & combine the two tbsp of the juice of the lime.

Keep the heat to med-high and then add to the pan the leftover two tbsp of oil Put the onion & sauté for 3 to 4 mins; add the oregano & garlic fry for around 1 min till it starts to brown. Whisk in the wine from the bowl and the remaining juice of shrimp. Cook till the liquid has completely evaporated. Switch the heat down to low & put half of the ready chipotle vinegar. Boil, stirring, for around 10 to 12 mins, till the paste thickens sufficiently to cover the back of the spoon.

Put the shrimp & take the pan from heat; mix gently. Cover & let sit till the shrimp become opaque & cooked completely, 2 to 4 mins. Stir in the coriander and the leftover juice of the lime. Taste, then sprinkle with salt, if needed.

Serve with slices of avocado, warmed tortillas, sour cream/Mexican cream & lime wedges. Enjoy

Nutrition

315 kcal calories, 35 grams' protein; 428 milligrams cholesterol; 15 grams' fat; 3 grams' carbohydrates.

Zesty Chicken with Artichokes

Preparation Time: 15 minutes Cook Time: 25 minutes' Total time: 40 Servings: 4

Ingredients

2 tsp thyme

1/4 tsp pepper

2 tsp grated lemon zest

1/4 tsp salt

Four chicken breast boneless

4 tsp olive oil

One chopped onion

Two chopped garlic cloves

14 oz. artichoke hearts

3/4 cup white wine

1/4 c sliced olives

Instructions

1. Mix the thyme, salt & pepper with the lemon zest; brush over the chicken. Brown chicken in two tsp oil in a big nonstick pan; remove & place away.

2. Sauté the onion in the leftover oil in the same pan till soft. Place garlic; fry one min longer. Mix in the wine, olives, & artichokes. Set the chicken back in the pan. Just get it to a simmer. Reduce heat; cover and cook for 6 to 8 mins.

3. Remove chicken. Simmer the exposed artichoke combination for 2 to 3 mins; serve with chicken.

Nutrition

260 kcal calories, 26 grams' protein; 63 milligrams cholesterol; 10 grams' fat; 13 grams' carbohydrates.

Curried Cream of Cauliflower Soup

Preparation Time: 15 minutes Cook Time: 50 minutes Total Time: 65 minutes Servings: 4

Ingredients

One chopped cauliflower

2 tbsp vegetable oil

1 tsp salt

1 tbsp butter

One chopped yellow onion

1 tsp chopped garlic

1 tsp curry powder

1 tsp cayenne pepper

1 tsp ground turmeric

1-quart chicken stock

1 cup heavy whipping cream

Salt to taste

Black pepper to taste

2 tbsp chopped parsley

Instructions

1. Oven preheated to 225 degrees C.

2. In a bowl, add one tsp of salt & vegetable oil to the cauliflower florets; place on a cookie sheet.

3. Roast the cauliflower for about 25 mins till browned in a heated oven.

4. Melt butter on med-high heat in a skillet. Sauté onions in warm butter till tender, around five min. Stir the onion with garlic & continue to cook for around two further mins till fragrant; sprinkle with cayenne pepper, curry powder, & ground turmeric. Fry the seasoned onion

combination, constantly stirring, for five minutes further.

5. Mix roasted cauliflower with onion combination. On the cauliflower combination, pour stock. Top the saucepan with a cover and carry the stock to a simmer. Remove the cover instantly, lower the heat & boil till the liquid has decreased significantly, around 10 minutes.

6. In a saucepan with such a stick blender, purée the combination till almost smooth. Stir in the broth with the cream; sprinkle with salt.
Top with parsley & ladle the broth into cups.

Nutrition

359 kcal calories, 5.4 grams' protein; 89.9 milligrams cholesterol; 32.7 grams' fat; 15 grams' carbohydrates.

1.50. Taco Cauliflower Rice Bowls

Preparation Time: 10 minutes Cook Time: 20 minutes Total Time: 30 minutes Servings: **4**

Ingredients

Taco meat

1 tsp olive oil

1 lb. ground beef

1 tsp paprika

1 tsp pepper

1 tsp chili powder

1 tsp garlic powder

1/2 tsp salt

1 tsp onion powder

1 tsp cumin

Cauliflower rice

1 lb. cauliflower rice

1 tsp olive oil

1/4 cup lime juice

1 tsp lime zest

2 tbsp chopped cilantro

Toppings

1 cup avocado sliced

1 cup Yogurt

1 c shredded cheddar cheese

1 c olives halved

1 c tomatoes halved

Instructions

Heat 1 tsp of olive oil in a skillet. Brown ground beef, when cooked nearly fully -around 10 minutes. Incorporate spices Plus cook for an extra ten min.

While the ground beef is roasting, heat the leftover olive oil in a separate skillet. Incorporate cauliflower rice plus sauté on low heat. Add the lime juice, cilantro, and lime zest. For five min, cook.

When you have cooked cauliflower rice Plus beef, assemble taco bowls with seasonings.

Nutrition

568 kcal calories, 38 grams' protein; 109 milligrams cholesterol; 14 grams' **fat; 17 grams**' carbohydrates.

1.51. Green bean and mushroom salad with poached eggs

Preparations Time: 5 minutes Cook Time: 15 minutes Total Time: 20 minutes Serving: 3

Ingredients

2 tsp olive oil

2.5 cup chopped green beans

3 cup sliced mushrooms

1/8 tsp salt

1/8 tsp pepper

1/4 cup chopped parsley

Juice 1/2 lemon

Zest 1/2 lemon

6 cup arugula

Four eggs

Instructions

Heat oil on med-high heat in a big sauté pan/ cast-iron skillet.

Put the green beans and sauté for around five min, till softened but still crunchy.

Place the mushrooms and sauté till they are browned, around three to four mins with pepper & salt, season. Add the lemon juice, lemon zest & parsley, & mix.

Poach eggs, one at a time: Put a one-quart water pot to a boil. Crack one egg into the little dish/ramekin. Keep it near to the water's edge and slip the egg into the water. Let cook for around 4 to 5 mins, till whites are ready. When frying, do not stir or enter the water. Remove the egg gently with a slotted spoon & drain on a towel.

In a wide plate or cup, put arugula to the plate & top with the green bean & mushrooms. Place eggs on the top.

Nutrition

145 kcal calories, 7.7 grams' protein; 0 milligrams cholesterol; 12 grams' **fat; 3.5 grams**' carbohydrates.

1.52. Crispy baked shrimp scampi

Preparation Time:10 minutes Cook Time: 15 minutes' Total time: 25 minutes Serving: 4

Ingredients:

1 kg shrimp

Pepper to taste

2 tbsp lemon juice

One chopped brown shallot

2 tbsp white wine

1/3 c melted butter

Salt to taste

1/3 cup breadcrumbs

Four chopped garlic cloves

2 tbsp grated parmesan cheese

1/2 tsp red pepper flakes

1/4 cup chopped parsley leaves

Lemon wedges

Instructions

oven preheated to 220 C. In a pan or baking bowl, mix the shrimp, white wine, lemon juice, shallots, melted butter, 1 tsp salt & 1/4 tsp pepper. Mix enough to cover shrimp.

Mix the leftover bread crumbs, melted butter garlic, red pepper flakes, parmesan cheese & 2 tbsp of minced parsley in a medium bowl; mix well.

Toss the breadcrumb combination on the shrimp & cook for twelve mins or till the shrimp is 'just' cooked completely, or until heated and bubbling. For another minute or so, adjust the oven settings to broil or roast until the surface is crispy & golden.

Sprinkle with the leftover parsley, a drizzle of lemon juice & serve with the wedges of lemon.

Nutrition

289 kcal Calories, 35 grams' protein; 448 milligrams cholesterol; 13 grams' **fat; 4 grams**' carbohydrates.

1.53. Turmeric Ginger Spiced Cauliflower

Preparation time: 5 minutes Cook time: 20 minutes Total Time: 25 minutes Servings: 4

Ingredients

1 tbsp Black mustard seeds

3 tbsp Vegetable oil

One head cauliflower (cut in florets)

One chopped jalapeno

1 tsp Turmeric

1 tbsp grated ginger

Salt to taste

Instructions

Heat oven up to 425 degrees F.

Mix the oil, jalapeno, mustard seeds, turmeric, and ginger in a small container.

Put cauliflower in a baking dish of medium size and toss with the spiced oil and sprinkle with salt. Cook until just tender and light golden brown for about 20 - 25 minutes. Enjoy hot.

Nutrition

139 kcal Calories, 0 milligrams cholesterol, 11 grams Fat, 9 grams Carbohydrates, 3 grams Protein.

1.54. Middle Eastern Meatballs with Dill Sauce

Preparation time: 30 Minutes Cooking time: 90 minutes' Total time: 120 minutes Serving: 10

Ingredients

50 g currants

1 tbsp lemon juice and zest

100g pack pine nuts

1 kg lamb mince

175 g breadcrumbs

Two chopped garlic cloves

2 tbsp chopped parsley

2 tbsp chopped dill

2 tbsp chopped coriander

Two chopped deseeded green chilies

2 tsp powdered cumin

1 tsp paprika

One beaten egg

150 ml olive oil

Two peeled and sliced butternut squash

For the sauce

Two chopped onions

2 tbsp olive oil

Two minced garlic cloves

2 tsp all spices in powdered form

1 tsp dried red chili flakes

3 x 400g tins chopped tomatoes

1 tbsp chopped thyme

One cinnamon stick

Two bay leaves

Instructions

Cook and prepare the sauce and meatballs the day before; store them apart (both freeze well, too). Heat the meatballs on greased baking trays, firmly sealed with foil, for 35-40 minutes at 190 ° C, 170 ° C fan, gas 5. Heat the sauce in a pot till it is hot and add hot water if required.

For 1 hour, soak the currants in the juice of a lime, then drain. Toast the pine nuts lightly and put aside to cool.

Using your hands, combine all the items till the paprika in the pine nuts and currants.

Sprinkle with freshly ground black pepper and 2 tsp of salt, then blend well with the egg. Taking a teaspoon of the mix and fry it to check the taste; change the seasoning accordingly.

Shape about 50 meatballs, walnut-sized with floured palms.

Heat two tbsp of oil in a wide frying pan put in a 1/3 of meatballs, and cook for around 5 minutes, till browned from all sides and tender in the center. Repeat for the remaining two lots. Drain fried meatballs on a sheet of paper.

Heat the oven to 200 ° C, gas to 6, fan to 180 ° C. Apply the remaining olive oil to the squash and season. Place on two wide baking trays and bake, stirring regularly, for about 35-40 minutes or till it's browned and soft.

In the meantime, prepare the sauce. Gently fry the onions in a wide pan with the oil till soft – about 15-20 minutes. Include the spice, garlic, and chili (if used) and simmer for about 5 minutes.

Add the tomatoes, cinnamon stick, bay leaves, and thyme to the sauce; simmer gently for about 30-35 minutes till thick. Taste and season. A little lemon juice and brown sugar could be required. Once the squash is baked, mix it in the sauce.

Include the meatballs, covering the pan, boil on low for another 15 minutes, or till cooked completely. Remove the cinnamon and bay leaves and serve with additional coriander leaves, pomegranate seeds, and toasted pine nuts.

Nutrition

396 kcal Calories: 17 g Fat, 28 g Carbohydrates, 0-milligram Cholesterol, 4 grams Protein

1.55. Creamy Lemon Chicken with Asparagus

Preparations Time: **5** minutes Cook Time: **25** minutes Total Time: **25** minutes Servings: **4**

Ingredients

Four boneless chicken breasts

1 tbsp Italian seasoning

1/2 tsp each red pepper, salt, pepper (crushed)

1 tbsp olive oil

2 tbsp butter

1-pound asparagus

1/2 cup chopped onion

Four chopped garlic cloves

1 cup heavy cream

2 tbsp lemon juice

1/4 cup Parmesan cheese if desired

Instructions

Sprinkle chicken with crushed chili pepper, Italian seasoning, pepper, and salt. Include a tablespoon of olive oil to a large frying pan on medium heat. Put the chicken in the pan and fry for 5 to 6 minutes per side. Take out from the pan and set aside.

Add in butter asparagus and onion to the pan and cook for about 2 to 3 minutes, till just tender. Include the garlic and fry for just below a minute.

Put in heavy cream, parmesan cheese, and lemon juice; mix to combine. Put the chicken in the pan again and cook on low heat for 3-4 minutes or till the sauce is thick. Taste to adjust the pepper and salt, if required. Add the fourth cup of water, broth, or chicken stock; if the sauce is still very thick.

Nutrition

607 kcal Calories: 55 grams Protein, 10 grams' carbohydrates, 39 grams Fat, 245 milligrams Cholesterol

1.56. Mahi Mahi with Zesty Basil Butter

Preparation Time: 10 minutes Cook Time: 30 minutes Total Time 40 minutes Servings: **2**

Ingredients

1.5 tbsp vegan butter

3/4 tsp lemon juice

2 tsp minced garlic

1/8 tsp black pepper

1 tbsp basil

1.5 tbsp olive oil

2 Mahi Mahi fillets (6 oz. each)

Instructions

Zesty Basil Butter

Mix the vegan butter, minced garlic, lemon juice, basil, and black pepper in a small pot.

Cook on low flame, stirring till the butter is heated.

Cover with lid and keep warm.

Mahi Mahi

Heat oven to 350 degrees Fahrenheit.

Grease a casserole dish with a nonstick cooking spray.

In the casserole dish, place the Mahi Mahi.

Dollop, a few tbsp of the lemony basil butter sauce on each fish.

Put in a heated oven for around 30 minutes. Moisten the fish with butter while baking every 10 minutes.

Serve the fish with leftover sauce before serving.

Nutrition

165 kcal Calories: 2 grams Carbohydrates, 1 grams Proteins, 17 grams Fat, 0 milligrams Cholesterol.

1.57. Sesame-Ginger Chicken

Preparation Time: 15 minutes Cook Time: 180 minutes Total Time 195 minutes Servings: **2**

Ingredients

1 tbsp sesame oil

Eight chicken thighs (2.75 lb.)

Cooking spray

1/4 cup soy sauce

1 tbsp brown sugar

1 tbsp orange juice

1 tsp hoisin sauce

1 tbsp chopped ginger

1 tsp minced garlic

1 tbsp cold water

1 tbsp cornstarch

2 tsp sesame seeds (toasted)

2 tbsp sliced green onions

Instructions

Heat a big nonstick pan on medium-high flame. Put oil in a pan; swirl to coat. Put in chicken; cook till golden or for 4 minutes on both sides. Move chicken to an electric slow cooker of 4-quart, which is coated with nonstick cooking spray.

Mix soy sauce and the next five ingredients (through garlic); drizzle over chicken. Cook covered, on low flame till chicken is tender or for 2 1/2 hours. Move chicken to a dish; keep warm.

Drain the cooking liquid into a small saucepan through a sieve to measure 1 1/4 cups. Remove solids. On medium-high heat, boil the cooking liquid. Mix cornstarch in a tablespoon of cold water in a small cup. Add this cornstarch mix to the sauce; keep stirring till well blended. Boil again. Cook for a minute stirring constantly or till sauce thickens. Drizzle sauce over chicken. Scatter with green onions and sesame seeds.

Nutrition

310 kcal Calories: 11.6 grams Fat, 36.7 grams Protein, 12 grams Carbohydrates, 148 milligrams Cholesterol.

1.58. Easy Fish Tacos

Preparations time: 10 minutes Cook time: 15 minutes' Total time: 25 minutes Serving: 4

Ingredients

½ lb. tilapia fillets

1 tbsp olive oil

1 tbsp chili powder

½ tsp cumin

½ tsp garlic powder

1 tsp paprika

½ tsp pepper

1 tsp oregano

½ tsp onion powder (tacos)

Eight corn tortillas (6 oz. each)

½ tsp salt

One sliced avocado

One sliced lime

Fish Taco Sauce as required

2 tbsp mayonnaise

3 tbsp sour cream

½ lime juice

½ tsp garlic powder

½ tsp cumin

½ tsp sriracha

Instructions

1. Heat oven to 400 degrees F.

2. Mix all the fish taco sauce items in a small container and set aside.

3. Mix rub ingredients and brush well into fish fillets. Put fish on a pan lined with parchment and drizzle lightly with olive oil.

4. Bake for at least 12 to 15 minutes or till cooked and flaky.

5. Prepare tortillas according to directions on the package.

6. Cut fish into big chunks and split between tortillas. Garnish as desired. Immediately serve.

Nutrition

163 kcal Calories, 27 grams Carbohydrates, 3 grams Protein, 5 grams Fat, 0 milligrams Cholesterol.

1.59. Sausage Stuffed Mushrooms

Preparations Time: 20 Minutes Cook Time: 25 Minutes Total Time: 45 Minutes Serving: 2

Ingredients

18 mushrooms without stems

3 tbsp butter

1/2 cup chopped onion

8 oz. mild Italian sausage

4 oz. cream cheese

1 tsp chopped garlic

1/4 cup grated parmesan cheese

1/2 cup shredded Monterey Jack cheese

1/4 cup chopped parsley

1/3 cup breadcrumbs

Instructions

Pre Heat the oven to 375 degrees F., Spray a sheet tray with cooking spray, and place the mushrooms on the tray.

In a pan, liquefy one tablespoon of butter on medium heat. Include the garlic and onion and cook until softened or for 3-4 minutes. Take out the cooked onion mix from the pan.

Include the sausage in the pan and cook for 5 to 6 minutes; break up the sausage meat into small pieces with a spatula's help.

Put the onion mixture, sausage, parmesan cheese, cream cheese, Monterey Jack cheese, and three tablespoons of parsley in a container. Mix to combine.

Fill the sausage mixture in the mushroom caps evenly.

In the microwave, heat the remaining butter and mix in the panko breadcrumbs.

Scatter the buttered panko on the mushrooms.

Bake until tops are browned for 20 minutes, and mushrooms are cooked thoroughly. Garnish with parsley, and serve.

Nutrition

109 kcal Calories, 2grams Carbohydrates, 4 grams Fat, 9 grams Proteins, 177 milligrams Cholesterol.

1.60. Chipotle lime shrimp

Preparations time: 10 Minutes Cook Time: 5 Minutes Total time: 15 Minutes Servings: 2 People

Ingredients

1 lb. shrimp

2 tbsp olive oil

Four chopped garlic cloves

1 tbsp honey

1.5 tbsp lime juice

½ tsp powdered Chili Pepper

¼ tsp salt

1 tbsp chopped parsley or cilantro

Lime wedges as required

Instructions

Wash the shrimp with tap water, and pat dry with kitchen towels. Put aside.

Heat a pan (cast-iron preferred) and add in the olive oil; add the garlic in the heated oil and stir a few times with a spatula. Add the shrimp into the pan, stirring and cooking. Put in the lime juice, honey, Chipotle Chili Pepper, and salt, mix well with the shrimp. Keep turning and stirring the shrimp so that both sides are evenly cooked.

Add the cilantro or parsley, stir to mix well. Turn the heat off and serve with fresh lime wedges immediately. Squeeze the lime juice on shrimp before eating.

Nutrition

209 kcal Calories, 47 grams Proteins, 12 grams Carbohydrates, 17 grams Fat, 572 milligrams

1.61. Homemade Sloppy Joes Recipe

Preparation Time: 5 minutes Cook Time: 25 minutes Total Time: 30 minutes Servings: 6

Ingredients

1 lb. ground turkey beef, turkey

1/2 cup chopped green bell pepper

1/4 cup diced onion

Two chopped garlic cloves

1/4 cup tomato paste

2 tbsp. brown sugar

1 tbsp yellow mustard

¼ tsp of pepper

2 tsp red wine vinegar

2 tsp Worcestershire sauce

1 cup beef broth

1/4 tsp of salt

Instructions

1. Chop onion and green bell pepper. Mince the garlic finely.

2. In a medium frying skillet, put in the ground beef (or pork or turkey) and decrease the heat to medium. As it cooks, separate the meat into smaller pieces. It will take around 7 minutes.

3. Mix in all of the ingredients; when the meat is cooked thoroughly, add water in last. Bring it to a simmer, then turn flame to medium-low and cook uncovered for around 15 minutes. Taste to adjust the seasonings.

4. Serve it on a bun.

Nutrition

233 kcal Calories: 15 grams Protein, 17 grams Fat, 5 milligrams of Cholesterol, 4 grams Carbohydrates.

1.62. One-Skillet Balsamic Chicken and Vegetables

Preparation time: 5 Minutes Cook time: 10 Minutes Total time: 15 Minutes Serving: 3

Ingredients

1/3 cup balsamic vinegar

2 tbsp honey

1 tbsp brown sugar

3 tbsp olive oil

2 tsp cornstarch

1/2 tsp pepper

2 cups broccoli florets

Four chicken breasts boneless (sliced)

1/2 tsp salt

1.5 cups sugar snap peas

4 tbsp. water if required

Instructions

1. Add balsamic vinegar, brown sugar, honey, one tbsp olive oil, salt, pepper, and cornstarch, mix into a mixing bowl or a large mixing cup to combine; put aside the sauce.

2. Add two tbsp of olive oil to a wide skillet, add in the chicken breasts, sprinkle with pepper and salt to taste, and simmer on medium-high heat for around 5 minutes or till around 75% of the chicken has cooked through, halfway into the cooking, flip chicken. Depending on the size of the chicken breasts and piece sizes, cooking time can differ.

3. Add in the sauce, noting that it may come to the surface in the first few seconds.

4. Include the vegetables and scatter them uniformly on the skillet, some of which would be on top of the chicken. Include two to four tablespoons of water to make the vegetable steam, if required. Due to the number of natural juices produced by the chicken when frying, adding water can differ.

5. Cover the skillet and steam the vegetables for around 3 to 5 minutes, or until the chicken is crisp-tender and cooked through. Stir to cover the vegetables with sauce uniformly.

6. Taste the sauce, to check the balance of the seasoning, make some required modifications before serving (more pepper, honey splash, salt, or balsamic vinegar, etc.)

Nutrition

407 kcal Calories: 41 grams' proteins, 102 milligrams cholesterol, 14 grams' **fat, 26 grams' carbohydrates.**

1.63. Easy lime crema recipe

Preparations time: 5 minutes Cook Time: 0 minutes Total Time: 5 minutes Servings: 8

Ingredients

8 oz. sour cream

1/4 tsp salt

1 tbsp of lime juice and its zest

One chopped garlic clove

Instructions

The lime juice is squeezed in a bowl after lime zest.

Add garlic, salt, and sour cream to a bowl and mix everything till creamy and well combined.

Use it at once or keep put in the fridge till ready for serving

Nutrition

58 kcal Calories: 1 gram's proteins, 15 milligrams cholesterol, 6 grams' **fat, 2 grams' carbohydrates.**

1.64. Fresh Pico de Gallo

Preparation time: 10 minutes Cook time: 0-minute Total time: 10 minutes Serving: 8

Ingredients

1 cup chopped white onion

¾ tsp salt

One chopped jalapeño or serrano pepper without seeds

¼ cup lime juice

1.5 lb. chopped tomatoes

½ cup chopped cilantro

Instructions

1. Combine the jalapeño, chopped onion, salt, and lime juice in a medium serving bowl. While you cut the cilantro and tomatoes, let it soak for around 5 minutes.

2. Add in the chopped cilantro and tomatoes to the bowl and mix to combine. Taste and adjust seasoning

3. For the greatest flavor, let the mixture soak for 15 minutes or, if possible several hours in the fridge. Serve as a dip, with a large serving fork to prevent transferring excessive watery tomato juice with your Pico.

Nutrition

26 kcal Calories: 1 gram proteins, 0 milligrams cholesterol, 0.2 grams' **fat, 6 grams' carbohydrates.**

1.65. Garlic ginger and spring onion chicken

Preparations Time: 5 minutes Cook Time: 10 minutes Total Time: 15 minutes Serving: 4

Ingredients

Sauce

1 tbsp oyster sauce

½ tsp salt

½ tsp sugar

1/3 cup water

½ black pepper

1 tbsp cornstarch

Chicken & Veg

1 tbsp cooking oil

6 oz. sliced chicken breast boneless

½ sliced onion

Two chopped garlic cloves

1 tbsp chopped ginger

Two sliced green onions

Instructions

1. Mix the oyster sauce, sugar, salt, pepper, water, and starch to a bowl and mix to combine. Put aside.

2. In a wok or a skillet, warm the oil over high heat. Put the chicken in and cook quickly for one to two minutes till it's no longer pink. Put the chicken on a serving plate and put aside.

3. To the same wok/skillet, Include the sliced onions. Add in a bit more oil if required and cook to soften the onion for a minute. Add in it the garlic and the ginger and cook for another minute.

4. Put the chicken back into the wok, also adding the green onions. Sauté a minute to finally cook the chicken.

5. Add to the wok the combined sauce and cook until it becomes thicker and saucy consistency.

6. Take off from the heat. It can be eaten over noodles or rice.

Nutrition

203 kcal Calories: 18 grams proteins, 54 milligrams cholesterol, 4 grams fat, 10 grams carbohydrates.

1.66. Pan-Seared Scallops Recipe over Wilted Spinach

Preparations Time: 5 minutes Cook Time: 15 minutes Total Time: 20 minutes Servings: 4

Ingredients

20 oz. scallops

Salt to taste

2 tsp butter

1 tsp olive oil

6 oz. spinach

Pepper to taste

Two minced garlic cloves

1 tbsp lemon juice

Instructions

1. With a paper towel, Pat dry sea scallops.

2. Season scallops lightly on the top and bottom with salt and pepper.

3. in a large skillet, heat one teaspoon of butter on medium heat.

4. place half of the scallops Carefully in the skillet, let them cook, untouched, for around 2 or 3 minutes on either side or till there is a light brown crust on the side touching the pan. When done, the sides will be nontransparent.

5. Transfer scallops to a serving plate and keeps them warm.

6. In the pan, add one teaspoon of butter and duplicate the process with the remainder scallops.

7. Include olive oil to the pan and whirl to coat.

8. Put spinach and garlic in the pan and stir for 1 to 2 minutes' till wilted.

9. Put scallops over spinach and serve. Press fresh lemon on the scallops before eating.

Nutrition

136 kcal Calories: 18 grams' proteins, 39 milligrams cholesterol, 3 grams' **fat, 6 grams' carbohydrates.**

1.67. Balsamic-Dijon Vinaigrette

Preparation time: 4 minutes Cook time: 4 minutes' Total time: 4 minutes Serving: 4

Ingredients

⅓ cup olive oil

kosher salt to taste

3 tbsp balsamic vinegar

2 tsp Dijon mustard

Black pepper to taste

Instructions

Shake or whisk together the vinegar, oil, mustard, ¼ teaspoon pepper, and ½ teaspoon salt in a small jar or bowl. Vinaigrette is ready.

Nutrition

86 kcal calories: 0 gram proteins, 0 milligrams cholesterol, 9 grams' fat, 1 gram carbohydrates.

1.68. Tuscan cream cheese spread

Preparation Time: 10 minutes Cook time: 0 minutes Total Time: 10 minutes Serving: 20

Ingredients:

2 * 8 oz. pkg cream cheese

2 tsp chopped garlic

1 tsp salt

14 ounce chopped artichoke

1⁄3 cup chopped black olives

Eight green chopped onions

3 oz. chopped sun-dried tomatoes

1⁄4 cup chopped parsley

1 tbsp chopped chives

Instructions

Mix cream cheese, salt, and; garlic in a medium-sized bowl, stir and mix in the artichokes and olives.

Add tomatoes, green onions, chives, and parsley; gently blend.

Keep in the fridge for several hours or at least overnight (if possible) to merge flavors.

Add in a little of the artichoke juice; if the mixture is very thick,

Serve with crispy bread or water crackers after Bringing to room temperature.

Or, to turn it into a dip, add more artichoke juice and eat with cut-up vegetables.

Nutrition

104 kcal calories: 2.7 grams' proteins, 25 milligrams cholesterol, 8.2 grams' **fat, 6.4 grams' carbohydrates.**

1.69. Vegan Stuffed Eggplant Provençal

Preparations time: 10 minutes, Cook time: 30 minutes, Total time: 40 minutes Serving: 4

Ingredients

For the eggplants

Three eggplants

Salt to taste

2 tsp olive oil

For the sauce

1 tbsp olive oil

½ chopped onion

Salt to taste

One chopped garlic clove

One bay leaf

Three chopped tomatoes

Pepper to taste

1/8 tsp dried thyme

1 tsp dried marjoram or 3/4 teaspoon dried
    oregano

1 tbsp tomato paste

For the stuffing

1 tbsp olive oil

One chopped onion

Two minced garlic cloves

Two chopped carrots

One diced red pepper

One chopped zucchini

3.5 oz. chopped mushrooms

2.5 oz. pine nuts

Black pepper to taste

2 tbsp. raisins

1 tsp dried marjoram

1/2 tsp dried thyme

Salt to taste

For the topping

1/2 cup breadcrumbs

Instructions

For the eggplants

1. heat the oven to 260 degrees Celsius (or 500
degrees Fahrenheit). Slice the eggplants into
halves and brush all cut sides with olive oil.

Season with salt. Put the eggplants on a greased
baking tray cut side down and bake them until
soft inside or around 20 minutes. Eggplants
should, however, be firm from outside and be
able to retain their form. Take out from the oven
and put aside.

For the sauce

1. in a medium-sized pan, heat the oil on
medium heat. Sauté the onions until colorless.
Add in the bay leaf and garlic and keep cooking
for a couple of minutes. Add in the tomatoes and
sprinkle salt, pepper, and herbs. Cook on low
heat for at least 15 minutes or till the tomatoes
have condensed and thickened. Lastly, include
the paste of tomato and cook for an additional 10
minutes.

For the stuffing

1. in a big pan, heat the oil on medium heat and
sauté the onions until colorless. Add in the garlic
and carrots and keep cooking till the garlic is
fragrant and soft. Include the rest of the
ingredients to be stuffed and cook till all the
veggies are tender or for upto15 minutes.

For the topping

1. on medium heat, heat a small pan and add the
breadcrumbs to it., Stirring frequently, Toast
until the color is golden brown.

For the stuffed eggplants

1. with the back of a spoon, push the eggplant's
flesh to the sides to Stuff the eggplant halves.
Fill in the stuffing with the help of a spoon and
cover the top with the toasted breadcrumbs. Top
with sauce and serve.

Nutrition

490 kcal calories: 11 grams' proteins, 0 milligrams cholesterol, 15 grams' **fat, 70 grams' carbohydrates.**

1.70. Super simple shrimp scampi

Preparations time: 10 minutes Cook Time: 10 minutes' Total time: 20 minutes Serving: 4

Ingredients

350 g cooked linguine

½ lb. shrimp

One chopped garlic cloves

6 tbsp butter

6 tbsp virgin olive oil

1 tbsp of lemon juice

1 oz. white wine

Lemon zest

¼ cup chopped parsley

Black pepper to taste

¼ tsp red chili flakes

1/2 cup chopped red bell pepper

Salt to taste

Instructions

1. In a sauté pan, heat the butter and the olive oil on medium heat.

2. Include the chopped garlic and sauté for about 30 seconds before adding one shrimp layer. Sprinkle with pepper and salt. Do not overfill your pan. Cook in smaller batches if there is a large number of shrimps to be cooked.

3. the shrimp should be cooked for only about one minute per side, according to the size. Do not overcook the shrimp.

4. Take out the shrimp off the pan and include the lemon juice/wine (or chili flakes if needed.)

5. Reduce the sauce down on medium heat to about half and put the shrimp back into the pan along with the red pepper, herbs, and lemon zest. Mix for a few more minutes before mixing in the cooked pasta.

6. garnish with lemon wedges. Serve.

Nutrition

842 kcal calories: 48 grams Proteins, 405 milligrams cholesterol, 42 grams' **fat, 65 grams' carbohydrates.**

1.71. Garlic Sautéed Spinach

Preparations time: 6 minutes Cook time: 4 minutes' Total time: 10 minutes Servings: 6

Ingredients

1 tsp olive oil

6 cups spinach

Five cloves garlic

1/8 cup feta cheese

4 tbsp chopped walnuts

Instructions

Sauté walnuts garlic in olive oil for around 5 minutes or till garlic is fragrant and tender.

Include around half of the spinach and mix till spinach is wilted on low heat.

Again add the remaining spinach and the cheese, keep stirring until all is wilted, for about 2 to 3 minutes more. Then It's ready to serve.

Nutrition

109 kcal calories: 3 grams' proteins, 5 milligrams cholesterol, 6 grams' **fat, 13 grams' carbohydrates.**

1.72. Rosemary and Garlic Simmered Pork Chops

Preparation Time: 10 minutes Cook Time: 45 minutes Total Time: 55 minutes Servings: 4

Ingredients

2 tsp dried rosemary

1 tsp powdered black pepper

½ tsp salt

2 tbsp butter

6 oz. boneless pork loin chops fat-free

Two chopped garlic cloves

1 cup beef broth

Instructions

1. Mix ground pepper, rosemary, and salt in a small cup; rub this mixture on pork chops generously.

2. in a large pan, melt butter on medium-high heat; mix the garlic into the melted butter and place the pork chops in the pan. Cook the pork

chops per side for 3 to 5 minutes, or till golden brown.

3. Decreasing the heat to low, transfer the beef broth in the pan, and simmer for at least 35 to 45 minutes, or till pork chops are cooked fully, and the meat thermometer reads 145 degrees F (63 degrees C) when inserted into the thickest part of the chop.

Nutrition

223 kcal calories: 22.2 grams' proteins, 68 milligrams cholesterol, 13.8 grams' **fat, 68 grams' carbohydrates.**

1.73. Roast Garlic Grilled Marinated Flank Steak

Preparation time: 10 minutes Cook time: 30 minutes' Total time: 40 minutes Serving: 6

Ingredients

1.5 lb. flank steak

1 tsp sea salt

½ cup olive oil

1 tsp Italian herb mix

¼ cup chopped garlic

1 tsp pepper

1 oz. lemon juice

1 tbsp garlic powder

zest of 1 lemon

Instructions

Place flank steak spread out, trim all skin with extra fat or silver.

Season the flank steak generously with pepper and salt.

In a bowl or (ideally) a big plastic container, incorporate the olive oil, herbs, lemon zest and juice, and the minced garlic, and blend well.

Put the steak into the bag and let it marinate for at least 40 minutes to two hours.

Start Grill or fire charcoal -aim for high heat (nearly 400 degrees).

Take out the steak from the bag and dust it with garlic powder.

On a really hot grill, cook the steak and flip it every 4 to 5 minutes.

Before placing the beef, brush a little olive oil over the grill grates.

The steak can cook for around 10 minutes for a medium-rare steak (this can change based on the barbecue, how hot it is outdoors, whether it is windy, etc., so be careful to monitor the steak and how rapidly it's cooking).

Cook the steak directly on the heat, turning twice, for 10 minutes as described, for a steak which is medium to well-cooked, and then move marginally away from the heat (the location where the fire isn't directly below) so that it continues to cook to your desired doneness without being too charred.

Remove from the grill when the steak is at your desired doneness.

Put a little foil around the steak to "tent" it and let it cook for 10 minutes while it rests.

When the steak has been sitting for at least 10 minutes (do not hurry-the steak juices would all drain out if you cut it straight off the grill), slice it width-wise (so that you have plenty of thin strips instead of only a few large strips) against the grain-which is important to prevent the steak from getting either chewy or stiff.

Serve and enjoy.

Nutrition

398 kcal calories: 32 grams' proteins, 90 milligrams cholesterol, 27 grams' **fat, 5 grams' carbohydrates.**

1.74. Crispy orange beef

Preparations Time: 20 minutes Cook Time: 15 minutes Additional Time:30 minutes Total Time: 65 minutes Servings: 6

Ingredients

1.5 lb. sliced beef top sirloin

1 cup long-grain rice

⅓ cup of rice wine vinegar

2 tbsp. of orange juice

1 tsp salt

¼ cup cornstarch

⅓ cup white sugar

1 tbsp soy sauce

1.5 tbsp minced garlic

2 cups of water

2 tsp orange zest

3 tbsp grated ginger

Eight broccoli florets

2 cups oil

Instructions

Arrange beef strips single layer on a baking sheet lined with paper towels and place in the fridge for 30 minutes. Take out the bowl, mix the salt, rice vinegar, orange juice, and soy sauce, sugar, Put aside.

In the Meantime, mix rice and water in a medium saucepan. Bring to a boil, decrease heat and simmer on medium-low heat for about 20 minutes, or till rice is cooked. Pour more water at the end if needed.

In a wok, heat oil on medium-high heat and mix dried beef in cornstarch to cover. Fry beef in small batches in the hot oil until golden brown and crispy; set aside. Remove all excess oil from the wok except about one tablespoon.

Add ginger, garlic, and orange zest, to the remaining oil, and cook for a while till fragrant. Include the soy sauce mix to the wok, bringing it to a boil, keep cooking until it's thick and syrupy, for about 5 minutes. Include beef, and heat thoroughly, stirring to cover the beef. Serve with steamed rice, and garnish with broccoli.

Nutrition

507 kcal calories: **27.4 grams**' proteins, 60.5 milligrams cholesterol, 19 grams' **fat, 59 grams**' **carbohydrates.**

1.75. Sloppy Joe Sliders

Preparations time: 10 minutes Cook time: 30 minutes' Total time: 40 minutes Serving: 4

Ingredients

1 lb. ground beef

1 tsp salt

½ chopped white onion

One chopped garlic clove

½ tsp pepper

¾ cup ketchup

1 tsp mustard

1 tsp Worcestershire sauce

2 tsp brown sugar

One pack dinner roll

½ cup shredded cheddar cheese

2 tbsp. butter

2 tbsp. Sesame seed

Instructions

Heat the oven to 180oC (350oF).

Add the ground beef in a saucepan on medium heat. and sprinkle it with pepper and salt

Mix up the meat with a spoon and stir until it is browned.

Add the garlic and onion and keep cooking till the onions are transparent.

Include ketchup, mustard, brown sugar, and Worcestershire.

Mix till the meat is completely cooked and until the sauce is uniformly mixed. Put Only set aside.

In a baking tray, split the dinner rolls into half and put the bottom half.

Layer with beef and cheese. Put the tops back on top of the rolls.

Use melted butter to brush the rolls, then scatter with sesame seeds.

Bake until the rolls are baked and the cheese is melted, or for 10 minutes.

Cut the sliders to serve.

Enjoy.

Nutrition

339 kcal calories: 23 grams' proteins, 0 milligrams cholesterol, 21 grams' **fat, 11 grams' carbohydrates.**

1.76. Southwestern Meat Loaf

Preparation time: 30 minutes Cook time: 95 minutes' Total time: 125 minutes Servings: 8

Ingredients

1/3 cup Ghee

Two chopped garlic cloves

½ -inch chopped ginger

1 tsp coriander seeds

½ tsp cumin seeds

½ tsp brown mustard seeds

½ tsp Pepper

½ tsp yellow mustard seeds

½ tsp turmeric ground

26 oz. Cauliflower

2 tsp Salt

2 tbsp Cilantro chopped

Instructions

Heat the ghee on medium-high in a broad nonstick skillet.

Include the ginger and garlic and sauté till fragrant.

Add all the spices and fry for 3 to 5 minutes, until "popping" sounds are made.

Include half of the cauliflower rice and combine gently with the ghee and spices. Before incorporating the remainder cauliflower rice, sauté for 3 minutes.

Add salt & pepper to taste.

Still cooking for another 8-10 minutes, proceed to mix the cauliflower rice till soft and cooked completely.

Take off the frying pan from the fire and add the coriander to the mixture.

Enjoy and serve.

Nutrition

143 kcal calories: 3 grams' proteins, 31 milligrams cholesterol, 13 grams' **fat, 8 grams' carbohydrates.**

1.77. Fragrant Cauliflower Rice

Preparation time: 10 minutes Cook time: 100 minutes' Total time: 110 Serving 4

Ingredients

¼ cup chopped onion

1 tbsp vegetable oil

1 cup long-grain rice

1 tbsp minced garlic

14.5 oz. beef broth

1 15 oz. black beans

2 lb. ground turkey

1 cup whole kernel corn

½ cup Picante sauce

0.5 cup crushed tortilla chips

1 tsp taco seasoning

Cilantro to taste (optional)

Shredded Mexican cheese (optional)

One chopped tomato (optional)

Jalapeño pepper as required (optional)

Instructions

Fry the onion in hot oil over medium heat in a large skillet for 5 minutes or till tender. Mix in the garlic and rice. For 5 minutes, cook and mix until the rice is brown. Include broth of beef. Get it to a boil; lower the flame. Simmer, covered, until the rice is soft, or for 10 to 15 minutes. Mix in the beans; put down for around 20 minutes to cool slightly.

Heat the oven to 350° F. Use parchment paper to line a 15x10x1-inch baking pan; set aside. Combine the turkey, Picante sauce, corn, taco seasoning crushed chips in a large mixing bowl. Stir in a mixture of rice. Lightly pat the turkey mixture into the 10x5-inch loaf in a prepared baking tray. Put in the oven for 1-1/4 to 1-1/2 hours or till the thermometer registers 165 degrees F when inserted in the loaf center.

Let the meatloaf rest for ten minutes. Sprinkle with tomato, cheese, coriander, and sliced jalapeño if needed, and serve with lemon.

Nutrition

343 kcal calories, 29 grams' proteins, 78 milligrams cholesterol, 11 grams' **fat, 33 grams**' carbohydrates.

1.78. Enchilada chicken roll-ups

Preparation Time:10 minutes Cook Time:45 minutes Total Time: 55 minutes Servings: 6

Ingredients

cumin 1 tsp

dried oregano 2 tsp

garlic powder 1 tsp

chili powder 1/2 tsp

Kosher salt 1 tsp

Freshly ground black pepper

mild red enchilada sauce one 10-ounce can

boneless, skinless chicken breasts, 1 ½ lb.

mild green chilies one 4-ounce can

reduced-fat cheese blend shredded Mexican 1 cup

avocado, yield 6-ounces, one large

Chopped cilantro, for garnish

Cooking spray

Instructions

1. Preheat the oven to 375 degrees F.

2. Combine the oregano, cumin, garlic powder, salt, chili powder, black pepper in a shallow cup. Rub each chicken portion on both sides.

3. Use cooking spray to spray a small oval or rectangular baking dish and add a thin coating of enchilada sauce on the lower side of the bowl.

4. Lay chicken on a work board, split side up. Cover each piece with around two teaspoons of chili and 1 1/2 tablespoons of cheese in the center.

5. Using foil to protect and bake for 30 minutes. Remove the foil and proceed to cook for another 10-15 minutes or until the chicken is finished.

6. With a few avocado pieces and cilantro, top each chicken roll-up and eat.

Nutrition

261 kcal calories, 8 grams' carbohydrates, 31 grams' protein, 11.5 grams' fat, 83 milligrams cholesterol

1.79. Spaghetti Squash Au Gratin

Preparation Time:15 minutes Cook Time:30 minutes Total Time: 45 minutes Servings: 6

Ingredients

halved and seeded one spaghetti squash

light margarine 3 tbsp

yellow onion, one small, sliced

red pepper flakes 1 tsp

garlic powder ¼ tsp

salt and black pepper to taste

fat-free sour cream ¾ cup

shredded light Cheddar cheese 1 cup

cooking spray

Instructions

In a covered bowl, put the spaghetti squash and add 1/4 of an inch of water. For 10 or 12 minutes, microwave. Scrape a fork within the squash and move it to a tiny bowl.

Heat margarine over medium heat in a medium skillet when cooking the spaghetti squash and cook the onion, garlic powder, red pepper flakes, salt, and pepper for 5 to 10 minutes until the onion is browned.

Preheat the furnace to 190 degrees C (375 degrees F), in nonstick cooking oil, grease a baking dish.

Stir together the spaghetti squash, onion blend, sour cream, and 1/2 of the Cheddar cheese. Switch to the baking dish that was packed and cover with the remaining Cheddar cheese.

Bake for 20 to 25 minutes in the preheated oven. For the last 2 or 3 minutes, turn on the broiler and broil until the gratin on top is golden brown.

Nutrition

115 kcal calories; 8 grams' protein; 10.5 grams' carbohydrates; 4.8 grams' fat; 9.6 milligrams cholesterol

1.80. Bibimbap bowls

Preparation Time: 15 minutes Cook Time: 20 minutes Total Time: 35 minutes Serving: 4

Ingredients

Rice

cooked jasmine rice ($0.75),

4 cups Spinach

cooking oil 1/2 Tbsp

fresh spinach, loosely packed, 6 cups

toasted sesame oil, 1 tsp

Pinch of salt

Chili garlic Beef

ground beef 1/2 lb.

chili garlic sauce 2 Tbsp

soy sauce 1 Tbsp

brown sugar 1 Tbsp

Vegetables

One carrot

onions two green

One cucumber

Toppers

eggs four large

kimchi 1/4 cup

sesame seeds 1 Tbsp

Instructions

1. If your rice isn't still cooked, start this first and, as the rice cooks, prep the rest of the bowl ingredients. You need four cups of cooked rice.

2. Next, cook the salted spinach. Over a medium flame, heat a wide skillet and sprinkle the cooking oil. To coat the skillet, stir and then apply the new spinach. Sauté the spinach, or only until it's wilted, for a few minutes. Drizzle on top of sesame oil and gently season with a pinch of salt. Remove the spinach from the skillet to a safe bowl.

3. To the pan used for preparing the spinach, add the ground beef. Add the soy sauce, chili garlic sauce, and brown sugar and cook the beef until fully browned. Stir and cook for around a minute, or until it is combined equally, and the beef is sauce coated. Turn off the sun.

4. Have the fresh veggies packed. Using a broad holed cheese grater, peel and grind the carrot. Slice the cucumber and slice the green onions thinly.

5. Fry the four big eggs

6. Create the bowls by adding 1 cup of cooked rice to the bowl first, accompanied by 1/4 of the cooked spinach, a few sliced cucumbers, 1/4 of the ground beef, shredded carrots, a cooked egg, and around a tablespoon of kimchi. Sprinkle the end of cut green onions and sesame seeds. No hard measures are needed for each ingredient per vessel; only break the ingredients equally or, however you see fit.

Nutrition

327.55kcal Calories: 20.83g Carbohydrates 12.58g Protein 11.45g: Fat: 3.13g Fiber

1.81. Lemon Chicken & Spaghetti Squash

Preparation time: 15 minutes Cook time: 60 minutes' Total time: 75 minutes Servings 4

Ingredients

spaghetti squash 1

sea salt, to taste

olive oil

black pepper, to taste

chicken breasts, 2, cut into 1-2 in (2-5 cm) pieces

Instructions

1. Preheat the oven to 200 ° **C (400 ° F).**

2. Poke multiple holes in the spaghetti squash around the middle of the squash lengthwise. Microwave for 5 minutes, on heavy.

3. Break the squash through the holes in two. With a spoon, extract the seeds and pulp. Drizzle the olive oil on the squash and season with pepper and **salt.**

4. Place the cut-side squash on the baking sheet and bake until soft, for 40 minutes. Only let it cool.

5. Heat a bit of olive oil over medium-high heat in a medium skillet. Add the breast and cook until the chicken is lightly browned and cooked through, for 6-8 minutes. Set aside and extract the chicken from the plate.

6. Apply a little more onion and oil and sauté for a few minutes before browning starts. Add garlic and fry, until fragrant, for 1 minute.

7. Connect the salt, tomatoes, pepper, and simmer before the tomatoes start leaking their juices for a few minutes.

8. Connect the lemon juice and chicken broth and boil for around 20 minutes until the liquid is reduced by half.

9. Add the chicken and cook over medium heat, then add the spinach and cook until wilted, for another 2 minutes. Taking the pain away from the sun.

10. Shred the spaghetti squash with two forks and shovel it out onto serving dishes.

11. Pour over the squash with the gravy. Immediately serve.

Nutrition

489 kcal calories, 24 grams' **fat, 40 grams'** carbohydrates, 28 grams' protein, 2 milligrams cholesterol.

1.82. Chicken Scarpariello

Preparation Time: 15 minutes Cook Time: 20 minutes Total Time: 35 minutes Serving: 2

Ingredients

1.25 lb. chicken breast boneless.

2 tbsp. chopped shallots

½ tsp crushed rosemary

1 cup of water

tbsp. olive oil

½ cup white wine

tbsp. flour

One pinch of powdered black pepper

One cube chicken bouillon

2 tsp. butter

Two chopped garlic cloves

¼ tsp salt

Instructions

Slice chicken pieces and coat with flour.

Cook chicken in heated butter and oil. Take out the chicken when turned brown from both sides and set aside.

Sauté, garlic and shallots in the same skillet and pour broth, water, and wine with continuous stirring. Cook until half of the liquid is evaporated.

Add chicken pieces and cook for 3 minutes.

Nutrition

580 kcal Calories, 68 grams' protein; 176 milligrams cholesterol; 21 grams' **fat; 14.3 grams**' carbohydrates.

1.83. Broccoli and shrimp stir fry

Preparation Time: 10 Minutes Cook Time: 10 Minutes Total Time: 20 Minutes Serving: 4

Ingredients

24 oz. broccoli

1 tbsp olive oil

One sliced green onion

1.5 lb. shrimp

1 tsp sesame seeds

For the sauce

1 tbsp rice wine vinegar

tbsp. soy sauce

1 tbsp chopped ginger

tbsp. oyster sauce

1 tbsp brown sugar

1 tsp cornstarch

Two chopped garlic cloves

1 tsp sesame oil

1 tsp Sriracha, optional

Instructions

Combine oyster sauce, vinegar, ginger, starch, soy sauce, sugar, garlic, sesame, and sriracha. Whisk well and keep it aside.

Cook shrimp in heated oil over high heat.

After 3 minutes of cooking, mix broccoli and cook for the next 3 minutes.

Add oyster sauce mixture and whisk for 2 minutes.

Garnish and serve.

Nutrition

287 kcal calories, 40 grams' protein; 321 milligrams cholesterol; 7.3 grams' **fat; 16 grams**' carbohydrates.

1.84. Citrus Shrimp and Spinach Salad

Preparation Time: 8 minutes Cook Time: 0 minutes Total Time: 8 minutes Serving: 5

Ingredients

⅓ cup Dijon mustard

1 lb. peeled and cooked shrimp

¼ cup honey

One sliced cucumber

¼ cup orange juice

1 tbsp balsamic vinegar

One sliced red onion

cups of lettuce leaves torn into pieces

⅓ cup toasted pieces of pecan pieces

cups of spinach leaves torn into pieces

Two chopped oranges

salt to taste

pepper to taste

Instructions

Whisk honey, vinegar, mustard, and orange juice in a bowl and refrigerate.

Make layers in serving dish. The first layer of lettuce leaves, followed by spinach. Onions, slices of cucumber, pieces of orange, and on the top place shrimp.

Sprinkle salt, pecans, and pepper

Pour mustard mixture and serve.

Nutrition

242 kcal Calories, 16 grams' protein; 114 milligrams cholesterol; 7 grams' fat; 32 grams' carbohydrates.

1.85. Shrimp Primavera

Preparation Time: 10 minutes Cook Time: 40 minutes Total Time: 50 minutes Serving: 2

Ingredients

1/2 lb. peeled shrimp

One spaghetti squash

1/2 lb. sliced asparagus

Olive oil

2-4 chopped garlic cloves

large chopped tomatoes

1 tbsp lemon juice

tbsp chopped basil

1/4 cup white wine

1/4 chopped onion

1/4 cup Parmesan cheese

Sprigs of basil for garnishing

Parmesan cheese for garnishing

slices of lemon for garnishing

Salt & pepper to taste

Instructions

Spaghetti squash

Cut spaghetti in halves.

In a pan, drizzle salt, oil, and pepper and place squash with cut side downwards.

Bake for 40 minutes at 375 degrees.

Shred using a fork and set aside

Shrimp Primavera

Heat oil in a skillet on high heat.

Stir fry onions for 3 minutes and mix garlic and cook for another minute.

Add asparagus and shrimp and cook from both sides for 2 minutes each side.

Mix in wine, tomatoes, and lemon juice and cook to heat tomatoes.

Add cheese, seasoning, and basil and mix well.

Pour over squash.

Garnish and serve.

Nutrition

399 kcal calories, 35 grams' protein; 294 milligrams cholesterol; 8 grams' **fat; 48 grams**' carbohydrates.

1.86. Rioja-Style Chicken

Preparation Time: 10 minutes Cook Time: 50 minutes Total Time: 60 minutes Serving: 5

Ingredients

Eight chicken breast and leg pieces

minced garlic cloves

Five oz., drained can peas

One chopped yellow onion

sliced red peppers

tbsp. olive oil

Three chopped parsley sprigs

1 cup chicken broth

1 cup white wine

Salt as required

Pepper as required

1 Spanish chopped sausage

Instructions

In a pan, heat oil and cook chicken until brown from both sides.

On medium flame, sauté garlic and onion in heated oil in a skillet.

Mix sausage, parsley, and peppers and cook for 10 minutes with stirring occasionally.

Add the sausage mixture to chicken and mix wine and broth while stirring.

Simmer for 40 minutes.

Add peas and turn off the flame after 7 minutes and serve.

Nutrition

456 kcal calories, 30 grams' protein; 75 milligrams cholesterol; 23 grams' fat; 25 grams' carbohydrates.

1.87. Stuffed chicken thighs with ham and cheese

Preparation Time: 25 minutes Cook Time: 45 minutes Total Time: 70 minutes Serving: 4

Ingredients

8 tbsp. Dijon mustard

16 slices of dill pickle

Eight chicken thighs boneless

8 oz. cheese

1 lb. of sliced bacon

Salt to taste

8 oz. sliced ham

Pepper to taste

Instructions

Remove the fat as much as you want and flatten the meat.

Place cheese, ham, 1 tbsp mustard, and pickles and tightly roll the thighs and drizzle pepper and salt outside the thighs.

Wrap the thighs using two strips of bacon from opposite ends and tie the strips.

Place the thighs on the pan in such a way that the skin side is upwards.

In a preheated oven at 400 degrees, bake for 40 minutes.

Nutrition

156 kcal calories, 73 grams' protein; 358 milligrams cholesterol; 91 grams' **fat; 7 grams**' carbohydrates.

1.88. Cheddar Ranch Popcorn Chicken

Preparation Time: 10 minutes Cook Time: 10 minutes Total Time: 20 minutes Serving: 4

Ingredients

One packet of ranch dressing

Four chicken breasts

Oil as required

cups buttermilk

2 cups cheese cracker

Instructions

Slice chicken in small size.

Mix ranch mixture, chicken, and buttermilk in a bowl and place for two hours in the refrigerator.

Smash cheese crackers in a bowl, coat each chicken piece, and fry in heated oil until turning brown.

Serve with any sauce

Nutrition

948 kcal calories, 33 grams' protein; 27 milligrams cholesterol; 72 grams' **fat; 40 grams**' carbohydrates.

1.89. Chicken cobb salad

Preparation Time: 15 minutes Cook Time: 25 minutes Total Time: 40 minutes Serving: 6

Ingredients

For Dressing

¼ cup lemon juice

1 tbsp Dijon Mustard

⅔ cup olive oil

tbsp. chopped shallot

½ tsp salt

½ tsp sugar

¼ tsp black pepper

For Salad

Four eggs boiled

1 cup chopped cucumber

One head of lettuce leaves

1 lb. chicken breast boneless

Six sliced tomatoes

Sliced radishes as desire

½ lb. cooked bacon

One sliced avocado

Instructions

In a large bowl, combine shallots, salt, mustard, sugar, pepper, and lemon juice with olive oil's gradual addition. The dressing is ready; keep it aside.

Coat chicken with oil and drizzle pepper and salt.

Over a high flame, heat oil and cook chicken in it from both sides for 5 minutes each. Cover and simmer for 10 minutes.

Cut chicken into small pieces.

Cut bacon and boiled eggs.

In a serving dish, place lettuce leaves, top it with chicken, bacon, tomatoes, eggs, cucumbers, avocado, and radishes.

Pour dressing and serve.

Nutrition

733 kcal calories, 42 grams' protein; 0 milligrams cholesterol; 59 grams' **fat; 7 grams**' carbohydrates.

1.90. Cheeseburger pie

Preparation Time: 15 minutes Cook Time: 25 minutes Total Time: 40 minutes Serving: 6

Ingredients

Two eggs

1 cup shredded cheese

One chopped onion

½ cup Original Bisquick mixture

1 lb. ground beef

½ tsp salt 1 cup milk

Instructions

Over medium flame, cook onion and beef for 10 minutes in a skillet.

When beef turns brown, add salt.

Take a pie plate and spread beef on it, and drizzle cheese.

Combine all the ingredients that are left in a bowl and spread over beef pie.

Bake in a preheated oven at 400 degrees for 25 minutes.

Nutrition

334 kcal calories, 25 grams' protein; 142 milligrams cholesterol; 20.8 grams' fat; 11 grams' carbohydrates.

1.91. Salmon Florentine

Preparation Time: 5 minutes Cook Time: 20 minutes Total Time: 65 minutes Serving: 2

Ingredients

1 lb. salmon

6 oz. sliced mushrooms

1/2 cup chopped onion

5 oz. chopped spinach chopped

1/4 cup white wine

1/2 tsp red pepper flakes

3/4 cup heavy whipping cream

garlic cloves

Salt

Instructions

Coat salmon with oil and place over a baking sheet with the skin side downwards.

Sprinkle pepper and salt and put in a preheated oven at 425 degrees for 18 minutes.

Sauté onion in heated oil in a saucepan.

Mix spinach, garlic, and mushrooms.

Cover and cook until spinach gets down.

Drain the liquid.

Add the wine to the same pan and simmer until it cools down.

Mix cream, flakes, and salt and cook for five more minutes.

Take out salmon on a plate and pour mushroom mixture over its top and serve.

Nutrition

713 kcal calories, 51 grams' protein; 247 milligrams cholesterol; 47 grams' fat; 14 grams' carbohydrates.

1.92. Maple Turkey Sausage Patties with Spaghetti Squash Hash Browns

Preparation Time: 10 minutes Cook Time: 55 minutes Total Time: 65 minutes Serving: 4

Ingredients

For Hash Browns

¼ tsp salt

4 oz. low-fat cheese

½ tsp powdered garlic

Three eggs

1 cup chopped scallions

One spaghetti squash

2 tsp. olive oil

½ tsp pepper

For Maple Turkey Sausage Patties

¼ tsp nutmeg

tsp. olive oil

¼ tsp dried thyme

¼ tsp ground pepper

1 lb. ground turkey

¼ tsp rosemary

½ tsp dried sage

¼ tsp salt

tbsp. maple syrup

Instructions

Cut spaghetti squash in half and place on dish keeping the cut face downwards and add water to submerge the squash.

Microwave the squash for 15 minutes.

Mix the ingredients of seasoning in a container and whisk with turkey.

Make patties out of turkey mixture.

Heat oil in a skillet and cook patties on it until turned brown.

Remove skin from squash and scrape into strands.

Squeeze strands to remove excessive water.

Mix scallions, salt, garlic, squash, pepper, eggs, and oil in a bowl and cook on high heat for 12 minutes.

Spread cheese and serve while hot.

Nutrition

330 kcal calories, 40 grams' protein; 0 milligrams cholesterol; 13 grams' **fat; 37 grams'** carbohydrates.

1.93. Asparagus and crab meat frittata

Preparation Time: 15 minutes Cook Time: 20 minutes Total Time: 35 minutes Serving: 6

Ingredients

¼ cup Parmesan cheese

½ tsp black pepper

Eight eggs

2 tsp. olive oil

1 tbsp basil

⅓ cup milk

¼ tsp salt

tbsp. water

¼ cup diced onion

1.5 cups sliced asparagus

6 oz. crab meat

chopped garlic cloves

2 tbsp parsley

⅓ cup roasted and chopped red sweet peppers

Hot sauce if required

Instructions

In a skillet, heat oil and sauté garlic and onions. After 2 minutes, combine water and asparagus.

Simmer for 5 minutes.

Drain the mixture and remove liquid from the skillet.

Place roasted peppers and crab over asparagus and add egg mixture over the asparagus.

Cook on medium flame.

Slowly stir the mixture so that the uncooked portion gets cooked.

Keeping of lifting egg mixture and cooking it until the mixture is done.

Put the skillet in a preheated oven at 400 degrees for 5 minutes.

Sprinkle parsley and cut into pieces and serve.

Nutrition

169 kcal calories, 16 grams' protein; 279 milligrams cholesterol; 9 grams' **fat; 5 grams'** carbohydrates.

1.94. Curry Roasted Cauliflower

Preparation Time: 10 minutes Cook Time: 15 minutes Total Time: 30 minutes Serving: 4

Ingredients

2 lb cauliflower

1.5 tbsp of olive oil

1.5 tsp. curry powder

1 tsp kosher salt

tsp. lemon juice

1 tbsp cilantro minced

Instructions

Separate leaves of cauliflower and cut in into small pieces discarding the core.

In a bowl, mix cauliflower, curry powder, oil, and salt.

Place and spread the mixture over the baking sheet and bake in a preheated oven at 425 degrees for 10 minutes.

Change the side and bake for seven more minutes.

Combine cilantro and lemon juice and serve.

Nutrition

110 kcal calories, 3 grams' protein; 0 milligrams cholesterol; 8 grams' **fat; 8 grams'** carbohydrates.

1.95. Garlic Parmesan Tilapia Over Cauliflower Rice

Preparation Time: 5 minutes Cook Time: 20 minutes Total Time: 25 minutes Serving: 4

Ingredients

Salt to taste

Pepper to taste

Four tilapia fillets

Topping

1 tbsp lemon juice

1/2 tsp powdered onion

1/4 cup parmesan cheese

1/2 tbsp parsley

1/4 tsp salt

1/2 cup low-fat yogurt

1/2 tsp powdered garlic

Rice

One diced onion

1/2 lemon juice

Salt to taste

12 oz. of cauliflower rice

Pepper to taste

Instructions

Put filets on a pan sprayed with oil and drizzle pepper and salt on it.

Combine all the ingredients of toppings and pour over filets.

Bake in a preheated oven at 425 degrees for 15 minutes.

Broil for 3 minutes.

Heat oil in a skillet at low, medium flame and sauté onions in it for 3 minutes.

Add rice to it and cook for 5 minutes.

Take the rice out on a plate and squeeze lemon juice with salt and pepper.

Place fish at the top of the rice and sprinkle parsley and serve.

Nutrition

175 kcal calories, 28 grams' protein; 63 milligrams cholesterol; 4.5 grams' **fat; 6 grams'** carbohydrates.

1.96. Crunchy Beet and Kohlrabi Salad

Preparation Time: 15 minutes Cook **Time:** 0 minutes Total Time: 15 minutes Serving: 4

Ingredients

Two peeled and chopped raw beets

One sliced apple

Two chopped green onions

Feta cheese

Salt to taste

One orange for juice

One peeled orange

Pepper to taste

One big kohlrabi

2 tbsp. parsley

One lime juice

¼ cup sunflower seeds toasted

1 tbsp. olive oil

Instructions

In a bowl, mix well salt, olive oil, pepper, orange juice, zest, lime juice, and set aside.

Put all remaining ingredients in a large bowl and mix.

Pour citrus dressing over the salad and mix well.

Nutrition

170 kcal calories, 4 grams' protein; 0 grams' cholesterol; 8 grams' fat; 23 grams' carbohydrates.

1.97. Chinese Chicken Salad

Preparation Time: 20 minutes Cook Time: 0 minutes Total Time: 20 minutes Servings: **3**

Ingredients

Dressing

¼ cup Rice vinegar

2 tbsp. Olive oil

1 tbsp. Calorie-free sugar

1 tsp Sesame oil

3 tbsp. Soy sauce

Salad

One can of Mandarin oranges, drained

One pkg Salad greens or shredded cabbage

2-3 cups chicken boiled and chopped

2 tsp Dried chives

½ cup Slivered almonds

Instructions

Whisk all ingredients for dressing together in a medium-sized bowl and keep aside

In another bowl, mix all ingredients for the salad together,

Pour dressing over salad while tossing.

Nutrition

412 kcal calories: 17.3 grams' carbohydrates; 72 milligrams cholesterol; 32.3 grams' protein; 23.3 grams Fats.

1.98. Left Over Chicken Salad

Preparation Time: 20 minutes Cook Time: 0 minutes Total Time: 20 minutes Servings: **3**

Ingredients

6 oz. chicken breast boiled and chopped

1 ½ cups lettuce

¾ cup chopped veggies (any) (tomatoes, cucumbers, broccoli, etc.)

Low-calorie Salad dressing

Instructions

In a large bowl, put salad greens.

Add chicken and vegetables.

Add dressing, toss and serve.

Nutrition

583 kcal calories: 8.35 grams' carbohydrates; 62 milligrams cholesterol; 16.65 grams' protein; 53.92 grams' fats.

1.99. Italian Chicken Salad

Preparation Time: 10 minutes Cook Time: 0 minutes Total Time: 10 minutes Servings: 4 Serving

Ingredients

Dressing

1 tsp Dried rosemary

¼ tsp Pepper

3 tbsp. Olive oil

¼ tsp Salt

3 tbsp. Balsamic vinegar

One clove of garlic chopped

Salad

4 cups Torn lettuce

½ tbsp. basil

1 cup white beans boiled

2 cups tomatoes chopped

2-3 cups chicken boiled and chopped

Instructions

In a bowl, mix dressing ingredients.

In another bowl, combine salad ingredients and pour dressing while tossing.

Nutrition

412 kcal calories: 17.3 grams' carbohydrates; 72 milligrams cholesterol; 32.3 grams' protein; 23.3 grams' fats.

1.100. Mediterranean Shrimp Salad

Preparation time: 7 minutes Cook time: 0 minutes' Total time: 7 minutes Serving: 4

Ingredients

8 cups sliced Romaine lettuce

3 oz. crumbled Feta

½ chopped onion

1 pound shrimp boiled and peeled

kosher salt to taste

Black pepper to taste

½ cup Kalamata olives

3 tbsp. olive oil

½ chopped cucumber

2 tbsp. vinegar red wine

2 cups pita chips

One 15.5-oz chickpea

Instructions

In a large bowl, toss the lettuce, shrimp, cucumber, chickpeas, onion, Feta, olives, and pita chips with the oil, vinegar, and ¼ teaspoon each salt and pepper.

Nutrition

473 kcal calories; 24 grams' fat; 191 milligrams cholesterol; 33 grams' **protein; 31 grams Carbohydrates.**

Mock Potato Salad

Preparation time: 5 minutes Cook time: 10 minutes' Total time: 15 minutes Serving: 4

Ingredients

1-2 chopped dill pickles

1 tbsp. mustard powder

2 tbsp. lemon juice

1/3 – 1/2 cup mayonnaise

1/4 cup red onion chopped

1/2 tsp celery seed

4 cups cauliflower

2 or 3 chopped eggs

1/2 cup celery

Salt to taste

1/2 cup crumbled bacon cooked

Pepper to taste

1 - 2 tsp sugar

Paprika

Instructions

Tenderize cauliflower by steaming and let it cool after drying it with a towel.

Blend all the ingredients (leave the eggs aside) in a big bowl.

Mix eggs and cauliflower in the mixture and gently combine them all.

Put the bowl in the refrigerator for 2 to 3 hours and serve after sprinkling paprika over the salad

Nutrition

242 kcal calories; 23.3 grams' fat; 63.4 milligrams cholesterol; 3.4 grams' **protein; 6.3 grams**' carbohydrates.

"PF Chang's" Lettuce Wraps

Preparation time: 15 minutes Cook time: 15 minutes' Total time: 30 minutes Serving: 4

Ingredients

One onion chopped

1/4 cup hoisin sauce

Two chopped cloves garlic

1 tbsp. olive oil

2 tbsp. soy sauce

One head butter lettuce

1 lb. chicken grounded

1 tbsp. ginger grated

1 tbsp. Sriracha

1 tbsp rice wine vinegar

Kosher salt to taste

Two green sliced onions

8-oz water chestnuts

Pepper to taste

Instructions

Heat olive oil in a saucepan over medium-high heat. Add ground chicken and cook until browned, about 3-5 minutes, making sure to crumble the chicken as it cooks; drain excess fat.

Stir in garlic, onion, hoisin sauce, soy sauce, rice wine vinegar, ginger, and Sriracha until onions have become translucent, about 1-2 minutes.

Stir in chestnuts and green onions until tender, about 1-2 minutes; season with salt and pepper, to taste.

To serve, spoon several tablespoons of the chicken mixture into the center of a lettuce leaf, taco-style.

Nutrition

297.9 kcal calories; 15.7 grams' **fat;** 98.8 milligrams cholesterol; 20.2 grams Carbohydrate; **22.3 grams' proteins.**

1.103. Double Garlic and Mustard Sauce

Preparation time: 10 minutes Cook time: 0 minutes' Total time: 10 minutes Serving: 4

Ingredients

150 g butter

4 tsp mustard (2 tsp each of French and Dijon)

¾ tbsp. chives chopped

Two minced garlic cloves

Instructions

First, melt the butter in a bowl and add all the ingredients and whisk until a thick sauce is formed.

Nutrition

271 kcal calories; 18 grams' **fat;** 112 milligrams cholesterol; 25 grams' **carbohydrate;** 30 grams' **proteins.**

Southwest BBQ Chicken Salad

Preparation Time: 10 minutes Cook Time: 20 minutes Total Time: 30 minutes Servings: **2**

Ingredients

2 tbsp. mayonnaise

BBQ sauce

1/2 cup chickpeas cooked

Ten dried chopped apricots

1/2 tsp cumin

pinch of salt

3 cups salad greens

Two ears of corn

Eight chicken tenders

1/2 chopped bell peppers (orange, red and green, each)

2 tbsp. honey

One diced avocado

2 tbsp. lime juice

Instructions

Brush the mayonnaise over the corn and dust cumin and kosher salt.

Grill them for 12 minutes until cooked.

After cooling it down, cut kernels and set aside.

Cut the bell peppers, apricot, and avocado into small pieces, drain boiled chickpeas, and set them aside.

Tenderized the chicken for 2 minutes each side on drill tenders 2 minutes per side, with occasional brushing the pieces with BBQ sauce.

After cooling the chicken, cut it into bite-sized pieces.

Take a bowl, pour honey, lemon juice, and salt in it and mix well and add salad green.

Add corn, apricot, chickpeas, BBQ chicken, and bell pepper and mix well.

Nutrition

518 kcal calories: 29.8 grams' protein; 49.6 grams' carbohydrates; 24.8 grams' fat; 75.4 milligrams cholesterol.

Taco Stuffed Pepper Casserole

Preparation Time: 15 minutes Cook **Time:** 45 minutes Total Time: 60 minutes Serving: 6

Ingredients

1.75 cups broth of beef

Three chopped bell pepper

Two chopped garlic cloves

1 lb. beef

1 cup cheddar cheese

8 oz. tomato sauce

One chopped onion

14 oz. chopped tomato (save its juice)

One pkg taco seasoning

2 cups instant rice

1/3 cup water

Instructions

In a pan on medium heat, cook onion, beef, and garlic till beef turned brown.

Mix pepper, taco seasoning, and water.

Simmer the mixture for 5 minutes or until ¾ of water is evaporated. Turn off the flame.

Add all other ingredients leaving cheese behind, and mix well in a baking pan.

Place the pan in a preheated oven at 375 degrees and bake for 35 minutes.

Spread cheese at the top and bake for 2 minutes until cheese melts and serve.

Nutrition

351 kcal calories, 26 grams' protein; 67 milligrams cholesterol; 11 grams' **fat; 37 grams'** carbohydrates.

Balsamic & Caramelized Onion Pork Chops

Preparation Time: 10 minutes Cook **Time:** 20 minutes Total Time: 30 minutes Serving: 4

Ingredients

2 tbsp. vinegar

Three chopped garlic cloves

Four pork chops

¼ cup chicken stock

1 tsp thyme

¼ tsp pepper

One chopped onion

1 tbsp honey

½ tsp salt

1 tbsp Dijon mustard

¼ cup chicken broth

½ tbsp. olive oil

Instructions

Drizzle pork chops with pepper and salt.

On a high flame, heat oil in a skillet.

Place pork chops on the skillet and cook both sides for 2 minutes each.

Take out the chops and keep aside.

Add and mix garlic, onion, and ¼ tsp salt and reduce the flame to medium and let it cook for 10 minutes.

In parallel, blend mustard, chicken broth, honey, and vinegar and get a smooth mixture.

Mix the sauce in onions and add chops in the pan and mix well.

Bake this layered structure (onion, chops, and onion again) at 150 degrees for 8 minutes.

Sprinkle thyme and serve.

Nutrition

296 kcal Calories, 30 grams' protein; 0 grams Cholesterol; 11 grams' **fat; 10 grams Carbohydrates.**

Braised Pork Loin with Rosemary

Preparation Time: 15 Minutes Cook **Time:** 120 Minutes Total Time: 135 Minutes Serving: 4

Ingredients

¾ cup white wine

2 tbsp. butter

One chopped garlic clove

Two sprigs rosemary

Kosher salt to taste

1 tsp Dijon mustard

½ chopped onion

2.25 lb. pork loin

6 tbsp. olive oil

1 tbsp wine vinegar

Instructions

Season the pork with pepper, salt, and rosemary.

Over medium flame, cook pork in butter for 10 minutes until both sides have turned brown.

Combine wine, garlic, salt, onion, pepper, and onion and simmer for 1.5 hours.

Place pork on a plate and let it cool.

Add and mix oil, pepper, mustard, and vinegar in the same pan and stir fry.

Spread sauce over the pork and serve.

Nutrition

428 kcal calories, 36.7 grams' protein; 110.5 milligrams cholesterol; 27.5 grams' **fat; 19 grams**' carbohydrates.

Pork Tenderloin with Mushrooms and Onions

Preparation Time: 1-minute Cook **Time:** 25 minutes Total Time: 26 minutes Serving: 4

Ingredients

2 cups onion

1 lb. pork tenderloin

12 oz. chopped mushroom caps

2 tbsp. thyme

¾ black pepper

2 tbsp. oil

1 tsp. kosher salt

Instructions

Drizzle salt (half tsp) and pepper (1/5 tsp) over pork and cook in a pan over medium flame.

Cook pork for 15 minutes or until it turned brown.

Take out the pork on the plate.

Mix leftover salt and pepper, mushroom, thyme, and onions in the same pan.

Cook for the next seven minutes.

Cut the pork into slices and serve with onions and mushrooms.

Nutrition

243 kcal Calories, 27 grams' protein; 74 milligrams cholesterol; 9.8 grams' **fat; 12 grams Carbohydrates.**

BBQ Pulled Pork

Preparation Time: 10 Minutes Cook **Time:** 5 hours and 10 Minutes Total Time: 5 hours and 20 Minutes Serving: 4

Ingredients

1 tsp onion salt

3 tbsp. olive oil

2.5 kg pork shoulder (boneless)

1 tsp garlic salt

2 tsp paprika

1 tbsp liquid smoke

2 tsp mustard

4 tbsp. BBQ

Instructions

Rub olive oil over the pork and cook in pan until turn golden.

Put the pork pieces over a wire rack.

Combine mustard powder, garlic salt, paprika, black pepper, and onion salt in liquid smoke.

Brush the mixture over pork

Take a roasting tin, add 1 cup of water and place pork rack, cover and cook for five hours.

Using a fork, shred pork.

Collect juice released for meat during cooking. Mix 4 tbsp BBQ sauce with 120 ml of juice and spread on meat, and serve.

Nutrition

251 kcal calories, 26 grams' protein; 0 grams' cholesterol; 16 grams' **fat; 0 grams'** carbohydrates.

Garden Herb New York Strip Steak

Preparation Time: 1-minute Cook **Time:** 40 minutes Total Time: 41 minutes Serving: 4

Ingredients

Salt to taste

Two strips steaks of boneless beef

For seasoning

Three chopped garlic cloves

2 tbsp. chopped thyme

1 tsp lemon peel grated

¼ tsp pepper

1 tbsp chopped oregano

Instructions

In a bowl, mix all the seasoning items and marinate beef pieces with this mixture. (save 1.5 tsp for the garnishing).

Place a grid over hot coals.

Put beef pieces over the grid.

Grill the streaks and cover it for 15 minutes. Don't forget to change sides at times.

Using a fork, carve the steak.

Garnish with leftover seasoning and serve.

Nutrition

219 kcal Calories, 31 grams' protein; 84 milligrams cholesterol; 9 grams' **fat; 1 grams Carbohydrates.**

Orange Pork and Broccoli

Preparation Time: 2 Minutes Cook **Time:** 20 Minutes Total Time: 22 Minutes Serving: 4

Ingredients

One wedge cut onion

2 tsp sugar

4 tsp cornstarch

Two pork tenderloins

Half broccoli bunch

One grated orange zest and juice

2 tbsp. oil

2 tbsp. white wine

Half cup chicken broth

Half tsp red pepper flakes

2 tbsp. soy sauce

Instructions

Combine cornstarch (two tsp), zest, red pepper, and meat in a bowl.

In another bowl, mix chicken broth, sugar, leftover cornstarch, orange juice, and soy sauce.

Heat oil in a skillet over a high flame.

Sizzle zest for a minute and stir in meat and onion and cook for 5 minutes.

Mix in broccoli and juice mixture and simmer for the next 5 minutes.

Nutrition

383 kcal Calories, 43milligrams Protein; 111 milligrams cholesterol; 14 grams' **fat; 19 grams Carbohydrates.**

Peppercorn Steak

Preparation Time: 5 Minutes Cook **Time:** 15 Minutes Total Time: 20 Minutes Serving: 2

Ingredients

¼ cup beef broth

Salt to taste

12 oz. T-bone steak

½ cup whipping cream

Oil as required

¼ cup brandy

2 tbsp. black peppercorns

½ chopped shallot

Instructions

Drizzle steak with salt.

Make a crust with peppercorns on steak (both sides).

On high heat, cook steak in a skillet for 5 minutes from both sides each.

Place steak on a plate and set aside.

Clean the skillet and add shallot.

Stir shallot for a minute and add brandy.

Reduce flame to low and mix in cream and broth.

Cook the mixture until desired consistency is achieved.

Drizzle salt and serve the sauce with steak.

Nutrition

552 kcal Calories, 31.5 grams' protein; 114.1 milligrams cholesterol; 34.8 grams' **fat; 6.6 grams Carbohydrates.**

Tomato Balsamic Pork

Preparation Time: 15 Minutes Cook **Time:** 25 Minutes Total Time: 40 Minutes Serving: 4

Ingredients

2 tsp olive oil

2 tbsp. chopped basil

1 tsp seasoning Italian herb

Salt to taste

Four chopped garlic cloves

4 (1.5 lb.) pork chops

¼ tsp pepper

1 cup chopped onions

¼ cup vinegar

1 tbsp grape tomatoes

Instructions

Marinate chops with salt, pepper, and half tsp of seasoning.

Over medium heat, cook chops in 1 tsp of olive over medium flame until turn brown.

Place cooked chops in baking pan.

Clean skillet and cook onions in 1 tsp of oil for two minutes.

Mix in seasoning and tomatoes and stir for the next two minutes.

Pour the onion mixture over chops in baking pan.

Pour vinegar over the chops and bake at 425 degrees for 15 minutes.

Garnish with basil and serve.

Nutrition

242.7 kcal Calories, 24.3 grams' protein; 67.2 grams Cholesterol; 13.3 grams' **fat; 6.3 grams Carbohydrates.**

1.114. Crustless Pizza

Preparation Time: 5 Minutes Cook **Time:** 15 Minutes Total Time: 20 Minutes Serving: 3

Ingredients

16 pepperonis

1.5 cups cheese (mozzarella)

¼ tsp Italian seasoning

1 tbsp chopped green pepper

Half cup pizza sauce

Half cup sausage

Instructions

Pour pizza sauce over skillet and heat until bubbles start forming in sauce.

Drizzle cheese over the sauce.

Place toppings on the sauce.

Spread cheese and seasoning

Bake in a preheated oven at 400 degrees for 10 minutes and serve.

Nutrition

339 kcal Calories, 20 grams' protein; 0 grams Cholesterol; 27 grams' **fat; 3 grams Carbohydrates.**

Tuscan Getaway Baked Chicken

Preparation Time: 15 Minutes Cook **Time:** 60 Minutes Total Time: 75 Minutes Serving: 4

Ingredients

One sliced red onion

Two chopped garlic heads

Sliced lemons (garnishing)

Three full chicken

Six pearl onions

Black and pepper to taste

Thyme and sage sprigs as required

For seasoning

1 tbsp. paprika

1 tbsp lemon zest

2 tbsp basil and parsley

2 tbsp. chopped garlic

1 tbsp black pepper and red pepper flakes

2 tbsp. chopped onion

1 tbsp thyme

2 tbsp. marjoram

Instructions

First, mix all the seasoning items in a blender and set aside.

Full dry the chicken and rub the seasoning mixture all over the chicken (in and out).

Place the covered chicken in the fridge for an hour to marinate.

In a baking pan, spread a layer of slices of red onion, sage, garlic, and thyme. Place chicken on them. Again spread pearl onion, sage, rosemary, garlic, and thyme over the chicken.

Bake chicken in a preheated oven at 425 degrees for an hour and brush seasoning over the chicken regularly.

After baking, keep chicken in a pan and let it cool for half an hour.

Garnish with sage and thyme and serve.

Nutrition

302 kcal calories, 172 grams' protein; 510 milligrams cholesterol; 50 grams' **fat; 45 grams**' carbohydrates.

Chicken with Acorn Squash and Tomatoes

Preparation Time: 15 minutes Cook **Time:** 25 minutes Total Time: 40 minutes Serving: 4

Ingredients

6 oz. chicken breast boneless

Four chopped garlic cloves

One sliced acorn squash

3 tbsp. olive oil

2 tbsp. oregano

Salt and pepper to taste

One tomato

Half tsp coriander

Instructions

Coat tomato, garlic, squash with oil (2tbsp.), pepper (1/4 tsp), and half tsp of salt over a baking pan. Set aside.

Stir fry vegetables for 25 minutes.

In a skillet, heat oil and add chicken, salt, pepper, and coriander.

Cook for 5 minutes from both sides until turned brown.

Drizzle oregano over chicken and serve with tomato sauce.

Nutrition

361 kcal Calories, 37 grams' protein; 94 milligrams cholesterol; 15 grams' **fat; 22 grams Carbohydrates.**

Chicken Cordon Bleu Pinwheels

Preparation Time: 10 Minutes Cook **Time:** 20 Minutes Total Time: 30 Minutes Serving: 4

Ingredients

¼ cup mustard (Dijon)

4 ounces of deli ham

6 oz. of 4 chicken breast

2 oz. of sliced cheese (Swiss)

2/3 cup bread crumbs

Instructions

Cut chicken into thin horizontal slices

Spread ham and Swiss cheese over chicken slices.

Roll chickens into a pinwheel shape and use a toothpick to secure it.

Rub mustard over chicken and coat with bread crumbs.

Bake for 20 minutes on preheated over at 400 degrees.

Nutrition

476 kcal calories, 47.8 grams' protein; 137 milligrams cholesterol; 23 grams' **fat; 15.8 grams'** carbohydrates.

Chicken with Spinach and Mushrooms

Preparation Time: 20 minutes Cook **Time:** 5 minutes Total Time: 25 minutes Serving: 4

Ingredients

1 lb. chopped button mushrooms

Two bunches of spinach

2 tbsp. olive oil

Pepper and salt to taste

Two chopped garlic cloves

Four boneless chicken breast (6 oz.)

One sliced red bell pepper

½ cup white wine

Instructions

Rub half tsp of pepper and salt over chicken.

Cook it for 7 minutes or turning brown over high in one tbsp of oil in a skillet.

Take out the chicken in a plate

Cook pepper and mushroom in 1 tbsp of oil in the same skillet.

Mix wine and garlic and further cook for 5 minutes.

Combine spinach and add pepper and salt.

For 5 minutes of cooking, serve with chicken.

Nutrition

295 kcal calories, 38 grams' protein; 94 milligrams cholesterol; 11 grams' **fat; 7 grams'** carbohydrates.

Cashew Chicken & Cauliflower Rice

Preparation Time: 15 Minutes Cook **Time:** 25 Minutes Total Time: 40 Minutes Serving: 4

Ingredients

¼ cup cashews

1 tbsp oil

1 tbsp rice vinegar

½ cup soy sauce (reduced sodium)

Two chopped green onions

1 tbsp chopped garlic

1.5 lb. chicken breast

1.5 tsp chili garlic sauce

2 tbsp of oyster sauce

½ tsp sesame oil

1 tbsp chopped ginger

Salt to taste

Pepper to taste

1 cup cauliflower rice

1 tbsp sugar

1 tbsp butter

One diced green bell pepper

Instructions

In a bowl, mix sesame oil, sugar, oyster sauce, vinegar, soy sauce, and chili sauce and dissolve sugar.

In a saucepan, melt butter and add rice.

Stir rice over medium flame for 7 minutes.

Over medium flame, heat skillet brushed with oil.

Drizzle salt and pepper over chicken, cook chicken on the skillet from both sides until it turned brown.

Add and mix ginger/ garlic, bell pepper for 5 minutes until bell pepper gets soften.

Bring the flame to low and combine sauce mixture in chicken.

Simmer until chicken gets tender as required.

Sprinkle cashew over chicken and rice and serve with onions

Nutrition

455 kcal Calories, 58 grams' protein; 152 milligrams cholesterol; 17 grams' **fat; 15.3 grams Carbohydrates.**

Cilantro Lime Chicken

Preparation Time: 15 Minutes Cook **Time:** 30 Minutes Total Time: 45 Minutes Serving: 6

Ingredients

¾ tsp of powder cumin

Four chopped cloves of garlic

¼ cup lime juice

Six chicken thighs

3 tbsp. olive oil

Lime slices to garnish

Salt to taste

Pepper to taste

2 tsp sugar

¼ minced cilantro

Cilantro leaves to garnish

1 tsp red chili flakes

Instructions

Mix cumin, flakes, sugar, lime juice, 2 tbsp oil, minced cilantro, and garlic in a bowl.

Combine chicken pieces in the marinade and refrigerate for 15 minutes.

In a skillet over medium flame, heat oil and cook chicken pieces from both sides until turned brown.

Place chicken pieces in a pan and bake for 20 minutes in a preheated oven at 425 degrees.

Serve with lime pieces and cilantro.

Nutrition

390 kcal Calories, 23 grams' protein; 141 milligrams cholesterol; 31 grams' **fat; 3 grams Carbohydrates.**

Mediterranean Roasted Chicken with herby pita salad

Preparation Time: 15 minutes Cook **Time:** 50 minutes Total Time: 65 minutes Serving: 4

Ingredients

One wedge cut onion

Two scallions sliced

6 tbsp. olive oil

1 tsp powder black pepper

¾ cup dill

2 tbsp. zaatar

¾ cup mint leaves

3 lb. chicken thighs and drumsticks

4 oz. of feta cheese

8 inches of 2 pita rounds

Four radishes sliced

2 tbsp. of lemon juice

Four cucumbers sliced

Instructions

Add onions, two tbsp of oil, and chicken on a baking sheet and mix to cat chicken.

Mix 1 tsp of salt, zaatar, and half tsp of pepper in a bowl and pour over chicken.

Bake for almost 40 minutes in a preheated oven at 400 degrees.

Blend ¼ tsp of salt, 2 tbsp of oil, and pita on a baking sheet. And bake for 10 minutes until turn golden.

Take a bowl, toss 2 tbsp oil, half tsp pepper, and salt with lemon juice, cucumbers, scallions and radishes, pita cheese, mint, and dill.

Serve chicken pita herby salad.

Nutrition

381 kcal calories, 32.9 grams' protein; 68 milligrams cholesterol; 18.5 grams' fat; 22 grams' carbohydrates.

Cinnamon Chicken

Preparation Time: 10 minutes Cook **Time:** 30 minutes Total Time: 40 minutes Serving: 4

Ingredients

3 tsp. salt

1 tsp powdered cinnamon

1 tsp powdered black pepper

1.5 tsp powdered garlic

Four boneless chicken breast

2 tbsp. Italian seasoning

Instructions

Marinate chicken with all the ingredients in a medium-sized bowl.

Bake marinated chicken in a preheated oven at 350 degrees for thirty minutes.

Nutrition

143 kcal Calories, 27.7 grams' protein; 68 milligrams cholesterol; 1.7 grams' **fat; 3 grams Carbohydrates.**

Chinese Five Spice Chicken

Preparation Time: 5 Minutes Cook **Time:** 45 Minutes Total Time: 50 Minutes Serving: 2

Ingredients

1 tsp powdered garlic

Two chicken breast

Pepper and Salt to taste

2 tsp. powdered five-spice (Chinese)

1 tbsp olive oil

Instructions

Marinate chicken with salt, five spices, garlic, and pepper and place in the fridge for two hours.

Place chicken in greased pan and pour olive oil over the chicken.

Bake chicken in a preheated oven at 350 degrees for 45 minutes.

Nutrition

436 kcal calories, 65.3 grams' protein; 177 grams' cholesterol; 16.2 grams' **fat; 4 grams'** carbohydrates.

1.124. Feta Chicken with Zucchini

Preparation Time: 15 minutes Cook **Time:** 20 minutes Total Time: 35 minutes Serving: 4

Ingredients

¼ tsp salt

One lemon

2 oz. crumbled feta

Two zucchini

2 tbsp. olive oil

Four chicken breast (boneless)

¼ cup chopped parsley leaves

13 tsp. black pepper

Instructions

Pour half tbsp of oil in a pan and thinly sliced lemon.

Put the chicken in the pan and drizzle salt over it.

Mix chopped pepper, zucchini, salt, lemon slices, oil, and parsley in a bowl and pour over chicken.

Spread feta over the chicken and cook for 20 minutes.

Shred the chicken into bite-sized pieces and serve.

Nutrition

270 kcal calories, 42 grams' protein; 110 milligrams cholesterol; 8 grams' **fat; 5 grams'** carbohydrates.

1.125. Chicken with Green Onion Cream Sauce

Preparation Time: 5 Minutes Cook **Time:** 25 Minutes Total Time: 30 Minutes Serving: 4

Ingredients

One whole onion (green)

Four chicken breast (boneless) (6 oz.)

8 oz. sour cream

2 tbsp. butter

½ tsp salt

Instructions

Melt butter in a skillet on medium flame.

Put the chicken in skillet.

Simmer chicken for 20 minutes: 10 minutes from each side on low flame.

Add chopped onions are cook for two more minutes, and turn off the flame.

Mix cream and salt and cover for minutes and serve.

Nutrition

400 kcal Calories, 38.4 grams' protein; 0 grams Cholesterol; 26 grams' **fat; 3.3 grams Carbohydrates.**

1.126. Cheesy Chicken Caprese

Preparation Time: 15 minutes Cook **Time:** 30 minutes Total Time: 45 minutes Serving: 4

Ingredients

250 g tomatoes

Two minced garlic cloves

2 tsp. lemon rind grated

1.5 tbsp. olive oil

10 g butter

2 tsp. chopped oregano

Four chicken thighs

2 tbsp. balsamic vinegar

1.5 cup risoni

½ cup cheese

1 tbsp brown

Three chopped eschalots

½ cup tomato puree

½ cup chopped parsley

Instructions

In a deep pan, add chicken in heated oil (1 tbsp) on high flame.

Cook chicken until turn brown from both sides.

Take chicken out of the pan.

Put half tbsp of oil and add garlic and eschalot in the same pan and stir fry them for two minutes.

Toss sugar and vinegar and cook for two more minutes.

Combine oregano and tomato puree with garlic mixture and let it boil.

Mix tomatoes and add chicken, pepper, and salt. Bake for 15 minutes in a preheated oven at 200 degrees.

Following instructions on the packet, cook risoni in a pan.

Drain risoni and place in the same pan with lemon rind, salt, pepper, and butter, and mix well and cover.

Mix chicken and spread cheese, and bake for another 5 minutes.

Garnish chicken with oregano and serve with risoni.

Nutrition

2533 kcal calories, 44.5 grams' protein; 166 milligrams cholesterol; 29 grams' **fat; 39 grams**' carbohydrates.

1.127. Pan-Seared Beef Tips with Mushroom gravy

Preparation Time: 10 minutes Cook **Time:** 20 minutes Total Time: 30 minutes Serving: 4

Ingredients

1.5 cups of beef broth

3 tbsp. butter

1 tbsp. parsley chopped

3 tbsp. flour

1 tbsp olive oil

2 tsp. soy sauce

1.25mlb. sirloin steak

8 oz. minced mushrooms

1 tbsp Worcestershire sauce

1 tsp chopped garlic

Salt to taste

Pepper to taste

½ cup onion chopped

Instructions

Drizzle pepper and salt over steaks and cook in olive oil on low flame for 5 minutes from each side.

Take out the steaks in a plate, and to keep it warm, cover it.

In the same pan, add butter and melt and add onions, mushrooms, pepper, and salt.

Cook for five minutes and add garlic.

Mix flour and cook for a minute with constant stirring.

Pour broth slowly with continuous stirring. Stir until a smooth mixture is formed.

Simmer the sauce for five minutes and add soy sauce and Worcestershire sauce, steaks, and whisk well.

Cook for the next two minutes.

Drizzle parsley before serving.

Nutrition

343 kcal calories, 32 grams' protein; 115 milligrams cholesterol; 18 grams' **fat; 4 grams**' carbohydrates.

1.128. Italian Dressing

Preparation time: 10 minutes Cook time: 0 minutes' Total time: 10 minutes Serving: 1

Ingredients

1 tsp oregano

2 tsp sea salt

1 tsp no-calorie sugar

1/4 cup lemon juice

1/2 tsp pepper

1 tsp basil

1 tsp mustard

3/4 cup olive oil

2-3 chopped garlic cloves

Instructions

In a medium-sized bowl, combine all the ingredients and add olive oil while mixing well and serving.

Nutrition

148 kcal calories: 16 grams Fat; 1 grams Carbohydrates; 1-gram Protein; 3 milligrams cholesterol.

Lemon Oregano Dressing

Preparation time: 5 minutes Cook time: 0 minutes' Total time: 5 minutes Serving: 1

Ingredients

1 1/2 tbsp. lemon juice

1/4 tsp garlic powder

1/4 tsp dried oregano

1/4 tsp salt

1 tbsp. olive oil

Instructions

Take a small bowl and combine all the ingredients well.

The prepared dressing can be poured over 2-4 cups of boiled stained

Nutrition

171 kcal calories; 18 grams' fat; 1-gram protein; 2 grams' carbohydrates; 0-gram cholesterol.

1.130. Lemon Poppy Seed Dressing

Preparation time: 5 minutes Cook time: 0 minutes' Total time: 5 minutes Serving: 1

Ingredients

1 tbsp. zero calorie sugar

1 tsp chives

3 tbsp. lemon juice

3 tbsp. olive oil

1/2 tsp poppy seeds

1 - 1 1/2 tsp wine vinegar

Instructions

Combine all the ingredients in a small-sized bowl.

Use this dressing to be poured over steamed vegetables, over salad, or a marinate fish or chicken.

Nutrition

139 kcal calories: 12.8 grams' fat; 6.7 grams' carbohydrate; 0.2-grams protein; 0-milligram cholesterol.

Pizza & Spaghetti Sauce

Preparation time: 2 minutes Cook time: 25 minutes' Total time: 27 minutes Serving: 3

Ingredients

12 oz. tomato sauce

12 oz. tomato paste

1 tsp garlic powder

1 tsp Italian seasoning

1 tbsp. zero calorie sugar

1 tsp onion powder

1/2 tsp lemon juice

2 tsp olive oil

1/8 tsp pepper

Instructions

Take a saucepan and place it on medium heat

Put all ingredients into a pan and mix well.

Boil them, and for the next 20 minutes,' place a pan on simmer while heat is reduced to low.

Nutrition

89 kcal calories; 5 grams' protein; 3.2 grams' fat; 10 grams' carbohydrate; 0 grams' cholesterol.

Taco Seasoning

Preparation time: 5 minutes Cook time: 0 minutes' Total time: 5 minutes Serving: 1

Ingredients

3/4 tsp garlic powder

1/4 tsp cayenne pepper

1/2 tsp onion powder

1/2 tsp dried cilantro

1 tsp paprika

1/2 tsp red pepper flakes

3 tbsp. chili powder

3/4 tsp oregano

3/4 tsp oregano

1 tsp cumin

1/2 tsp black pepper

1/2 tsp salt

Instructions

Take a small bowl and combine all the ingredient well in it

Can store it in an airtight container for later use.

Tip: You can add red chili flakes, cumin, chili powder, and cayenne for hotter flavor

Nutrition

5 kcal calories: fat 0.2 gram; protein 0.2 grams; carbohydrate 0.9 gram; cholesterol 0 grams.

Tarragon Dressing

Preparation time: 5 minutes Cook time: 0 minutes' Total time: 5 minutes Serving: 1

Ingredients

2 tbsp. olive oil

Pepper to taste

Salt to taste

1 tsp zero calorie sugar

1 tsp dried tarragon

1/2 tbsp. chives

One garlic clove

1 tbsp. balsamic vinegar

1 tbsp. lemon juice

Instructions

In a small-sized bowl, whisk all the items well.

Can store for later use.

It can be poured as dressing over steamed veggies.

Nutrition

166 kcal calories, 0-gram carbohydrate; 0-gram cholesterol; 0-gram protein; 18 grams' **fat.**

Teriyaki Sauce

Preparation time: 5 minutes Cook time: 10 minutes' Total time: 15 minutes Serving: 10

Ingredients

3 tsp. cornstarch mixed in ¼ cup of water

1 tsp sesame oil

Two chopped cloves of garlic

1/2 cup soy sauce

3 tbsp mirin

1 tbsp. honey

2 tbsp. sugar

1 tsp chopped ginger

Instructions

In a saucepan at high flame, add all the ingredients and boil.

Reduce the flame to low and cover the pan and simmer for 4 minutes.

Cool it and can store it in the fridge for a week almost.

Nutrition

48 kcal calories, 10 grams' carbohydrate; 0-milligram cholesterol; 1-gram protein; 0 grams' **fat.**

Tomato Basil Sauce

Preparation time: 10 minutes Cook time: 25 minutes' Total time: 32 minutes Serving: 4 cups

Ingredients

1 tsp sugar

½ tsp black pepper

228 oz. crushed tomatoes

1/4 cup olive oil

1 tsp kosher salt

1 tsp basil

Five chopped garlic cloves

¼ tsp of red pepper flakes

Instructions

At medium flame, add olive oil in a large bowl.

Stir fry garlic in it until turn brown.

Mix sugar, pepper flakes, salt, black pepper, and tomatoes.

Cook until a thick solution is formed.

Add basil, mix and turn off the flame.

Store in the freezer in an air-tight container.

Nutrition

130 kcal calories; 14 grams' fat; 3 grams' carbohydrates; 1-gram protein; 1-milligram cholesterol

White Wine Vinaigrette

Preparation time: 5 minutes Cook time: 0 minutes' Total time: 5 minutes Serving: 5

Ingredients

1 1/2 tsp balsamic vinegar

1/2 cup white cooking wine

1/2 tsp rosemary

1 tsp powdered garlic

1/8 tsp pepper

1 tbsp. lemon juice

1/4 tsp salt

Instructions

Combine well all the ingredients in a small-sized bowl.

Nutrition

117 kcal Calories; o milligram cholesterol; 0.1-gram protein; 2.5 grams' carbohydrates; 12.1 grams' fat.

Creamy Layered Squares

Preparation time: 15 minutes Cook time: 225 minutes' Total time: 240 minutes Serving: 20

Ingredients

3 cups cold milk

cups graham crumbs

½ cup of sugar

Two pkg cheese cream

3 cups cool whip whipped topping

Six tbsp. melted butter

Two pkg jello instant pudding

Instructions

Blend sugar, butter, and crumbs.

Pour the mixture into the pan and press firmly.

Whisk ¾ sugar, ¼ milk, and cream cheese and spread it over the mixture.

Whisk well ¾ milk and pudding mixture for 5 minutes.

Pour it in the pan over the cream layer. Set aside for 5 minutes.

Spread cool whip topping and refrigerate for 3 ½ hours. And serve.

Nutrition

200 kcal Calories; 13 grams' **fat;** 35 milligrams cholesterol; 20 grams Carbohydrates; 3-gram Protein.

Sugar-Free Jell-O Jigglers

Preparation time: 5 minutes Cook time: 10 minutes' Total time: 15 minutes Serving: 8

Ingredients

2 1/2 cups boiling water

0.3 oz. jello

Instructions

First, dissolve gelatin in boiling water.

Pour it into pan and place in the refrigerator for 1 hr.

Cut the jelly into different sizes and put into the refrigerator to chill and serve

Nutrition

20 kcal Calories; 0 milligrams cholesterol; 5 grams Carbohydrates; 0 milligrams Cholesterol.

Vanilla Spiced Nuts

Preparation time: 10 minutes Cook time: 20 minutes' Total time: 30 minutes' Serving: 16

Ingredients

2 tsp vanilla bean paste

1/2 tsp all spices

3/4 cups sugar

4 cups nuts (almonds, cashews, walnuts)

1/2 tsp cinnamon

One egg white

1/4 tsp salt

Instructions

Take two bowls.

In one bowl, mix egg white and vanilla bean paste, then add nuts into it and mix well

In the second bowl, mix salt, sugar, ground cinnamon, and spices. Mix sugar mixture with the second bowl mixture.

Transfer the batter to a baking pan and place in a preheated oven at 350 degrees for 20 minutes.

After 10 minutes, take the pan out of the oven and let it cool and use airtight containers for storage.

Nutrition

253 kcal calories; 18 grams' fat; 18 grams' carbohydrates; 6 grams' protein; 0-milligram cholesterol.

Black Bean Soup

Preparation time: 5 minutes Cook time: 20 minutes' Total time: 25 minutes Servings: 6

Ingredients

4 tbsp. sour cream

One chopped onion

1 tbsp. chili powder

15 oz. black beans

1 tbsp. canola oil

1 tsp cumin

1/2 cup prepared salsa

1/4 tsp salt

1 tbsp. lime juice

3 cups of water

2 tbsp. chopped cilantro

Instructions

In a saucepan, heat oil and add onion

Cooked onion for 3 minutes

Add cumin and chili powder while stirring.

Then, add salt, water, salsa, and beans and boil at low heat for 10 minutes.

Turn off the heat and add lime juice.

Later, blend the mixture in a blender and make a puree.

Afterward, slightly cook the puree in a pan for 5 minutes.

Serve it with cilantro or sour cream

Nutrition

191 kcal calories; 4 grams' fat; 9 grams' protein; 31 grams Carbohydrates; 5 grams Cholesterol.

Cold Tomato Summer Vegetable Soup

Preparation time: 20 minutes Cook time: 0 minutes' Total time: 20 minutes Serving: 8

Ingredients

1/2 tsp black pepper

Two minced zucchini

Two chopped stalks of celery

2 tsp sugar

Two chopped garlic cloves

2 tbsp. olive oil

One chopped cucumber

Six chopped tomatoes

1/2 chopped onion

tsp salt

One chopped red bell pepper

1 tsp chopped dry oregano

1 tsp Worcestershire sauce

1/4 cup sherry vinegar

3 cups tomato juice

1.5 cups vegetable broth

1 tbsp. chopped dill

Hot sauce if needed

Instructions

Take a big bowl

Add all the ingredients and mix them all.

To adjust the consistency to the desired level, use extra tomato juice.

Add spices to the taste and serve the next day

Nutrition

Calories 88.6 kcal; Fat 0.6 grams; Cholesterol 0.0 milligrams; Carbohydrate 18.4 grams, Protein 3.2 grams.

Egg Flower Soup

Preparation time: 5 minutes Cook time: 20 minutes' Total time: 25 minutes Serving: 6

Ingredients

1/8 tsp black pepper

1 tsp rice vinegar

4 cups chicken broth

1/2 cup chicken boiled and shuddered

2 tbsp. soy sauce

2 tsp chives

2 tsp olive oil

1/2 cup mushrooms sliced

Two eggs

1/2 cup water chestnuts chopped

Instructions

Beat eggs and oil in a bowl.

On a medium-high flame, boil the broth and slowly add the egg mixture to it.

Add all other ingredients and bring it to boil while stirring

Turn off the flame and serve.

Nutrition

Calories 109 kcal; Carbohydrates 10 grams; Protein 7 grams; Fat 4 grams; Cholesterol: 87 milligrams.

Baked Salmon with Tomatoes, Spinach & Mushrooms

Preparation time: 10 minutes Cook time: 25 minutes' Total time: 35 minutes Serving: 4

Ingredients

1 lb. skin-on salmon fillets

2 cups spinach leaves chopped

One chopped tomato

1 cup mushrooms sliced

1/3 cup Kraft Sun-Dried Tomato Vinaigrette Dressing

Instructions

Preheat oven at 375°F.

Take a baking dish and grease it with oil

Put fish in the baking pan and brush all the ingredients over fish

Place the pan in the oven and bake for 25 minutes

Serve with rice

Nutrition

200 kcal Calories, Fat 9 grams; Cholesterol 55 milligrams; Carbohydrates 5 grams; Protein **25 grams.**

Caribbean Lime Fish

Preparation time: 8 minutes Cook time: 20 minutes' Total time: 28 minutes Serving: 6

Ingredients

1 lb. white fish

2 tbsp. olive oil

1/4 cup lime juice

2 tsp Mrs. Dash Caribbean Citrus seasoning

Instructions

In a bowl, mix all the ingredients and pour it over the fish in a baking pan.

Place the pan in a preheated oven at 350 degrees for 20 minutes.

Use fresh cilantro and lime while serving.

Nutrition

230 kcal calories, 26 grams' protein, 12 grams' **fat, 3 grams**' carbohydrates, 80 milligrams cholesterol.

Cilantro Lime Fish

Preparation time: 10 minutes Cook time: 20 minutes' Total time: 30 minutes Serving: 6

Ingredients

1/4 tsp red pepper flakes

1 tbsp. cilantro

Salt to taste

1/3 cup lime juice

Pepper to taste

1 tbsp. olive oil

2 lb. white fish fillets

Instructions

Take a pan and put fish on it.

Drizzle pepper and salt over the fish.

Combine all the ingredients in a bowl and spread over the fish

Place pan in a preheated oven at 350 degrees for 20 minutes.

Nutrition

Calories 557 kcal, Fat 17 grams; Cholesterol 221 milligrams; Carbohydrate 27 grams; Protein 76 grams

Lime Garlic Cilantro Shrimp

Preparation time: 10 minutes Cook time: 15 minutes' Total time: 25 minutes Serving: 4

Ingredients

One chopped onion

Salt to taste

2 lb. peeled shrimp

Pepper to taste

Six chopped garlic cloves

½ cup chopped cilantro

2 tsp olive oil

½ lime, juiced to taste

Instructions

Stir fry garlic, pepper, salt, and onion in a skillet on a medium flame for five minutes.

Add shrimps to the mixture and sauté them till turned pink. Fry from both sides.

Sprinkle pepper and salt over shrimps

In the end, drizzle lime juice and cilantro and coat shrimps, and serve.

Nutrition

228 kcal Calories; Protein 38.1 grams; Carbohydrates 7.4 grams; Fat 4.4 grams; Cholesterol 345.6 milligrams.

Grilled Tuna with Tomato Salsa

Preparation time: 25 minutes Cook time: 10 minutes' Total time: 35 minutes Serving: 4

Ingredients

One chopped garlic clove

½ cup olive oil

¼ cup fresh lemon juice

Four fresh tuna steaks

zest of 1 grated lemon

One small chopped shallot

1 cup chopped arugula

2 tsp. oregano

2 tbsp. chopped capers

Two chopped tomatoes

1 tsp honey

Pepper to taste

kosher salt to taste

Instructions

Combine the lemon juice, shallot, oil, lemon zest, honey, garlic, ½ teaspoon salt, oregano, and ¼ teaspoon pepper in a bowl.

In a baking pan, position tuna steaks and drizzle ½ cup of the vinaigrette on it and turn tuna upside down to coat well and put in the refrigerator for 15 minutes.

Next, blend tomatoes, arugula, and capers in leftover the vinaigrette and keep it aside.

Grill the tuna at medium flame for 4 minutes on each side.

Spread the tomato sauce over grilled tuna and serve.

Nutrition

470 kcal Calories; Fat 29 grams; Cholesterol 82 milligrams; Protein 44 grams; Carbohydrates 8 grams.

Herbed Halibut

Preparation time: 10 minutes Cook time: 20 minutes' Total time: 30 minutes Serving: 6

Ingredients

2 tsp soy sauce

1 tsp rosemary

3 tbsp. wine vinegar

1 lb. halibut steaks

Three chopped garlic cloves

1/2 tsp mustard

Instructions

Take a baking pan and place foil at the bottom

Put fish over it

Mix all the ingredients in a bowl and spread over the fish.

Place the pan in the repeated oven at 350 degrees for 20 minutes.

Nutrition

270 kcal Calories; Protein 47.8 grams; Carbohydrates 3.9 grams; Fat 6.5 grams; Cholesterol 72.6 milligrams.

Italian Tilapia

Preparation time: 10 minutes Cook time: 20 minutes' Total time: 30 minutes Serving: 8

Ingredients

1/3 cup Italian dressing

1 tbsp. lemon juice

1/4 tsp paprika

1/4 tsp pepper

1 lb. Tilapia fillets

Instructions

In a baking pan, cover the bottom with foil and place fish in it.

Mix all the ingredients in a small-sized bowl and spread them over fish

Put the pan in a preheated oven at 350 degrees for 20 minutes.

Nutrition

215 kcal calories: 4 grams Fat; 86 milligrams cholesterol; 12 grams Carbohydrate; 36 grams Protein.

Lemon Tarragon Fish

Preparation time: 5 minutes Cook time: 20 minutes' Total time: 25 minutes Serving: 4

Ingredients

1/4 cup white wine

2 tsp tarragon

1/4 cup olive oil

1/2 tsp dried lemon peel

1/4 cup lemon juice

2 lb. white fish

1/4 tsp pepper

Instructions

Take a baking pan and place foil at the bottom

Put fish over it

Mix all the ingredients in a bowl and spread over the fish.

Place the pan in the repeated oven at 350 degrees for 20 minutes.

Nutrition

Calories 207.6 kcal; Fat 13.1 grams; Cholesterol **106.7 milligrams; Carbohydrate** 0.6 grams; Protein **21.2 grams**

Mesquite Grilled Shrimp

Preparation time: 120 minutes Cook time: 12 minutes' Total time: 132 minutes Serving: 6

Ingredients

2 tbsp. garlic chopped

1/4 cup lemon juice

1 tbsp. chili powder

1 tbsp. paprika

1 tbsp. mesquite liquid smoke

1/2 cup olive oil

1 tbsp. basil

1 tbsp. onion powder

2 lb. shrimp peeled

1 tbsp. chili powder

1 tsp salt

Red pepper flakes to taste

black pepper to taste

1/2 cup olive oil

Instructions

Mix well all the ingredients and shrimps in an air-tight container and place it in the refrigerator for 1hr.

Preheat the grill pan at medium heat, put shrimps without marinade on the grill, and cook until shrimp color changed to pink.

Serve hot with sauce.

Nutrition

Calories 231 kcal; Fat 7.7 grams; Cholesterol 121 milligrams; Carbohydrates 17.2 grams; Protein 21.3 grams

Sautéed Scallops

Preparation time: 5 minutes Cook time: 12 minutes' Total time: 17 minutes Serving: 4

Ingredients

1 tbsp. dried chives

24 oz. bay scallops

1/2 tsp lemon pepper

3/4 tsp basil

Two chopped garlic cloves

1 tbsp. lemon juice

One bay leave

1/2 cup white wine

Instructions

Boil scallops along with lime, wine, and lemon at high flame.

Put all the ingredients and reduce the flame to low.

Cover the pan for 5 minutes and leave it to simmer.

Take shrimps and serve with sauce.

Nutrition

Calories 254 kcal; Carbohydrate 6 grams, Protein 17 grams; Fat 16grams; Cholesterol 56mg.

Shrimp Scampi

Preparation time: 5 minutes Cook time: 10 minutes' Total time: 15 minutes Serving: 4

Ingredients

1lb cooked and peeled shrimp

Two chopped garlic cloves

3/4 tsp basil

1/2 tsp lemon pepper

1 tbsp. lime juice

1 tbsp. lemon juice

1 tbsp. chives

1/2 cup white wine

One bay leaf

Instructions

Boil shrimps along with lime, wine, and lemon at high flame

Put all the ingredients and reduce the flame to low.

Cover the pan for 5 minutes and leave it to simmer.

Take shrimps and serve with sauce.

Nutrition

285 kcal Calories; 28 grams' protein; 5 grams Carbohydrates; 15 grams' fat; 80 grams Cholesterol.

Super bowl Shrimp

Preparation time: 15 minutes Cook time: 20 minutes' Total time: 35minutes Serving: 30

Ingredients

2 tbsp. olive oil

2 Tbsp. lime juice

1 lb. shrimp cooked and peeled

1 tsp chives

Pepper to taste

1/4 tsp rosemary

tsp red pepper flakes

Salt to taste

Instructions

Combine rosemary, oil, and lime

Take a pan and put shrimps in it and drizzle pepper and salt over it.

Then spread the lime mixture over shrimps and leave them for 5 minutes.

Take shrimps and place them on a preheated skillet at 400 degrees without marinade.

Cook each side for 2 minutes or till they turn pink.

Drizzle chives and serve

Nutrition

466 kcal Calories: 31 grams Protein; 7 grams' fat; 72 grams Carbohydrates; 321 grams Cholesterol.

Sweet & Sour Shrimp

Preparation time: 10 minutes Cook time: 10 minutes' Total time: 20 minutes Serving: 3

Ingredients

tbsp. Ketchup

1 lb. shrimp boiled and peeled

1 tbsp. sugar

1/2 tsp red pepper flakes

tbsp. Hoisin sauce

tbsp. Worcestershire sauce

1/3 cup water

1/4 cup Sweet BBQ Wing Sauce

1/4 tsp vinegar

Instructions

Combine ingredients.

Take a skillet and put shrimps.

Pour sauce over the shrimp

For 2 minutes, cook each side of shrimp

When turned pink and starts curling, remove the skillet and serve.

Nutrition

288 kcal Calories; 11 grams' **fat;** 381 milligrams cholesterol; 12 grams Carbohydrates; 32 grams' **protein.**

Teriyaki Fish

Preparation time: 8 minutes Cook time: 20 minutes' Total time: 28 minutes Serving: 5

Ingredients

1/2 cup soy sauce

1/4 cup balsamic vinegar

1/3 cup maple syrup

1 tsp ginger

2 tbsp. sugar

Two chopped cloves of garlic

1 1/2 - 2 lb. white fish fillets

Instructions

Dissolve sugar in soy sauce in a bowl.

Add all the ingredients except for fish in a sugar solution and whisk well.

Place fish in baking pan and pour the mixture over it

Put the pan in a preheated oven at 356 degrees for 20 minutes.

Nutrition

276 kcal Calories: 10 grams Fat; 78 milligrams cholesterol; 13 grams Carbohydrates 13g; 29 grams Protein.

West Indies Shrimp

Preparation time: 5 minutes Cook time: 15 minutes, Total time: 20 minutes Serving: 18

Ingredients

1 cup green bell pepper chopped

12 cups water

1 tsp salt

2 tsp Old Bay seasoning

2 lb. shrimp

1 1/2 tbsp. vegetable oil

1 cup onion chopped

2/3 cup cider vinegar

1/4 tsp black pepper

Instructions

Place shrimps in boiling water for 3-4 minutes.

Take shrimps out of the water and cool

Take an air-tight bag and add shrimps along with all the ingredients, and put in the refrigerator for 30 minutes.

Take out the shrimps and peel the skin

Coat shrimps while tossing with the marinated mixture.

Nutrition

57 kcal calories: 1.8 grams' fat; 9 grams' protein; 2.1 grams' carbohydrate; 57 milligrams Cholesterol.

Cauliflower latkes

Preparation Time: 25 Minutes Cook Time: 30 Minutes Total Time: 55 Minutes Serving: 3 to 5

Ingredients

Eggs, two large one

Egg whites, 2

Onion, 1/2 cup

Cauliflower, 32 ounces should be frozen

White flour, 2 tbsp. multipurpose

Pepper, 1/8 teaspoon

Cooking spray, nonstick

Canola oil, 2 tbsp

Instructions

Steam frozen or new cauliflower. Squeeze out the liquid.

Put onions and large eggs in the food processor and blend until mixed. Add fresh cauliflower, white flour, and black pepper and pulse until finely diced (but don't over-process).

Clean the frying pan using the clean cloth soaked in oil, and then coat the clean frying pan with the cooking spray (should be nonstick).

Heat on low flame until the pan is hot. Pour batter into the frying pan by a tablespoon.

Brown latkes on both ends, spinning once. Enjoy.

Nutrient

79 kcal Calories, 5 grams' protein; 53 milligrams cholesterol; 3 grams' **fat; 8 grams Carbohydrates.**

Instant pot chicken tikka masala

Preparation Time: 15 Minutes Cook Time: 50 minutes Additional Time: 15 minutes Total Time: 85 Minutes Serving: 5

Ingredients

boneless chicken breasts 1 pound, cut 2-inch pieces

plain yogurt 1 cup

garam masala one tablespoon

lemon juice one tablespoon

cayenne pepper1 teaspoon

ground ginger one pinch

Sauce

can tomato sauce 1 (15 ounces)

minced garlic, cloves 4

garam masala 1 ½ tablespoons

paprika one teaspoon

ground turmeric ½ teaspoon

salt ½ teaspoon

heavy cream 1 cup

Instructions

In a dish, mix chicken, cream, curry powder, ginger, and cayenne pepper; toss until thoroughly covered. Cover and chill for one hour.

Switch on a multipurpose pressure cooker and pick Sauté. Include chicken and marinade; cook until soft, stirring periodically, around 5 minutes.

Put tomato sauce, garlic, curry powder, paprika, turmeric, and salt in the bowl; mix until well blended. Cover the lid, then lock it. Pick high pressure as instructed by the manufacturer;

set the timer for ten min. Leave for ten to fifteen minutes to build up the pressure.

Carefully release pressure using the quick-release system as per the manufacturer's guidance for about 5 minutes. Remove the lid and choose the Sauté function. Drop-in some cream; mix well. Boil until the sauce becomes thickened for around 4 minutes.

Nutrient

08 Calories kcal, 28.5 grams' protein; 143.7 milligrams cholesterol; 26.5 grams' fat; 16.4 grams Carbohydrates

Cheesy chicken cauliflower skillet

Preparation Time: 10 Minutes Cook Time: 5 minutes Additional Time: 5 minutes Total Time: 20 Minutes Serving: 4

Ingredients

sliced mushrooms 1½ cups (4 oz.)

the bag is frozen riced cauliflower 1, 12-oz.

minced garlic, cloves 2

olive oil 2 tsp

chicken broth ½ cup

shredded chicken breast 1, 12-oz

shredded mozzarella cheese reduced-fat, 8 oz.

dried oregano ½ tsp

chopped two scallions

Instructions

Cook the mushroom with cauliflower and garlic using oil for 4 minutes. Pour in the broth, bring to the boil.

Add meat, decrease heat and cook for about 5 minutes or till vegetables are tender and meat is cooked. Stir in the Oregano and mozzarella, cover with scallions.

Nutrient

295 kcal Calories, 22 grams' protein; 78 milligrams cholesterol; 20 grams' **fat; 5 grams Carbohydrates.**

Zucchini spinach manicotti

Preparation Time: 30 Minutes Cook Time: 25 minutes Additional Time: 5 minutes Total Time: 40 Minutes Serving: 4

Ingredients

Zucchini 2 large

skim ricotta 1 ½ cups

egg 1

frozen spinach 1 cup, patted dry

shredded mozzarella, 1 ½ cups

grated parmesan ¼ cup

salt 1/8 Tsp

nutmeg Pinch

tomato sauce (low-sugar) 1 cup

Instructions

Preheat an oven to 375 degrees

Cut the zucchini into 1/8-inch thick pieces by using the mandolin slicer and put them aside.

Combine ricotta, egg, parmesan, spinach, 1/2 cup mozzarella, salt, and nutmeg into a medium-sized dish.

Place three slices of zucchini in line, such that they are somewhat overlapping each other. Put a big, spoonful mixture of ricotta starts from one end of turquoise slices and roll up the turquoise. Put the stuffed zucchini in a finely greased baking dish 9*9 inches next to each other. Now Sprinkle tomato sauce over zucchini, then sprinkle some cheese and bake for 25 minutes.

Nutrient

330 kcal Calories, 30 grams' protein; 17 grams Carbohydrates; 17 grams' **fat, 0 mg Cholesterol.**

Cheese stuffed portabella mushrooms

Preparation Time: 10 Minutes Cook Time: 15 minutes Additional Time: 15 minutes Total Time: 35 Minutes Serving: 2

Ingredients

Portobello mushrooms 2

Olive oil spray

Diamond Crystal kosher salt 1/4 teaspoon

black pepper 1/4 teaspoon

garlic powder ¼ teaspoon

cayenne pepper 1/8 teaspoon

shredded sharp cheddar 2 oz.

Instructions

Place an oven rack into the center of the oven. Cover the broiler safely with a rimmed baking sheet greased with oil.

Wipe mushrooms with a wet paper towel. Gently curl the stem of each mushroom. Keeping each mushroom in one palm, use a spoon to carefully scrub the gills. Spray olive oil on mushrooms. Now Season with salt, vinegar, garlic, and cayenne vinegar.

Place all the mushrooms onto the prepared baking dish. Broil each side for 5 minutes before tender.

Drain, then put the gill side down onto the paper towels for about 10 minutes to fully drain.

Cover the cheese with mushrooms. Broil until cheese is molten, just underneath the sun, for 1-2 minutes.

leave on paper towels for another 5 minutes, then serve

Nutrient

195 kcal calories, 9 grams' protein; 16 grams' **fat; 5 grams**' carbohydrates, 0-milligram cholesterol.

Mini pepper nachos

Preparation Time: 30 minutes Cook Time: 10 minutes Total Time: 40 Minutes Serving: 6

Ingredients

mini bell peppers 2 pounds (2 bags are worth)

93% lean ground turkey 1 pound

taco seasoning one package (gluten-free)

water 3/4 cup

drained corn 1 cup

black beans 1 cup drained and rinsed

shredded cheddar cheese1 cup 2% milkfat

jalapeños 4

green onions 1/4 cup, chopped

Instructions

Pre-heat an oven to 400F. Place a slice of parchment paper on the sheet plate. Wash the little bell peppers. Break the stems, and the ends off. Cut the peppers in half and extract the seeds. Place the chopped peppers onto the prepared sheet plate, outside edge facing the plate. Flatten the pepper out by splitting it slightly if necessary. Cook the turkey with a medium skillet on medium heat until cooked. Chop the turkey into the crumbs before frying.

Add water with taco seasoning and start cooking over low heat for another 5 minutes. Stir it continuously. Add the beans and the corn into the turkey mixture. Mix well.

Start the layering process: make a small layer of cheese at the bottom of each pepper (this stops the other ingredients from falling out). Add the mixture of beef and bean to the top of the pepper before the pepper is filled. Top of the cheese. Repeat for all of the peppers. Heat in the oven for about 10 minutes or till the cheese has melted. Garnish with jalapenos, green onions, or you may use low-fat sour cream.

Nutrient

197 kcal calories, 28.41 grams' protein; 96 milligrams cholesterol; 21.97 grams' fat; 6.58 grams Carbohydrates

Vietnamese chicken pho

Preparation Time: 20 minutes Cook Time: 15 minutes Total Time: 35 minutes Serving: 4

Ingredients

small size organic whole chicken 1

oil 1 Tbsp

1 inch sliced ginger,

finely chopped onion 1,

fish sauce 2 Tbsp

whole star anise 3

cinnamon stick 1

coriander seeds1 Tbsp.

Black peppercorns 1/4 tsp.

Five-spice powder Chinese 1/4 tsp.

Coconut sugar 1 tsp.

salt1 Tsp.

400g/14oz dried flat rice noodles

To garnish

mung bean sprouts 2 cups

spring onions 4

lime wedges 6

fresh coriander (cilantro) 1 cup

Thai basil (optional) 1 cup

fresh mint (Vietnamese mint) 1 cup

chili freshly chopped 1 (optional)

Instructions

Put oil in a shallow saucepan and sauté the onion with ginger gently for few minutes or until they get a golden color. Set it aside.

Wash and rinse the chicken with cold water, strip extra fat, and break into four sections.

Place the chicken inside a big pot fill enough cold water in the pot to cover the chicken. Add onion, ginger, cloves, fish sauce, and salt. Bring to boil and cook for 25 min, over low heat. Discard some stuff that falls to the top.

Check that if a chicken is cooked, then remove the tongs and put aside and start shredding into bite-sized bits.

Add chicken bones back to the water and simmer (don't let them boil) for another 60 minutes.

In the meantime, plan some fresh vegetables to cook with the rice noodles according to the package's directions, do not overcook them.

When the broth has been prepared, discard the bones, then strain the broth via the sieve. Taste then season with even more fish sauce if necessary.

Insert the fried noodles into cups. Cover with the shredded chicken. Place the chicken broth on each bowl equally. Top with broccoli, mung beans, fresh herbs, and fresh chili as needed.

Serve with a lemon slice and chili sauce.

Nutrient

501 kcal calories, 20 grams' protein; 71 milligrams cholesterol; 8 grams' fat; 87 grams' carbohydrates

Tropical chicken medley

Preparation Time: 30 minutes Cook Time: 25 minutes Total Time: 55 Minutes Serving: 4

Ingredients

raw chicken breast skinless, boneless, 2 lb. cut into strips

raw chopped broccoli, 3 cups

chopped red bell pepper 1 ½ cups

chopped bell pepper yellow 1 ½ cups

light lime vinaigrette dressing ½ cup

onion powder 2 tsp

garlic 1 tsp and herb seasoning 1tsp blend

pine nuts ½ oz.

Instructions

Coat the chicken breast pieces with the sauce of the salad. Sprinkle the spice mixture with the onion powder on the chicken strips. Allow marinating for 30 minutes (preferably 1 to 2 hours).

After chicken is marinated, sauté the peppers and the broccoli in a big, lightly coated sauté-pan until the tender-crisp texture is made. When cooking the peppers, often apply a little water so that the peppers may not burn. Place aside the sautéed peppers and the broccoli.

Add the chicken to the skillet and cook it until it is no longer pink. In the meanwhile, put the pine nuts on the tray in a toaster oven. Toast them until brown.

Once the chicken is done, insert peppers, broccoli, and pine nuts and serve hot.

Nutrient

370 kcal Calories, 55 grams' protein; 12 grams' fat; 16 grams Carbohydrates, 0 mg cholesterol.

Philly cheesesteak stuffed peppers

Preparation Time: 20 Minutes Cook Time: 30 minutes Additional Time: 5 minutes Total Time: 55 Minutes Serving: 6

Ingredients

bell peppers3, cut in half, ribs and seed removed any color

olive oil one tablespoon

yellow thinly sliced onion 1

mushrooms sliced 8 ounces

steak such as flank 1 pound, thinly sliced

salt and pepper as per taste

provolone cheese 12 slices

chopped parsley one tablespoon

Instructions

Preheat an oven to 400 degrees. Place the peppers sliced sideways in the baking dish, season with pepper and salt.

Bake for approximately 20 minutes. When the peppers are frying, plan the filling of the cheesesteak.

Start heating the olive oil into a wide pan over medium heat.

Add the onions into the pan and simmer for 5 minutes or till the onions are soft.

Add mushrooms and simmer for another 5 minutes before the vegetables are golden brown and soft. Add a pinch of salt and pepper for seasoning.

Add steak to skillet and cook for about 3 minutes.

Put one slice of the cheese within each half of the pepper, then apply a combination of cheesesteaks to each pepper. Add another piece of cheese to the end of each of the peppers.

Broil peppers for 3 min. or until the cheese becomes golden brown and fully melted. Sprinkle with parsley, and serve

Nutrient

354 kcal calories, 32 grams' protein; 84 milligrams cholesterol; 21 grams' **fat; 7 grams**' carbohydrates

Spinach and pepper jack breakfast burrito

Preparation Time: 15 minutes Cook Time: 15 minutes Total Time: 30 minutes Serving: 4

Ingredients

spinach stems cut 1 bushel

finely chopped leaf cilantro1

butter 3 tbsp

eggs 8

Roma tomatoes sliced 1/2

diced red onion 1/2 cup

diced green onion 1/4 cup

Monterey Jack shredded cheese 1/2 cup

tortilla shell size burrito three flour

salt and black pepper as per taste

cayenne and garlic pepper as required

Instructions

Wash and slice all the vegetables

In a cup, mix the eggs rapidly with cayenne pepper, garlic powder, salt, and black pepper until well mixed; let at room temperature for 7 minutes.

Heat the butter till it is sizzled in a broad skillet over medium heat (or spray the pot with some vegetable spray).

Bring the red and green onion to boil over medium heat for around 5 minutes (do not caramelize)

Add spinach and mix with the tongs before it wilts for 3 to 5 minutes.

Drop the heat and put aside

Nutrient

314 kcal Calories, 34 grams' protein; 6 grams' fat; 29 grams Carbohydrates

Savory cilantro salmon

Preparation Time: 35 Minutes Cook Time: 30 minutes Additional Time: 18 minutes Total Time: 85 Minutes Serving: 2

Ingredients

fresh cilantro leaves 1 1/2 cups

fresh lime juice one tablespoon

ground cumin 1/2 teaspoon

salt 1/2 teaspoon

hot pepper sauce dash 1

salmon fillets 10 ounces

yellow bell pepper medium, sliced and seeded 1

medium-size red bell pepper, sliced and seeded 1

Instructions

Inside a food processor, add cilantro, juice, cumin, cinnamon, hot sauce with 1/4 cup of water to create the marinade puree until it's smooth.

Move marinade to a gallon-sized lined plastic bag; substitute salmon. Sealing the bag, pushing out the warmth, changing to the salmon suit. Refrigerate for 1 hour; turn the bag periodically.

Preheat the oven to 400F. Spray a baking dish using a nonstick spray.

On a prepared plate, put the pepper slices in a thin layer, bake for 20 min, change the peppers once.

Drain the salmon and remove the marinade. Put salmon on top of the pepper slices, bake, and turn salmon once, 12-14 minutes before the fish flakes are quickly checked with the fork.

Nutrient

207.3 Calories, 29.8 grams' protein; 72.9 milligrams cholesterol; 5.4 grams Fat.

1.168. Chicken and shrimp gumbo

Preparation Time: 35 Minutes Cook Time: 20 minutes Additional Time: 5 minutes Total Time: 60 Minutes Serving: 8

Ingredients

canola oil, divided, six tablespoons

boneless skinless chicken thighs ¾ pound

all-purpose flour ¾ cup

frozen or fresh sliced okra 3 cups

chopped onion 2 cups

poblano Chile chopped seeded 1 ½ cups

chopped celery 1 cup

chopped garlic cloves, 10

dry white wine 1 cup

unsalted chicken stock 4 cups

water 2 cups

ground red pepper two teaspoons

kosher salt one ¾ teaspoons

diced can eat unsalted tomatoes petite, drained1 (14.5-ounce)

medium-size shrimp, deveined and peeled ¾ pound

red wine vinegar one tablespoon

fresh ground black pepper ½ teaspoon

precooked brown rice three packages (8-ounce)

green onions thinly sliced ⅓ cup

Instructions

Begin by heating one tablespoon of oil inside a Dutch oven with medium-high heat.

Add the chicken; cook for 2 minutes on either side. Remove from the pan; let stand for 10 minutes. Slice the entire grain.

Reduce the heat and apply the remaining five teaspoons of oil to the tub. Stir in flour; cook for 25 minutes, constantly stirring with a fork until the half-sweet chocolate's color has dissolved.

Stir in the okra, then apply the next four ingredients. Increase the heat to medium-high; simmer for 3 minutes.

Stir in the wine; simmer for 2 minutes. Add the stock and the remaining four ingredients; bring to a simmer.

Reduce heat; boil for 15 minutes. Now add chicken with shrimp; cook for 3 minutes.

Mix in vinegar, some black pepper & rice; simmer for 1 minute. Top with some green onions.

Nutrient

430 kcal calories, 23 grams' protein; 94 milligrams cholesterol; 15 grams' **fat; 48 grams'** carbohydrates.

Skinny chicken queso

Preparation Time: 10 minutes Cook Time: 30 minutes Total Time: 40 minutes Serving: 4

Ingredients

Buttermilk 1 cup

chicken breast four boneless

taco seasoning two teaspoons

pepper and salt as per taste

chilies and ro-tel tomatoes 10 ounces

queso 1 cup

pepper jack and cheddar cheese 1 cup

Instructions

Put the chicken inside a zip lock bag containing buttermilk and then let it sit overnight or at least 30 min. Drain it, then pat dry it.

Preheat the oven to 375oC.

Spray chicken with taco seasoning, salt, and pepper. Put it in a crystal baking dish.

Drain the chilies and tomato, put half on chicken, now cover with the queso, but rest of the tomatoes on top, and then cover with a mixture of grated cheese.

Bake now for 25-30 minutes, until instant thermometer shows 155o. They would continue to cook until extracted from the oven.

Nutrient

595 kcal calories, 65 grams' protein; 225 milligrams cholesterol; 30 grams' fat; 10 grams' carbohydrates.

Shrimp cucumber bites

Preparation Time: 20 Minutes Cook Time: 30 minutes Total Time: 50 minutes Serving: 6

Ingredients

For the shrimp

extra-virgin olive oil 1/3 tbsp.

lime juice ¼ tbsp

honey 2 tbsp

minced garlic cloves, 2

Cajun seasoning1 tsp.

Kosher salt as per taste

shrimp, 1 lb. tails discarded peeled and deveined

For the guacamole

Avocados 2

lime juice 2 tbsp.

finely minced red onion, 1/2

finely chopped jalapeno, 1

freshly chopped cilantro 2 tbsp. keep some more for garnish

sliced 1/2 " thick cucumbers, 2

Instructions

In a big cup, mix the oil and lime juice with sugar, garlic, and Cajun seasonings. Season to taste with salt.

Add the shrimp and toss until thoroughly covered, cover and chill in the fridge for 30 minutes or 1 hour.

Cook shrimp around 2 minutes each side in a wide saucepan over medium heat until they are pink and fully opaque. Remove from the heat.

Mash the avocados in a medium dish. Apply lime juice, red onion, jalapeno, and cilantro and mix to blend. Season as per taste with salt.

Put a teaspoon of guac on each piece of cucumber. Cover with shrimp and garnish with a little more cilantro.

Nutrient

49 kcal Calories, 4 grams' protein; 51 milligrams cholesterol; 2 grams' **fat; 1 grams Carbohydrates.**

Cauliflower nachos

Preparation Time: 15 Minutes Cook Time: 27 minutes Additional Time: 3 minutes Total Time: 45 Minutes Serving: 4

Ingredients

olive oil or avocado oil 1 Tablespoon

garlic powder 1/2 teaspoon

onion powder 1/2 teaspoon

ground cumin 1/2 teaspoon

paprika 1/2 teaspoon

chili powder 1/4 teaspoon

sea salt 1/2 teaspoon

cauliflower florets 5 cups, cut ½-inch slices

refried beans1/3 cup

Mexican shredded cheddar cheese 3/4 cup

sliced jalapeno, 1

chopped cherry grape tomatoes 1/2 cup

diced red onion 1/4 cup

fresh cilantro chopped 1/4 cup

sliced or chopped avocado1, (optional)

Instructions

Preheat your oven to 425 ° F. Spray some olive oil or avocado oil on a large baking dish.

Cut into 1/2-inch strips of cauliflower.

Mix oil and garlic and onion powder, cumin, chili, and salt in a wide cup. Add chopsticks and toss to cover softly.

On the baking sheet, put seasoned colic on the bread and separate the panels to roast rather than steam.

Bake for 20 minutes, until tender and brown, becomes the cauliflower starts.

Take the pan out of the oven, then push the cauliflower in the middle of the pan together. Now Sprinkle cheese and put Jalapeño slices on top.

Cover cauliflower with chips of beans. Again put in an oven and bake for about 6-7 minutes or until the beans have heated and the cheese is melted.

Top diced tomato on cauliflower, red onion, and cilantro. Serve straight from the pan. Add avocados (if desired).

Nutrient

150 Calories, 5 grams' protein; 10 grams' fat; 10 grams Carbohydrates: o milligram cholesterol.

Mushroom bun sliders

Preparation Time: 10 Minutes Cook Time: 15 minutes Additional Time: 2 minutes Total Time: 27 Minutes Serving: 4

Ingredients

Portobello mushroom caps 12

vegan butter 2 tbsp

olive oil 1 tbsp

vegan butter 1 tbsp

Italian seasoning 1 tsp.

pepper and salt according to taste

slider buns 12

Instructions

Cut the stems first from mushrooms and dust off the soil.

Heat the butter with some oil in a medium-sized saucepan over medium heat.

When the oil and butter are hot and bubbly, use a spatula to scatter oil uniformly in the skillet, add the mushrooms.

Sprinkle with the Italian seasoning, pepper, and salt on the mushrooms and roast for around 5 to 7 minutes. Then Cook for another 7 minutes or till the mushrooms are tender.

If you include vegan cheese, place a slice over each mushroom, then cook until it melts. You may place a cover on the pan to speed up the operation.

Place a mushroom on a bun and finish it off with your favorite topping.

Nutrient

137 kcal calories, 4 grams' protein; 5 grams' **fat; 19 grams'** carbohydrates; 0-milligram cholesterol.

Mushroom tofu stroganoff with zucchini pappardelle

Preparation Time: 10 minutes Cook Time: 15 minutes Total Time: 25 minutes Serving: 4

Ingredients

zucchini chopped 1

mushrooms chopped 1/2 lb.

garlic roughly chopped two cloves

fettucini/spaghetti or pappardelle pasta 8 oz.

marinara sauce 2 cups

olive oil extra-virgin 2 tbsp

pepper and salt as per taste

parmesan cheese optional

Instructions

Boil the pasta as per instructions in salted water until it's fully cooked

In the meantime, sauté the mushrooms, the zucchini, and the garlic in 2 teaspoons of olive oil with salt and pepper as per taste in a large skillet.

Now stir and remain undisturbed to encourage vegetable water to evaporate such that the vegetables are orange. (approx. 5 minutes)

Apply the marinara sauce to the vegetables, stir, and cook.

Drain the pasta, add sauce, and stir.

Serve with cheese parmesan and seasoning.

Nutrient

270 kcal Calories, 12 grams' protein; 48 milligrams cholesterol; 3 grams' **fat; 51 grams Carbohydrates.**

Grilled fajita bowl

Preparation Time: 10 Minutes Cook Time: 35 minutes Additional Time: 2 minutes Total Time: 47 Minutes Serving: 8

Ingredients

skinless, boneless three chicken breast pieces (1 1/4 lb.)

vegetable oil two tablespoons

fajita seasoning mix one package (1 oz.)

cut in slices one large onion,

red bell pepper 1, slices in quarters

green bell pepper 1, slices in quarters

Soft Tortilla Bowls 8 Old El Paso, cooked as per directions on the package

Instructions

Heat the grill with gas or charcoal.

Rub chicken with 1 tbsp of oil; cover with a fajita spice mix.

Now use a medium size dish, toss the remaining bell peppers and onion with oil. Set aside.

Place chicken to medium heat, directly on the grill.

Cover the grill; cook for about 15 to 18 minutes, and regularly rotate until the chicken juice becomes transparent (at least 165 ° F) when the middle of the thickest section is sliced.

Add the vegetables and Cook for 5 to 7 minutes, rotating once or twice, or until crisp.

Remove from the grill and allow to rest for 5 minutes, then slice into thin pieces. Break thin slices of bell peppers; split the onions into circles.

In warmed pans, spoon the grilled chicken and vegetables. Serve with toppings that keep it fresh.

Nutrient

220 kcal calories, 18 grams' protein; 45 milligrams cholesterol; 9 grams' **fat; 17 grams**' carbohydrates.

Crockpot chili

Preparation Time: 15 minutes Cook Time: 120 minutes Total Time: 135 Minutes Serving: 10

Ingredients

lean ground beef 1 lb.

Italian sausage, 1 lb.

Diced medium-size yellow onion 1

red bell pepper 1, seeded and chopped

minced garlic cloves 2

kidney beans 30 oz. rinsed and drained

pinto beans 15 oz rinsed and drained

diced tomatoes 29 oz. with juice.

Tomato paste 3 oz.

Worcestershire sauce 2 tbsp

beef broth 1 cup

hot sauce 1 tsp

chili powder 2 tbsp

ground cumin 1 tsp

smoked paprika 1 tsp

cayenne 1/4 tsp

salt 1/2 tsp

ground black pepper 1/2 tsp

granulated or brown sugar 1 tbsp

tomato sauce 8 oz.

Instructions

Start with Browning the ground beef and the sausage over medium flame in a large skillet and cook till it's almost done. A little pink is alright.

To mix, add the bell pepper, diced onion, garlic, and stir. Cook until the onion gets transparent, over medium heat. Move beef to 6-quart crockpot or slow cooker.

Add Kidney and pinto beans at this stage.

Garnish with chopped onions, Worcestershire sauce, tomato paste, chili sauce, and beef broth.

The seasonings are then applied (chili powder, cumin, paprika, cayenne, garlic, sugar, and pepper).

In the end, pour tomato sauce, then stir to mix.

Put the cover on the cooker and steam for 4 to 6 hours over low heat or 2 to 3 hours over high heat, stirring periodically.

Serve with the toppings of your choice, such as melted cheese, ice cream, maize chips, tortilla chips, etc.

Nutrient

433 kcal Calories, 29 grams' protein; 62 milligrams cholesterol; 17 grams' **fat; 40 grams Carbohydrates.**

Lemon chicken spaghetti squash with spinach and tomatoes

Preparation Time: 15 Minutes Cook Time: 35 minutes Additional Time: 2 minutes Total Time: 55 Minutes Serving: 4

Ingredients

spaghetti squash 1

Olive oil 2tbsp

Sea salt, as per taste

Black pepper, as per taste

1-2 inch pieces' chicken breast 2,

medium size diced yellow onion, 1

minced garlic cloves 4

cherry tomatoes, 3 cups

sea salt 1/2 teaspoon

black pepper 1/4 teaspoon

½ lemon

chicken broth 1 cup

baby spinach 8 ounces

Instructions

Preheat the oven to 375 F or 200 C. Through the spaghetti squash, place many holes. Now Microwave for 4 minutes, on high.

Break the squash halfway through the holes. With a spoon, extract the seeds. Drizzle the olive oil with the squash, sprinkle salt and pepper.

Place the squash upside down on the baking tray and start to bake until tender for about 40minutes. Then let it cool.

Cook chicken breast with some olive oil for 8-10 minutes over medium-high heat, using a pan, till the chicken becomes golden brown and fully cooked.

Take the chicken out of the pan and put it aside. Now Sauté for a few minutes with the onion.

Stir in the garlic, then simmer for a couple of minutes. Stir in the tomatoes and simmer for another few minutes. Cook till you have transparent onions.

Add lemon juice with chicken broth and cook it for around 20 minutes or till the liquid is partially reduced.

Add the chicken and cook for roughly 2 minutes. Include the spinach and simmer for roughly 2 minutes.

Shred the interior of the squash with the help of a fork.

Over the squash, spill sauce. Serve hot.

Nutrient

489 kcal calories, 28 grams' protein; 24 grams' **fat; 40 grams**' carbohydrates; 0-milligram cholesterol.

Broccoli Cheese Soup

Preparation Time: 5 minutes Cook Time: 15 minutes Total Time: 20 minutes Serving: 6

Ingredients

1 tbsp butter

Salt & pepper

1 c carrots diced

1 ½ c light cream

3 c fresh broccoli

2 c chicken broth

One small onion diced

1 c sharp cheddar cheese shredded

½ tsp each thyme & garlic powder

2 tbsp flour

⅓ c parmesan cheese fresh

Instructions

Cook the onion, carrots, and butter in a saucepan until the onion softens (3 minutes) over medium heat. Chicken broth, broccoli, and seasonings are added. Simmer for 8 minutes until the broccoli is softened.

Remove 1 cup of chop coarsely, vegetables, and set aside. Blend the remaining vegetables and broth using a stick blender.

Place the flour in a bowl. Add a little bit of cream at a time, stirring until smooth. Bring a blended mixture of vegetables to a boil and whisk in a mixture of cream. Continue whisking for about 4 minutes until thick and bubbly.

Remove from the heat, stir in the cheeses and chopped vegetables and serve immediately.

Nutrition

333 kcal Calories, 10 g Protein, 28 g Fat, 94 mg Cholesterol, 2 grams Carbohydrates

Oven-Roasted Asparagus

Preparation Time: 10 minutes   Cook Time: 15 minutes   Total Time: 25 minutes

Ingredients

One thin asparagus spears, trimmed

1 tbsp lemon juice

One clove garlic, minced

1 tsp sea salt

1 ½ tbsp grated Parmesan cheese

½ tsp ground black pepper

3 tbsp olive oil

Instructions

Preheat the oven to 220 degrees Celsius (425 degrees F).

Place the asparagus and drizzle with the olive oil into a mixing bowl. Sprinkle with the Parmesan cheese, salt, garlic, and pepper and toss to coat the spears. Arrange the asparagus in a single layer over a baking sheet.

Bake in the oven until tender, depending on the thickness, for 14 minutes. Sprinkle just before serving with lemon juice.

Nutrition

123 Calories; 3.3 g Protein; 5.2 g Carbs; 10.8 g Fat; Cholesterol 1.7 mg

Pork and apple winter salad

Preparation Time: 20 minutes Cook time: 0 minutes Total Time: 25 minutes Serving: 4

Ingredients

200g green beans

1 x 300g sliced lean pork fillet

1 tbsp Dijon mustard

1 x 200g sliced kale

1 tbsp chopped sage

One red-skinned three apples

2 tbsp cider vinegar

2 tsp olive oil

100g red cabbage, finely shredded

Instructions

Bring it to a boil with a pan of salted water. Bash medallions between 2 sheets of baking paper with a rolling pin to flatten them to 2 cm thick, then season.

Heat a frying pan, adding oil (1 tsp.). Sear the pork on each side before it has cooked through (4 minutes). Remove and leave it to rest on a plate. Let the heat off the pan.

Meanwhile, for 4 minutes, blanch the beans (green) in boiling water. For a minute, add the kale and then cool the greens underwater (cold). Using kitchen paper, drain it well, and pat dry.

Add the vinegar, sage, mustard, and one teaspoon of oil to the frying pan with the pork juices and whisk; season to make the dressing.

In a large dish, add the cabbage, blanched greens, and apple together. Before pouring this over the salad, slice the pork and pour any juices into the pan dressing. Toss well with the pork to serve and top.

Nutrition

170 kcal: Calories, 6 g: Fat, 7 g Carbs, 5 g fiber, 20 g Protein, 0 mg Cholesterol.

Greek Broccoli Salad

 Preparation Time: 15 minutes Cook time: 0 minutes Total Time: 15 minutes Servings: 4

Ingredients

Broccoli salad

¼ cup sliced almonds

1.25 lb. chopped to bite-sized broccolis

¼ cup chopped shallot/red onion

⅓ cup sun-dried tomatoes chopped

¼ cup crumbled feta cheese/thinly sliced Kalamata olives

Dressing

½ tsp Dijon mustard

¼ c olive oil

1 tsp honey or maple syrup or agave nectar

Pinch red pepper flakes

One clove garlic, pressed or minced

2 tbsp lemon juice

½ tsp dried oregano

¼ tsp salt, more to taste

Instructions

Toss the broccoli, red onion, sun-dried tomatoes, olives, and almonds in a serving bowl.

Whisk together all of the ingredients in a bowl until blend. Drizzle over the salad with the dressing and toss well.

Let the salad rest 30 minutes before serving the best flavor so that the broccoli marinates in the lemony dressing.

Nutrition

272 kcal: Calories, 8.3 mg: Cholesterol, 16.9 g: Carbs, 8 g: Protein, 2 g Fats

Winter Greens Salad with Pomegranate & Kumquats

Preparation time: 5 minutes Cook Time: 35 minutes Total Time: 40 minutes Servings: 12

Ingredients

6 tbsp pomegranate juice

1 ½ tsp cornstarch

1 ½ tsp sugar

⅛ tsp garlic salt

1 c pomegranate arils/raspberries

¼ c extra-virgin olive oil

1 ½ tbsp orange juice

Two heads of Belgian endive without

¼ c toasted walnuts

5 c baby bitter greens

½ c kumquats, thinly sliced/ orange segments

One small head torn radicchio

½ tsp orange zest

¼ c toasted pepitas/pistachios

Instructions

In a small saucepan, combine the orange zest, sugar, pomegranate juice, orange juice, cornstarch, and garlic salt, and whisk well. Heat over medium-high heat, constantly stirring, before the mixture starts to boil, darkens, and becomes cooler, around 5 minutes. Remove from the heat and leave to cool for 20 minutes at room temperature. Whisk the oil in.

On a plate, arrange radicchio, endive, and baby greens. Cover with oranges and raspberries and drizzle with the dressing. Sprinkle with pistachios and walnuts.

Nutrition

337 kcal calories, 29.7 g Protein, 27.9 g: Carbs, 13 g: Fat; 62 mg: Cholesterol

Easy Edamame Salad

Preparation time: 25 minutes Cook time: 5 minutes Total Time: 30 Minutes Serving: 8

Ingredients

8 c torn green leaf lettuce leaves

One bunch sliced asparagus

1 c sliced radishes

1 c shelled edamame

½ c extra-virgin olive oil

¼ cup torn fresh mint leaves

One chopped hard-boiled egg

One sliced fennel bulb

½ tsp granulated sugar

¼ c fresh lemon juice

½ tsp kosher salt

Instructions

Bring the medium saucepan to a boil of salted water.

Add the asparagus and cook for 1 minute or until soft and crispy.

Plunge immediately into ice water; drain properly.

Toss the lettuce leaves, radishes, mint, asparagus, fennel, edamame, and egg together in a large bowl.

Whisk the olive oil, lemon juice, salt, and sugar together in a small bowl.

Drizzle the amount desired over the salad and toss.

Nutrition

180 kcal Calories, 4 g Protein, 6 g Carbs, 16 g Fat, 20 mg Cholesterol

Spring Asparagus Salad with Lemon Vinaigrette

Preparation Time: 35 minutes Cook time: 0 minutes Total Time: 35 minutes Servings: 4

Ingredients

1/2 lemon juiced & zested

Two scallions chopped

1 1/2 lb. asparagus spears

3 tsp white wine vinegar

Black pepper

1 1/2 tsp mint finely diced

1/3 c sliced almonds toasted

1 c grape tomatoes quartered

4 tbsp olive oil

Sea salt

1/2 c shaved Parmesan/Manchego cheese

Instructions

In a bowl, combine the lemon zest and scallions, vinegar, lemon zest & juice, and salt and pepper to taste. Stir and let sit for 15 minutes.

In a frying pan, toast the sliced almonds over medium-low heat for 5 minutes, often stirring, until golden brown. Remove and cool from the stovetop.

To thinly slice the asparagus into strips, use a vegetable peeler. Pace the sliced spears with the quartered tomatoes in a large bowl.

Drizzle the oil in a thin and steady stream into the lemon-vinegar mixture, whisking constantly. Season with salt and pepper to taste.

Toss half of the cheese, asparagus, almonds, and mint, and tomatoes in the dressing. If desired, season with pepper and salt again. Allow the salad to sit before serving for 10 minutes, then top with the remaining cheese.

Nutrition

288 kcal calories, 12 grams' **carbohydrate, 11 grams'** protein, 23 grams' fat, 8 milligrams cholesterol

Peas-lime mint puree with goat's cheese and raw ham

Preparation time: 12 minutes Cook time: 8 minutes Total Time: 20 minutes, Servings: 4

Ingredients

Four thick slabs of soft goat cheese

50-g frozen pea

50-g mixed leaf lettuce

3 tbsp crème Fraiche

Eight paste raw ham

One lime

2 tbsp virgin olive oil

1 tsp thyme

1 cup mint

Dressing

125-g cherry / Christmas

Instructions

Heat a grill for the oven. For 6 minutes, cook the peas and drain them.

Place the ham and goat cheese sandwich slices side-by-side on the baking sheet and pour over the goat cheese with a little olive oil.

Use crème Fraiche, fresh mint, lime juice, and pepper and salt to purée the peas. If a smooth puree is formed, add a trickle of olive oil.

Serve a scoop of peas puree of goat's cheese. Sprinkle and lay the roasted ham on it with the thyme.

Mix the dressing and the salad and serve the salad.

Nutrition

590 kcal calories, 35 grams' **fat, 31 grams'** protein, 32 grams' carbohydrates, 2 milligrams cholesterol.

Lemon Mint Lamb Chops with Pea Purée

Preparation Time: 15 minutes, Cook Time: 10 minutes, Total time: 25 minutes Servings: 4

Ingredients

1 tsp cumin

1 tsp of lemon juice

Two cloves garlic

1 tsp salt

1 tsp lemon zest

2 tbsp fresh mint chopped

Eight lamb loin chops without fat

1/2 tsp pepper

Pea Purée

2 tbsp Greek feta cheese

1 tsp extra virgin olive oil

One minced small shallot

1 tsp lemon zest

1/2 c vegetable stock

One chopped garlic

1/2 tsp chopped mint chopped

2 tbsp 4 % plain Greek yogurt

Salt & pepper to taste

Garnish

Mint leaves torn

3 tbsp feta crumbled

Instructions

Mix 2 tbsp. Oil, mint, salt, lemon zest, cumin, juice, garlic, and pepper in a big plastic bag. Add the chops of lamb; refrigerate to marinate for 1 hour.

In a skillet, heat oil and add shallot and garlic; simmer for 5 minutes until softened. Stir in peas and stock over heat, bring to a simmer, and reduce heat to medium-low. Cover the pan and cook until the peas are soft but still green, for fresh peas (6 minutes) and frozen peas (4 minutes).

Transfer the peas together with lemon zest, mint, yogurt, feta, salt, and pepper to a food processor. Purée until it is very smooth.

Return the pan to the stove; over medium heat, add 2 tsp (10 mL) of the oil. Remove the lamb and wipe out pieces of mint or garlic from the marinade. Add the lamb to the pan; cook on each side for 3 minutes or until golden brown at a 145 ° F temperature for a medium-rare duration. Let them rest for a minute.

Top with crumbled feta cheese and torn mint leaves; serve with puree and lamb chops.

Nutrition

620 kcal calories, 73 grams' protein, 29 grams' **fat, 14 grams**' carbohydrates, 219 milligrams cholesterol

Zucchini Hash Browns

Preparation time: 15 minutes Cook time: 40 minutes' Total time: 55 minutes Serving: 4

Ingredients

Two zucchinis

Salt to taste

½ c parmesan cheese grated

⅓ c fresh chives

¼ tsp black pepper

1 tsp dried oregano

¼ tsp garlic powder

One egg

Instructions

Heat the oven to 400 degrees F/200 degrees C.

Grate the zucchini on the coarse side using a box grater.

In a bowl, transfer the grated zucchini and sprinkle it with salt. The zucchini while the salt draws moisture, mix the zucchini, and put it aside for 20 minutes.

To a large kitchen towel, transfer the zucchini and strain the extra liquid into a bowl.

Add the zucchini to the bowl and toss in the egg, chives, black pepper, parmesan, oregano, and garlic powder and mix until well combined.

On a parchment-lined baking sheet, portion the zucchini mixture into six hash brown patties.

Bake until golden brown, for 35 minutes.

To set, cool the hash browns for 15 minutes.

Serve with the desired sauce for dipping.

Nutrition

45 kcal Calories, 2 g Fat, 2 g Carbs, 3 g Protein, 0 mg cholesterol

Zucchini Pickles

Preparation Time: 30 minutes Cook Time: 5 minutes' Total time: 35 minutes Serving: 3 quarts

Ingredients

2 cup white sugar

2 lb. sliced zucchini

½ lb. sliced onions

1 tsp ground turmeric

¼ cup of salt

2 cup apple cider vinegar

2 tsp mustard seeds

1 tsp celery seed

1 tsp prepared yellow mustard

Instructions

Place the onions and zucchini in a bowl, cover it with water, and stir in the salt until it dissolves. Allow the vegetables to soak for 2 hours in salted water; drain and then transfer to a heatproof bowl.

Bring the celery, mustard, sugar, vinegar, mustard seeds, and turmeric to a boil in a saucepan; over the zucchini and onions, pour the mixture. Let the mixture rest for two more hours. Add the tomatoes, zucchini, and spicy pickling liquid to a large pot and bring it to a boil (3 minutes).

As the vegetables are soaked in the pickling liquid, lids it in boiling water (5 minutes) for sanitizing the jars. In the heat, sterilized jars, pack the onion and zucchini, filling the jars with pickling liquid within the tip (1/4 inch). Once they have been filled, over the jars'

insides with a knife to remove any air bubbles, then wipe the jars' rims to remove food residue, wipe the jars' rims with a paper towel (moist). The end of the screw-on lids and rings.

On the stockpot, place a rack and fill half water in it. Boil it and lower the jars using the holder into the boiling water. Leave a space (2-inch) between the jars. Cover the pot and boil for a process (10 minutes).

The stockpot removes the jars and put them on a cloth-covered (inches apart) until cool. To ensure the seal is tight, press a finger on each lid after cooling. Store it in a cool place and wait before opening (24 hours).

Nutrition

20 kcal calories; 0.2 g Protein; 4.8 g carbs; 0.1 g fat; 0 mg cholesterol

Sautéed Zucchini and Cherry Tomatoes

Preparation time: 15 minutes Cook time: 0 minutes Total Time: 15 Minutes Servings: 4

Ingredient

2 tbsp olive oil

1 tsp salt

One chopped red onion

1 tbsp chopped basil

1-pint cherry tomatoes

1-lb zucchini

Two chopped garlic cloves

1/4 tsp powdered black pepper

Instructions

Heat the olive oil in a saucepan. Add red onions and cook until soft and pale purple, frequently stirring, for 8 minutes. Don't transform brown.

Add the tomatoes, zucchini, garlic, pepper, and salt and cook for 4 minutes, frequently stirring until tomatoes have started to create a little bit of sauce. Stir in the basil, then, if necessary, taste and adjust the seasoning. Transfer to a serving dish and garnish with more fresh basil. (if needed)

Nutrition

104 kcal Calories, 7 g: Fat, 9 g: Carbs, 3 g: Fiber, 2 g: Protein, 0 mg: Cholesterol

Zucchini and Avocado Salad with Garlic Herb Dressing

Preparation Time: 20 minutes Cook Time: 25 minutes Total Time: 45 minutes Serving: 4

Ingredients

Chickpeas

15 oz. chickpeas

Salt to taste

1 tbsp olive oil

Black pepper to taste

Salad

Four medium zucchinis

One jicama

Two large avocados

Kale

Arugula

Basil

Microgreens

Chopped parsley

1/2 c chopped green onion

Dressing

1/2 c tahini

1/2 c cilantro

One lemon juiced

1.2 cup parsley without stem

Pepper to taste

1 tbsp apple cider vinegar

1 tbsp honey

Salt to taste

Water

Instructions

Chickpeas

Preheat the oven to 400 ° F. Toss the dried and rinsed chickpeas with salt, pepper, and olive oil in a medium bowl. Spread the chickpeas over the baking sheet evenly and roast for around 30 minutes, or until crispy. Remove from the oven and cool aside.

Meanwhile, shave the zucchini thinly while the chickpeas are roasting. Slice the jicama and cube the avocado into thin matchsticks. Just set aside.

Arrange the greens in a large salad bowl — arugula, kale, microgreens (if required), chopped green onions, and fresh herbs. To combine, toss. On top of the greens, arrange the zucchini ribbons, jicama, and avocado and top it with cooled roasted chickpeas.

Dressing

In a blender, add all ingredients and process until creamy and smooth. Add water if required and any necessary seasoning.

Drizzle and serve with your preferred amount of dressing garlic herb. The dressing will last up to 3-4 days in the refrigerator.

Nutrition

775 kcal Calories, 74 g Carbs, 21 g Protein, 49 g Fat, 20 mg Cholesterol

Parmesan Garlic Shrimp Zucchini Noodles

Preparation Time: 10 minutes Cook Time: 8 minutes Total Time: 18 minutes Serving: 4

Ingredients

16 oz. shrimp

3 tbsp olive oil

1 c cherry tomatoes

1 tsp dried oregano

8 c zucchini noodles

2 tbsp minced garlic

1/2 tsp salt

1/2 c grated Parmesan cheese

1/2 tsp chili powder

1/2 tsp pepper

Instructions

To 400 degrees, preheat the oven. Line with foil in a large sheet pan.

Place the frozen shrimp and run cool water for 5 minutes over them to melt in a colander.

Stir the chili powder, parmesan cheese, oregano, salt, and pepper together.

Using a paper towel, drain the shrimp and pat them dry. Place it in a bowl. Top the shrimp with one tablespoon of oil and one tablespoon of garlic and stir to cover.

Sprinkle the shrimp with 1/2 of the cheese mixture and stir to coat. Sprinkle on top with the remaining cheese and stir again. Into the prepared pan, pour the shrimp and spread out until they lay flat. Place the mixture in the oven for 9 minutes.

In a skillet, pour in the remaining oil and garlic. Heat for a minute then stirs in the tomatoes and zucchini noodles. Toss it to coat it. Continue to stir and toss the noodles for 7 minutes while they sauté.

Right away, serve the hot veggies and shrimp. Sprinkle, if necessary, with extra parmesan cheese.

Nutrition

333 kcal: Calories, 250 mg: Cholesterol, 14 g: Carbs, 3 g: Fiber, 33 g: Proteins

Zucchini Lasagna

Preparation Time: 10 minutes Cook Time: 40 minutes Total Time: 50 minutes Serving: 4

Ingredients

1 lb. lean ground beef

1 c chopped yellow onion

pepper to taste

Three minced garlic cloves

24 oz. marinara sauce

salt to taste

1 c chopped green bell pepper

One large thinly sliced zucchini

8 oz. fresh sliced mushrooms

1/2 c shredded Parmesan cheese

1 1/2 c shredded mozzarella cheese

Instructions

Preheat the oven to 350 ° C. Set a 13x9 inch baking dish or a similar size aside.

Brown the ground beef over medium heat in a skillet, crumbling as you go. Add the onion, garlic, green pepper, and sauté for 5 minutes until the vegetables are tender.

Stir in the sauce with the marinara and bring it to a boil. Season with salt and pepper (to taste). Reduce the heat and stir in 1/4 cup of parmesan cheese. Remove from heat.

Place a tiny (about 1/2 cup) layer of the sauce in the baking dish. Layer the zucchini over the

sauce with the mushrooms and mozzarella cheese.

Repeat, alternating sauce layers, then mushrooms and zucchini, and mozzarella. Sprinkle with the remaining Parmesan cheese and complete with a layer of mozzarella cheese on top.

Bake the lasagna for 15 minutes, coated with foil, in a preheated oven. Remove the foil after 15 minutes and bake for an additional 15 minutes, until the cheese is melting and bubbly and the lasagna edges are golden brown.

Nutrition

209 kcal Calories, 10 g Carbs, 21 g Protein, 9 g Fat, 55 mg Cholesterol.

Creamy cucumber salad

Preparation Time: 25 Minutes Cook time: 0 minutes Total Time: 25 Minutes Serving: 4

Ingredients

2 English cucumbers

1/3 c sour cream

1/4 c finely chopped red onion

1/4 c chopped dill

1/3 c plain yogurt

2 tsp sea salt

1 tbsp white wine vinegar

1/2 tbsp honey

Pepper

Instructions

In zebra patterns, wash the cucumbers and peel lengthwise.

To slice the cucumbers into around 1-2 mm thick rounds in a large bowl, use a mandolin.

To the cucumber slices, add sea salt, mix well with your hands, and put them aside in the bowl for 20 minutes before most of their water is released.

In the meantime, chop the red onion and remove the dill's stalk and chop the dill leaves.

Mix the salad dressing in a bowl and whisk in the sour cream, sugar, vinegar, and yogurt.

Tip the cup on one side and pour the liquid out of the bowl as the hands carry the cucumber slices. If you keep the water in there, the dressing will water down, and gradually it becomes more like a broth than a salad.

Add dill and onion to the cucumber, pour dressing over it, and give it a good stir.

Nutrition

86 kcal calories, 11 grams' carbohydrates, 3 grams' protein, 4 grams' fat, 11 milligrams cholesterol.

Israeli Salad

Preparation Time: 10 minutes Cook time: 0 minutes' Total time: 10 minutes Servings: 8

Ingredients

One chopped green/yellow bell pepper

1 tsp salt

Three medium tomatoes

One med peeled cucumber

3 tbsp olive oil

2 tbsp lemon juice

1 tsp fresh powdered pepper

Instructions

Chop all the vegetables into small cubes (chop them larger too if you want). Add the olive oil, lemon juice, pepper, and salt. Mix. Enjoy

Nutrition

65.2 kcal Calories, 5.6 g Fat, 0.0 mg Cholesterol, 4.4 g Carbs, 0.8 g Protein.

1.194. Homemade Marinated Mushrooms

Preparation Time: 5 Minutes Cook Time: 5 Minutes Total Time: 10 Minutes Servings: 4

Ingredients

8 * 12 oz. white button mushrooms

5 tbsp virgin olive oil

3 tbsp white vinegar

Three chopped garlic cloves

½ chopped red bell pepper

1/2 tsp dried basil

1/4 tsp dried thyme

1/4 Tsp dried oregano

1/2 Tsp sugar

1/8 Tsp salt

1/2 Tsp red pepper flakes

1/2 tsp Garlic Herb

Instructions

Slightly cook the mushrooms by heating them in a microwave for 5 minutes.

Whip up Marinade # 5 and emulsify with a whisk.

Pour hot mushrooms over them and seal them in a bag or covered bowl.

In the fridge, let your mushrooms rest 24 hours marinating.

Whatever floats the boat, enjoy cool or at room temperature.

Serve with toothpicks since food on a stick is even more enjoyable.

Nutrition

230 kcal Calories, 18 g Fat, 4 g Carbohydrates, 2 g Protein, 0 mg Cholesterol.

Green Chile mushroom burger with Monterey jack cheese sauce

Preparation Time: 10 minutes Cook Time: 14 minutes Total Time: 24 minutes Serving 4

Ingredients

Burger

1.5 lb. lean ground beef

1/2 tsp salt

1/2 c Paisley Mushrooms

1/3 c finely chopped green chilies

Butter

1/3 c chopped onions

1/2 c seasoned breadcrumbs

½ tsp pepper

Cheese Sause

3/4 c milk

3 tsp flour

dash of salt

1/2 c shredded cheese Monterey Jack

1/4 tsp black pepper

Instructions

In a bowl, combine all the ingredients for the burger (except butter). Form it into six patties.

In a skillet, melt the butter until hot. Place the burgers in the skillet and cook for seven minutes. Flip and cook for an extra 7 minutes. The burgers will be cooked, and the inside won't be pink. With your spatula, resist the urge to squeeze them down. Keep it inside with the juices!

To check if you are concerned, use a meat thermometer. Ground beef is not completely done until it has reached 156 degrees F. Get the cheese sauce prepared when the burgers are cooking. In a saucepan, add the milk, salt, and starch. Whisk until the flour has been incorporated and no lumps are present. Bring to a boil and then bring it to a simmer to reduce heat. Whisk until the liquid thickens or for around 4 minutes. Taking it off the heat and add the pepper and cheese. Whisk before you've melted the cheese.

Place the burger on a roll or bun, top it with cheese and serve it. Add the desired condiments.

Nutrition

381 kcal calories, 117 mg cholesterol, 20 g fat, 12 g carbs, 38 g protein

Steak with Marinated Mushroom & Asparagus Medley

Preparation Time: 30 minutes Cook Time: 5 minutes Total Time: 35 minutes Serving: 4

Ingredients

1 lb. asparagus, trimmed and cut into 1 1/2-"pieces

3 tbsp + 2 tsp extra virgin olive oil, divided

3/4 lb. assorted mushrooms, sliced

2 tbsp balsamic vinegar

2 tsp reduced-sodium soy sauce

1 tsp lemon zest, plus 3 tbsp fresh lemon juice

Five cloves garlic, thinly sliced

1/4 c sliced Kalamata olives

1/3 c + 1 tbsp fresh thyme leaves, divided

1 1/4 tsp ground black pepper, divided

2 lb. top sirloin steak (3/4-"thick), trimmed

1 1/2 tsp garlic powder

1/2 tsp coarse sea salt

2 tbsp shredded Parmesan cheese

Instructions

The oven rack is positioned 3 inches below the heating element. Preheat the oven to broil.

To a boil, bring a pot of water. Add the asparagus, then cook for three minutes. Meanwhile, fill it with ice and water in a large bowl. Drain the asparagus and plunge the asparagus into ice water immediately; set aside to cool.

Heat 2 tsp of oil over medium heat in a large, heavy skillet. Add the mushrooms, stirring regularly, for 5 minutes, until softened. Set aside.

Whisk three teaspoons of vinegar, lemon zest, oil, soy sauce, and juice in a small bowl. Set aside for the use of the Meal Plan 2 tbsp of dressing; refrigerate.

Drain the ice water from the asparagus bowl, combine the asparagus, garlic, cooked mushrooms, and olives in the same dish. Add 1/3 cup of thyme and 1/2 tsp of pepper to the remaining dressing; toss to coat. Cover the bowl and allow to marinate in the refrigerator.

6. With foil-lined baking sheet, and top with a metal rack. Set the steak on a rack. Combine the garlic powder, 3/4 tsp of pepper, and salt in a small bowl; rub over the steak's top. Broil the steak for 10 minutes. Flip the steak over after 3 minutes and sprinkle the remaining 1 tbsp of thyme over the top.

Cut the steak into 4-oz pieces to serve and put on serving plates. Divide the marinated vegetables among plates. Sprinkle the vegetables with cheese.

Nutrition

417 kcal Calories, 13 g Carbs, 109 mg Cholesterol, 20 g Fat, 50 g Proteins.

10 Minute Lean & Green Tofu Stir-Fry

Preparation time: Cook Time: 10 minutes Total Time: 10 minutes Servings: 2

Ingredients

1/4 c chopped onion

1/4 c chopped button mushrooms

8 oz. chopped extra-firm tofu

3 tsp nutritional yeast

1 tsp Braggs liquid aminos

4 c baby spinach

4–5 chopped grape tomatoes

Cooking spray

sriracha/another hot sauce for garnishing

Instructions

Over medium heat, spray a pan with cooking spray and heat. Add the mushrooms and onion and sauté until the onions and mushrooms are translucent and softened (about 4 minutes).

To the skillet, add tofu. Mix to combine and cook for an extra 2 minutes.

Add the nutritional yeast and the amino liquids to the pan. Stir until it's all well coated.

Add the tomatoes and spinach. Cook for four more minutes before the spinach begins to wilt a little bit. Plate, top and serve with sriracha.

Nutrition

202 kcal Calories, 11 g Fat, 7 g Carbohydrates, 5 mg cholesterol, 18 g Protein

Baked Chicken and Mushrooms

Preparation Time: 5 minutes Cook time: 30 minutes Total Time: 35 Minutes Serving: 4

Ingredients

Six chicken breast halves (boneless)

1/2 c chicken broth

1/2-pound sliced fresh mushrooms

1 tbsp butter

Three chopped green onions

3/4 cup shredded mozzarella cheese

One chopped garlic clove

1/2 tsp salt

1/4 tsp paprika

1/8 tsp pepper

Instructions

Arrange the 13x9-in chicken. Coated baking dish with spray for cooking. Use paprika to sprinkle. Bake, uncovered, for 15 minutes at 350 °.

Meanwhile, sauté the mushrooms for 5 minutes in butter in a nonstick skillet. Add the salt and pepper, broth or sherry, garlic, and green onions. Just get it to a boil. Pour chicken over it.

Bake for 15 minutes longer, before 165 °. Cheese on top. Bake until the cheese is melted, for 5 minutes.

Nutrition

215 kcal calories, 8 g fat, 77 mg cholesterol, 604 mg sodium, 28 g Protein.

Orange-Scented Green Beans with Toasted Almond

Preparation time 5 minutes Cook time 15 minutes Total Time: 20 minutes Servings: 4

Ingredients

1-lb trimmed green beans

½ tsp grated orange zest

1 tsp olive oil

1/4 cup sliced almonds, toasted

¼ tsp salt

Freshly powdered pepper to taste

Instructions

Place a basket steamer in a large saucepan, add water (1 inch), and boil it. In the basket, put the green beans and steam for 6 minutes, until tender. Toss the green beans with the oil, almonds, orange zest, salt, and pepper in a large bowl.

Nutrition

83 kcal calories; protein 3.3 g; carbohydrates 10.1 g; carbs 0.5 g; fat 4.3 g.

Citrus Green Beans with Pine Nuts

Preparation time: 5 minutes Cook time: 18 minutes Total Time: 22 Minutes Servings: 4

Ingredients

1-lb trimmed green beans

1 tsp grated orange rind

2 tsp olive oil

3/4 c sliced shallots

1 tbsp orange juice fresh

1 tbsp toasted pine nuts

1/4 tsp black pepper

1/8 tsp salt coarse sea

Instructions

Cook the green beans for 2 minutes in boiling water. Drain under cold running water. Drain well.

Over medium-high heat, heat a nonstick skillet. In a pan, add oil; swirl to coat. Add shallots; sauté for 2 minutes or until soft. Garnish with green beans; stir well. Add juices, rind, salt, and pepper; sauté for 2 minutes. Spoon it into a dish; sprinkle it with nuts.

Nutrition

86 kcal Calories 3.8 g Fat 2.5 g Protein 12.8 g Carbohydrate   0.0 mg Cholesterol

Herbed Tuna in Tomatoes

Preparation Time: 20 minutes Cook time: 0 minutes Total Time: 20 minutes Serving: 6

Ingredients

Six tomatoes large

One lemon zest

3 * 6-ounce tuna

3 tbsp roughly chopped capers,

1 c fresh roughly chopped parsley leaves

¼ c fresh lemon juice

1 tbsp olive oil

¼ tsp black pepper

Instruction

Remove the stem tip from each tomato with a paring knife. Scoop the seeds out and dump the pulp into a bowl.

In a bowl, add the capers, tuna, parsley, juice, lemon zest, oil, pepper, and mix.

Spoon the mixture into the rusted-out tomatoes with care.

Nutrition

149 kcal calories, 6 g fat, 45 mg cholesterol, 9 g carbohydrates, 23 g Protein.

Chapter 2: Recipes for fuelings

Refueling Recipes

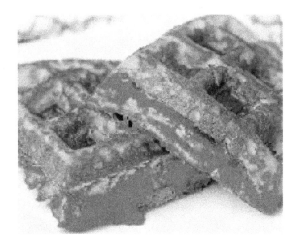

Pudding Pies

Preparation Time: 10 Minutes Cook Time: 25 Minutes Total Time: 35 Minutes Serving: 8 Serving

Ingredients

For the crust

5 1/3 tbsp unsalted butter

65 vanilla wafers

For the pie

Two bananas

For the pudding

2 tsp vanilla extract

½ cup of sugar

¼ tsp salt

1/3 cup flour

2 cups of milk

Four egg yolks

For the whipped cream

1 tsp vanilla extract

2 tbsp confectioner's sugar

1 cup cream

Instructions

Crust making

Crush vanilla wafers in a blender and blend with butter. Save some wafer powder for topping.

Take a pie plate and spread the dough on it, and bake in a preheated oven at 350 degrees for 12 mins

Let it cool

Making pudding

Mix flour, salt, and sugar in a saucepan on medium heat.

Add milk to the mixture and mix till it becomes thick.

Separate egg yolk in a bowl and pour 3 tbsp of milk mixture while hot and mix.

Pour this egg mixture into a saucepan and stir till it gets thickened.

Turn off the flame and add vanilla while stirring.

Assembly

Divide bananas into two portions.

Organize the first one-half of banana slices on the crust.

Pour pudding mixture (half) over the layer of bananas.

Spread leftover powdered wafers over the pudding and topped it with leftover bananas.

Then again, pour the pudding over the top of the second layer of bananas.

To fully cool it, place the pot in the fridge.

Whipped cream

Blend vanilla, sugar, and heavy cream and make it frothy.

Spread the frothy cream over the chilled pudding and serve.

Nutrition

567 kcal: Calories; 65 g: Carbohydrates 165 mg Cholesterol; 16 g Fat; 6 g Protein; 1g: fiber.

Pancake Cinnamon Roll

Preparation Time: 30 Minutes Cook Time: 10 minutes Additional Time: 15 minutes Total Time: 55 Minutes Serving: 8

Ingredients

Pancakes

Two tablespoons white vinegar

One teaspoon baking powder

1 cup flour

½ teaspoon baking soda

1 ½ teaspoons vanilla extract

Two tablespoons sugar

½ teaspoon salt

¾ cup milk

Two tablespoons butter

One egg

Cinnamon Swirl Filling

1 ½ teaspoons cinnamon

¼ cup butter

5 ½ tablespoons sugar

Cream Cheese Icing

¾ cup confectioners' sugar

2 oz. cream cheese

¼ cup butter

½ tsp vanilla extract

Instructions

Sour the milk by adding vinegar to it. Keep it aside for a few minutes.

Combine butter, vanilla extract, and eggs in sour milk.

Take a large bowl, add sugar, baking powder, salt, baking soda, and flour and mix them well.

Gradually pour sour milk solution into the dry mixture and mix until a smooth batter is formed.

Take another bowl, mix cinnamon, butter, and sugar in it.

Put this mixture in a cone-shaped container and refrigerate.

In a small bowl, blend cream cheese and butter until they get smooth.

Then add confectioners' sugar and half tsp of vanilla into the mixture and mix. Icing is ready.

On medium heat, place skillet sprayed with cooking oil and place two-third of batter on it.

Cook the batter. After 3 minutes' bubbles begin to rise.

Take out the cone-shaped container from the fridge and swirl the mixture over the pancake. Be careful that the mixture should not touch the skillet.

Turn the pancake upside down and cook the other side for the next three minutes.

Spread the icing on the pancake and serve.

Nutrition

Calories 327 kcal; 3.9 g Protein; 37.9 g Carbohydrates; 18.1 g Fat; 71 mg Cholesterol

Chocolate Chip Coffee Cake Muffins

Preparation Time: 20 Minutes Cook Time: 25 Minutes Total Time: 45 Minutes Serving: 15 muffins

Ingredients

1 cup of chocolate chips

1/2 cup sugar

2 cups flour (all-purpose)

2 tsp baking powder

2 tsp coffee granules (instant)

1 tsp cinnamon (powdered)

1/4 tsp salt

One egg

1/2 cup brown sugar

1 cup milk

1 tsp vanilla extract

1/2 cup butter

Topping

1/4 cup brown sugar

1/4 cup butter

1/2 tsp cinnamon (powdered)

6 tsp flour (all-purpose)

Instructions

In a medium-sized bowl, whisk vanilla, butter, egg, and milk.

In another large bowl, mix sugar, baking powder, coffee, salt, cinnamon, and flour and add with mixing the egg mixture. Spread chocolate chips and toss,

In greased muffins molds, fill the batter

Combine sugar (brown), cinnamon, and flour in a bowl and add butter and whisk until a smooth thick, smooth solution is formed. Topping is ready

Spread it on the batter.

Put the baking pan with batter in it in a preheated oven at 375 degrees for 25 minutes.

After baking, let it cool and serve.

Nutrition

Calories 291 kcal, Fat 14 grams, Cholesterol 41 milligram, Carbohydrate 41 grams

Zucchini Bread

Preparation Time: 20 Minutes Cook Time: 50 Minutes Total Time: 70 Minutes Serving: 24

Ingredients

1 cup walnuts (sliced)

3 cups flour

3 tsp vanilla extract

1 tsp baking soda

1 tsp cinnamon

Two ¼ cups sugar

1 tsp salt

2 cups zucchini

Three eggs

1 tsp baking powder

1 cup oil

Instructions

Whisk baking powder and soda, cinnamon, salt, and flour in a container.

Whisk oil, sugar, egg, and vanilla in a large container. Add dry ingredients and whisk well. Put nuts with zucchini and mix well.

Pour smooth without lumps batter in baking pan.

Place the pan in a preheated oven at 325 degrees for 50 minutes.

After baking, cool it and serve.

Nutrition

Calories 255 kcal; 3.3 grams' protein; 13.1 grams' fat; 23.3 grams Cholesterol; 32.1 grams Carbohydrates.

Cinnamon Blondies

Preparation Time: 25 Minutes Cook Time: 40Minutes Total Time: 65 Minutes Serving: 16 blondies

Ingredients

Making Blondies

1 3/4 cups dark brown sugar

2 tbsp. milk

1 tsp baking powder

1/2 cup butter

1/2 teaspoon kosher salt

Four tsp cinnamon

Two eggs

2 cup flour

1/4 tsp baking soda

1 tbsp vanilla extract

Topping

1/4 cup sugar

1 tbsp butter

1 tsp cinnamon

Instructions

Whisk sugar and butter in a bowl, add egg one by one with beating, add vanilla and milk, and add salt and cinnamon.

Sift flour, baking soda, and powder over the mixture and stir until a smooth mixture is formed.

Pour the batter into the pan

Place the pan in a preheated oven at 350 degrees for 40 minutes.

Mix cinnamon and sugar in a bowl and spread it on the top of blondies, and serve.

Nutrition

217 kcal Calorie; 4 grams' fat; 41 milligrams cholesterol; 2 grams' fiber; 36 grams' carbohydrates.

Haystacks

Preparation Time: 10 minutes Cook Time: 0 minutes Total Time: 10 minutes Serving: 15 cookies

Ingredients

4 cups chow mien noodle

12 oz. chocolate chips

11 oz. butterscotch chips

Instructions

In a bowl, whisk butterscotch chips and chocolate chips and use a microwave to melt them to make a smooth flowy liquid.

Put noodles in the liquid and toss so that they are coated with chocolate chip syrup.

Pour full spoon batter over butter paper and place the tray in the fridge to cool them for 20 minutes and serve.

Nutrition

267 kcal Calories; 2 grams' protein; 38 grams Carbohydrates; 11 grams Fat; 3-milligram Cholesterol

Banana Cheesecake Chocolate Cookies

Preparation Time: 20 Minutes Cook Time: 25 Minutes Total Time: 45 Minutes Serving: 14 cookies

Ingredients

Crust

2 tbsp. butter

12 Oreo cookies

Cheesecakes

1 tsp vanilla extract

1/2 cup sugar

2 tbsp flour

1/2 cup chocolate chips

1/2 cup banana

1/4 cup cream

One egg

2 * 8 oz. cream cheese

Chocolate Whipped Cream

1/4 cup cocoa powder

1/2 cup powdered sugar

2 Tablespoons mini chocolate chips

1/2 teaspoon rum extract

1 cup heavy whipping cream

One yellow banana, sliced

Instructions

Blend cookies in a blender.

Pour and press the cookies mixture firmly in cupcake molds.

Whisk sugar and cream cheese and add flour, vanilla, and cream and whisk again well.

Then, add egg and banana and beat. Put chips and mix softly.

Pour the mixture in molds over cookies mixture.

Bake in a preheated oven at 350 degrees for 25 minutes.

After baking, cool it down at room temperature and place it in the fridge for 4 hours.

Whisk cocoa powder, whipping cream, vanilla extract, and sugar until a frothy mixture is formed.

With the help of a piping bag with tip ahead, swirl the cream on cheesecake and serve with chips sprinkled over it.

Nutrition

351 kcal Calories; 72 mg Cholesterol; 31 g Carbohydrates; 25 g Fat; 4 g Protein.

Cheesecake Ice Cream

Preparation Time: 20 Minutes Process Time: 20 Minutes Total Time: 40 Minutes Serving: 1.5 quarts

Ingredients

1 cup milk

2.5 cups cream

Two eggs

1 tsp vanilla extract

12 oz. cream cheese

1-1/4 cups sugar

1 tbsp lemon juice

Instructions

Mix milk and cream at high flame and dissolve sugar.

Beat eggs in a bowl and add 2 tbsp of hot milk

Pour egg solution in a saucepan with continuous stirring

Reduce the heat and continue stirring for few more minutes

Turn off the flame and add and mix cream cheese.

Place the bowl in ice-chilled water to cool the mixture immediately. Add vanilla extract and lemon juice.

Place the bowl in the refrigerator with a lid on it overnight.

Put the chilled mixture in an ice cream machine and freeze for 2 hrs. And serve.

Nutrition

272 kcal calories; 6 grams' protein; 94 grams' cholesterol; 16 grams' fat; 24 grams' carbohydrates

Vanilla Custard

Preparation Time: 10 minutes Cook Time: 20 minutes Total Time: 30 minutes Serving: 4

Ingredients

1/3 cup sugar

1 cup milk

1 Vanilla Bean

1 tbsp corn-flour

Four yolks of egg

1 cup cream

Instructions

Take a saucepan, add cream, vanilla beans, and its seeds and milk in it and cook on medium flame with continuous stirring until it boils and remove beans for it.

In a bowl, mix cornflour, egg yolk, and sugar.

Pour hot milk solution over an egg mixture with constant stirring.

Place the bowl on low flame and cook with continuous stirring until the solution gets thickens.

Cool it down and serve with pancakes or fruits.

Nutrition

1570 kcal Calories; Protein 5 grams, Carbohydrates 23 grams; Fat 29 grams, 0-milligram Cholesterol.

Chocolate Cheesecake Shake

Preparation Time: 10 Minutes Cook Time: 0 Minutes Total Time: 10 Minutes Serving: 4

Ingredients

Six scoops of ice cream (chocolate flavor)

8 oz. cream cheese

2 cups of milk

Instructions

Make a smooth solution of milk (one cup) and cream cheese in a blender.

Then make a smooth mixture of ice cream and milk (one cup).

Fill the serving glass with milk and cream solution and then pour ice cream smoothie and serve.

Nutrition

Calories 227 kcal; 15.6 grams' **fat; 7.3 grams**' protein; 51.3 grams Cholesterol; 15.3 grams Carbohydrates.

Pistachio Milk-Shake

Preparation Time: 5 Minutes Cook Time: 0 Minutes Total Time: 5 Minutes Serving: 4 glasses

Ingredients

1 tsp vanilla extract

5 cups ice cream (pistachio)

4 tbsp pistachios

Pinch of salt

1 cup milk

Instructions

Blend salt, ice cream, vanilla extract, and milk in a blender to make a smooth, fluffy thick solution.

Garnish with pistachios and serve.

Nutrition

400 kcal Calories; 26 grams' fat; 140 milligrams cholesterol; 31 grams Carbohydrates; 9 grams Protein.

Chocolate Crunch Cookies

Preparation Time: 15 Minutes Cook Time: 10 Minutes Total Time: 25 Minutes Serving: 35 cookies

Ingredients

1 ½ cups chocolate chips

One teaspoon baking soda

1.5 cups butter

2 cup of sugar

One teaspoon vanilla

One teaspoon salt

One teaspoon baking powder

½ cup pecans

2 cups oats

Two eggs

2 cups flour

2 cups Krispies Rice

Instructions

Blend eggs, vanilla, butter, and sugar.

In a large bowl, combine salt, baking powder, flour, and baking soda.

Then add Krispies rice, pecans, chips, and oats to the bowl and mix well.

Pour batter into a greased baking pan and bake for 10 minutes in a preheated oven at 350 degrees.

Nutrition

271 kcal Calories; 38.5 milligrams cholesterol; 14.2 grams' fat; 34.3 grams Carbohydrates, 48 grams Protein

Peanut Butter and Cream Cheese Stuffed Brownies

Preparation Time: 30 Minutes Cook Time: 25 Minutes Total Time: 55 Minutes Serving: 12

Ingredients

Base for Brownie

1/4 tsp baking soda

1/2 cup maple syrup

1 tsp vanilla extract

One egg

2 tsp coconut oil

6 tbsp cocoa powder

1 cup peanut butter

Filling for Peanut Butter Cheesecake

2 tsp. vanilla extract

2/3 cup maple syrup

6 oz. cream cheese

1 cup peanut butter

For the Topping

7 oz. peanut butter

For the Fudge Sauce

2 tbsp. cocoa powder

3 tbsp. maple syrup

Instructions

Brownie Base

Take a large bowl, combine all the ingredients for the brownie base and whisk well.

Bake for 25 minutes in a preheated oven at 325 degrees. And let it cool.

Fudge Sauce

Mix the cocoa powder and maple syrup on medium flame.

Peanut Butter Cheesecake Filling

In a blender, blend all the ingredients until a smooth mixture is obtained.

Refrigerate the mixture for 10 minutes.

At the top of the brownie, spread the filling and place the brownie in the refrigerator overnight with plastic wrap covering.

After refrigeration, with peanut butter cubes, garnish the top and pour randomly chocolate sauce and serve.

Nutrition

552 kcal calories; 45-gram carbohydrates; 40 milligrams cholesterol; 14 grams' protein; 37 grams' **fat.**

Chocolate Mint Soft Serve Brownie Bottoms

Preparation Time: 75 Minutes Cook Time: 0 Minutes Total Time: 75 Minutes Serving: 12

Ingredients

7 oz. of whipped cream

8 oz. cream cheese

One brownie mix in addition to ingredients written on the box

1/2 cup sugar

One pkg crushed mint Oreos

2 tsp mint extract

1/4 cup milk

Chocolate syrup (as required)

Green food color

Instructions

Ice cream

Mix food color, sugar, mint extract, cream cheese, and milk and make a smooth mixture in a mixer.

Later pour whipping cream in it and gently fold them all.

Brownie

By following the instructions on the brownie box, make brownie dough and bake it.

After baking, completely cool it.

Assembly

Place a brownie layer as the first layer in a pan covered with parchment paper (paper should be covering the sides; this will help take the final cake out).

Cover the top of the brownie with the Oreo layer, later pour chocolate sauce over it.

Then add a layer of mint ice cream.

Place the second layer of brownie with Oreos covering it.

Pour the second layer of chocolate sauce and add an ice cream layer over it.

Freeze the cake completely.

Using parchment paper, place the ice cream cake in the serving dish and top the upper layer with leftover Oreos and chocolate sauce before serving.

Nutrition

540 kcal Calories; 5.6 grams' protein; 43 milligrams cholesterol; 23.4 grams' **fat; 79.6 grams Carbohydrates.**

Grilled Cheese Tomato Sandwich

Preparation Time: 20 Minutes Cook Time: 25 Minutes Total Time: 45 Minutes Serving: 15 muffins

Ingredients

2 tsp. mayonnaise

Two slices tomatoes

One pinch pepper

Two slices of Swiss cheese

2 tbsp. butter

One pinch salt

Two slices of bread

One pinch of powdered garlic

One pinch of Italian seasoning

Instructions

Spread mayonnaise over the bread slices.

Top one bread with slices of tomato.

Drizzle Italian seasoning, salt, and pepper.

Place cheese on the tomatoes and place the second bread slice over it.

Take a skillet and heat butter and garlic powder on it.

Slightly spread butter over both sides of bread and grill both sides until cheese melts and turns brown.

Nutrition

559.4 kcal calories; 30.5 grams' carbohydrates; 19.6 grams' protein; 40.3 grams' fat; 112.6 grams' **cholesterol.**

2.16. Peanut Butter Crunch Bars

Preparation Time: 3 minutes Cook Time: **1-minute Total Time:** 4 minutes Serving: 20 bars

Ingredients

3 cups of rice cereal

1/2 cup maple syrup

1 cup peanut butter

1 1/2 cups chocolate chips

1/4 cup coconut oil

Instructions

Melt all the ingredients except rice cereal in a microwave oven and mix well.

Pour the melted mixture over rice cereal in a bowl and toss gently.

Spread the mixture in a baking pan lined with butter paper and refrigerate for an hour.

Cut into pieces and serve.

Nutrition

142 kcal Calories; 16 grams Carbohydrates; 4 grams' protein; 15 grams Cholesterol, 0.2 grams Fat

Mousse Treat

Preparation Time: 5 Minutes Cook Time: 20 Minutes Total Time: 25 Minutes Serving: 8

Ingredients

8 oz. chopped baking semisweet chocolate

Four egg yolks

2 ½ cups whipping cream

¼ cup of sugar

Instructions

Blend egg yolks in a blender with slow addition of sugar.

At medium flame, heat whipping cream and pour half of the hot whipping cream in the egg mixture and mix well.

Pour the egg mixture back to hot whipping cream in a saucepan at low flame and cook for the next five minutes.

Add and mix chocolate and cook until chocolate melts.

Refrigerate for two hours till it gets chilled.

Using a beater, beat cream, and mix in a chocolate mixture.

Put one spoon of mixture in each serving dish.

Nutrition

430kcal Calories; 175 milligrams cholesterol; 5 grams' protein; 33 grams' **fat; 27 grams Carbohydrates.**

Tiramisu Milkshake

Preparation Time: 7 Minutes Cook Time: 0 Minutes Total Time: 7 Minutes Serving: 2

Ingredients

2 tsp. espresso powder

4 scoops Vanilla Ice Cream

1 cup whipped cream

Four ladyfingers cookies

4 tsp. cocoa powder

1/2 cup milk

Instructions

In a blender, put espresso powder, ice cream, and milk and blend to get a smooth, fluffy mixture.

Pour the shake into glasses and add whipping cream at the top and drizzle cocoa powder.

Use ladyfinger cookies for garnishing and serve.

Nutrition

257 kcal calories; 6 grams' protein; 83 milligrams cholesterol; 11 grams' fat; 32 grams' carbohydrates.

Garlic Potato Pancakes

Preparation Time: 10 minutes Cook Time: 15 minutes Total Time: 25 minutes Serving: 12 muffins

Ingredients

Five baking potatoes

8 tbsp. butter

Two chopped cloves of garlic

2 cups of milk

3 tsp. salt

Pinch of black pepper

1 tsp oil

Instructions

Add peeled cubes of potatoes in boiling water with salt dissolved in it.

Boil potatoes for ten minutes.

Cool boil potatoes and mashed them in a container. Add milk to get the required consistency.

Stir fry garlic in oil till they turn golden brown.

Add fried garlic along with salt and pepper into mashed potatoes.

Give the batter a pancake shape.

Cook both sides of pancake in butter in a skillet over medium flame until they get crispy.

Nutrition

429.7 kcal Calories; 8 grams' protein; 25.5 grams' fat; 44.2 grams Carbohydrates; 67.2 grams Cholesterol.

2.20. Mashed Potato Buns

Preparation Time: 140 Minutes Cook Time: 20 Minutes Total Time: 160 Minutes Serving: 32

Ingredients

1-3/4 cups milk (warmed)

1/4 cup oil

One pkg active yeast

1/4 cup butter

6 tbsp. sugar

One egg

1/4 cup warm water (warmed)

1/2 cup boiled and mashed (with milk and butter) potatoes

1 tsp baking powder

6 cups flour

1-1/2 tsp. salt

1/2 tsp baking soda

Instructions

For making dough, in warm water, add yeast and stir.

Then add egg, potatoes, milk, butter, sugar, and butter and stir well.

Later add baking soda and powder and flour.

Knead the flour mixture for 10 minutes to form an elastic, smooth dough.

Place it in at a warm place for two hours to rise.

Knead again for 2 minutes.

Make small sized balls out of dough and place on a baking dish, and leave for thirty minutes.

Place the pan in a preheated oven at 375 degrees for 20 minutes.

Nutrition

Calories 137 kcal; Protein 3 grams; Cholesterol 13 milligram; Fat 4 grams; Carbohydrates 22 grams.

Bread Pudding

Preparation Time: 30 Minutes Cook Time: 45 Minutes Total Time: 45 Minutes Serving: 12

Ingredients

¾ cup of sugar

1 tsp cinnamon

Four eggs

2 tbsp. butter

2 cups of milk

½ cup raisins

Six slices bread

1 tsp vanilla extract

Instructions

Combine and beat vanilla, cinnamon, egg, sugar, and milk in a bowl and make a smooth mixture.

Spread over the bread pieces placed in the baking pan.

Put the pan in a preheated oven at 350 degrees for 45 minutes.

Serve when cooled down a little.

Nutrition

Calories 165 kcal; Fat 4.8 g; Cholesterol 70.3 g; Carbohydrates 26.5 g; Protein 4.6 g.

Maple Pancakes

Preparation Time: 5 Minutes Cook Time: 12 Minutes Total Time: 17 Minutes Serving: 6

Ingredients

One egg

1-1/2 tsp. baking powder

1 cup milk

1 tbsp maple syrup

2 tbsp. oil

1 cup flour

1/2 tsp. salt

Instructions

Beat oil, milk, egg, and syrup in a bowl.

Add and mix salt, baking powder, and flour in another bowl and add egg mixture slowly while stirring.

Drop spoonful batter on a heated pan. Cook until bubbles formed and then flip the side and cook another side till turned golden brown.

Serve with syrup.

Nutrition

Calories 486 kcal; Carbohydrate 60 g; Protein 14g; Fat 21 g; Cholesterol 123 mg

Pizza Bread

Preparation Time: 5 Minutes Cook Time: 40 Minutes Total Time: 45 Minutes Serving: 4

Ingredients

Four chopped garlic cloves

One large loaf of Italian bread

2 oz. Parmigiano-Reggiano

4 tbsp. olive oil

3 tbsp. butter

1/2 tsp oregano

1/4 cup parsley

pinch of red pepper flakes

14.5 oz. tomatoes mashed

Kosher salt

8 oz. mozzarella cheese grated

Instructions

In a saucepan, melt butter, add olive oil, stir fry garlic and oregano, and red pepper flakes.

Later add salt and parsley and turn off the flame.

Take cut bread pieces and press to reduce its height to two-third, and spread garlic paste (cooked in step one) over the cut side of bread with the help of a brush.

Afterward, cook tomatoes and leftover garlic paste in a saucepan at medium flame.

Reduce the flame to low at put a pan on simmer for 15 minutes and add salt later.

Place mozzarella cheese over bread (prepared in step three) and bake until cheese melts. It will take almost 6-8 minutes.

When the sauce is cooked, spread over baked bread, place leftover mozzarella cheese, and bake for the next 8-10 minutes until cheese melts. Drizzle parmigiana-Reggiano after taking it out of the oven. Sprinkle leftover parsley and olive oil and serve when cool down.

Nutrition

152 kcal calories; 7 grams' protein; 14 milligrams cholesterol; 5 grams' fat; 18 grams' carbohydrates

Silky Peanut Butter Cookies

Preparation Time: 20 minutes Cook Time: 12 minutes Total Time: 32 minutes Serving: 5 dozen cookies

Ingredients

1 tsp Kosher Salt

1 cup Sugar

1 cup Crisco

1 tsp Vanilla

2 tsp. Baking Soda

1 cup Peanut Butter

3 cups Flour

2 Eggs

36 Chocolate

Instructions

Combine sugar, peanut butter, and Crisco cream in a bowl and beat until smooth, fluffy mixture is obtained.

Then beat egg one by one and add vanilla, and mix.

In another bowl, combine salt, baking soda, and flour,

Add the content of the second bowl to the first bowl and gently toss all together.

Make dough balls and place them on the butter sheet.

Bake in a preheated oven at 350 degrees for 12 minutes.

Sprinkle chocolate kisses on cookies and let them cool and serve.

Nutrition

415 kcal Calories; 8 grams' protein; 25 grams' fat; 42 grams Carbohydrates; 42 grams Cholesterol.

Greek Yogurt Cookie Dough

Preparation Time: 4 Minutes Cook Time: 0 Minutes Total Time: 4 Minutes Serving: 1

Ingredients

1 tbsp honey

1 tbsp peanut butter

1 cup of greek yogurt

0.5 tsp vanilla extract

1 tbsp of chocolate chips

Instructions

In a small bowl, combine all the ingredients and
serve.

Nutrition

280 kcal Calories; Protein 22 grams; Fat 12
grams; Cholesterol 11 milligrams; Carbohydrates
37 grams.

Chapter 3: Recipes for snacks

Snacks Recipes

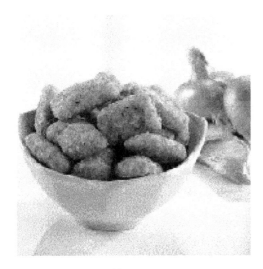

Mini Veg Puffs

Preparation Time: 35 Minutes Cook Time: 10 minutes Baking time: 25 minutes Total Time: 70 Minutes Serving: 6

Ingredients

Vegetable filling

¼ cup chopped beans

1 tsp mustard

2 tbsp. chopped coriander

2 tbsp. peas

1 tbsp. oil

½ tsp lemon juice

½ tsp garam masala

Salt as required

¼ cup chopped carrot

½ tsp cumin

¼ tsp turmeric powder

½ cup potatoes boiled and chopped

¼ cup onion chopped

½ chili powder

1 tsp garlic/ginger paste

Puff roll

1.5 tsp vinegar

1 tsp salt

2 cups flour

¾ cup margarine

1.5 tsp gluten

2 tbsp. milk

Instructions

Vegetable Filling

In a pan, stir fry cumin and mustard seeds.

Add ginger/garlic paste and onions and stir fry.

Mix garam masala, turmeric powder, and chili powder.

Combine beans, peas, and carrots with 1 tbsp water and mix well.

Cook for 2-3 minutes.

Mix lemon juice, coriander, and potatoes and cook for 5 minutes.

Set aside and cool.

Puff roll

In a bowl, mix salt, gluten, vinegar, and flour.

Knead the mixture using water for 15 minutes until a stiff dough is formed.

On a flat surface dusted with flour, place the kneaded dough and, using a rolling pin, roll it to a rectangular shape.

Place margarine over the flattened dough surface

Fold the sheet and again, using a rolling pin, roll it to a thin sheet.

Cut this big rectangular sheet into six small sheets and fill them with prepared vegetable fillings.

Pack the sheet to form a small bite-sized rectangular shape. Press all the sides. Brush milk all over the surface.

Bake in a preheated oven (350 degrees) for almost 25 minutes.

Serve.

Nutrition

170 kcal Calories; 5.1 grams' protein; 31 grams Carbohydrates; 2.9 grams Fat; 0-milligram Cholesterol

Candied Corn Puffs

Preparation Time: 15 Minutes Cook Time: 35 Minutes Total Time: 50 Minutes Serving: 8

Ingredients

8 oz. corn puffs

Salt as required

1 cup butter

1 cup peanuts

1 cup of sugar

1 tsp baking soda

1.2 cup of corn syrup

Instructions

Mix peanuts and corn in a bowl.

Mix corn syrup, sugar, and butter, and boil.

Turn off the flame and add baking soda and mix well.

Pour the syrup over corns.

Place in a preheated oven at 250 degrees for 35 minutes.

Cool and serve.

Nutrition

631 kcal Calories; 6.2 grams' protein; 62 grams Carbohydrates; 42.2 grams Fat; 62.1-milligram Cholesterol

Puffed Rice Balls

Preparation Time: 10 Minutes Cook Time: 15 Minutes Total Time: 25 Minutes Serving: 6

Ingredients

1/8 tsp cardamom powder

½ cup jaggery

1/8 cup water

2 cups puffed rice

1/8 tsp ginger powder

Instructions

Melt the jaggery in a pan using water. (jaggery should be immersed in water).

Remove impurities from jaggery and place the pan on low flame and heat it to form a thick jaggery syrup (you should be able to make a firm ball out of it).

Pour syrup over puffed rice.

Mix ginger powder and cardamom. Toss them.

Make bite-sized balls or of your requirement.

Store in an airtight jar.

Nutrition

24 kcal calories; 1.82 grams' protein; 40.18 grams' carbohydrates; 0.91-gram Fat; 0-milligram cholesterol

Rosemary Garlic Popcorn

Preparation Time: 6 minutes Cook Time: 0 minutes Total Time: 6 minutes Serving: 6

Ingredients

1/8 tsp salt

½ cup popcorn kernels

1 tsp rosemary

2 tbsp. olive oil

Pinch of pepper

Two chopped garlic cloves

Instructions

In a pan at medium flame, heat the olive oil and stir fry garlic.

Turn off the flame and mix rosemary in garlic.

Strain oil in a bowl and put popcorns in it.

Combine everything well and drizzle pepper and salt and serve.

Nutrition

122 kcal Calories; 2.7 grams' protein; 17 grams Carbohydrates; 5.4 grams Fat; 0-milligram Cholesterol

Salami and cream cheese roll

Preparation Time: 10 Minutes Cook Time: 0 Minutes Total Time: 10 Minutes Serving: 20

Ingredients

¼ cup capers (baby)

6 oz. salami sliced

8 oz. cream cheese

2 tbsp. parsley

Crackers as required

Instructions

Wrap cream cheese with cling wrap and bring it in a rectangular shape with a rolling pin.

Remove the cling sheet

Place sliced salami on cheese and roll it using a rolling pin after covering with the sheet again.

Then turn it upside down

Drizzle parsley and capers and firmly roll up the cheese sheet.

Cover the roll with cling wrap and refrigerate for about 4 hrs.

Cut into slices.

Put the slices on the serving dish along with crackers.

Nutrition

45 kcal Calories; 1.4 grams' protein; 0.4-gram Carbohydrates; 4.2 grams' fat; 13 milligrams Cholesterol

Taco beef and cheese

Preparation Time: 15 Minutes Cook Time: 240 Minutes Total Time: 255 Minutes Serving: 4

Ingredients

8 oz. butter

4 oz. green chilies chopped

1 cup chopped onion

10 oz. kernel corn

1.25 oz. taco seasoning

1 cup chopped red bell pepper

1 lb. lean beef grounded

Instructions

On medium flame, cook onion, bell pepper, and beef in skillet until beef turned brown.

Drain off the excess fat.

Shift beef in a cooker and add all other ingredients and cook for 4 hrs at low flame.

Mix and serve.

Nutrition

530 kcal calories; 39 grams' protein; 27 grams' carbohydrates; 30 grams' fat; 10 milligrams cholesterol

Grilled Chicken Breast

Preparation Time: 5 minutes Cook Time: 20 minutes Total Time: 35 minutes Serving: 4

Ingredients

1 tsp. powdered garlic

¼ cup vinegar

2 tbsp. lemon juice

1 tbsp. salt

Four chicken breast pieces boneless

1 tbsp. pepper and sugar

2 tbsp. Italian seasoning

1/3 cup oil

3 tbsps. Worcestershire sauce

2 tbsp. Dijon mustard

Instructions

Take a large bowl.

Add chicken and mix all the ingredients.

Set it aside for 3-4 hrs.

On medium flame, place chicken on preheated grill and cook both sides for 8-10 minutes until chickens' tenders.

Slice it and serve

Nutrition

238 kcal Calories; 24 grams' protein; 2 grams Carbohydrates; 14 grams Fat; 72-milligram Cholesterol

Cucumber Guacamole

Preparation Time: 15 Minutes Cook Time: 0 Minutes Total Time: 15 Minutes Serving: 8

Ingredients

½ tsp salt

Two chopped onions

One pitted avocado

½ cup of water

1 tbsp. lime juice

½ chopped cucumber

Instructions

Blend all the ingredients in a blender until a smooth mixture is obtained.

Nutrition

60 kcal calories; 0.9-grams protein; 3.8 grams' carbohydrates; 5.2 grams' fat; 0-milligram cholesterol

BLT Lettuce Wrap

Preparation Time: 10 minutes Cook Time: 0 minutes Total Time: 10 minutes Serving: 1

Ingredients

Pepper to taste

One chopped tomato

1 oz. avocado

Three lettuce leaves (iceberg)

Four slices of boiled and chopped bacon

1 tbsp mayo

Instructions

Mix mayo, pepper, and tomatoes in a bowl.

On a serving plate, place lettuce leaves.

Put shredded lettuce on lettuce leaves and put tomato mixture followed by bacon and wrap the leave.

Serve.

Nutrition

161 kcal Calories; 11 grams' protein; 8 grams Carbohydrates; 10 grams Fat; 20-milligram Cholesterol

Celery and Peanut Butter

Preparation Time: 6 Minutes Cook Time: 0 Minutes Total Time: 6 Minutes Serving: 4

Ingredients

¼ cup peanut butter

Four celery stalk

Instructions

Slice celery stalks.

Put peanut butter over celery pieces and serve with dipping sauce.

Nutrition

103 kcal Calories; 4 grams' protein; 5 grams Carbohydrates; 8 grams Fat; 0-milligram Cholesterol

Oven-Baked Kale Chips

Preparation Time: 10 Minutes Cook Time: 10 Minutes Total Time: 20 Minutes Serving: 4

Ingredients

¼ tsp salt

One bunch of kale

1 tbsp. olive oil

Any flavorings (optional)

Instructions

Wash and cut kale into medium-sized pieces.

Spread oil thoroughly over the kale pieces and drizzle salt.

Make a layer of kale leaves over the baking pan.

Bake the loaves in a preheated oven at 300 degrees for 10-12 minutes.

Note: watch leaves carefully after 8 to 10 minutes of baking. Don't let them turn brown.

They will become crispier when cool down. Drizzle flavorings after baking.

Nutrition

65 kcal Calories; 2.1 grams' protein; 7.4 grams Carbohydrates; 3.5 grams Fat; 0-milligram Cholesterol

Pork Rinds

Preparation Time: 15 Minutes Cook Time: 90 Minutes Total Time: 105 Minutes Serving: 4

Ingredients

Olive oil as required

1 lb. pork skin

kosher salt to taste

¼ onion and garlic powder (optional)

¼ tsp pepper/ paprika (optional)

Instructions

Cut pork into medium-sized pieces leaving a thin layer of fat on it.

Place the skin on a baking sheet at a distance.

Spray oil over the skin and drizzle salt and other spices if using any.

Bake the skin in a preheated oven at 325 degrees for 2 hrs.

Cool it and serve.

Nutrition

152 kcal Calories; 17 grams' protein; 0-gram Carbohydrates; 7 grams Fat; 0-milligram Cholesterol

Meatballs

Preparation Time: 15 Minutes Cook Time: 25 Minutes Total Time: 40 Minutes Serving: 5

Ingredients

1 lb. meat

½ cup milk

One chopped garlic clove

Pepper to taste

One egg

½ cup breadcrumbs

½ cheese grated

2 tsp. salt

½ cup onions chopped

2 tbsp. parsley

Instructions

In a bowl, combine and whisk well salt, pepper, cheese, parsley, and egg.

Take another bowl, add breadcrumbs and milk, and mix. Set aside.

Combine meat in the egg mixture and mix well.

Mix breadcrumbs (soaked), onion, and garlic with meat mixture.

Make bite-sized balls out of the meat mixture.

Now you can either bake the meatballs in a preheated oven at 360 degrees for 25 minutes or can fry in a saucepan until they turn brown.

Nutrition

215 kcal calories; 24 grams' **protein; 9.8 grams'** carbohydrates; 8.8 grams' fat; 0-milligram cholesterol.

Turkey Roll-ups

Preparation Time: 5 minutes Cook Time: 25 minutes Total Time: 30 minutes Serving: 15

Ingredients

16 pieces of cheese (Swiss)

½ lettuce

Two tomatoes

8 oz. cream cheese

Eight tortillas

16 pieces of deli turkey

¼ cup cranberry sauce

Instructions

Whisk cranberry sauce and cream cheese in a bowl and set aside.

On a flat surface, place tortillas and spread cheese mixture over them.

Place lettuce leaves (3) over tortillas.

Place turkey deli (2 slices) and Swiss cheese (4 slices) over lettuce and put few tomato slices.

Start wrapping tortilla from one side. Wrap tightly.

Refrigerator the tortillas for a few hours.

Cut each tortilla into several pieces as desired and serve.

Nutrition

287 kcal calories; 16.9 grams' protein; 16.6 grams' carbohydrates; 17.1 grams' fat; 60.8 milligrams cholesterol.

French Onion Dip

Preparation Time: 10 minutes Cook Time: 25 minutes Total Time: 35 minutes Serving: 2 ¼ cups

Ingredients

¼ cup egg mayonnaise

¾ tsp. salt

4 oz. cream cheese

½ tsp. pepper

2.5 cups chopped onions

½ cup sour cream

¼ tsp cayenne pepper

3 tbsp. butter

½ tsp powdered onion

Instructions

In a pan, at medium flame, melt butter and add cayenne pepper, pepper, salt, onion, and powdered onion.

Stir onions for five minutes.

Then reduce the flame to low and cook onions for 20 minutes.

Turn off the flame and let it cool.

Whisk well mayonnaise, sour cream, and cream cheese in a container.

Add cooked onions to cream mixture and mix well.

Place the bowl in the refrigerator for a few hrs. To develop flavor and serve.

Nutrition

162 kcal Calories; 2.1 grams' protein; 6.3 grams Carbohydrates; 14.8 grams Fat; 35-milligram Cholesterol.

Granola Bars

Preparation Time: 10 Minutes Cook Time: 5 Minutes Total Time: 15 Minutes Serving: 10

Ingredients

1.5 cups roasted oats

¼ cup maple syrup

1 cup dates

1 cup roasted almonds

Banana chips, dried fruits, chocolate chips (you can also add ingredients as per desire)

¼ cup peanut butter

Instructions

Blend dates in a blender.

Mix almonds, oats, and blended dates in a bowl and set aside.

Melt butter and syrup in microwave and pour over oats mixture.

Spread the mixture over the sheet and press firmly.

Place the sheet in the freezer for 20 minutes to harden.

Cut into bars of the required size and serve.

Can store in an airtight container for one week.

Nutrition

231 kcal Calories; 5.8 grams' protein; 34 grams Carbohydrates; 10 grams Fat; 0-milligram Cholesterol

Red pepper hummus in cucumber cups

Preparation Time: 20 Minutes Cook Time: 20 Minutes Total Time: 40 Minutes Serving: 20 pieces

Ingredients

3 tbsp. Olive oil

1/3 cup tahini

7 oz. chopped cooked red pepper

¼ cup lemon juice

Two cucumbers thick sliced

Salt and pepper to taste

2 cups chickpeas

One chopped garlic

¼ tsp powdered cumin

Instructions

Blend tahini, red pepper, olive oil, salt, cumin, pepper, chickpeas, 1 tbsp hot water, and

lemon juice in a blender to get a smooth mixture.

Using a small spoon, scoop out the seeded portion from thick slices of cucumber.

Fill the center of cucumbers with the blended mixture and serve.

Nutrition

54 kcal Calories; 2 grams' protein; 6 grams Carbohydrates; 5 grams Fat; 0-milligram Cholesterol

31.8. Chocolate orange oats

Preparation Time: 5 Minutes Cook Time: 0 Minutes Total Time: 5 Minutes Serving: 1-pint jar

Ingredients

1 tsp vanilla extract

½ cup oats

¼ cup yogurt

1 tbsp maple syrup

Juice of one orange

1.5 tbsp. cocoa powder

1/3 cup milk almond flavor

Instructions

In a jar, put all the ingredients.

Shake the jar energetically to mix them

Refrigerate the jar for three hours and serve.

Nutrition

303 kcal Calories; 8 grams' protein; 58 grams Carbohydrates; 5 grams Fat; 1-milligram Cholesterol

3.19. Easter Deviled Eggs

Preparation Time: 15 Minutes Cook Time: 25 minutes Additional Time: 30 minutes Total Time: 70 Minutes Serving: 24

Ingredients

Four drops of green, blue and red food color

Hot sauce as required

12 eggs

Salt to taste

3 cups of water

Pepper to taste

¼ cup salad dressing

¼ tsp mustard powder

Instructions

add eggs and add water to immerse them in a deep pan.

Bring water to boil and boil for three minutes.

Turn off the flame and let eggs be cooked in hot water for the next 20 minutes.

Peel the eggs.

Cut the eggs in half and separate yolks.

Smash the separated egg yolks in a bowl and mix in salad dressing, hot sauce, mustard powder. Salt and pepper to get a smooth mixture.

Add food color one in each container and pour water (1 cup) in each of them. Dip eight egg white in each bowl and give them all three colors.

Let the egg white to cool.

Put a spoonful of egg yolk mixture over colored egg whites.

Chill egg whites for 30 minutes before serving.

Nutrition

87 kcal Calories; 6.2 grams' protein; 1.1 grams Carbohydrates; 6.3 grams' fat; 188 milligrams Cholesterol

Cream Cheese wontons

Preparation Time: 20 Minutes Cook Time: 10 Minutes Total Time: 30 Minutes Serving: 6

Ingredients

Oil as required

8 oz. cream cheese

One egg

24 wontons wrappers

½ tsp sugar

2 tsp. chopped chives

½ tsp onion powder

Instructions

Whisk onion powder, sugar, and cream cheese together.

Put wrappers over flat surface and place spoonful cream mixture in the center.

Brush egg on the corners of the wonton wrapper.

Join the opposite sides and press.

Take a deep pan and heat oil in it.

Fry wontons for 4 minutes or until they turn brown.

Drizzle chives and serve.

Nutrition

228 kcal Calories; 6 grams' protein; 19 grams Carbohydrates; 14 grams' fat; 71 milligrams Cholesterol

Cucumber and Ranch Dressing

Preparation Time: 5 Minutes Cook Time: 0 Minutes Total Time: 8 Minutes Serving: 4

Ingredients

¼ tsp pepper and salt each

½ tsp dill

Two sliced cucumbers

½ cup ranch dressing

½ chopped onion

Instructions

Take a bowl, mix well all the ingredients.

Set aside for thirty minutes and serve.

Nutrition

232 kcal Calories; 2 grams' protein; 11.8 grams Carbohydrates; 21 grams' fat; 13.2 milligrams Cholesterol

Dill Pickles

Preparation Time: 15 Minutes Cook Time: 5 Minutes Total Time: 20 Minutes Serving: 2 mason jars

Ingredients

1 cup of water

1 cup cider vinegar

1.5 lb. cucumbers

½ tsp red chili flakes

1.5 tbsp. pickling salt

2 tsp. dill seeds

Four chopped garlic cloves

Instructions

Cutaway the stem end of the washed dried cucumber and bring it to pieces of the desired size.

Take a boiled dry jar and add chili flakes, garlic, and dill.

Place cucumbers pieces in the jar and airtight the jar.

In a pan boil salt, water and vinegar in it.

Pour this vinegar solution into a cucumber jar. The jar should be filled to the top, leaving an inch space at the top.

Remove the air bubble by tapping the jar for few times.

Airtight the jar.

After it gets cooled down, place the jar in the refrigerator.

Best to use after 48 hrs.

Nutrition

91 kcal Calories; 2.9 grams' protein; 16.6 grams Carbohydrates; 0.7 grams Fat; 0-milligram Cholesterol

Leftover cheeseburger mac and cheese

Preparation Time: 5 Minutes Cook Time: 25 Minutes Total Time: 30 Minutes Serving: 4

Ingredients

2 cups cheese

1 tsp salt

2 cups pasta

½ tsp pepper

1 tsp garlic and onion powder each

Three patties of leftover chopped cheeseburger

3 cups of milk

Instructions

Take a deep pan and boil onion powder, garlic powder, pasta, 2 cups milk, pepper, and salt.

Boil until all the milk is evaporated.

Mix leftover milk and cheese and boil.

Simmer for 5 minutes

Add leftover burger pieces and simmer it for the next 3 minutes.

Stir and Serve.

Nutrition

530 kcal Calories; 27 grams' protein; 48 grams Carbohydrates; 25 grams Fat; 78-milligram Cholesterol.

Baked cheese crisp

Preparation Time: 5 Minutes Cook Time: 7 Minutes Total Time: 12 Minutes Serving: 4

Ingredients

¾ cup shredded cheddar and parmesan cheese

1 tsp Italian seasoning

Instructions

Whisk both the cheese together.

Put a spoonful of cheese mixture over the baking sheet. Remember to keep sufficient distance between each spoon dropping. Drizzle seasoning over cheese mixture

Bake in a preheated oven at 400 degrees for 8 minutes.

Let them dry on paper towels and serve.

Nutrition

152 kcal calories; 11 grams' protein; 1 gram carbohydrates; 11 grams' fat; 0-milligram cholesterol.

Beef jerky

Preparation Time: 15 minutes Cook Time: 180 minutes Total Time: 195 Minutes Serving: 6

Ingredients

1 tsp powdered onion

1 tbsp honey

¾ Worcestershire sauce

2 tsp. Black pepper

2 lb. sliced beef

1 tsp red chili flakes

¾ cup soy sauce

1 tsp garlic powder

1 tbsp paprika

Instructions

Mix powdered onion, soy sauce, pepper, flakes, paprika, Worcestershire sauce, honey, and garlic powder in a medium-sized bowl.

Combine sliced beef in the bowl and mix well with all the ingredients.

Marinate it for almost three hours.

Dry beef slices over paper towels and place the pieces over a baking sheet.

Place the sheet over a wire rack and put in preheated at 175 degrees for three hours.

Cut the slices into bite-sized portions and serve.

Nutrition

286 kcal calories; 32.7 grams' protein; 13.9 grams' carbohydrates; 10.5 grams' fat; 81 milligrams cholesterol.

Conclusion

The optavia program offers diet plans assisting you to lose weight quickly and later to maintain it too. Its low calorie and rich protein meals allow you to meet your weight loss goals giving you fulfillment.

The collection of three main diet courses, optavia, permits users to choose and follow conveniently what best suits them according to their needs. For instance, if someone wants a flexible diet plan, then optavia has a 4-2-1 program in which the user can have four fuelings, two lean and green, and one snack. In the 5-1 strategy, the customer will eat five fuelings and one lean and green in one day with 2 to 3 hours of interval. This program is adjustable to accommodate a wide range of targets such as patients with diabetes and old aged people. Optavia program has meal plans that help you lose weight (4-2-1 and 5-1 diet plans) and guide you to maintain the weight you desire to keep through a 3-3 meal plan. Initially, it restricts you to 100 calories a day, which causes weight reduction because your stored food is burned to meet the energy requirements. Once you are on your required weight, the transition period starts in which food that was not allowed previously is allowed now to increase your calorie intake, but it is again under strict surveillance as to eat only that much calories which you can burn easily during your daily work out. Thus, someone wants a quick reduction in weight by following simple and easy meal schedules to go for optavia diet plan. In addition to following the optavia program, talk to the dietitian; you can guide your eating habits and lifestyle to bring necessary changes to keep living a healthy life.

CARNIVORE DIET

The Dietetic Plan Based on the Prehistoric Man Eating Habits. Discover How to Lose Weight Enjoying 127+ Meat-Based Dishes Avoiding Carb and Hard-to-Digest Foods

John Ramsey

Introduction

Congratulations on purchasing *Carnivore Diet: A New Powerful Diet for Weight Loss with a Healthy Meat-Based Meal Plan That Exceeds the Use of Plant-Based Products,* and thank you for doing so.

You are already taking a big step towards improving your life and health for the better just by wanting to get to know about the carnivore diet. Do you ever think about losing a couple of pounds but can't find the perfect method? Do you suffer from any pains or illnesses, either physically and mentally? Do you want to know the most efficient and fast method to gain muscle and get ripped? If your answer is yes to any of those questions, then you've come to the right place. This book will be your guide to smoothly transitioning to a new diet that strictly restricts anything that is not meat!

The following chapters will discuss and go into detail about the carnivore diet, what it is, and how it affects the human body. The book will also include more than twenty delicious recipes with pictures that follow all the rules of the carnivore diet. It even includes a Seven-day meal plan, the best ways to save money, and tips and tricks to follow when transitioning.

This book guide will not only get you familiar with the carnivore diet but also excited for all the delicacies that you will be eating and enjoying as well as the countless benefits that come with the diet!

There are plenty of books on this subject on the market, thanks again for choosing this one! Every effort was made to ensure it is full of as much useful information as possible. Please enjoy!

Chapter 1: What Is The Carnivore Diet

The Carnivore diet is a diet based on consuming only meat, fish, and animal-based products such as certain dairy foods and eggs, but that is only if you are a beginner. A more advanced level requires only the consumption of meat, no dairy, or eggs! This means that you are mostly getting your energy from fat and protein while living on almost zero carbohydrates a day. Those who have adopted such a diet have experienced a faster weight loss process, improved athletic performance, healthier digestion, brighter mental clarity, and prevention or reduction in countless diseases.

There are many people in the past who lived off only by eating meat, such as the Inuit, Chukotka of the Russian Arctic, Sioux of South Dakota, Brazilian Gauchos, and many other tribes or countries. The Inuit, in particular, are a tribe of indigenous people from Northern Canada, Greenland, and parts of Alaska. As you can imagine, the weather there is very cold, and the plants are unable to grow, making their main source of food comes from animals such as fish, seal, walrus, and other animal products. Their diet mostly relied on what they can hunt, with little or no carbohydrate intake. Traditionally, these people had low rates of diseases such as heart disease, diabetes, and obesity. But being introduced to a western diet, which contained vegetables, grains, and fruits, it spiked their rates higher than usual.

But how exactly did this diet travel all over the western and eastern countries? Vilhjalmur Stefansson, born in 1879, was a Harvard educated man and an Arctic explorer. When exploring the Arctic, he adopted the Inuit diet, which consists of eating mostly meat. At first, Stefansson only ate meat in order to survive but returning back to his homeland, he picked up the all-meat diet once again, making him realize how healthy he felt during his time in the Arcticup He was the first to introduce the no-carb diet to the world, writing an article where he discusses his months traveling, including what today is known as the carnivore diet. Not just eating the meat parts of the animal, but also the liver, chops, brains, boiled short-ribs, also contain plenty of nutrients that helped him throughout the days.

It sounds a bit risky not eating any fruits or vegetables because those provide us with our everyday vitamins, but it is scientifically proven that you will not have nutritional shortages. Red meat is well known for containing a lot of vitamins such as zinc, vitamin D, vitamin B, protein, selenium, and many more. However, it does lack Vitamin CUP, But due to the low intake of carbohydrates, less and less vitamin C is needed for the body. When you are on the carnivore diet, eating meat and consuming very little cabs will not result in scurvy which is a disease that is caused by the lack of vitamin CUP When your carbs are low, very little or sometimes none vitamin C is required to prevent scurvy because it has a higher bioavailability due to all the nutrients coming from within the meat.

Why and how does this diet work exactly? Eating animal source foods restricts calories and acts as if the body is fasting. We often feel full after eating a huge steak, and when you are adopting an all-meat diet, your body adjusts to the high intake of meat and fatty foods, which then stops you from often feeling hungry. The high-fat foods fill you up easily making you eat less frequently, which is why many carnivores eat only two to three meals a day. It is also because when eating the same foods over and over again, the brain completely stops your cravings and hunger, so you start to eat less.

The carnivore diet is also known as a low residue diet because of its lack of high fiber foods like whole grains, seeds, fruits, nuts, and veggies. It is often designed to ease symptoms such as bloating, abdominal pain, gas, and diarrhea, but it can also help cure people who are suffering from IBD (inflammatory bowel disease). Since the carnivore diet strongly lacks high fiber since meat is mostly made out of fat and protein, it is unable to inflame or irritate the gut and stomach.

Ketogenic diets are diets filled with high-fat and moderate-proteins that can often cure a wide variety of conditions such as diabetes, epilepsy, sclerosis, glycogen storage disease, polycystic ovary syndrome, can prevent tumor growth, breast cancer, and many more. The carnivore diet is also often ketogenic with its ability to be in the state of ketosis, which is when the body lacks carbs and burns fat instead. If you are mostly eating a lot of meat fat about once or twice a day, then your body is most likely in the ketosis state, enabling you to fight against such diseases. But to have a ketogenic diet, you must be eating plenty of meat so that the energy within your body comes from sixty to Seventy percent of fat, twenty to thirty percent from protein, and five to ten percent from carbohydrates.

In 2014, a research study put a couple of volunteers on a carnivore diet, which resulted in drastic changes in the gut microbiota, which are the microorganisms found inside the human body. They are responsible for the proper function of the body. The carnivore diet managed to decrease the levels of those microbes in less than 48 hours. The significant increase in the abundance of bile-tolerant organisms and change in gut microbiota has been connected to a lot of chronic inflammatory diseases, and it became fascinating how a change in diet can serve such strong and significant connections to health in such a small period of time.

There are three main levels of a carnivore diet. Level one is the beginner level. It is the most basic level to get used to the new diet and changes within your body. You are allowed to eat any type of meat and fish. You can eat eggs, butter, heavy whipping cream, and cheese. You can also drink coffee and tea! When starting off this diet, your body is not very used to breaking down the meat and extracting all the nutrients

out, so it is recommended that you take any supplements such as electrolytes, pink Himalayan salt, or any other supplements if you have digestive issues.

Level two carnivore is a step further into the all-meat diet. Although level 1 carnivore can give fair results, level two can push you closer towards achieving your goals. This time you can only eat meat and drink water. This means that you can't have any 'side' ingredients like coffee, eggs, tea, butter, teacup. Supplements are allowed if you are jumping straight into level two carnivores, but if you are not, then it is advised that you don't take any and let your body digest and extract the nutrients on its own.

Level three is the ultimate diet that not many follows. You can only drink water and eat beef; ideally, it should be grass-fed. Cut out all the meats that are not grass-fed. It may be expensive, but if you decide upon moving to this diet, then try to at least have a thirty-day streak in order for you to really see changes. If you can't afford grass-fed beef, then just buy normal beef but still eliminate other meats such as pork and seafood.

Of course, you can always go beyond level three by testing what suits you best. Only attempt it after you have completed a thirty-day streak at level 3. This is where you test the foods that you have previously eliminated. Start by adding other meat or seafood, see how you feel after two to three days of eating that along with beef and water. Notice how it affects your body, observe if you gain weight or lose weight. But remember to keep track of your weight before you attempt to experience with your diet. Try different things like adding eggs, dairy, coffee, tea, or other meats. Give each a couple of days in order to see clear results. This will show you what is best for your body as well as help you maintain your appetite.

Everyone who is starting off the carnivore diet should begin with level 1 unless they have a balanced meat intake throughout at least a few weeks and do not drink coffee if that is the case, then you can move on to level 2. However, it is not healthy, starting at level 3 without having completed at least thirty days of level 1 or 2. It can really affect your health poorly if your body is not yet used to the all-meat diet.

Chapter 2: What To Eat When On Carnivore

Our diets as a species have undergone huge changes in the past few centuries, and it's no surprise that as our lives got easier and more focused on convenience – we forgot that nutrition has always been the most important. Particularly around the end of the twentieth century, America had developed a booming fast-food industry that catered to the needs of busy families with busy America lives.

It seemed like the perfect solution to heating up frozen TV dinners when you couldn't make time to cook. But as food production skyrocketed, we started to realize that all over the country, people were demanding foods from thousands of miles away that couldn't withstand the journey. In order to combat the natural process of decay, the food packaging industry began using ingredients that could hold up in all conditions – ingredients that were synthetic, unhealthy, and highly manipulated. In a process called hydrogenation, fats and oils can be heated up to a temperature that somewhat solidifies their molecular structure, allowing them to last longer on the shelves before going bad.

However, hydrogenated fats and oils are not the same as the healthy fats and oils that they started out to be (like the ones you will be eating on a carnivore diet). Instead of offering our bodies that coveted fatty acid fuel source that produces high energy ketones, these hydrogenated fats and oils are now what you know to be saturated or trans fats. Saturated fats are no longer the healthy monounsaturated sources you began with, and they will increase your harmful low-density lipoprotein cholesterol levels while actively reducing your good cholesterol. Saturated fats and oils are most often found in processed foods, but if you think about the amount of fat in meat that doesn't get processed, you will understand why a carnivore diet tends to eliminate unhealthy processed ingredients.

Although you will have to balance the amount of dairy like cream that you ingest, the outlines of the macronutrient portions in a carnivore diet will easily help you know when you have eaten enough. The final benefit of a carnivore diet that relates to an unhealthy development in agricultural farming is the lack of pesticides you will ingest when you are only eating animal-sourced products. Plants are much more susceptible to natural predators like insects, and when you have huge wheat fields prime and ready for eating, it is no wonder agricultural scientists spent years using too harsh of pesticides.

Our plants are often covered in chemicals that are designed to keep them sealed off from bugs, but this often means using a spray that is poisonous to the insects when ingested. While most of these chemicals have passed heavy regulatory standards, it still doesn't seem like the healthiest idea – even when almost all of us are raised to wash our vegetables before we eat them. When was the last time you had to wash a steak? It is not necessarily the fault of the convenience culture for changing our nutritional values and manipulating ingredients, but they are to blame for keeping so much of the information inaccurate or under wraps. Now that you know what unhealthy ingredients can be lurking in processed foods, it's much more unlikely that you will find yourself in the Taco Bell drive-through. Natural animal products are just as delicious and fulfilling as an unhealthier diet, without the negative side effects and weight gain.

Let's start off with the basics, what you can and can't eat while pursuing the all-meat diet. Red meat is the primary food that you must have. It is recommended that you eat it at least once a day due to its high nutritional benefits, which can keep your energy levels high. Red meats such as beef, lamb, venison, veal, goat, and pork are very beneficial to the body. Anything that is high in fat such as eggs, butter, fish, and bacon, can actually help the body lose fat because consuming low carb and high-fat foods with little sugar and glucose can cause the body to release ketones which acts as a fuel for the brain, making sure that your body doesn't go hungry and has the energy to carry on with your day to day activities. This is why most carnivore people stick to strike three meals a day after their bodies get used to the new change in diets. It also primarily relies on the fat within the body and the fat that you consume from the meat, instead of eating the sugar and high carb foods. The body manages to burn the excess fat and lose the bad fats, almost like exercising, but instead, the body is doing all the work for you and in return, you are just eating specific healthy foods. You are also allowed to eat foods such as bone marrow, lar, organ meats, bone broth, water, and poultry.

You can't eat foods such as:

- **Sugar:** regular white sugar, sweets, brown sugar, maple syrup, candy, and many others.

- **Nuts and seeds:** pumpkin seeds, almonds, sunflower seeds, any type of nuts, and pistachios.

- **Vegetables:** broccoli, cauliflower, potatoes, green beans, black beans, peppers, and many others.

- **High-lactose dairy:** yogurt, milk, soft cheese, etcup

- **Alcohol:** wine, beer, liquor, etcup

- **Fruits:** berries, apples, bananas, kiwis, grapes, oranges, and many others.

- **Grains :** rice, spaghetti, wheat, quinoa, pasta, bread, cereal, etcup

- **Beverages:** any type of juices, sodas, tea, coffee, etcup (you CAN drink water)

- **Legumes:** lentils, beans, etcup

Aim for the fattiest meat you can find, steak, 80/20 ground beef, porterhouse, ribeye, NY strip steak, and T-bone. Fish such as salmon, mackerel, catfish, trout, and sardines are also allowed. Replace vegetable oil with olive oil, or even better tallow, lard, or animal-based fats such as bacon juice fats, which you can save and store after you cooked the bacon. Eating meat every single day can become boring for some people, however adding salt and pepper, as well as herbs and spices, are always allowed while on the carnivore diet. It is encouraged that you experiment with different tastes and flavors while cooking, and know which suit your taste more. But remember to stick to simple ingredients, make sure to avoid foods that contain sugar or high amounts of carbohydrates. Dairy products are allowed but many people tend to avoid them because they cause acne and have lactose which is sugar. You cannot eat plant-based foods, make sure to avoid any fruits or vegetables as well as seeds, legumes, nuts, grains, or any starches such as bread, potatoes, pasta, beans, and rice. Stay away from sugar; in other words, anything that is sweet.

For some of us, it is very difficult to stay away from coffee, but many people who pursue the carnivore diet still drink it. For the first month, try drinking only water for thirty days, resist the urge to grab a cup of coffee or tea, but if you find yourself giving in to the temptation, then try again the next day. This goal is for you to notice what and how your body reacts to only drinking water. Don't give up on yourself. Maintaining an all-meat diet is what really matters but if you can also only drink water, then that's a level up for you.

The point of the carnivore diet is to eat only animal-sourced foods, which are defined as any product derived from an animal product (a bit redundant, but the point is the same). Animal sourced foods are considered to be your classic dairy options, including milk, cheeses, yogurt, and, obviously, meat. When it comes to your main fatty intake, you will want to focus on eating mainly beef – in any and all possible ways.

The fun thing about a carnivore diet is that you don't necessarily have to worry about particularly fatty cuts, although you should still make sure they come from as unprocessed a source as possible. Any style of beef is up for grabs, from the ground chuck in your hamburger to a prime rib. Sirloin steaks, ribeye steaks, porterhouse steaks, New York strip, as well as brisket, will serve you well on a carnivore diet. Although you will want to stick to beef first and foremost, some digestive systems take easier to a carnivore diet with a more colorful distribution of chicken, beef, pork, bison, venison, lamb, turkey, and fish.

Chicken thighs are a bit higher in fat content but have a delicious and more robust taste than the regular breast (and if you've been into your fitness for a while, you know how boring those can be). You won't be able to match the protein content of turkey, and it's a much healthier option for nights when you don't feel like eating heavy red meats. Pork of any style is on the table, from ribs, roasts, and pork belly, to shoulder butt, and bacon. Lamb chops and lamb shanks are equally as tasty of dark meat, and a good lamb roast can feed you for days. When it comes to fish, you are going to want to stick to the healthiest styles you can find – seafood like scallops, mussels, and shrimp, as well as crab, lobster, salmon, trout, and sardines.

Anchovies are often high in salt, but they can be great as well. Beyond meats exclusively, you can incorporate whichever low carbohydrate dairy products you can find; but the catch here is to be wary of the sugar content. Plenty of dairy products, if you'll recall, contain high amounts of processed sugars, and those harmful carbohydrates will affect your ability to reach ketosis. However, you are perfectly able to eat as much milk and cheese as you want if you're careful. Coffee and tea are allowed, as are water

and bone broth. Bone broth can be a great way to increase your micronutrient counts as well – these styles of broth tend to be packed with calcium, magnesium, iron, and selenium, on top of numerous vitamins. All you have to do is boil the bones, connective tissue, and marrow of either a chicken, cow, pig, or fish – or some combination of all three. Salt and pepper are your best bets for seasoning, and if you have to add some sort of sauce or condiment just for variation, try and stick with the lowest carb zero calorie sauce that you can find.

Don't forget, when you're calculating carbohydrate content, you have to subtract the amount of dietary fiber from the number of total carbohydrates in order to get your net carbohydrates, the only carbs your body will actually digest. This can help you determine exactly how healthy and unhealthy. A sauce can be. You'll also want to switch out as many animal products as you can for vegetable products, like switching out coconut and olive oil with tallow which is derived animal fat.

What You Should Avoid

It comes as no shock that any ingredient that is not an animal product shouldn't be eaten on a carnivore diet. But there are some more nuanced rules and regulations to the proper cuts, fat content, and distribution of proteins and fats that you choose to eat while eating carnivore.

Vegetables and fruits of all sorts are off-limits, and you will want to make sure you are also cutting out nuts, legumes, grains, and seeds. Anything that isn't meat, likely shouldn't get eaten. You will also, unfortunately, want to avoid all types of alcohol, as they can be packed with sugars and carbohydrates that will ruin your chances of reaching ketosis. It's also worth it to note that alcohol is never considered healthy, and likely, if you are beginning a diet in the first place, you shouldn't even think about drinking if you want to lose weight.

Any sort of fruit juices that you may enjoy likely won't comply with a carnivore diet, and if you wake up with lemon juice every morning, it might be time to stop. Other sneaky foods that you aren't allowed to consume during the carnivore diet are any sort of seasonings or spices beyond just salt and pepper, any oils or dressings, sauces, condiments, or garnishes. Salt and pepper are the only two taste enhancers that you are allowed to use, but they do the best job of seasoning natural meats anyway. Condiments and sauces might be harder, especially if you like a good Worcestershire sauce every now and again. Condiments are frequently packed with hidden sugars and added chemicals that will doubtlessly sabotage your weight loss and ketosis.

Chapter 3: How It Works

If you will recall back to chapter one, we discussed a little bit about the scientific mechanisms involved in the carnivore diet that make it easy for you to eat healthy animal fats while also losing weight. In order to properly execute an effective carnivore diet, you need to understand the processes that your body goes through in order to get you to the coveted state of fat-burning ketosis. First, we'll tackle your metabolism and what happens when you switch from catabolizing carbs to catabolizing fats, and then we'll discuss the components of the Krebs cycle that make your body biologically primed for weight loss. Once you understand how your body needs to be fueled on a carnivore diet, you can maximize your gains, productivity, and weight loss based on only your fuel source. Theoretically, you will lose weight on the carnivore diet even without an exercise plan, because the science is designed to cut your body fat no matter what. But don't worry – we'll give you all the tips to make your caveman eating work best for your lifestyle.

Metabolic rate is a term whose definition often gets mistaken for something else – at a huge detriment to your weight loss. Your metabolism is defined as all the chemical processes in your body that you have to perform every day to stay alive. Metabolism is not just how effectively your body loses weight – but that incorrect mindset can lead to fueling your body with more protein than your gains can support. An incorrect balance of fuel that attempts to control your weight loss only tends to miss the point of a functioning metabolism. When your body is operating regularly, you catabolize glucose first and foremost. Glucose breakdown and process by which our bodies extract energy from sugar occurs inside our cells, specifically in the cytoplasm. The cytoplasm of the cell is the soup-like material that supports your cell's organelles, and one of those organelles, the mitochondria, needs glucose present inside your cells in order to break it down for energy. The difficulty with this is that glucose molecules are too large to diffuse across our cell membranes themselves, which means they need a helping hand in order to provide us energy. This helping hand is called insulin, and you have doubtlessly heard of it before. Insulin is a renaissance man of a chemical, providing our bodies with support almost all over. However, one of insulin's main functions is to operate as a key that fits into your cell walls to allow large glucose molecules to make it to the mitochondria. Insulin is secreted by the pancreas, and when it's functioning to regulate our sugar intake, it simply makes sense that your pancreas would release more insulin into your bloodstream at mealtime.

Now, what does this have to do with your metabolism and your diet? Many Americans have one, both, or even more of the following conditions that are considered "metabolic" disorders: Type 2 and Type 1 diabetes, obesity, heart disease, and glucose-galactose malabsorption disorder. While there are thousands of metabolic disorders by their technical definition, we are going to focus on just these which relate specifically to glucose catabolism and handling.

The reasons most Americans have one of these disorders is because of processed sugars, saturated and trans fats, and hydrogenated oils. Most of these unhealthy ingredients started out healthy and then were chemically altered to change their molecular structure. While this most often occurs in order to make foods last longer on grocery store shelves, it also occurs in order to enhance the taste of nutritionally devoid meals.

When processing and adding chemicals to your food, there's a give and take of adding what will satisfy the customer without actually offering any nutritional value. On a carnivore diet, you are going to be eating mostly natural animal fats, which often contain no chemical additives or preservatives, have not been processed, and still maintain their healthy whole construction. While dairy is more likely to be processed, you will still be avoiding almost all of the unhealthy, modified glucose molecules that most Americans have no idea they're eating.

It's worth it to note that a carnivore diet often doesn't include more ingredients than simply meat and spice, and so you will effectively avoid the complicated and technical nutritional labels that sometimes tell us nothing. When you fuel your body with only healthy fats, you offer your metabolism nearly three-fold the energy that you could with that same amount of carbohydrates. Extra energy – without the extra stored sugar, if you recall. This means that your metabolism suddenly has an endless supply of energy, without the energy-impacting side effects of eating too much glucose.

It's no wonder your metabolism benefits from a diet that fuels you for optimization in almost every aspect – from weight loss to cardiac function and digestive regularity, a carnivore diet affects every single aspect of your metabolism, and not just the "weight loss" side. Optimizing your metabolism to work better for longer, without the repercussions, makes a carnivore diet the perfect lifestyle change to take on, and sustain, for years to come. However, there are a few nuances to your body's fat-burning mechanism that can make it difficult for some individuals to achieve their best weight loss. Let's take a closer look at what happens during cellular respiration to make healthy fats so beneficial before we get into what makes the carnivore diet so beneficial for you.

You already know that cellular respiration takes place in the cytoplasm of your cells, but there's a smaller process that occurs within cellular respiration that's going to change the way you eat for the rest of your life. The Krebs cycle, also known as the "citric acid" cycle, is one of the oldest catabolic pathways in your body, and the bodies of thousands of other eukaryotic and prokaryotic cells (that's everything from a buck to the bacteria living in your gut!).

The Krebs cycle normally runs with glucose, but since it occurs in the middle of your cellular respiration, glucose has already been altered to form pyruvate, which your body will feed into the Krebs cycle as acetyl-CoA. When you only fuel your body with healthy fats, your cellular respiration has to run with triglyceride molecules instead of glucose, which you then turn into the fatty acids that will enter the Krebs cycle. Triglyceride is just a fancy name for a fat molecule, but once they've been turned into fatty acid, triglycerides provide your body with almost three times the amount of energy per each turn of the Krebs cycle than glucose.

Now, energy production is not the only reason that fat catabolism can be better than sugar; catabolizing fats also helps your body burn weight without any effort. Think back to what happens when you digest too much sugar – it gets stored as glycogen in your liver cells, muscle cells, and fat cells when you're really unlucky. Ironically, healthy fats won't get stored on your person, both because they can't and because your body doesn't want to. When you eat too much fat, you produce an acidic bi-product during the Krebs cycle called a "ketone body". The word "ketone" should sound familiar because it's the basis of the keto diet that is so close in style to your carnivorous eating. A ketone body is made up of three acids, acetone, acetoacetate, and beta-hydroxybutyrate.

While these three divisions can cause some adverse side effects, which we will discuss later on, they provide fuel for your brain and body that is not glucose-based. This is key to your carnivore diet because our bodies love glucose, and when you are not supplying it orally, your metabolism is going to search everywhere in your structural self to find extra glucose. When you fully switch over to catabolizing only fats, and never carbohydrates, your body will have all the ketone body energy it needs, and more, to fuel a scientific internal weight loss.

Remember all the glucose stored as glycogen on your person? There is sugar hidden in your muscle cells, your liver cells, and, most importantly, your fat cells. Fat cells can clump everywhere from your love handles to visceral fat around your internal organs, and it is not always easy to get rid of without help. We've all experienced those hard to reach fatty areas at the gym, but what if you could rewire your body to target and break down THAT fat so that you wouldn't have to do the work?

On a glucose-free diet, your metabolism will go into glucose starvation mode, and your body will begin to seek out and burn those more difficult deep-tissue fatty sections that are so embedded in our physique. On a low carb, high-fat diet, you will almost always be able to achieve this fat-burning state called "ketosis" as long as you make sure to keep your carbohydrate intake below fifty grams per day. While this is difficult for some people because of the starches and sugars hidden in many healthy fruits and vegetables, individuals eating on a carnivore diet barely have to think to ensure they don't consume any sugars. Since you will be eating only animal-sourced foods like eggs, cheeses, and fatty meats, it's almost an afterthought to consider how much glucose you're consuming since your diet makes it almost non-existent.

Thinking about and maintaining ketogenic eating is one of the hardest parts of the keto diet, and it's one of the main reasons that most people don't make it through to the fat-burning stage. You will be more likely to give up a carbohydrate diet if you're still consistently eating the sugary fruits and starchy vegetables that your body's glucose metabolism loves.

If you're still eating carbs, you can be sure you will also continue to experience carbohydrate withdrawal side effects. Eating a carnivorous diet in order to promote fat burning ketosis is easy and mindless, which makes for the most flexible and maintainable style of diets. Is that about fighting illnesses? e classic description of the Atkin's diet, which was developed in the nineteen twenties, is a low carbohydrate diet that is designed to combat seizures in epilepsy patients. The theory behind a low carbohydrate diet for epilepsy patients relies on the ability of fats to be broken down without stimulating seizures.

When children at a young age diagnosed with epilepsy fasted intermittently or ate on a low carb diet (both eating patterns that trigger ketosis), scientists found that their seizures didn't occur when their bodies ran on ketone bodies, but began to reoccur when proteins and carbohydrates were present in their diets. For adults, the Atkin's diet was designed similarly to help adults manage epilepsy as well as high blood pressure, heart disease, and diabetes.

Let's start with the carnivore diet and high blood pressure in relation to heart disease. When you eat too much unhealthy glucose, you raise your levels of bad low-density lipoprotein cholesterol and lower your levels of good high-density lipoprotein cholesterol. If you weren't aware that cholesterol could be good, it can! Cholesterol is a necessary fat-like steroid hormone that is designed to clear out the arteries around your heart. Good high-density lipoprotein cholesterol breaks down and removes plaque from difficult and clogged arteries so that your heart won't have to pump extra hard in order to properly circulate your blood. Atherosclerosis, or the tightening of your heart muscles as a result of high blood pressure, is one of the most common disorders affecting everyday Americans – and stress can also have a huge impact on your swelling levels. Eating a fatty diet high in animal-sourced foods will allow you to control your cholesterol levels more accurately than if you were attempting to regulate them with only a regular diet and medication. Most patients eating on a low carbohydrate diet can take themselves off their blood pressure medication after approval from their doctor and months of clean, carnivorous eating. Low carb diets also directly after the inflammation that you experience as a result of atherosclerosis, and here's a benefit of the carnivore diet that really comes full-circle.

The reason those dead cells building up in your tissues become so harmful is that they cause inflammation in your tissues, and you would be surprised at the manifold diseases caused by mere inflammation. Depression and anxiety are often linked to high levels of inflamed tissues, which are much less obvious symptoms of a tissue disorder. Arthritis or swelling of the joints due to autoimmune disorders, as well as simple muscle soreness after a hard workout, can all benefit immensely from eating a diet that cleans and clears out tough inflammation. But inflammation is not the only area that a carnivorous diet can improve. When you fuel your body with ketones, you shouldn't be surprised if, alongside a decrease in your anxious or depressed tendencies, you experience a sharper mind with more focused concentration because of the neurological benefits of the carnivore diet.

The Neurological Effects of Meat Eating

Although depression and anxiety have proven to be amplified by inflammation, the neurological sources of each disorder can be occasionally unknown. However, autoimmune disorders that deal specifically with the neurons of the brain like multiple sclerosis, Alzheimer's, and Parkinson's disease have all shown scientifically correlated improvements in patients eating low carbohydrate diets. It all comes back to ketones and autophagy for your neurological benefits as well, and if you have been waiting for a discussion on increase brain function and cognitive processing, we have now arrived.

One of the most important benefits for busy individuals eating on a low carbohydrate diet is the incredible mental clarity that comes with fueling your brain off a power source three times more potent than you're used to. When you eat high fat and low carbohydrate diet, your fuel source (when it finally reaches your brain) is like powering a lightbulb. with a nuclear reactor. Many dieters that chose to switch to catabolizing fats report that they've never been as focused or as productive as they are when they're eating for ketosis. Your neurons are able to fire faster, work more efficiently, and repair themselves twice as better when your brain is functioning on ketones.

This is a fairly big deal for individuals with autoimmune diseases that tend to target and break down their neural pathways. Parkinson's disease, Alzheimer's, and Multiple Sclerosis are only three examples of diseases related to the myelin sheath of your neurons that a carnivore diet can combat. While all autoimmune diseases have a time limit and no real cure, you can manage the symptoms well enough with a low carbohydrate diet to improve your quality of life and life span.

The process of autophagy stimulated by your ketosis fat burning won't just clear out dead cells causing inflammation in your tissues – it will also seek out and clean the pathways in your brain that become clogged with sticky proteins. Focus and a sharper mindset are one thing, but combatting the symptoms of often debilitating autoimmune diseases can be a huge benefit of choosing meat over vegetables.

Low Carbohydrate Diets and Type 2 Diabetes

It's been a moment since we talked about insulin, but it is high time that we brought the body's favorite renaissance hormone back into the picture. While type 2 diabetes does fall under the category of a metabolic disorder, the specific biological mechanisms that undergo damage in patients with type 2 diabetes can be functionally repaired by a low carb diet. Type 2 diabetes is often caused by an unhealthy diet, obesity, or high blood sugar.

The disease results in an inability to produce or regulate your insulin levels. If you remember back to our first conversation on insulin, you will recall that the pancreas releases insulin into the bloodstream when it senses a mealtime has supplied us with new glucose stores. The more insulin that is present in your bloodstream, the more sugar you will be able to take into your cytoplasm to fuel cellular respiration. However, if your blood sugar is consistently high, you run the risk of over-working your pancreas and developing a dangerous inability to produce insulin. No insulin means a high concentration of glucose trapped in your bloodstream. Now, let's think about all this information in the context of your carnivore diet. When you choose to fuel your body only with animal-sourced fats and protein, there won't be any glucose available to spike your blood sugar.

Materials like healthy fats and proteins also tend to slow down your digestion, which allows your body to absorb your nutrients without slowly and safely spiking your blood sugar. It's worth mentioning that processed foods and foods high in sugary additives run right through your digestive system, spiking your blood sugar and wreaking havoc on your digestion. This is simply another way that a meat-only diet can regulate your insulin levels, but it's worth it to note that the effects of ketosis can actually help reverse the effects of type 2 diabetes.

When you have high blood sugar, it's likely that you have high cholesterol, as well as some form of excess body weight leading to an overweight or obese state. Once your body begins to entirely metabolize fats instead of carbohydrates, remember your metabolism will seek out tough stored sugar inside your fat cells. For individuals with type 2 diabetes contracted as a result of alcohol abuse, this can be an incredible benefit for anyone with a condition known as a "fatty liver". Burning the fat off of your liver's stored glycogen is not something you can do in a gym, and if you have got the internal damage, chances are – there's external damage as well.

Don't forget that a ketogenic diet low in carbohydrates also stimulates your autophagy, which will begin to slowly clean out those inflamed tissues you have aggravated in your heart. Plus, healthy fats contain plenty of monounsaturated fat molecules, which will clear arterial plaque and lower your levels of low-density lipoprotein cholesterol. Before long, you will be able to slowly ween yourself off medication and should see a drastic improvement in both your day to day life and weight and your long-term health.

Chapter 4: Falsehood Of The Carnivore Diet

Following the carnivore diet means elimination everything that is not meat with the exception of fish, eggs, and low lactose dairy products. It is a strict diet and requires a lot of dedication. Your daily energy comes from your consumption of high-fat meat. In order to maintain the energy, you must eat fatty cuts of meat rather than, for example, just scrambled eggs for breakfast. Every time you eat something, it has to contain meat, not only for your daily energy needs but it also prevents you from getting hungry in-between feeding time. You make up your own rules when it comes to your serving sizes, calorie intake, amount of meat and meals you eat per day. Most advocates of this diet suggest eating as often as you wish.

On average, Seventy percent of people who steadily maintain a carnivore diet eat two meals a day. Twenty percent of carnivores eat one meal a day, and ten percent eat three meals a day. There is nothing wrong with eating three meals a day and it doesn't mean that if you eat less often, then you will be able to achieve your goals faster. Remember, each body is different from everyone else. Some people might have a very slow metabolism so they eat as much as they can in one or two meals and it is often enough to make them last the entire day without going hungry. If you happen to get hungry in between your scheduled meals, then you should add more meat into your diet or more mealtimes.

Many of those who attempt the carnivore diet have a goal in their minds, and most of the time, its weight loss. Scientifically, many studies have proven that the intake of high-protein and low carb foods can lead to weight loss. This is because of protein that comes from the meat that you'd eat every day which helps you to feel full after a meal. This is mainly the reason why many carnivores eat anywhere from one to three meals a day. With their high intake of meats, they are able to prevent their bodies from often getting hungry. A reduce in calories within the body can lead to weight loss and an increase of protein can lead to a higher metabolic rate, which can help you burn more calories. Not only that but your body is able to go into a state called ketosis which was previously mentioned in this chapter.

Caloric restriction results in weight loss when the intake of calories drops, the insulin growth factors, and the hormone growth factors are significantly decreased. This leads to autophagy, which is when your body reaches a certain point when it starts to eat its own tissues, thus losing weight. It is also an internal cleaning process of old cells and even repairs new ones which are why many people who go on carnivore find themselves healed from many diseases and illnesses in their bodies due to the fact that many of their cells are being replaced with new healthy ones. Many diseases such as rheumatoid arthritis, autoimmune, inflammation in the body, decrease the risk of cancer, gut issues, and many more. Together with the reduction of calories, an increase in protein, and an increase in fat can lead to weight loss.

In fact, a three-month study was conducted in hopes of comparing the effects of two different energy-restricted diets with around 132 overweight adults. Their diets contained varying amounts of protein and carbs that helped lead to weight loss. The subjects who ate a high-protein diet with around 0.9 to 1.3 grams per kilogram (0.4 to 0.6 grams per lb..) of their body weight per day had resulted to a significant weight loss to those who ate 0.6 to 0.8 grams per kilogram (0.3 to 0.4 grams per lb..) of their body weight per day. There are also many other studies that conclude that a reduction of carbs and an increase in protein lead to weight loss.

The carnivore diet entails eating, on average 200 to 300 grams of protein per day. Chewing meat really works your jaw muscles but it can also increase satiety and overcome your strong appetite and cravings. Do you sometimes get hungry when chewing gum? This is because the chewing action often tricks your brain and body into thinking that food is coming down to your stomach which then prepares the gastric juices to break down the food and with lack of food in your stomach, you become hungry. This relates to the chewing of meat since it takes slightly longer than average food; thus, it tricks your body once again that food is coming down which completely gets rid of your urge to eat something that is out of your carnivore diet.

Insulin is responsible for all of your metabolic malfunctions but it is also held accountable for the weight loss your receive when you are on the carnivore diet. A decrease of carbs keeps the insulin levels on the low which increases the speed of weight loss. High levels of insulin can lead to heart disease, obesity, and even cancer.

A lot of bodybuilders and people whose goals are to gain muscle and get ripped follow the carnivore diet. The carnivore diet can increase testosterone levels, which leads to muscle gain, increased libido, fat loss, increase in energy, and many more. The most important one that we are going to focus on is muscle gain and how that happens. A study conducted of forty-three men, all between the ages of nineteen and fifty-six. They were split into two groups. Group A followed a diet that consisted of forty-one percent of calories from fat which also came from saturated sources. Group B followed a diet of nineteen percent of calories coming from fat which were also polyunsaturated sources meaning the polyunsaturated fats were liquid at room temperature. Both groups consumed a strict identical number of calories, similar foods, and an equal amount of protein to ensure compliance. At the end of a ten-week period, it was concluded that high fat and low fiber diet could increase testosterone. Group A had an increase in thirteen percent higher than Group B. Although the research proved that the carnivore

diet does, in fact, increase testosterone levels, it is simply not enough for muscle gain.

However, combined with exercise, at least a few times a week can change your course of muscle gain and getting ripped. Exercising can help boost your testosterone levels by about fifteen percent post-workout. Combined with a carnivore diet, it strongly guarantees an increase in muscle growth and a more toned body shape. Resistance training such as weight lifting, weight machines, suspension equipment or even your own body weight is the best way to boost your testosterone in both the long and short term. Exercising can also prevent multiple diseases such as asthma, heart disease, diabetes, arthritis, cancer, back pain, dementia, and many more.

Stress can strongly affect your testosterone levels by elevating the hormone cortisol but it can also promote weight gain due to an increase in appetite. So start worrying less, and take some time off for yourself in order to relax. Always make sure you are not overworking; it is very important to maintain a healthy balance between your work-life and personal life. When feeling stressed, take a moment to calm yourself by breathing in and out deeply for a minute or two, meditating, or simply getting enough sleep can improve your testosterone levels. What you don't know is that a plant-based diet can lower your testosterone levels and can slow the process of weight loss compared to the carnivore diet.

Nutrient deficiencies can lead to some serious problems, both physically and mentally. However, there is nothing to worry about when it comes to the carnivore diet. Meat is known to be an excellent source of micronutrients, which is a vitamin chemical required for the correct development of many living organisms. Many people think that plants provide us with many nutrients that our body needs, but what they don't know is that animal source food is even better at that job. In fact, the carnivore diet can provide many vitamins and nutrients that are higher in quantity.

100 grams of *white fish* has around 576 milligrams of Potassium, 669 milligrams of Omega-3, and 107 milligrams of Magnesium.

100 grams of *chicken liver* can provide you with 3296 micrograms of Vitamin A, 588 micrograms of Folic acid/B9, and 17.9 milligrams of Vitamin CUP

100 grams of *eggs* has 225 milligrams of choline and 353 micrograms of Lutein.

100 grams of *beef* (rib-eye) gives 5.6 milligrams of Vitamin B3/Niacin, 0.4 milligrams of Vitamin B6, and 3.1 micrograms of Vitamin B12.

100 grams of *fish eggs* has 2434 milligrams of omega-3 and 10 micrograms of Vitamin B12.

Combined together and consumed at least once a week can lead to a guaranteed healthy diet; therefore, we don't need to eat plant-based foods. In fact, every single plant species, whether it is a fruit or vegetable that is regularly eaten every single day, is so much different from what it used to be decades and decades ago, and more than half of them didn't exist back then. This is all because of chemicals and artificially breeding. Seeds are constantly laced with chemicals to provide the most nutrients, enhance size, and taste. Those plants that do not meet the qualifications are not to be sold. Nowadays, the plant food that you see undergoes artificial selection, forced chemical fertilizers, and engineering in order to get the best quality and quantity in order to stand a chance in the competitive market.

Before the use of chemicals and machines, there was no wheat, or corn, or even rice, which currently makes up about fifty percent of the calories eaten all around the world. Take grains as an example, which come from natural grasses, and each grain plant is only able to provide just a few seeds, making them easily fall and scatter. Humans would have never eaten these without the help of agriculture and artificial selection.

Nowadays, these crops are being cultivated into staple foods for calories. Not only it is a massive change in the regular diet to which our bodies are so used to but it's also low in fat, low in protein, and low in minerals and vitamins. But it is also high in chemical toxins which are not good for the body.

Take a moment and walk up to your kitchen, look inside, and pick out a product that comes in a box or bag. Read the list all the ingredients inside the product and there is a very good chance that you don't know more than half of those ingredients that are used to change the product entirely such as a flavor enhancer, artificial flavors, food coloring materials, antifoaming agents, artificial sweeteners, antioxidants, and so many more. Many of those ingredients even biochemists, don't recognize. Although they are claimed to be 'safe' and 'health tests' approved, are they really? How would such chemicals mix with other chemicals from other foods? What about any medication that you are taking, or how would they react inside the human body, which also releases plenty of natural chemicals? There are so many possibilities that we don't know of and many of those possibilities haven't been tested yet.

Over the years of the world's development, our brains actually started shrinking, over ten percent, we started developing diseases, and many of those have no cure, bone lesions, and degenerative conditions also became part of this new evolving world. Compared to the early ancestors, the guts and stomach transformed so drastically that they can barely compare. In the past, humans' beings mainly relied on hunting, their main source of food came from animals, making them evolve over time in order to absorb the natural nutrients to provide energy and fuels for the large brains. But over time, as the diet began to change, the bodies no longer receive such nutrients and energy that it began to revolve around the modern plant-based diet. Damage in cell membranes, can disrupt its functions and even cause inflammation.

Inflammation comes from omega-3 fatty acids that come from vegetable oils. The ancestors who relied on meat to survive had an intake of omega-3 fatty acids. Omega-3 and omega-6 used to be a balance with each other, either increasing or decreasing inflammation, giving the body balance since there used to be a little intake of plants. With such a huge drastic increase in eicosanoids which are hormone-like compounds highly involved in inflammation due to oils such as corn and soybean that became available widespread for cheat, the scale of balance between omega-3 and omega-6 has been tipped. Although we need inflammation to heal our wounds and repair tissues, too much of it can lead to chronic systemic inflammation and diseases such as autoimmune disease, heart disease, cancer, IBS, joint pain, and neurological problems. There is plenty of evidence indicating that such an imbalance of the ratio of six to three can cause depression, anxiety, violent behavior, and aggression.

Oxalate is a naturally occurring molecule found within plants and humans, but too much of it can cause some serious damage. Many foods like cauliflower, broccoli, and kale have a high concentration of oxalate and if the kidney fails to eliminate the excess oxalate, it eventually forms oxalate crystals within the body, causing hyperoxaluria, kidney stones, bone disease, and blood, skin, heart problems. It is very toxic as it steals essential vitamins and minerals within the body.

Another toxic substance that is found in plants is a neurotoxin called glycoalkaloids, which are enzyme inhibitors. Mostly found in potatoes, one of the main enzyme inhibitors is often called acetylcholinesterase inhibitor which prevents the breakdown of acetylcholine which is a neurotransmitter. If the acetylcholine doesn't break down but starts to build up instead, it can cause some serious damage like muscular paralysis and sometimes even death to many of its predators and pests. However, for human beings, health dangers are numerous and often insidious. It can cause many mental health problems such as anxiety, insomnia, and restlessness. Physically, people with a high level of acetylcholine can become paralyzed, get convulsions, respiratory arrest, and even death in some cases. It can't necessarily be identified as the main 'root' of the problem since if your body has a healthy GI tract, then the acetylcholine won't make it into your bloodstream, although when eaten regularly, they can build-up, impacting your body poorly.

But you might be wondering, how can an all plant-based diet can be bad if many people saw good and improving results? Think about it this way, the people who are vegan or adopted the plant-based diet are eating much healthier than others who stick to the modern average diet consisting of junk food and sugar. They are switching from a horrible diet to a slightly less horrible, showing results as 'improvement' from before they picked up that new diet. But removing even plant-based products from the diet and replacing it for natural meats can show even more improvements and cures to health problems.

Chapter 5: Benefits Of The Carnivore Diet

Apart from major weight loss, the carnivore diet has other benefits that will improve your lifestyle. Since the diet excludes carbs, your body will be free from the sodas, cakes, cookies, and many other high-carb foods, which will finally let you live a healthy and balanced lifestyle. Many high-sugar foods are a cause for diabetes since they are known to spike blood sugar levels drastically. In fact, the elimination of sugary foods and carbs is recommended for those who suffer from diabetes. Many people claim and believe that an all-meat lifestyle is able to change the body from within, using the energy that is naturally provided within instead of looking and breaking down the chemicals within foods. Many even claim that it is able to solve countless illnesses, diabetes among them. Now of course, there has been little studies on diabetes and an all-meat-diet, do consider consulting your doctor before jumping into a diet that may or may not fit your body, after all, everyone is different and unique in their own way.

Having an all-meat diet can reduce inflammation, which happens when the body is undergoing an injuring or illness causing it to activate the immune system. Many studies show that high levels of certain chemicals like C-reactive protein and cytokines are associated with Several diseases including cancer and obesity. One study, in particular, was conducted at Boston University. The research consisted of fifty-five obese women and men, split into two groups. Group one had a diet consisting of about fifty-five percent calories which come from fat, thirty-five percent calories from protein and ten percent of calories from carbs. However, group two had a diet of twenty-five percent calories from fat, fifteen percent of calories came from protein and sixty percent calories from carbs. Eating sugar can increase the C-reactive protein levels so the diet was adjusted to fit accordingly.

Both diets were specifically made to allow both of the groups to lose one pound per week for about twelve weeks. At the beginning and end of the study, the scientists were able to measure the body composition, weight, and blood levels of C-reactive protein. At the end of the twelve-week period, group one was able to see a thirty percent reduction of C-reactive protein levels in their blood, while group two only saw a drop of three percent. This means that the fewer carbs you eat and the more protein you eat leads to a decrease of inflammation within your body, leaving you with more beneficial health.

There are many health benefits to having a carnivore diet, many of which are mental. Food is the fuel for our brains, and bad food can sometimes worsen the conditions of our brains, in terms of both physically and mentally. Like solving autism, which is a mental disorder that is difficulty in communicating and interacting with people with a restrictive pattern of behavior and thoughts. And it so happens that a carnivorous diet can solve it. A person receives high levels of cysteine when consuming meat. Cysteine is an amino acid that can aid people who suffer from autism. N-acetyl cysteine is a supplement form cysteine which can help by releasing cysteine which resolves and reduces the symptoms associated with autism. Meat also carries a high level of carnitine. Study research found out that children who suffer from autism have a lower carnitine level and another study proved that carnitine supplements could reduce symptoms of autism. This is the only diet that is high enough in cysteine but an increase consumption of fatty acids can also improve the symptoms. Adding foods such as salmon, sardines into the diet is very beneficial for those with autism.

Carnivore diet can also cure anxiety and depression. There are many studies that have linked a non-celiac gluten sensitivity to depression and anxiety. The carnivore diet strictly eliminates glute and other potential triggers that affect anxiety or depression, which is why many people claim that their insane anxiety or stress has completely vanished after just a couple of weeks on a carnivore diet. In a different study, scientists have discovered that people who have a low vitamin B12 had depression and through supplements, they were able to reduce the symptoms. Red meat possesses a high content of vitamin B12 and can help cure depression and improve your mood. This also because of the restriction of carbohydrates. Studies have shown that when the body is in ketosis, ketones are released and they have neuroprotective properties, making the brain prefer fats over carbohydrates when it comes to energy.

A study of a carnivore ketogenic diet said that eating meat can reduce tumors in many cancers, which were tested on animal models. A well-designed study found out that some cancers respond well to ketosis and can even potentially cure them but there were also some cancers that can worsen on the carnivore diet. You must consult a doctor before attempting the diet on your own. There are currently not enough studies and evidence that the carnivore diet can fully treat cancer but many reported having a lot of their symptoms disappear.

Many people also encountered their blood pressure, heart rate, and cholesterol drastically decrease. Others say that eating only meat decreased their risk of a heart attack and even removed plaques in the blood vessels. Saturated fats which found high levels in meat was claimed that it is the main risk factor for heart attack or heart disease, that was what people believed until 2019. A meta-analysis proved that there is absolutely no correlation between saturated fat consumption and heart disease. People started believing that eating meat is bad for health because of the lab rat studies where many of the rats who were being fed meat died or became very sick. The researchers were using high-fat diets to increase triglycerides,

cholesterol but induce nonalcoholic liver disease. The reason the results turned out negative was that the rats were being fed too much meat and they are very different from the human body in terms of the immune system, brain, and digestion. They weren't meant to eat too much meat since their ancestors didn't also, meaning their digestion system is not used to high intake of meat.

However, in the human body, ketogenic diets can decrease triglycerides and cholesterol levels and can even reduce blood pressure proven in countless studies with people who are suffering from obese. The experiments usually last at least 24 weeks to 56 weeks, given enough time to reduce the symptoms of obese through a carnivore ketogenic diet.

Carnivore diet can clear brain fog and make you more focused mentally. Many people experience autoimmunity triggered in plant-based products like wheat, milk, vegetables, and nuts. The antibodies that protect from the proteins that come from those foods can also cross-react, meaning that they can turn against each other and attack their own brain tissues, causing brain fog and mental illnesses. A meat-based diet comes high with zinc which can prevent autoimmunity and increase regulatory T cells which can help stop the damage of the tissues. Not only that but zinc supplements have even said that they are able to improve autism for some people.

Many vitamins like vitamin B is present in the meat and can help improve symptoms of an autoimmune condition called lupus. Vitamin B6 can even decrease the risks of inflammation and correct the immune functions for many people who suffer from lupus.

During the first week of your new carnivore diet, you might start to feel a bit off focus, distracted and restless as your body adjusts itself to the new way of digesting. It is important that you do plenty of exercise during those days to help you sleep better, for instance, go for a jog at least two hours before you go to bed. It will help you fall asleep faster and better. Eventually, your focus will go back to normal and even improve, and so will your sleep quality. Be advised to drink plenty of water throughout your first week, especially when you go hungry in between meals. It can help you feel full but also you won't have to move your scheduled meal time unless drinking water doesn't help. Don't starve yourself and wait until it's time to eat; this is not how the carnivore diet works. You can even do more harm than good just by not eating.

In many ways, the carnivore diet is very similar to the keto diet and is sometimes considered as an improved version of the keto because it provides you with protein and fat without including veggies to your diet. Another difference except for the involvement of plant-based food in keto is the fact that the keto diet allows an intake of twenty grams of carbs while the carnivore diet has no exceptions, leaving the diet at a stable zero carb intake. The animal source food is known to be a much better choice than the keto because it eliminates the plant foods which are bad for the bodies. Cyanogenic Glycosides are natural toxins that are found in plants. If the capacity to produce hydrogen cyanide exceeds its average number that your body can detoxify, it will become extremely toxic up. You can suffer from a drop in blood pressure, headaches, stomach pain, dizziness, rapid respiration, rapid pulse, twitching, convulsions, mental confusion, diarrhea, vomiting, and it some cases, even death.

A lot of the people are being led to believe the carnivore diet is bad, but that is because the market doesn't want all the concentration and money flow into one product so they made up fake 'facts' about health and diseases to scare the people into believing that meat is bad and it is all because of money. If half the world population adopted the carnivore diet, then there would be a drastic decrease in products such as pasta, junk food, sugary food, and many others. Such a decrease in money would put a lot of people out of business and the economy income would go down since all you'd have to buy is animal-based products and the consumption of food would decrease since meat makes you less hungry. Now obviously, that would be bad for the economy. The leaders like to have tight control over the people and their money. The meat is, however, currently expensive since not a lot of people buy it, and there are not a lot of animals because they don't need that many. After all, what would the world do if it had so many chickens and cattle? But if the meat demand increases, the supply would have to increase too.

Vegans and vegetarians would argue otherwise because animals have 'feelings,' but you know who else has feelings? Humans and the countless diseases they suffer from eating processed foods that are bad for the body instead of filling themselves with natural nutrients from animal products. Animals are being put down the correct way, without pain, but many children, adults, and families suffer from the physical or mental traumas that even a couple of pain killers can't solve. The animal and human brains are very different, although both can feel pain, the human brain is able to think back to the pain while the animal's brains are simply not that developed in terms of intelligence. The consumption of meat provides countless health benefits both physically and mentally while plant-based food is toxic for our bodies.

In the past, such a thing as heart disease did not exist, but then again, in the past, people mostly relied on animal-based products to survive. Then the concept of meat causes heart disease has been introduced due to saturated fats. Due to this misleading association, the demand for meat dropped while the consumption of vegetable oil increased, but so did heart disease. The real concept is that polyunsaturated fat and trans fats are the most toxic fats in the entire world, but it's not a surprise that they are found in almost all processed foods such as pizza, peanut butter, baked goods, frozen food, fast food, and many others. Always consuming high amounts of such fats can build up within your body, causing numerous health issues.

Animal fat is very high when it comes to monounsaturated and saturated fatty acids. Vegetable seed oils are very high in polyunsaturated fatty acids which originated in plant seeds and underwent artificial selection and chemical boosts. These vegetable oils mostly are found in foods like corn, sunflower oils, and soybean. After further hydrogenation or processing of the food, these fats can become solid at room temperature, such as margarine that is spread on your bread or even used as shortening to keep the baked goods tender, nice, and moist. Undergoing hydrogenation turns fats into completely unnatural like the notorious trans fats which are very dangerous.

Fat is a fundamental component of every single cell in the body, it is absolutely vital in hormone production, the brain is made out of fat, and it's needed for vitamins and minerals. Now the thing about how these natural fats turn into toxic and chemical like molecules will react in the body. It is no surprise that the brain has started shrinking through an evolution since less and less natural and healthy fat is being consumed by the body. In fact, these unnatural molecules have the power to fool our bodies. They are so similar to actual natural fats that they pass through our bodies and into our cells and tissues without being noticed. But they are not natural and lack the correct functions to operate properly. They manage to cause inflammation, damage cell membranes, and disrupt the functions. They are what is really connected to heart disease, cancer, and neurological problems.

With help from the agricultural revolution, many foods such as vegetable oils and grains now possess poisons and toxins that are harmful to the human body. These foods make out more than fifty percent of our daily food staples, but so does sugar. Carbohydrate consumption increased over the years as sugar entered the world. It first came to Europe and was a luxury that was only reserved for the wealthy since it was so new and expensive. Around this time, carbohydrates came from the intake of refined starches and grains. Everything changes during the 1900s when the industrial processing decided to spice things up. Sugar became cheaper and more available thus becoming a great part of the daily diet which now makes up a bit over twenty-five percent of our diets.

Our bodies were not made to take in such a substance that every single time we eat something unnatural, we create a metabolic panic that stresses out the pancreas whose job is to unload insulin and re-establish homeostatic blood sugar. Such a massive blood sugar spike and unnatural carbohydrates can cause some serious problems. Metabolic hormones become dysregulates, cells give up, pancreas wears off causing type two diabetes. There is a disturbance in the immune system, water balance, damage in vision, nerves, and kidneys, all leading to cancer, vascular damage, cardiovascular diseases, obesity, diabetes, hypertension, dementia, and many other health problems. All because of the increase in sugar consumption, they can also take on direct damage to the tissues.

One disadvantage that you might be thinking about is that plants have fiber, which is needed for the human body, but the question is, is it really necessary? Fiber is a non-digestible carbs which is found in plant foods. It promotes healthy bowel movements and gut-health. Many people say that a lack of fiber can lead to a weak immune system but carnivores believe otherwise. In 2012, a research study was conducted to test the theory if fiber is crucial for gut health and healthy digestion. Instead, they found out that decreasing fiber consumption in people with chronic constipation undergone vital improvements in their symptoms like bloating, straining, and gas. However, the group that ate a high fiber diet saw no change in their symptoms. This proves that fiber is not a necessity in the human body and can easily be replaced by many nutrients from meat and animal-based products.

Let's talk about the negative drawbacks of eating an all-meat diet. The truth is, there aren't many long-term studies conducted with a large group of individuals on the carnivore diet for a meaningful length of time since this diet is fairly new. Although the fatty cuts of meat do provide many vitamins and minerals required for the body, it does lack a few main ones. Vitamin C is an antioxidant that supports the immune cells' functions and it's essential for stimulating collagen synthesis. Vitamin E is also an antioxidant that blocks the oxidation of lipoproteins and lipids. It is also a mineral needed for healthy bones, nerve transmission, and muscle contraction. A fat-soluble vitamin that decreases the amount of calcification of blood vessels. Vitamin A is important for mining immune defenses and for a proper vision for it is not found in meat. Vitamin B is essential for cell growth, methylation, and metabolism. It is present in meat but it is not enough to maintain a healthy lifestyle.

Although it may be true that those vitamins are not present inside the meat, they are, however, foods such as liver, organ meats, and eggs can fix that. In 1953, it was discovered that organ meats such as liver, adrenal, brain, contain a high concentration of vitamin CUP Liver contains high amounts of vitamin B, vitamin C, and vitamin A. Note that vitamin C is heat-sensitive, so only the very fresh and gently cooked organ meats will have some good amounts. Egg yolk is a good source for vitamin E and even has hints of vitamin B. Not only does liver and eggs provide high nutritional value, but they are also part of the carnivore diet! Many carnivores spent years following this diet and reported not having any nutrient deficiencies which makes them

wonder, is the claim of nutrient requirements for an 'average person' true?

However, be advised that you can always take supplements or vitamins to get the correct amount of nutrition if eating organ meats is not up to your appetite. If you do decide to, make sure to pick out the most organic form of the supplement.

Although you already know that you can get all of your necessary micronutrients from eating solely animal-sourced foods, there's a bit of a catch in that logic that makes it necessary for you to supplement your diet. When we as humans consume another animal, the benefit is that we also get to consume all of the nutrition that that animal had. However, think about how our bodies work – once you eat something, your intestines tend to work as quickly as possible to make sure you absorb the nutrients. When you eat meat, the micronutrient content in your meals will automatically be less, since you are not consuming each nutrient from its actual source.

Instead, you are getting what acts as a kind of second-hand nutrition, which does ensure that you check all your nutrition boxes, but it doesn't always ensure the correct amounts. There's no way for you to know how much iron is in your flank steak if you didn't know what the cow had eaten during its lifetime. Silly, but necessary. It's worth it to note, however, that your carnivore diet already predisposes you to high levels of protein, and you probably won't need as high a content of your micronutrients since you will only be running digestion on mostly fats and protein.

Micronutrients act as a helping agent for your macronutrients, but you need a higher concentration if your digestion is not so limited (in a good way). When you eat on a carnivorous diet, most of the things you will find that you lack can be taken in a male multi-vitamin targeted to your age group. In order to get the proper amounts of your daily micronutrients on a caveman diet, you are going to want to make sure you get these vitamins and minerals in your multi-vitamin: Vitamin C, Vitamin A, Vitamin B12, Vitamin D3, Vitamin K, selenium, zinc, magnesium, calcium, and thiamine. (If you've always been a skeptic when it comes to multi-vitamins, consider that sailors used to get scurvy on the sea because of the lack of vitamin C in their diets).

While we won't go through what each of these micronutrients does for your body individually, boosting your levels of each of these vitamins is not just a healthy choice to support your carnivore diet. Almost all Americans, regardless of sex or age, tend to be critically deficient in their vitamin B12, vitamin D3, and calcium. A regular American diet packed with processed foods even including sugary vegetables and fruits still won't provide you with the proper nutrients you need – which is all the more reason to eat exclusively animal-sourced foods.

Chapter 6: Tips And Tricks

When on the carnivore diet, you don't need to watch your calories in order to lose weight. Just by adding exercise into your schedule can improve your health. Try different types of exercises to find out which fits you the best, find something that you enjoy doing so you can go with it in the long run. Many people prefer cycling instead of running or weight lifting rather than bodyweight exercises such as pushups, squats, or pullups. Make time to exercise at least three times a week; turn it into a sport or a habit.

The exercises that will be mentioned below will target a muscle group with compound exercises instead of isolation exercises. Compound exercises are known to use secondary muscle groups, which works to help you get bigger and stronger. There are many benefits from compound exercises. The main ones include building a lot of different muscles, burn more calories, increase in strength, and improvement of coordination, balance, and reaction. Repetition is key when it comes to building muscles. To increase muscle mass, you have to increase the number of reps you are performing with moderate weight. A good rep example is when training with moderate weights, do eight to twelve reps and when training with heavy weights, do two to four reps. The weights shouldn't be too heavy or too light. You have to be able to feel the burn with every rep you perform. Below are some tips to follow when exercising.

Performing supersets can work more than one muscle at a time. Supersets are when you perform two or more exercises in a row, making you use more muscles and providing you with the intensity of a burn. Examples of superset exercises are just any combination exercises such as dumbbell chest press and dumbbell flies. Below are some exercises that can help you build muscle in certain areas of your body.

Exercises for Chest and Back

Barbell bench press for two sets x fifteen to twenty reps

Barbell deadlift for three sets x twelve to sixteen reps

Barbell bench press for five sets x eight to twelve reps

Incline barbell bench press for four sets x eight to twelve reps

Barbell bent-over row for three sets x twelve to sixteen reps

Dips with assistance for three sets x eight to twelve reps

Dumbbell fly's for three sets x eight to twelve reps

Wide grip lat pulldown for three sets x twelve to sixteen reps

Exercises for Shoulders, Traps, and Abs

Overhead press for two sets x fifteen to twenty reps

Overhead press for four sets x ten to fifteen reps

Behind-the-Neck Press for three sets x eight to twelve reps

Crunches for five sets x ten to fifteen reps

Dumbbell side lateral raise for four sets x ten to fifteen reps

Hanging leg raise for five sets x ten to fifteen reps

Oblique crunches for four sets x ten to fifteen reps

Bent-over lateral raise for four sets x ten to fifteen reps

Dumbbell shrug for four sets x eight to twelve reps

Warmup crunch hold for three sets x ten to fifteen seconds

Lying oblique leg raise for five sets x ten to fifteen reps

Exercises for Calves and HIIT Cardio

Warmup standing calf raise for two sets x fifteen to twenty reps

Standing calf raise for four sets x ten to fifteen reps

Seated calf raise for five sets x ten to fifteen reps

Calf press on leg press for four sets x twelve to sixteen reps

Treadmill or bike for ten to sixteen minutes on medium level

Exercises for Arms

Triceps pushdown for four sets x ten to fifteen reps

Bar bicep curl for two sets x fifteen to twenty reps

Bar bicep curl for four sets x eight to twelve reps

Seated triceps dumbbell extension for four sets x eight to twelve reps

Incline dumbbell curl for four sets x eight to twelve reps

Standing triceps press for four sets x eight to twelve reps

Standing biceps cable curl for four sets x ten to fifteen reps

Standing triceps press for two sets x fifteen to twenty reps

Exercises for Legs

Warmup squats for two sets x fifteen to twenty reps

Squats for five sets x ten to fifteen reps

Leg extension for four-set x fifteen to twenty reps

Lying leg curl for four sets x fifteen to twenty reps

Lunge for four sets x ten to fifteen reps for each leg

Leg press for four sets x ten to fifteen reps

When first starting to exercising, it is important that you start off slow, don't put too much pressure all at once because you can do more harm than good. Start with a little amount if you are a beginner and then gradually increase your dumbbell weight or continue by doing more sets. If you are a pro when it comes to workout, try exploring different exercises or just by adding more sets or days to workout can make a drastic

change. Below are some frequently asked questions that beginner carnivores might have.

Another helpful tip is to manage your time and organize your diet. One of the main reasons that individuals tend not to last on a carnivore diet is because they can't withstand that variable energy levels. While most regular ketogenic dieters will experience more variation in energy levels than carnivorous dieters, you will still want to know the following tips and tricks to keep yourself bright and chipper during a diet that might not always make you feel so. When you're eating carnivorously, you will be holding your body in a maintained state of ketosis – which, for all its energy-boosting qualities, can be a tad tricky to maintain sometimes. If you accidentally eat any sort of carbohydrate sugar, you could slip up and drop out of that fat-burning state you want to be in.

Any diet that takes this much work is bound to exhaust you, but it is worth it to note that keto, in general, gets to be draining on the body after long periods of time. Many keto dieters work intermittent fasting into their low carbohydrate diets because the mechanism you trigger when you fast is the same Krebs cycle fat seeking mechanisms you use when eating meat.

Fasting for sixteen hours per day and then eating during an eight-hour window between noon and eight p.m. is one of the most common intermittent fasts that can help boost your ketone levels and energy during the day, and let your body recover and regenerate overnight. While you shouldn't necessarily fast immediately alongside your carnivore diet, plenty of fitness gurus and athletes combine a carnivore or keto diet with fasting in order to balance their energy levels.

Another great way to combat the dips in energy you might experience is with something called bulletproof coffee, which sounds a lot less appetizing than it actually is. Bulletproof, or "keto" coffee, is made with full-fat butter, natural whole coffee beans and some sort of added oil like medium-chain triglycerides (which we'll explain in a second). Butter in your coffee or tea might sound a bit off-putting, but you will barely notice anything more than a bit creamier texture.

Coffee that is packed with healthy fats first thing in the morning will help jumpstart your ketogenic mechanisms and charge your body with a fatty acid-filled Krebs cycle. If you aren't partial to coffee, you can feel free to use hot chocolate, and you should get a similar boost in energy from your fat content (although caffeine does the job a bit better). But remember, coffee is only suited for those who are starting off at level 1 Carnivore and slowly making their way up to level 3.

Medium-chain triglycerides are a common additive found in fitness and dieting communities, and it can really have an impact on how effective your ketosis is. Medium-chain triglycerides are short, easy to digest fats that are typically found in natural sources but are man-made to act as an additive. Medium-chain triglycerides support the quick recovery of muscles during and after a workout, efficient weight loss, and increased energy levels alongside a high concentration of fat.

While it isn't necessary to add medium-chain triglycerides in order to benefit from just the coffee and butter, it is always important to add as much healthy fat to your carnivore diet as possible in order to balance your high protein intake and manage your ketosis. The time-tested recommendation for higher energy levels is, of course, drinking more water, but if you drink too much, you can also begin to experience negative side effects that may lead to an energy slump.

Plenty of water tends to flush out your sodium content alongside bodily toxins, which can cause weakness, fatigue, and even fainting. Sprinkling some extra salt on your salmon every once in a while will help your body maintain its sodium levels so that you can lose weight – and if you

still feel tired, you can always purchase electrolyte boosters to help rebalance your fluids.

Below are some frequently asked questions that many newcomers have on the Carnivore Diet.

Can I Drink Alcohol?

It is recommended that you stay away from any alcoholic beverages because it will slow down the weight loss process. Your liver metabolism will change due to depleted glycogen, meaning it will break down protein and fat to form glucose and energy. This means that if you were to drink alcohol, instead of burning the protein and fat, the liver would transform the alcohol into energy, thus slowing down the weight loss process. However, there are many people who find it hard to stay away from certain beverages; thus, a lot of carnivores still manage alcohol in their system.

How Does Exercise Affect the Carnivore Diet?

When exercising, you are using up more energy than when you don't, so in order to not feel weak while exercising, you have to eat more than your usual daily dosage of meat, especially if you are planning on working out later during the day. Your fat is being used up for energy, so when your body is performing some type of exercising activity, such as raising dumbbells or doing yoga, the muscles work twice as hard and your fat is being burned twice as much as when you were not on the carnivore diet. Even if you choose to not exercise, your muscles are still going to be used more frequently in your day-to-day activities, making you appear much stronger and more toned.

Can I Have Cheat Days?

You shouldn't have cheat days. The carnivore diet should become like a habit to you. At first, it may be hard to adjust to but then it will just become easier and easier. Cravings for certain foods or beverages will stop as well as your urge to drink alcohol. If you do, however, decide to have a cheat day, don't consume foods with a high intake of carbs and don't stray too far from your diet because it might become difficult to get back up.

What If I Am Gaining Weight While on a Carnivore Diet?

If you find yourself gaining weight instead of losing it, then know that it is perfectly fine. This is your body's way of repairing itself from a broken and deranged metabolism. Before you were not getting the nutrients that you needed, so don't panic because your body is healing itself. What matters is that you stay consistent. Once the healing process is over, the weight will drop off quickly and even your appetite will shift accordingly.

Can Children Eat a Carnivore Diet?

Do not force your child to go through a carnivore diet without consulting a doctor because there is little evidence of children who grew up eating carnivore. If you force your child to a carnivore diet, they would feel all the symptoms of fatigue and keto-flu, which their under-developed guts and bodies won't be able to handle. So instead, eliminated processed foods from their diets, add a bit of meat every now and then and most importantly, consult with your doctor to check the child's health.

Did You Experience Digestive Problems?

No, you might feel a stomach ache, but it will go away the next day as long as you drink plenty of water. However, stomach pain becomes extreme and doesn't go away within two days, consult with a doctor.

What About Bowel Movement Regularity?

Many people don't have to go number two for anywhere in between two to twelve days on average since everyone's body is different. A lot of carnivores experienced even a longer period than that. Unless you find yourself experiencing smelly stole, discomfort, or pain, then you should consult a doctor.

Who Should and Should Not Follow the Carnivore Diet?

If you think or know that you have a food intolerance, then you can adopt the carnivore diet for the short-term to uncover which foods don't agree with your immune system. Follow the carnivore diet for six weeks before slowly reintroducing foods into your diet, one at a time to see what fits you and what doesn't. If you are trying to lose weight or get in shape, then this diet is for you.

Those suffering from disordered eating, chronic diseases like diabetes or heart disease should consult a doctor before attempting to follow this diet. But if you have any level of kidney disease, this diet is not for you.

The health benefits of the carnivore diet for regular individuals can't really be overstated, but there are specific medical conditions and biological predeterminations that make a meat-only diet dangerous. Although patients with type 2 diabetes can and should eat a low carbohydrate diet to manage their health, patients with the genetic form of the disease, type 1 diabetes, should never cut out carbohydrates. Type 1 diabetes differs from type 2 diabetes in that your body cannot produce insulin at all, and so you have to offer yourself intravenous injections to maintain stable blood sugar.

Diabetics who are afflicted with type 1 tend to be more at risk of falling into a hypoglycemic coma, which occurs because of an insulin shock when your levels dip too low. A diet that is high in healthy fats like a carnivore diet will already drastically reduce the amount of insulin in your bloodstream, and if you don't take the proper care to maintain your own blood sugar, your body won't be able to. Other patients who should avoid a carnivore diet are individuals with a history of disordered eating, mostly when it relates to limitation and starvation. The carnivore diet is designed to regulate your eating without limiting your nutrition, but any diet plan has the potential to trigger unhealthy habits. If you have a history of a heart condition as well, either a stroke, heart attack, or heart murmur, et cetera, you should consult with your doctor before beginning a carnivore diet.

Many people who are on 'strict' and balanced diets manage to gain weight instead, and that is because of the quality of the food, which matters strongly. Many people believe that fruits and vegetables are healthy, and although they do contain plenty of natural vitamins and minerals, unhealthy amounts of it can become very bad for the body. Since there are plenty of forced vitamins and chemicals on the food, eating so many portions of it can often put the gut under pressure from trying too hard to get rid of so many bad substances inside that it can slow down the metabolism leading to a slow rate of weight loss.

In the following chapters, we will be covering many different ways to cook meat with unique and delicious recipes that will suit your appetite. The nutritional facts mentioned with each recipe are estimated per serving unless stated otherwise.

Chapter 7: Carnivore Meal Plan

Meal preparation has been a staple in the fitness and bodybuilding communities for a long time because of its easy, helpful, and organized style. Diets can be hard to stick to if you are running around between the gym, work, home, and whatever activities you surely also do. If you find yourself hungry in the middle of the day without a proper snack, it can be a huge energy drain to go hungry while you wait for your next healthy opportunity. Preparing your meals and snacks ahead of time and packaging them up will help you better track what you are eating, how much you are eating, and when you are eating.

The idea behind meal prepping is that each weekend before you begin your workweek, you will take the time to prepare portioned out entrees for either lunch, dinner, or both that can be refrigerated and heated up for nutrition on command. Most meal preppers do their grocery shopping and cooking on Sundays to make sure that their meals are as fresh as possible for the week ahead, but you can choose Saturday as well.

When it comes to meal prepping specifically for a carnivore diet, we'll go over a few cooking tricks in the recipe section, but usually, you'll want to prepare between three and four portions of each entrée. Once you have each portion separated out evenly in Tupperware, make sure to use masking tape and a sharpie to write the date you cooked each one. Meal prepping is essentially a tool for mastering your diet organization, and keeping track of dates will help you know if a meal has gone bad or is still worth it to eat. Most of the time, cooked meats, fish, and poultry can all last in the refrigerator for up to five days.

When you meal prep for a carnivore diet, you'll be better prepared for making use of your finance than individuals who choose to eat the produce. Meats last almost twice as long in the freezer, and they tend to cost less when you buy in bulk for organic ingredients. Although matching Tupperware might seem like a waste of your money, purchasing tight-sealing glass Tupperware will actually help keep your meals fresher for longer. And, similar Tupperware makes it incredibly easy to eyeball when one of your portions is larger than the others.

Especially if you are operating on a calorie deficit to maximize your weight loss, portion control is essential to keeping your body consistent. Plus, there are few ways to actually save you time during the week ahead that can result in time spent elsewhere – meal prepping frees up all the time you would have spent cooking, to go to the gym, or visit with friends. Because your work will be clustered on a Saturday or Sunday when we likely have more than a few free hours anyway, you won't have to worry about missing a training session either on the weekend or during the week. Meal prep is also highly beneficial for those of you that want to track your macronutrients in order to make sure you're getting the right portions of fat and protein. In order to track your macronutrients, you need to meal prep each of your entrees with every portion together like one large meal.

Using a food scale and a large, dry plastic container, zero out your scale and weigh how much the entire meal prepped course weighs. If you don't already use MyFitnessPal or a similar fitness tracker, you can utilize an online calculator to enter the amount of each ingredient in the dish and the weight of the dish to estimate the calorie content, protein content, and fat content of each meal. A simple division by three or four depending on your portions, and you have effectively created your own nutritional label for a home-cooked meal.

But if you're like the rest of us, you probably don't eat every single meal at home, and you probably also noticed that there are more than four days in the workweek. Typically, meal preppers won't cook a meal for their Thursday or Friday in case they have exciting weekend plans with friends. But for a carnivore diet, it might be tricky trying to eat at a restaurant. Let's look at some of the best ways to make use of your non-meal prep days so that you can stay social while you eat carnivore.

When you aren't at home, it can be a bit more difficult to eat a healthy carnivore diet that is high in unprocessed meats and low carbohydrate dairy. However, when you're traveling or spending the holidays with non-carnivorous eaters, there are a few easy changes you can make that are similar to the switches you would make during a fancy night out. When you're traveling, one of the first things that can sabotage your weight loss isn't your breakfast foods, which can often be high in fruits, vegetables, and grains – but your lunch and dinner meals that you'll likely be eating out.

During breakfast, you can make easy egg-based switches that will account for a decent amount of your thirty-five percent protein before breakfast. Choosing items like omelets filled with natural cheeses and avoiding pastry items will fill you up on proteins that won't have you feeling hungry around mid-morning. Breakfast is also a great place to build up your healthy fats with meats like ham and bacon that are available at almost any buffet, even continental hotel spreads. Coffee is your best friend while you are away from a constant source of meat-based nutrition, and if you can't find another decent snack around lunchtime, now's the time to stock up on frozen meat snacks to keep in your hotel fridge. Turkey sausages come frozen and organically processed, so you can minimize your calorie count and still stay full while you're on the road. One of the most important skills you can develop while eating a carnivore diet is learning to pick up healthy meat and animal-sourced snacks that don't require a lot of cooking. Beef jerky is delicious and very portable and can be a great source of protein.

Just make sure to avoid any jerkies with extra seasonings beyond what you're allowed to eat. Pepperoni sticks can be great options as well, but you'll want to make sure that the nutritional labels don't indicate a high amount of unhealthy carbohydrate sugars added to enhance the taste. Prepackaged cheeses can also fit in easily accessible places and won't break your carnivore diet. When you're eating for a holiday meal at someone else's home, you'll want to make sure that you make preparations in advance. If you're eating with friends and family, most of the time, no one will argue if you offer to bring something – be it a side dish, appetizer, or entrée.

If you plan ahead and prepare your own entrees to share that will be delicious and nutritious for you, and also a kind gesture for your loved ones, you can keep with your diet and still celebrate socially. Plenty of traditional holiday recipes can be adapted to be either vegan or vegetarian, and if you can adapt a dish to have no meat, you can adapt a dish to have no vegetables. If you aren't able to bring your own dishes to a holiday meal, it's just as easy to survey your options a decided from what is available. Party platters will often be packed with cubed cheeses, skewed meats, and deli slices for eating with charcuterie boards. It might be a bit like crafting a picnic, but your creativity is essential to lasting through the holidays and long vacations if you want to keep to a carnivore diet.

That being said, don't forget about the importance of eggs for more than just breakfast. You can hard boil a protein-filled egg snack in less than twenty minutes for a boost of energy or a nicely laid out salt and pepper deviled egg plate. The options are endless if you're dedicated enough, but you won't always be dealing with holidays or vacations getting in the way of your eating; sometimes, you need a few more tips to deal with eating a meat-only diet around non-carnivore friends and restaurants.

Meat can sometimes be very expensive, so let's talk about the budget. Not everyone can afford a juice fat steak every single day and this diet appears quite pricey if you don't know the tricks to save money. Ground beef is going to be your best friend throughout this journey. It is the most inexpensive good quality meat, and not to mention it tastes delicious when cooked right. The fattiest ground beef is 75% lean and 25% fat (75/25). Research of any pasture-raised farms in your area to help you save a few bucks. The bones can be used to make bone broth for many delicious recipes. Bulk meat in Costco and Sam's club is a bit expensive but sometimes buying more expensive meat with a higher quantity can last you for weeks and will save a lot of money in the long run. You can store it in the freezer for up to months and it won't go bad. Uncooked ground meat can stay frozen for three to four months while frozen cooked meat for two to three months. Refrigerators are often not cool enough to keep the meat from going bad, so it is important that you put it in the freezer. Some meat like raw steak can even be frozen for up to a year!

However, you have to watch out for the 'use by date'. This means that products after the date indicated are it is not safe to consume. So if you are planning on buying meat and storing it for quite some time, look at the date indicated first before purchasing it, which then brings the next tip for carnivore on a budget, shop the sales. When the 'sell-by date' is approaching, many employers provide discount offers for those meats that are close to the expiration date in order to sell it faster. This is a great way to save money and you can immediately cook it up for the day. Ground beef can be stored only for one to two days after the sell-by date while beef can be stored three to five days.

Another tip is to do your research, visit your local supermarkets and compare the prices of different meats that are affordable, this way you can always save money buying meat for cheaper but before you go buying a ton of meat, try it out first to see if it's good because many supermarkets sell poor quality meat for cheaper that can often make you feel sick.

Additionally, look for coupons and sign up for a card for the supermarket of your choice in order to get groceries cheaper. If you don't have an intolerance to eggs, then that is the way to go. Take a break from always eating meat by preparing yourself scrambles or hard-boiled eggs which serve as a great light snack. They are cheap and have a lot of fat too, not to mention delicious and go with plenty of recipes.

One thing you should keep in mind is your shopping list. In your food journal, brainstorm what you are planning on making for the following week. Look at the recipes and determine how much meat you'd need for example looking at the three recipes that require chicken and adding how many pounds you'd need will determine how much you'd need to buy, this way you'd only need to make a stop at the supermarket once or two times a week. It is always a smart move to go out and buy plenty of spices and herbs, which will be used for weeks and months to go.

When living with non-carnivores, it can appear tough since they might not share the exact same viewpoints as you, but what matters is that both sides are able to open their minds to accept and understand one another. Show respect to both parties and silently acknowledge your differences, both of you have goals in your mind that you wish to achieve, instead of disrespecting each other, show love and support for one another. If the person living with you has a similar diet, you can even cook together but adding meat into your dish.

When ordering your dish in the restaurant, make sure you order foods that have plenty of meat and fat. You shouldn't worry too much about what oil it is cooked in unless you are on level 3 carnivore. However, do know that it won't affect your body that much since you've already begun your streak of only animal source foods. When going to restaurants like a steakhouse, you can request; however, you want your steak or meat to be cooked but do not stress too much about it since you will less likely be going to a restaurant every single day.

When starting off, try eating three times a day in order to know when precisely you get hungry and whether you are eating enough. Adjust this diet especially for you, don't follow someone else's carnivore diet and meat intake because it will probably not work for you, instead focus on your own body and making sure you are eating right and being healthy. There is a main rule in this diet that always applies whatever level you are on, always eat until full. It means until you think that you have eaten plenty and can't eat another bite. Don't force yourself to eat a certain amount without knowing what is your limit. On average, people eat 2-4 lbs.. a day, and many people can't eat 2 lbs.. of meat in one meal time which is why they divide it into three meals a day. Everything always depends on your metabolism, weight, height, exercise, genetics, the kind of meat or fat it is, so eat until you feel satisfied. This is a high-fat diet; therefore, fatty cuts of meat are strongly advised.

Meal preparation can take a while. It is advised that when you are cooking or preparing a meal, you make double or triple the usual amount you'd make for yourself. Especially foods that can be stored in the fridge and microwaved a couple of hours or days later, it will be easier to pick a two to three days during the week when you can prepare a few different meals that can last you for a couple of days throughout the week. It is more time-efficient if you have a tight schedule, that way you won't have to cook every single day since you'll have to cook a lot of meat. Always remember to eat until you are full, that way you won't get hungry as much. It will be hard at first, always making sure you are eating enough and saving money because meat can be quite expensive, but once you get used to it, things will only become easier.

Don't expect to lose weight straight away, although many people on the carnivore diet lost a lot of pounds during the first couple of weeks, remind yourself that each body is different. If you are moving from a keto diet, which is fairly similar to the carnivore, then it is likely you experience not a noticeable change due to the similarities of the diets. But if you are moving from an unhealthy diet filled with junk food and sugar, then it is more likely you'd drop a couple of pounds in the first two weeks. But be aware of the difference in genetics, immune systems and metabolisms in everyone's bodies, don't be disappointed if you don't lose weight straight away, your body is still adjusting.

The meal plan below is designed to help you save money and time shopping for correct foods. It is also only for beginners who are starting off the diet with Level 1 Carnivore. The recipes to all of the delicious delicacies mentioned below will be included in the following chapters!

The first week is always the hardest, but do not force yourself to eat too little or too much. This is also a perfect time to experiment, so set a specific time of the day when you will be having breakfast, lunch, and dinner and stick to it, write in your food journal so you won't forget. Record how much meat you are eating the first day, and if you find yourself getting hungry in between your meal times, then it means you are not eating enough meat. Always eat until you are full. Feel free to make yourself a small snack if you get hungry. Remember to increase your meat consumption the next day and record time and meat intake in your food journal. However, if you find yourself not feeling hungry when it's time to eat, then you might be one of the carnivores that eat only two meals a day, change up your schedule and meat intake if that is the case.

Day 1
Breakfast - scrambled eggs with bacon, make enough to be able to fill you up

Lunch - Meatloaf with ground pork, ground veal, ground beef, and bacon. Cook a large size meatloaf since the preparation time and cooking time is quite long. Save some for

Dinner - Crispy tandoori chicken drumsticks. Although you can reheat them when hungry, they taste better when fresh.

Snack - Garlic bacon wrapped chicken bites

When first starting, try not to eat too much meat at once unless you have been preparing for the transition beforehand by slowly removing certain foods from your diet. Drink plenty of water, recommended at least thirty minutes before and after mealtime. You can make more serving sizes, so when you finish eating, you still have some as a snack for later in the day, or for the next day. This way, you won't have to cook as much often.

Day 2
Breakfast - Chicken bacon meatballs can also be eaten as a light snack.

Lunch - Finish the meatloaf made from day 1.

Dinner - Poached chicken with egg, eat when fresh.

Snack - Garlic bacon wrapped chicken bites or chicken bacon meatballs from breakfast.

You can make plenty of snacks to store up so you can eat them any time you want. You can also make a high quantity of food so you won't have to cook the next day since cooking meat can be rather time-consuming. Make sure to explore with different herbs and spices. You can do that by making a large quantity of meat and adding different flavors to each individual meat that you made.

Day 3
Breakfast - Sausage egg muffins, easy and fast to make.

Lunch - Roasted leg of lamb.

Dinner - Baked lemon butter tilapia, can be reheated and used for Day 4.

Snack - Chicken and prosciutto spiedini, enough for the next day.

Day 4
Breakfast - Beef stew is soup, you can make a lot, reheat it, and use it for the next day.

Lunch - Baked lemon butter tilapia from Day 3.

Dinner - Mozzarella-stuffed turkey meatballs, make a lot to fill you up.

Snack - Chicken and prosciutto spiedini.

Day 5
Breakfast - Beef stew from Day 4.

Lunch - Meatazza (meat crust pizza), make a few large burger patty sizes, enough to fill you up.

Dinner - Marinated grilled flank steak, enough for one day.

Snack - Chicken and prosciutto spiedini.

Day 6
Breakfast - Garlic shrimp, enough for one day.

Lunch - Mexican shredded beef, enough for one day.

Dinner - Baked lemon butter tilapia, save some for the next day.

Snack - Pinchos Puerto Rico marinated grilled chicken kebabs, enough for the next day.

Day 7
Breakfast - Chicken and bacon patties

Lunch - Baked lemon butter tilapia from the previous day.

Dinner - Roasted bone marrow, enough for one day.

Snack - Pinchos Puerto Rico marinated grilled chicken kebabs from the previous day.

Chapter 8: Carnivore Breakfast

Scrambled Eggs With Bacon

This recipe requires 5 minutes of preparation time, 15 minutes to cook, and will make 4-6 servings.

Net Carbs: 2 grams

Protein: 12 grams

Fats: 16 grams

Calories: 201

Sodium: 238 milligrams

What to use

- Bacon (8 slices)
- Eggs (8 average-sized)
- Butter (2 tbsp.)
- Parmesan cheese (0.3 cups)
- Fresh chives (2 tbsp.)
- Salt (0.5 tsp.)
- Light cream (3 tbsp.)
- White pepper (0.13 tsp.)

How it's made

1. Cook the bacon. Place the bacon strips on the cold and dry frying pan, make sure the strips do not overlap. Turn on the heat and fry the bacon over medium heat, let it cook in its own grease. Do not move the bacon until it releases easily from the pan. Check the side, and if it's goldish brown, use tongs to flip the bacon to the other side. Cook the bacon until its crispy.

2. Drain the cooked bacon. Place the bacon aside on top of a paper towel to drain the excess grease. Remove ¾ of the bacon juice from the frying pan. Do not wash the pan.

3. In a wide bowl, beat the eggs, salt, cream, and white pepper.

4. Cook the eggs, Using the same frying pan, melt the butter over medium heat before adding the egg mixture. Stir the eggs with a heat-proof spatula to form large curds. Cook until eggs are almost ready.

5. Add bacon and cheese into the pan.

6. Finish by adding chives. Make sure it is chopped into small pieces before adding.

7. Serve and enjoy

Sausage Egg Muffins

This recipe requires 20 minutes of preparation time, 20 minutes to cook and will make 12 servings.

Net Carbs: 1.6 grams

Protein: 8.7 grams

Fats: 12.6 grams

Calories: 155

Sodium: 251 milligrams

What to use

- Eggs (12 average sizes)
- Pork sausage (0.5 pounds)
- Green chili peppers (4 ounces)
- One onion

- Garlic Powder (1 tsp.)
- Shredded cheddar cheese (0.5 cups)
- Salt and Pepper (optional)

How it's made

- Grease twelve muffin cups and preheat oven to 175 degrees C (350 degrees F).
- Cook the sausages.
  In a frying pan over medium heat, cook the sausages until they are evenly brown. Drain the grease by placing them over a paper towel and set aside.
- Prepare the egg mixture.
  Beat the twelve eggs in a bowl. Chop the onion and green chili peppers into small pieces. Mix the chopped onion, green chili peppers, cheddar cheese, garlic powder, the cooked sausages, and a pinch of salt and pepper into the egg mixture. If sausages are too big, chop them enough to fit the muffin cups.
- Use a cup to measure 0.25 of the egg mixtures before filling each muffin cup with it.
- Bake in the oven for 15 to 20 minutes until the egg mixture has set. Poke a toothpick into the muffins. If it comes out dry, then it's ready.
- Serve and enjoy!

Meatazza (Meat Crust Pizza)

This recipe needs 5 minutes of preparation time, 20 minutes to cook, and will make 2 servings.

Net Carbs: 1 gram

Protein: 36 grams

Fats: 26 grams

Calories: 417

What to use

- Parmesan cheese (75 g)
- Pepperoni (20 grams)
- Chicken mince (250 grams)
- HK's Keto Basil Pesto (1 tbsp.)
- Mushrooms (10 grams)
- Garlic bread seasoning (1 tsp.)
- Olive oil (1 tsp.)
- Pinch of salt and pepper

How it's made

- In a bowl, mix the chicken mince with salt, pepper, and seasoning of choice.
- Using a cold pan, coat it with olive oil. Shape the mince into a pizza base shape before putting it on the pan.
- Fry the mince on high heat until it starts to turn brown.
- When almost fully cooked, remove from pan and put on a wire rack.
- Smear the pesto on top, add cheese, mushrooms, and pepperoni or any toppings of your choice in whichever order you'd like.
- Turn the broiler setting on before putting the rack inside the oven. Bake at the highest temperature.
- Cook for ten minutes or until the cheese is melted and golden brown.
- Serve and enjoy!

Chicken and Bacon Patties

This recipe requires 10 minutes of preparation time, 20 minutes to cook, and will make 12 servings.

Net Carbs: 3 grams

Protein: 40 grams

Fats: 21 grams

Calories: 370

What to use

- Pinch of salt and pepper
- Ground chicken (1 lb..)
- Bacon (2 slices, cooked)
- Italian seasoning (2 tbsp.)
- Garlic powder (2 tsp.)
- Onion powder (2 tsp.)
- Egg (1 average size)

How it's made

- Cook the bacon, drain and chop into small pieces (refer to scrambled eggs and bacon recipe for more guidance).
- Preheat oven to 220 degrees C (425 degrees F), or you can also fry the patties on the frying pan.
- Mix all the ingredients together.
- Using your hands, shape 12 thin patties from the mixture (½ inch thick).
- Use foil over the baking tray when placing the patties on top.
- Bake for 20 minutes.
- Serve and enjoy!
- You can store in the fridge or freezer and they can be used to reheat the next day in the frying pan or microwave.

Beef Stew

This recipe requires 5 minutes of preparation time, 4-5 hours to cook, and will make 4 servings.

Net Carbs: 1 gram

Protein: 39 grams

Fats: 18 grams

Calories: 322

What to use

- Beef stew meat (1 lb..)
- Sea salt (1 tsp.)
- Bone broth (4 cups)

How it's made

- Using an instant pot or a slow cooker, add the bone broth, sea salt, and stew beef to the pot.
- If you use an instant pot, set the settings to 'meat/stew' and turn the top knob to 'stewing'.
- If you use a slow cooker, blend the same ingredients, and cook for 4-6 hours until the meat is brown.
- Serve and enjoy!

Garlic Shrimp

This recipe requires 10 minutes of preparation time, 5 minutes to cook, and will make 2 servings.

Net Carbs: 6.1 grams

Protein: 34.7 grams

Fats: 19.5 grams

Calories : 363

Sodium: 1424.4 milligrams

What to use

- Pinch of salt and pepper

- Parsley (finely chopped)
- Lemon (half)
- Chicken broth (0.25 cup / 60 ml)
- Garlic cloves (2)
- Virgin olive oil (2.5 tbsp.)
- Shrimp (300 grams / 10 oz)

How it's made

- In a bowl, place the shrimp, garlic, and olive oil (1.5 tbsp.). Use your fingers or spoon to mix gently. Set aside for exactly 20 minutes.
- Use the remaining 1 tbsp. of olive oil in a large frying pan over high heat. When you see bits of smoke emerge, add the shrimp. Shake the pan to spread out the layer, don't overlap the shrimp.
- Cook the shrimp for 1 minute, tossing and turning.
- Pour chicken broth over the shrimp. Shake the pan. The broth will bubble and sizzle. Cook for about one minute until most of the chicken broth is evaporated.
- Sprinkle a pinch of salt and pepper.
- When done, finish by sprinkling parsley and squeeze some lemon juice over the shrimp.
- Serve and enjoy!

Chicken and Bacon Meatballs

This recipe needs 15 minutes of preparation time, 30 minutes to cook, and will make 8 servings.

Net Carbs: 1 gram

Protein: 13 grams

Fats: 25 grams

Calories: 280

What to use

- Egg (1 average size, whisked)
- Onion powder (1 tbsp.)
- Ground chicken breast (1 lb.. / 450 g)
- Bacon (8 slices, cooked and crumbled)
- Cloves of garlic (2, peeled)
- Liquid smoke (2 drops)
- Olive oil (4 tbsp.)

How it's made

1) Cook the bacon until crisp and brown, drain on a paper towel, and crumble into small pieces.

2) In a big bowl, mix all the ingredients but the olive oil.

3) Using the mixture and your hands, frame 20-24 small meatballs.

4) Set the olive oil into a frying pan. With medium heat, fry the meatballs until they turn a brownish-goldish color. Flip the sides occasionally to not burn the meatball.

5) Serve and enjoy!

Carnaffles

Prep Time: 15 mins. Cooking Time: 5 mins.

Number of Servings: 4

Nutritional Values (Per Serving):

Calories 340kcal

Fat: 26.9g

Saturated Fat: 10.8g Polyunsaturated Fat: 1.3 g Monounsaturated Fat: 8.4 g Carbohydrates: 0g

Fiber: 0g

Sodium: 299.9 mg

Protein: 21.7 g

What to use

- 8oz grass-fed ground beef 5 duck eggs
- Tallow or Ghee
- Raw honey as a topping (optional)

How it's made

- In a saucepan, add the meat and cover it with water. Bring to a gentle boil, then let it simmer for about 10-15 mins or until the meat changes color.
- Strain the water and keep it as the fat of the meat will separate when cooking with water.
- Put the strained water in the freezer until the fat rises to the top, then skim the fat off and add it back to the meat.
- Heat your waffle iron.
- Transfer the meat in a blender, then add the eggs in and blend until it combines in a smooth batter.
- Use the tallow to grease your waffle iron.
- Pour enough batter for a waffle onto your iron and cook until ready.

- Repeat until you use up all the batter
- Serve plain or top with butter (high fat low lactose) or honey.

Eggs and Bacon Breakfast Meat Sandwich

Prep Time: 10 mins. Cooking Time: 10 mins.

Number of Servings: 2 sandwiches

Nutritional Values (Per Serving):

Calories: 1134 Fat: 87.5g

Saturated

Fat: 36.3g Trans Fat: 10g Carbohydrates: 0g Fiber: 0g

Sodium: 809mg Protein: 83g

What to use

- 6oz ground beef Salt
- 2 eggs
- 2oz cheddar cheese (or other high fat low lactose cheese) 1 tsp tallow or bacon grease
- 2 slices of fatty bacon

How it's made

1. In a bowl, mix the meat with 1 egg and salt to taste until well combined.
2. Form the mixture into four patties about half an inch thick each
3. Get a non-stick skillet, let it get very hot, then melt your tallow and add the patties.
4. Cook until they are well-done and brown, around 3 minutes, then flip and repeat.

5. When the patties are done, cook the bacon slices until crispy.

6. Use the same pan to incorporate all the right flavors and cook the two eggs sunny side up. If you like a moist sandwich, keep the yolk runny.

For each sandwich:

1. Using a spatula, put one patty on a dish that will serve as the bottom "bun."

2. Top with one slice of bacon, cheese, and one egg then finish with another patty.

Carni Muffins

Prep Time: 6 mins. Cooking Time: 20 mins.

Number of Servings: 12

Nutritional Values (Per Serving):

Calories: 491 Fat: 26.1g

Saturated Fat: 10.1 g Trans Fat: 1.2g
Carbohydrates: 0g Fiber: 0g

Sodium: 758mg Protein: 60.1g

What to use

- 2lbs grass-fed venison, ground

- 2lbs grass-fed venison liver, grounded

- 2 tsp salt

How it's made

1. Line a muffin tin with muffin liners.

2. Preheat your oven at 350F.

3. In a bowl, combine the two kinds of ground meat and mix until they're well incorporated.

4. Add salt to taste.

5. Divide the dough evenly among the 12 liners.

6. Bake for around 20 minutes.

Carncakes

Prep Time: 35 mins. Cooking Time: 4 mins.

Number of Servings: 8

Nutritional Values (Per Serving):

Calories: 411

Fat: 19g

Saturated Fat: 6.4g

Trans Fat: 0.4 g

Carbohydrates: 0g

Fiber: 0g

Sodium: 207 mg

Protein: 55.7 g

What to use

- 1lb free-range chicken, ground

- 10 eggs

- Ghee for the skillet

- 1 cup heavy cream for topping, whipped (optional)

How it's made

1. In a saucepan, add the meat and cover it with water. Bring to a gentle boil, then let it simmer for about 30 mins or until the meat changes color.

2. Heat a non-stick skillet until it gets very hot.

3. Transfer the meat in a blender, then add the eggs in and blend until it combines in a smooth batter.

4. Use the ghee to grease your skillet.

5. Pour enough batter for a pancake in your skillet and cook until it bubbles, then flips to the other side, about 2 minutes on each side.

6. Repeat until you use up all the batter

7. Serve plain or top with butter (high fat low lactose) and whipped cream.

Fish muffins

Prep Time: 30 mins. Cooking Time: 15 mins.

Number of Servings: 12

Nutritional Values (Per Serving):

Calories: 299

Fat: 24.4g

Saturated Fat: 13.9g

Trans Fat: 1.2g

Carbohydrates: 0g

Fiber: 0g

Sodium: 549mg

Protein: 20.3g

What to use

- 16oz cod
- 16oz salmon fillet 8oz ghee
- 1 egg
- 5oz parmesan cheese
- 2 tsp salt
- 2tsp pepper

How it's made

1. Line a muffin tin with muffin liners

2. Preheat your oven at 350F.

3. Cut the cod and salmon into tiny chunks and transfer to your food processor or blender.

4. Blend until they're well incorporated.

5. Add the cheese and egg to the mixture and mix with a spoon.

6. Add salt and pepper to taste.

7. Using a spoon, divide the dough among the liners.

8. Bake for around 15-20 minutes.

Lamb Scotch Eggs

Prep Time: 15 mins. Cooking Time: 20 mins.

Number of Servings: 6

Nutritional Values (Per Serving):

Calories: 280

Fat: 21.6g

Saturated Fat: 9.1g

Trans Fat: 0.8g

Carbohydrates: 0.1g

Fiber: 0g

Sodium: 1203 mg

Protein: 18g

What to use

- 1lb lamb sausage meat, ground
- 6 large hard-boiled eggs, peeled
- Salt to taste

How it's made

1. Preheat your oven to 350F
2. In a bowl, mix the meat with the salt and knead until thoroughly combined
3. Form 6 balls with your hands. Try to make them the same size.
4. Line a rimmed baking dish with wax paper
5. Arrange the balls on the dish and press flat. Use a rolling pin if necessary.
6. In each meat disc, place an egg.
7. Carefully wrap the meat around the eggs, making sure they are entirely covered without holes.
8. Place in the oven and bake for about 10 minutes or until the top side looks cooked.
9. Flip and bake the other side until crispy.
10. Serve hot

Meatballs Surprise

Prep Time: 5 mins. Cooking Time: 20 mins.

Number of Servings: 8

Nutritional Values (Per Serving):

Calories: 481

Fat: 25.1g

Saturated Fat: 10.3g

Trans Fat: 1g

Carbohydrates: 0g

Fiber: 0g

Sodium: 797mg

Protein: 59.1g

What to use

- 16oz grass-fed beef, ground
- 16oz grass-fed beef heart, ground
- 2 tsp salt

How it's made

1. Line a 16x16 baking dish with wax paper
2. Preheat your oven at 350F.
3. In a bowl, combine the two kinds of ground meat and mix until they're well incorporated.
4. Add salt to taste.
5. Using a scoop, take enough dough and form it into a ball by rolling it with your hands.
6. Place onto the prepared dish and repeat until you run out of dough.
7. Bake for around 20 minutes.
8. The meatballs will ooze out their juices while baking. Save

it and serve it over the warm meatballs as a "sauce."

Offal Pie

Prep Time: 5 mins. Cooking Time: 20 mins.

Number of Servings: 8

Nutritional Values (Per Serving):

Calories: 450

Fat: 17.9g

Saturated Fat: 6.8g

Trans Fat: 0.1g

Carbohydrates: 0g

Fiber: 0g

Sodium: 146mg

Protein: 64g

What to use

- 1lb goat meat, ground
- 1/2 goat lungs, ground
- 1lb goat liver, ground
- 1lb goat heart, ground
- 6 eggs
- Tallow, melted Salt

How it's made

1. Preheat your oven to 350F
2. Grease a pie dish with tallow
3. In a bowl, add all of your meats, then add the eggs. Knead thoroughly until evenly combined.
4. Season with salt
5. Combine all ingredients in a mixing bowl. Salt to taste.
6. Transfer the mixture into the pie dish
7. Bake for about 20 minutes
8. Take it out of the oven and let it slightly cool before serving.
9. It can be eaten warm or cold.

Bacon Cups

Prep Time: 5 mins. Cooking Time: 20 mins.

Number of Servings: 12

Nutritional Values (Per Serving):

Calories: 365

Fat: 32.9g

Saturated Fat: 11.3g

Trans Fat: 1g

Carbohydrates: 0g

Fiber: 0g

Sodium: 541mg

Protein: 15.3g

What to use

- 12 slices bacon
- 12 eggs
- Salt & pepper to taste
- 1/2 cup cheddar cheese, shredded

How it's made

1. Preheat your oven to 400F
2. Line a muffin tin with muffin liners
3. Arrange the bacon slices in the liners, making a circle with each one
4. Put in the oven for around 10 minutes
5. Take out of the oven and crack one egg in each muffin slot in the center of the bacon circle
6. Season with salt and pepper to taste then top with the cheese
7. Bake for another 10 minutes.
8. Serve immediately

Eggs in a Basket

Prep Time: 10 mins. Cooking Time: 25 mins.

Number of Servings: 8

Nutritional Values (Per Serving):

Calories: 388

Fat: 34.1g

Saturated Fat: 14g

Trans Fat: 0.2g

Carbohydrates: 0g

Fiber: 0g

Sodium: 472mg

Protein: 18.4g

What to use

- 2lb grass-fed beef, ground Salt
- Pepper
- 4 tbsp tallow
- 8 eggs
- 8 slices cheddar cheese 8 slices bacon, cooked

How it's made

1. Form the beef into 6 patties
2. Using a shot glass, cut a hole in the middle of each patty like a ring shape
3. Use the excess meat to form two additional patties and also cut out the centers
4. Season with salt and pepper to taste
5. Melt the tallow in a large non-stick pan over high heat
6. Place the patties in the pan and cook for two minutes
7. Flip and crack an egg in the middle of the ring
8. Season egg with salt and pepper then cover the pan and let it cook until the egg white is set, about 5 minutes
9. Remove from heat and take off the lid
10. top each basket with a cheddar slice, then replace the lid to allow the cheese to melt
11. Finish with a crispy bacon slice on top

Oat Pancakes

Prep Time: 10 mins Total Time: 20 mins

Servings per Recipe: 4

Calories 207 kcal

Fat 9.3 g

Carbohydrates 24.6g

Protein 6 g

Cholesterol 48 mg

Sodium 605 mg

What to use

- 1/2 CUP all-purpose flour
- 3/4 CUP buttermilk
- 1/2 CUP quick cooking oats
- 1 tsp vanilla extract
- 1 tbsp white sugar
- 2 tbsp vegetable oil
- 1 tsp baking powder
- 1 egg
- 1/2 tsp baking soda
- 1/2 tsp salt

How it's made

1. In a food processor, add the flour, oats, sugar, baking powder, baking soda, salt, buttermilk, vanilla, oil and egg and pulse till smooth.

2. Heat a lightly greased griddle on medium-high heat.

3. Add about 1/4 CUP of the mixture into the griddle and cook till browned from both sides.

4. Repeat with the remaining mixture.

5. Serve hot.

Buttermilk Oat Pancakes Wednesday's

Breakfast Pancakes Prep Time: 20 mins
Total Time: 50 mins

Servings per Recipe: 4

Nutritional value

Calories 548 kcal

Fat 29.5 g

Carbohydrates 57.2g

Protein 17 g

Cholesterol 163 mg

Sodium 1079 mg

What to use

- 1 Cup. whole wheat flour
- 5 1/3 tbsp cold unsalted butter 2/3 Cup. all-purpose flour
- 2 1/2 Cup. buttermilk
- 1/3 Cup. wheat germ
- 2 eggs, beaten
- 1 1/2 tsp baking powder
- 3 tbsp unsalted butter
- 1/2 tsp baking soda
- 2 tbsp brown sugar
- 1 tsp salt

How it's made

1. In a food processor, add the whole wheat flour, white flour, wheat germ, baking powder, baking soda, brown sugar and salt.

2. With a knife, cut the cold butter into small pieces into the flour-mixture and mix till a sand-like mixture form.

3. Make a well in the center of the flour mixture.

4. Add the buttermilk and eggs into the well and stir till well combined.

5. Grease a frying pan with 1 tbsp of the butter and heat on medium heat.

6. Add the desired amount of the mixture into the pan to form a 4-inch pancakes and cook till the bubbles form on the surface.

7. Flip and cook for about 2 minutes.

8. Repeat with the remaining mixture.

December's german

Prep Time: 25 mins Total Time: 45 mins

Servings per Recipe: 6

Nutritional value

Calories 283 kcal

Fat 11 g

Carbohydrates 40.7g

Protein 6.8 g

Cholesterol 62 mg

Sodium 246 mg

What to use

- 2 eggs shredded
- 2 tbsp all-purpose flour
- 1/2 CUP finely chopped onion
- 1/4 tsp baking powder
- 1/4 CUP vegetable oil
- 1/2 tsp salt
- 1/4 tsp pepper
- 6 medium potatoes

How it's made

1. In a large bowl, add the eggs, flour, baking powder, salt, and pepper and beat till well combined.

2. Stir in the potatoes and onion.

3. In a large skillet, heat oil on medium heat.

4. Add the mixture by heaping tbsps. into the skillet and press to flatten.

5. Cook for about 3 minutes per side.

6. Transfer onto a paper towel-lined plate to drain.

7. Repeat with the remaining mixture.

December's German Pancakes

Prep Time: 5 mins Total Time: 25 mins

Servings per Recipe: 4

Nutritional value

Calories 318 kcal

Fat11.9 g

Carbohydrates 43.7g

Protein 9 g

Cholestero75 mg

Sodium 1119 mg

What to use

· 1 1/2 CUP all-purpose flour cooking spray

- 3 1/2 tsp baking powder
- 1 tsp salt
- 1 tbsp white sugar
- 3 tbsp butter, melted 1 egg
- 1 1/4 CUP milk

How it's made

1. In a large bowl, sift together the flour, baking powder, salt, and sugar.

2. Add the melted butter, egg, and milk and beat till just combined.

3. Keep aside the mixture for about 5 minutes.

4. Grease a large skillet with the cooking spray and heat on medium-high heat.

5. Add about 1/4 CUP of the mixture and cook for about 2-3 minutes.

6. Flip and cook for about 1-2 minutes.

7. Repeat with the remaining mixture.

Country

Cottage Waffles Prep Time: 10 mins Total Time: 20 mins

Servings per Recipe: 1

Nutritional value

Calories 312.1

Fat 12.6g

Cholesterol 94.0mg

Sodium 540.3mg

Carbohydrates 38.6g

Protein 11.1g

What to use

- 4 tbsp unsalted butter, melted

- 1 CUP milk
- 1 3/4 CUP all-purpose flour
- 2 large eggs
- 2 tsp baking powder
- 2 1/2 tbsp honey
- 1/4 tsp baking soda
- 1/2 tsp salt
- 1 CUP cottage cheese

How it's made

- Set your waffle iron and lightly grease it.
- In a bowl, add the flour, baking powder, baking soda, and salt and mix well.
- In another bowl, add the honey, eggs, milk, and cottage cheese and beat until just combined.
- Slowly add the flour mixture and mix until just combined.
- Add the butter and stir to combine.
- Add the desired amount of the mixture to the waffle iron and cook as suggested by the manufacturer.
- Repeat with the remaining mixture.
- Enjoy warm.

Country Cottage Waffles Banana

Waffles with Extras Prep Time: 1 hr. Total Time: 1 hr.

Servings per Recipe: 1

Nutritional value

Calories 215.8

Fat 13.0g

Cholesterol 65.2mg

Sodium 130.1mg

Carbohydrates 22.0g

Protein 3.9g

What to use

- 1/2 CUP pecans, lightly toasted
- 3 tbsp sugar
- 1 1/2 CUP flour
- 1 tbsp light brown sugar
- 1/2 CUP yellow cornmeal
- 1 small banana, sliced into discs
- 1 tbsp baking powder maple syrup, warmed
- 1/4 tsp salt
- 1 1/4 CUP milk
- 3/4 CUP unsalted butter, melted 3 large eggs, separated
- 2 large ripe bananas, quartered lengthwise and chopped

How it's made

1. Set your oven to 350 degrees F before doing anything else.

2. In the bottom of a baking sheet, place the pecans in a single layer.

3. Cook in the oven for about 10 minutes.

4. Remove from the oven and keep aside to cool completely.

5. After cooling, chop the pecans roughly. And set aside.

6. In a bowl, add the cornmeal, flour, baking powder, and salt and mix well. In another bowl, add the butter, milk, and egg yolks and beat until well combined.

7. Gradually, add the butter mixture into the flour mixture until just combined. Gently fold half of the banana pieces.

8. In a glass bowl, add the egg whites and with an electric mixer, beat on medium speed until fluffy.

9. Now, beat on high speed until firm peaks form.

10. Add both sugars and beat until stiff.

11. Gently fold the whipped egg whites into the flour mixture.

Banana Waffles with Extras 25

12. Set your waffle iron and lightly grease it.

13. Add the desired amount of the mixture to the waffle iron and cook for about 6 minutes.

14. Repeat with the remaining mixture.

15. Enjoy warm with a topping of the banana slices, pecans, and maple syrup.

Sweetened Flax Waffles

Prep Time: 5 mins Total Time: 45 mins

Servings per Recipe: 1

Nutritional value

Calories 165.2

Fat 5.7g

Cholesterol 0.0mg

Sodium 238.0mg

Carbohydrates 24.4g

Protein 4.7g

What to use

- 1 1/2 CUP white flour
- 3 CUP of soy milk

- 11/2 CUP whole wheat flour
- 1 large banana, mashed
- 1/4 CUP flax seed
- 1/4 CUP canola oil
- 2 tbsp sugar
- 2 tsp vanilla extract
- 1 tbsp baking powder
- 1 tsp salt

How it's made

1. In a bowl, add the flours, flaxseed, sugar, baking powder, and salt.

2. In another bowl, add the remaining ingredients and beat until well combined.

3. Add the flour mixture and with a hand mixer, beat on a low setting well combined.

4. Heat waffle iron and spray with oil.

5. Add the desired amount of the mixture to the waffle iron and cook as suggested by the manufacturer.

6. Repeat with the remaining mixture.

7. Enjoy warm.

Victorian Waffles Yam

Prep Time: 10 mins Total Time: 40 mins

Servings per Recipe: 12

Nutritional value

Calories 141.6

Fat 4.6g

Cholesterol 31.6mg

Sodium 157.6mg

Carbohydrates 20.7g

Protein 4.8g

What to use

- 1 CUP whole wheat flour
- 1 CUP pureed cooked sweet potato
- 1 CUP all-purpose flour
- 3 tbsp oil
- 4 tsp baking powder
- 2 tsp grated orange rind
- 1/2 tsp cinnamon
- 1 tbsp granulated sugar
- 1/4 tsp clove
- 2 eggs, separated
- 1 1/2 CUP skim milk

How it's made

1. In a bowl, add the flour, spices, and baking powder.

2. In another bowl, add the oil, milk, egg yolks, orange rind, and sweet potato and beat until well combined.

3. Add the flour mixture and mix until just combined.

4. In a glass bowl, add the egg whites and, with an electric mixer, beat until soft peaks form.

5. Add the sugar and beat until stiff peaks form.

6. Gently fold the whipped egg whites into the flour mixture.

7. Add the desired amount of the mixture to the waffle iron and cook for about 5 minutes.

8. Repeat with the remaining mixture.

9. Enjoy warm.

Almond Waffles

Prep Time: 5 mins Total Time: 10 mins

Servings per Recipe: 6

Nutritional value

Calories 299.6

Fat 25.4g

Cholesterol 0.0mg

Sodium 414.4mg

Carbohydrates 15.6g

Protein 5.0g

What to use

- 1 large banana, mashed
- 1/4 tsp salt
- 1 3/4 C. soy milk
- 1/2 C. chopped almonds
- 1/2 C. vegetable oil
- 1 tbsp honey
- 2 C. gluten-free flour
- 4 tsp baking powder

How it's made

1. Set your waffle iron and lightly grease it.
2. In a bowl, add the oil, soy milk, honey, and bananas and with an electric mixer, beat until well combined.
3. Add the baking powder, flour, and salt and mix until just combined.
4. Gently fold in the almonds.
5. Set your waffle iron and lightly grease it.
6. Add 2/3 C. of the mixture to waffle iron and cook for about 5 minutes.

7. Repeat with the remaining mixture.
8. Enjoy warm.

Vegan Almond Waffles Crispy

Prep Time: 15 mins Total Time: 22 mins

Servings per Recipe: 1

Nutritional value

Calories 148.5

Fat 7.0g

Cholesterol 24.5mg

Sodium 135.8mg

Carbohydrates 17.4g

Protein 3.6g

What to use

- 2 eggs, beaten
- 1 (1/4 oz.) package yeast, dissolved in
- 1/4 C. 1 tsp saltwater
- 1 tbsp sugar
- 3 1/4 C. flour, sifted
- 1/2 C. vegetable oil
- 2 C. warm milk

How it's made

1. In a bowl, add the oil, eggs, sugar, and salt and mix well.
2. In another bowl, add the flour, yeast mixture, and warm milk and mix until well combined.

3. With a plastic wrap, cover the bowl and place it in the fridge for the whole night.

4. Set your waffle iron and lightly grease it.

5. Add the desired amount of the mixture to the waffle iron and cook as suggested by the manufacturer.

6. Repeat with the remaining mixture.

7. Enjoy warm.

Crispy Waffles

Prep Time: 30 mins Total Time: 35 mins

Servings per Recipe: 4

Nutritional value

Calories 904.4

Fat 50.3g

Cholesterol 261.5mg

Sodium 534.2mg

Carbohydrates 103.3g

Protein 12.2g

What to use

- 1 (1/4 oz.) package yeast
- 1 C. softened butter
- 1/3 C. lukewarm water
- 1 C. pearl sugar
- 1 1/2 tbsp granulated sugar
- 1/8 tsp salt
- 2C. flour
- 3 eggs

How it's made

1. In a bowl, add the sugar, yeast, salt, and water and mix until well combined.

2. Keep aside for about 13-15 minutes.

3. In another bowl, add the flour and, with a spoon, create a well in the center.

4. Add the yeast mixture in the center with your hands, knead until well combined.

5. Slowly add the eggs, 1 at a time alongside 2 tbsp of the butter, and mix well.

6. Keep aside in a warm place until dough rises in bulk.

7. Add the pearl sugar and gently stir to combine.

8. Keep aside for about 13-15 minutes.

9. Set your waffle iron and lightly grease it.

10. Add 3 tbsp of the dough to in waffle iron and cook for about 4-5 minutes.

11. Repeat with the remaining mixture.

12. Enjoy warm.

Zesty Waffles

Prep Time: 50 mins Total Time: 1 hr 5 mins

Servings per Recipe: 1

Nutritional value

Calories 308.3

Fat 11.9g

Cholesterol 131.7mg

Sodium 442.8mg

Carbohydrates 41.6g

Protein 9.5g

What to use

- 1 3/4 C. all-purpose flour, sifted
- 1 3/4 C. low-fat milk
- 2 tsp baking powder
- 1/4 C. melted butter
- 1/2 tsp baking soda
- 3 eggs, separated
- 1/4 tsp salt
- 2 tbsp icing sugar
- 1 lemon, zest, grated

How it's made

1. In a bowl, add the flour, baking soda, baking powder, and salt and mix well.

2. Now, sift the flour mixture into another bowl.

3. Add the lemon zest and mix well.

4. In another bowl, add the egg yolks, butter, and milk and beat until well combined.

5. With a spoon, create a well in the center of the flour mixture.

6. Slowly add the flour mixture to the well and mix until just blended.

7. With a plastic sheet, cover the bowl, and 8. keep aside for about 30 minutes.

9. Set your waffle iron and lightly grease it.

10. In a glass bowl, add the egg whites and beat until fluffy.

11. Slowly add the icing sugar, beating continuously until soft peaks form.

12. Gently fold the whipped egg whites into the flour mixture.

13. Add the desired amount of the mixture to the waffle iron and cook as suggested by the manufacturer.

14. Repeat with the remaining mixture.

15. Enjoy warm.

July's Zesty Waffles

Prep Time: 10 mins Total Time: 40 mins Waffles

Servings per Recipe: 6

Nutritional value

Calories 249.5

Fat 8.9g

Cholesterol 36.9mg

Sodium 301.7mg

Carbohydrates 33.7g

Protein 8.5g

What to use

- 1 large egg, beaten
- 1 1/2 tsp cinnamon
- 2 egg whites, beaten
- 1/2 tsp nutmeg
- 4 tbsp brown sugar
- 1/4 tsp ginger
- 1 C. evaporated skim milk
- 1/4 tsp clove
- 2 tbsp vegetable oil
- 1/2 C. apple, diced

- 1/2 C. pumpkin puree, canned
- 1/4 C. toasted walnuts
- 2 tsp vanilla
- 1 C. all-purpose flour
- 2 tsp baking powder
- 1/4 tsp salt

How it's made

1. Set your waffle iron and lightly grease it.

2. In a bowl, add the flour, baking powder, and salt and mix well.

3. In another bowl, add the pumpkin, sugar, oil, milk, egg, egg whites, and vanilla and beat until well combined.

4. Add the flour mixture and mix until just combined.

5. Gently fold in the walnuts and apple.

6. Add 3/4 C. of the mixture to waffle iron and cook as suggested by the manufacturer.

7. Repeat with the remaining mixture.

8. Enjoy warm.

Apple, Walnuts, and Pumpkin Waffles Florida

Duplex Waffles with Prep Time: 25 mins Total Time: 45 mins Vanilla Syrup

Servings per Recipe: 8

Nutritional value

Calories 429.2

Fat 12.5g

Cholesterol 83.4mg

Sodium 325.8mg

Carbohydrates 72.0g

Protein 8.8g

What to use

- 2C. all-purpose flour
- 1/2 C. light corn syrup
- 1 tbsp sugar
- 1/4 C. water
- 2 tsp baking powder
- 1 (5 oz.) cans evaporated milk
- 1/2 tsp salt
- 1 tsp vanilla extract
- 3 eggs, separated
- 1/2 tsp ground cinnamon
- 2 C. milk
- 1/4 C. vegetable oil Syrup
- 1 C. sugar

How it's made

1. In a bowl, add the sugar, flour, baking powder, and salt.

2. Add the oil, milk, and egg yolks and mix until just combined.

3. In a glass bowl, add the egg whites and beat until a stiff peak form.

4. Gently fold the whipped egg whites into the flour mixture.

5. Add the desired amount of the mixture to the waffle iron and cook as suggested by the manufacturer.

6. Repeat with the remaining mixture.

7. In the meantime, for the syrup: in a pot, add the corn syrup, sugar, and water over medium heat and cook until boiling.

8. Cook until the desired thickness of the syrup.

9. Remove from the heat and immediately stir in the milk, cinnamon, and vanilla.

10. Enjoy the waffles alongside the syrup.

Willie mae's

Buttermilk Waffles Prep Time: 10 mins
Total Time: 25 mins

Servings per Recipe: 4

Nutritional value

Calories 176.9

Fat 4.5g

Cholesterol 2.4mg

Sodium 700.1mg

Carbohydrates 26.8g

Protein 6.8g

What to use

3/4 C. all-purpose flour

2 egg whites

1/4 C. cornmeal

1 tbsp vanilla

1 tsp baking soda

1/2 C. wheat germ

1/2 tsp salt

1 C. buttermilk

1 tbsp canola oil

How it's made

1. Set your waffle iron and lightly grease it.

2. In a bowl, add the flour, cornmeal, baking soda, and salt and mix well.

3. In another bowl, add the oil, buttermilk, and vanilla and beat until well combined.

4. Add the flour mixture and mix until well combined.

5. In a glass bowl, add the egg whites and beat until a stiff peak form.

6. Gently fold the whipped egg whites into the flour mixture.

7. Add the desired amount of the mixture to the waffle iron and cook as suggested by the manufacturer.

8. Repeat with the remaining mixture.

9. Enjoy warm.

Burger Patties

This recipe requires 15 minutes of preparation time, 10 minutes to cook, and will make 8 servings.

Net Carbs: 9.1 grams

Protein: 21.5 grams

Fats: 17.8 grams

Calories: 288

Sodium: 196 milligrams

What to use

- Ground beef (2 pounds)
- Egg (1 average size)
- Evaporated milk (3 tbsp.)
- Worcestershire sauce (2 tbsp.)
- Garlic (2 cloves, minced)
- Cayenne Pepper (0.13 tsp.)
- Dry bread crumbs (0.75 cups)
- Burger buns (8, optional)

How it's made

1) Preheat grill on high heat.
   You can also use the frying pan, however, reduce the thickness of the patties.

2) Make the mixture.
   Using a large bowl, mix the egg, bread crumbs, ground beef, cayenne pepper, garlic, evaporated milk, and Worcestershire sauce. Using your hands, shape the mixture into hamburger patties.

3) Lightly oil the pan or the grill, fry or grill the patties until well done.

4) Serve (with burger buns) and enjoy!

Poached Chicken and Egg

This recipe needs 7 minutes of preparation time, 25 minutes to cook and will make 2 servings.

Net Carbs: 1 gram

Protein: 29 grams

Fats: 7 grams

Calories: 201

What to use

- Chicken breasts (2)
- Clove garlic (1)
- Onion slices (2 large)
- Chicken broth
- Bay leaf (1)
- Sprinkle Rosemary and parsley (optional)
- Sprinkle of salt and pepper (optional)
- Peppercorn (1 tbsp.)
- Egg (1 average size)
- Vinegar or apple cider vinegar (1-2 tbsp.)

How it's made

1) Using a shallow pan, place the chicken, any spices or herbs, garlic, onion, peppercorn, and bay leaf inside.

2) Pour in the broth, enough to cover the chicken (halfway).

3) Bring a different pot to a boil.

4) Bring to a boil, then reduce the heat. Simmer uncovered for about 5 minutes.

5) Turn off the heat and allow to rest for 15 minutes. Make sure to cover it with a lid.

6) While waiting, let the other pot simmer after it reached the boiling pot. Reduce the heat, but make sure there are still some small bubbles.

7) Pour 1-2 tbsp. Of vinegar or apple cider vinegar.
You will not be able to taste the vinegar. Make sure you do NOT add salt in the water.

8) Crack an egg over a mesh sieve, let the liquidy whites leak through over the sink or a bowl, you do not need those.

9) Stir the water inside the pot, and quickly pour the egg inside while the water is flowing around. Set a timer for three minutes.

10) Serve you and enjoy!

Mozzarella-Stuffed Turkey Meatballs

This recipe requires 35 minutes of preparation time, 35 minutes to cook, and will make 12 servings.

Net Carbs: 26 grams

Protein: 38.3 grams

Fats: 25.3 grams

Calories: 486

Sodium: 1621 milligrams

What to use

- Egg (1 average size)
- Garlic cloves (4, minced)
- Chopped onion (1 cup)
- Milk (0.25 cup)
- Salt (1 tbsp.)
- Fresh ground black pepper (2 tbsp.)
- Fresh mozzarella (2 cups, 1 lb..)
- Extra virgin olive oil (3 tbsp.)
- Marinara sauce (2 jars, 24 ounces)
- Prepared pesto (0.25 cup)
- Fresh flat-leaf parsley (0.5 cup, chopped)
- Italian style breadcrumbs (1 cup)
- Ground turkey (6 cups, 3 lbs..)
- Parmigiano Reggiano cheese (0.5 cup)
- Prepared pesto (0.25 cup)

How it's made

1) Preheat the oven to 190 degrees C (375 degrees F).

2) Cut the mozzarella into small cubes.

3) Create the meatballs.
In a large bowl, mix the onion, garlic, the egg, Parmigiano Reggiano cheese, pesto, ground turkey, bread crumbs, parsley, salt, milk, and black pepper. Gently mix until its evenly blended. Using your hands, form 1.75-inch meatballs.

4) Put the cheese in.
With your finger, make a hole inside the meatballs. Place the mozzarella cube inside, seal the meatball. Make sure the mozzarella cannot be seen. The meatball has to cover it whole.

5) Place the mozzarella meatballs on top of a nonstick baking sheet. Lightly drizzle the olive oil over the mozzarella meatballs.

6) Bake in preheated oven for 30 minutes until the meatballs are evenly brown, not pink.

7) Using a saucepan, heat the marinara sauce over low heat. Bring it to a simmer, and leave the meatballs inside the sauce for 2 minutes.

8) Serve and enjoy!

Meatloaf

This recipe requires 10 minutes of preparation time, 1 hour and 20 minutes to cook and will make 8 servings.

Net Carbs: 15 grams

Protein: 10 grams

Fats: 22 grams

Calories: 352

Sodium: 821 milligrams

What to use

Meatloaf

- Medium onion (0.5 cup, chopped)
- Ground beef (2 cups, 1 lb..)
- Bacon (6 slices)
- Ketchup (0.5 cup)
- Quick-cooking oats (0.3)
- Yellow mustard (1 tbsp.)
- Ground veal (1 cup, 0.5 lb..)
- Ground Pork (1 cup, 0.5 lb..)
- Worcestershire sauce (1 tbsp.)
- Salt and pepper (each 0.5 tsp.)

Topping

- Ketchup (0.5 cup)
- Worcestershire sauce (1 tbsp.)
- Dark brown sugar (2 tbsp.)

How it's made

- Preheat the oven to 350 degrees F (177 degrees C).

- Cook the bacon until crisp. Drain on paper towels. Make sure to reserve 1 tbsp. drippings in the frying pan. Chop the bacon into tiny pieces and set aside.

- Cook onion. Using the same frying pan with the bacon drippings, cook the onion over medium heat. Stir occasionally, until its tender.

- In a big bowl, mix the cooked onions and all the remaining ingredients except the bacon. Apply the cooking spray on the broiler rack before putting the mixture inside. Shape the mixture into a 10 x 5-inch loaf and bake for 50 minutes.

- In a smaller bowl, mix all the topping ingredients. Spread all over the top and the sides of the loaf. Sprinkle the cooked bacon over the top.

- Bake for 20-25 minutes longer. Let it stand for 5 minutes before slicing.

- Serve and enjoy!

Mexican Shredded Beef

This recipe requires 20 minutes of preparation time, 5 hours to cook and will make 12 servings.

Net Carbs: 1.9 grams

Protein: 29.51 grams

Fats: 27.82 grams

Calories: 416

What to use

- Liquid smoke (2 tbsp.)
- Bacon fat or lard (0.25 cup)
- Pinch of salt and pepper
- Chuck roast (8 cups, 4-5 lb.)
- Can diced tomatoes (1.8 cups, 15 ounces)
- Water (1 cup)
- Chipotle powder (1 tsp.) OR chili powder (1 tbsp.)
- Garlic cloves (4 minced)
- Ground cumin (1 tsp.)

How it's made

1) Preheat oven 300 degrees F (149 degrees C).
   Place an oven rack at the second-lowest position from the bottom. Sprinkle liberally the meat with salt and pepper.

2) Cook the meat.
   In a Dutch oven, use the bacon fat or lard to cook the roast over medium heat. Once warmed up, add the chuck roast. Make sure it is nice and brown on all sides before you proceed. Add water, liquid smoke, cumin, diced tomatoes, garlic, chipotle powder or chili powder. Stir gently.

3) Put the pot in the oven.
   Make sure the water is at a simmering stage before transferring it. Cook for 5 hours or until it is tender and can be poked with a fork easily.

4) When done, use two forks to tear the meat into small pieces. Use the juice at the bottom of the pot and gently pour over the roast.

5) You can also use a slow cooker or an instant pot to make this.
   Using a slow cooker, brown the meat before adding it to the crockpot. Proceed to add the rest of the ingredients. Cook on low for 8 hours.
   For an instant pot, press the sauté function to cook the roast, add the ingredients, and then press the stew/meat button. Cook for 70 minutes.

6) You can wrap it with foil and freeze for up to one month or store in a refrigerator for up to three days.

Pan-Fried Pork Tenderloin

This recipe requires 3 minutes of preparation time, 20 minutes to cook and will make 2 servings.

Net Carbs: 0 grams

Protein: 47 grams

Fats: 15 grams

Calories: 330

What to use

- Coconut oil (1 tbsp.)
- Pinch of salt and pepper for flavor
- Pork tenderloin (1 lb..)

How it's made

- Chop the pork tenderloin (1 lb..) in half, creating two equal halves.
- Prepare the frying pan on medium heat, add coconut oil.

- Place the two pork pieces on the frying pan, but only after the coconut oil is done melting.

- Cook the pork on one side. Using tongs, flip it to cook on the other side. Keep turning until the pork is nice and golden brown in color.

- Make sure to cook all the sides of the pork and give it an even color or until the meat thermometer reads 63 degrees C (145 degrees F).

- Know that the pork will still be cooking itself a bit even when you take it out of the pan, so let it sit for a few minutes before slicing it into one-inch pieces. Be careful not to cut your hands.

- Serve and enjoy!

Cheesy Wings

Prep Time: 10 mins. Cooking Time: 60 mins. Number of Servings: 4

Nutritional Values (Per Serving):

Calories: 398

Fat: 36g

Saturated Fat: 15g

Trans Fat: 1g

Carbohydrates: 0g

Fiber: 0g

Sodium: 531mg

Protein: 25g

What to use

- 2 pounds of chicken wings
- 1/4 cup parmesan grated
- 1/2 tsp salt

- 1/2 tsp ground black pepper 1/8 cup ghee

How it's made

1. Preheat your oven to 350F

2. Prepare a baking sheet by lining it with wax paper.

3. In a wide microwave-safe bowl, melt the ghee.

4. In a separate bowl, mix the parmesan cheese, the salt, and the pepper.

5. Dip each wing in the fat and then in the cheese mix bowl until they're well-covered.

6. Set on the baking sheet and repeat until you have done the same to all wings.

7. Bake until they're nicely crispy, about an hour.

8. Serve warm.

Grilled Shrimp

Prep Time: 20 mins. Cooking Time: 5 mins.

Number of Servings: 2

Nutritional Values (Per Serving):

Calories: 341 Fat: 27g Saturated Fat: 3g Sodium 1354mg Trans Fat: 0g

Carbohydrates: 2g Fiber: 1.5g

What to use

- 1/2lb jumbo shrimp, deveined and peeled
- Salt and pepper for seasoning
- 1/2 cup ghee

How it's made

1. Season the shrimp with salt
2. Combine all other ingredients in a bowl
3. Leave the shrimp in the mixture to marinate. It needs at least one hour but is better overnight
4. Turn on your grill and bring it to medium-high heat
5. Thread skewers through the shrimp and place on grill.
6. Turn on your grill and bring it to medium-high heat.
7. Grill for about 3-5 mins until no longer pink, flipping halfway through.

Lengua Carnitas

Prep Time: 5 mins. Cooking Time: 8 hours.

Number of Servings: 8

Nutritional Values (Per Serving):

Calories: 253 Fat: 18g Saturated Fat: 8g Trans Fat: 1g

Carbohydrates: 0g Fiber: 0g

Sodium: 78mg Protein: 17g

What to use

- 2lbs Grass-fed beef tongue (1 tongue)
- Sea Salt

How it's made

1. Heavily season the tongue with salt and place in a crockpot.
2. Cover the tongue with water.
3. Set the heat on low and let the tongue cook for about 8 hours or until the tongue is tender. You should be able to poke through it easily.
4. Save the broth for later.
5. Let the tongue to cool.
6. When the tongue is cool enough to handle, slit the skin a little with sears or a knife, then begin peeling it off with your hands.
7. Using two forks, scrape on the tongue's surface, so it shreds and starts looking like pulled meat.
8. Use the desired amount of broth as a sauce and to keep the meat moist.
9. Enjoy!

Sea Bass in Paper

Prep Time: 15 mins. Cooking Time: 15 mins.

Number of Servings: 4

Nutritional Values (Per Serving):

Calories: 324

Fat: 9g

Saturated Fat: 3g

Trans Fat: 0g

Carbohydrates: 27g

Fiber: 0g

Sodium: 560mg

Protein: 56g

Protein: 38g

What to use

- 2lb sea bass, filleted
- Salt
- Pepper
- 2 tablespoon grass-fed butter

How it's made

1. Preheat your oven to 350F
2. Line a baking dish with wax paper and place the sea bass, skin side down on it
3. Season the fillets with salt and pepper to taste
4. Make sure the fillets are a little lower than the center of the paper, then add a tbsp of butter to each
5. Lightly water the edges of the paper fold into a packet
6. Bake for 10-15 minutes.
7. Serve hot.

Oxtail Stew

Prep Time: 20 mins. Cooking Time: 60 mins.

Number of Servings: 6

Nutritional Values (Per Serving):

Calories: 391

Fat: 24g

Saturated Fat: 8.5g

Trans Fat: 0.9g

Carbohydrates: 0g

Fiber: 0g

Sodium: 235mg

What to use

- 3-4lbs oxtail Salt
- Pepper
- ½ pint beef broth
- 4 tbsp lard or other animal fat of your preference

You will also need a pressure cooker

How it's made

1. In a skillet over high heat, place the oxtail, 4 tbsps. of lard, salt, and pepper to taste
2. Sauté for 3 minutes on either side or until it becomes golden brown.
3. Place the meat in a pressure cooker and set it over medium-high heat.
4. Add the broth and close the lid.
5. Turn the valve to the proper pressure indicator and let the meat simmer on low heat for 60 minutes.
6. Serve with pepper, salt, and lard.

Pasta

Prep Time: 30 mins. Cooking Time: 2 hours.

Number of Servings: 4

Nutritional Values (Per 1 Cup):

Calories: 177

Fat: 8.3g

Saturated Fat: 4.1g

Trans Fat: 0.3g

Carbohydrates: 0g

Fiber: 0g

Sodium: 827mg

Protein: 17g

What to use

- 1 beef shank, cleaned and cut into pieces 1 beef belly, cleaned and cut into pieces
- Water
- 1 tbsp Tallow
- Salt and pepper to taste

How it's made

1. It's better if you ask your butcher to clean and cut the shank and belly, but if you have experience with it, you may also do this yourself.

2. Wash the meat thoroughly and place in a pot

3. Pour in water until it covers the beef halfway.

4. Add the tallow and bring it to a boil, letting it cook for about an hour.

5. Remove from heat

6. Using a skimming spoon, remove the pieces of meat and let them cool. Leave the broth in the pot.

7. When the meat cools enough to handle, pull it off the bones and then cut all parts into small pieces

8. Place back into the pot and season with salt and pepper to taste.

9. Cover the pot with a lid and boil for another hour.

10. Serve hot with more tallow if you like.

Turkish Kokoreç

Prep Time: 60 minutes + 90 minutes hands off Cooking Time: 2 hrs. 30 minutes.

Nutritional Values (Per Serving):

Calories: 490

Fat: 24g

Saturated Fat: 11g

Trans Fat: 1g

Carbohydrates: 0g

Fiber: 0g

Sodium: 242mg

Protein: 61g

Number of Servings: 8

what to use

- 4lbs lamb intestines thoroughly cleaned Salt
- 1 lamb caul fat
- 1 lamb pluck including sweetbreads
- Pepper

You will also need

- A 12x16 baking tray fitted with a rack
- Two 12" steel skewers

How it's made

1. Wash intestines thoroughly inside and out.

2. In a large bowl, add 2oz of water and 2 tbsp of salt.

3. Let the intestines soak for 10 minutes, then rinse

4. Drain and discard water, then place intestines in a bowl and let it chill in the refrigerator for about 2 hours.

5. In a separate bowl, add the caul fat and rinse thoroughly using warm water.

6. Let pluck soak in the water for 30 minutes.

7. Drain and set aside.

8. While the caul fat soaks, wash the lamb pluck thoroughly

9. Chop into small pieces around 2" thick

10. Place in a bowl and sprinkle with pepper.

11. Do not add salt yet as it will toughen the meat.

12. Let it marinate for 1 hour.

13. Preheat the oven to 390F on the Fan setting.

14. Take one skewer and begin threading the pluck in the following order lungs, heart, liver, sweetbreads. Keep going in the same order until you're out.

15. Season with salt and pepper to taste.

16. Take the caul fat and cat a large enough piece to cover the whole skewer and nicely wrap it around the meats.

17. Begin wrapping the intestines around the meat. Cover the whole skewer and tie it up at the edge of the skewer. The process is quite time-consuming and will need a lot of intestines!

18. Using wax paper, wrap the skewer, then cover again with tin foil

19. Transfer to the tray

20. Roast for 2 hours, then remove the tin foil and paper.

21. Roast again until golden, approximately 30 minutes.

22. Serve hot, seasoned with salt and pepper to taste.

Greek Magiritsa

Prep Time: 25 mins. Cooking Time: 5 mins.

Number of Servings: 8

Nutritional Values (Per Serving):

Calories: 300

Fat: 12g

Saturated Fat: 4g

Trans Fat: 0g

Carbohydrates: 0g

Fiber: 0g

Sodium: 712mg

Protein: 26g

What to use

● 2lbs lamb pluck cleaned 1/2lb lamb intestines, cleaned Salt

● 1 tbsp black pepper

● 4-5 tablespoons tallow

● 2 pints water

● 1 pint+ 2 fl oz beef broth

For the egg finish:

● 2 eggs

● salt pepper

How it's made

- Fill a pot with water and set over high heat.

- Bring to a boil, then add the lamb pluck, intestines, salt, and pepper.

- Let it boil for about 15 minutes, skimming the foam off the top often.

- Drain the water and discard it. Let the meats cool.

- When cooled, finely chop them into small pieces.

- Return the pot to high heat and add the tallow.

- Add the meats to the pot and sauté for 8-10 minutes.

- Deglaze with the 2fl oz of broth, then add the rest of the broth and the water. Cover the pot with a lid and let it boil over medium heat for about an hour.

For the egg finish:

- In a bowl, add the eggs, salt, and pepper and whisk until the egg froths slightly.

- Slowly add 5-6 ladlesful of the hot stock, whisking continuously, so the egg doesn't cook.

- When you feel the bowl becoming warm, add the mixture to the pot.

- Shake the pot so that it distributes evenly and remove from the heat.

- Season with salt and pepper to taste.

Serve with tallow and black pepper.

Pork Belly Fry

Prep Time: 30 mins. Cooking Time: 10 mins.

Number of Servings: 6

Nutritional Values (Per Serving):

Calories: 756 Fat: 47.1g

Carbohydrates:0g

Fiber: 0g

Sodium: 2458mg

Protein: 69.g

What to use

- 2lb pork belly, boneless

- 2-3 tablespoons lard Salt

- Pepper

- 1-2 tsp beef or chicken broth

Directions:

- Cut the pork belly into small ¼ inch cubes.

- Place the meat in a bowl and add the lard, salt, and pepper.

- Mix well to coat the pieces evenly and set aside to marinate

- Place a large skillet over high heat and leave it to get very hot.

- Add the pork belly to the skillet and let it cook until it is crispy and golden, about 3 minutes on each side.

- Don't stir much to ensure the meat cooks properly and doesn't boil.

- Deglaze with 1-2tsp of broth and mix.

- If your skillet isn't big enough, you can do this in two batches.

- Serve with salt and pepper to taste on their own or on <u>carnivore "bread"</u> pieces.

Rotisserie chicken

A very quick and easy meal to prepare and then cook on the barbecue. You can either serve it as the main part of the meal or as a starter.

Prep: 15 mins Cook: 1 hr 30 mins Total: 1 hr 45 mins

Servings: 6

Nutritional value

Calories: 155

Total fat: 10.9 g

Cholesterol: 50.2 mg

Sodium: 518.8 mg

Total carbs: 2.7 g

Dietary fiber: 0 g

Sugar: 1.8 g

Protein: 11.8 g

What to use

- 1.36 Kg Whole Chicken
- 57gram Butter (Melted)
- 1 Tablespoon Salt
- 1 Tablespoon Paprika
- ¼ Tablespoon Ground Black Pepper

How it's made

1. Season the inside of the chicken using a pinch of salt. Then spear it with the rotisserie skewer before then placing it on your preheated barbecue. Make sure that the heat is as hot as possible, and then allow the chicken to cook for 10 minutes.

2. Whilst the chicken is cooking in a bowl, mix together the melted butter, salt, paprika, and pepper. Once the mixture is ready and the 10 minutes have elapsed, reduce the heat and baste the chicken with the mixture you have just prepared.

3. Once all the chicken has been basted, you can close the lid and cook the chicken for 1 to 1 ½ hour. Whilst it is cooking, don't forget to regularly baste it with the mixture, as this will help to prevent the meat from drying out. You know when the meat is ready when the juices run clear after inserting a skewer into the thickest part of the chicken body or when you insert a meat thermometer, the internal temperature of the chicken has reached 180 degrees Fahrenheit.

4. After the meat has cooked, you now remove it from the barbecue and allow it to rest for 10 to 15 minutes before then carving it up and serving. Whilst it is resting, make sure that you keep the meat covered up.

Shish taouk grilled chicken

Bored with your chicken kebabs always tasting the same, then give this particular recipe a whirl.

Prep: 30 mins Cook:10 mins Additional: 4 hrs. Total: 4 hrs. 40 mins

Servings: 6

Nutrition Facts

Calories 299

protein 34.3g

Carbohydrates 9.8g 3%

fat 13.4g 21%

What to use

- Onions (Cut Into Large Chunks)
- 907gram Chicken Breast (Cut Into 2 Inch Pieces)
- 60ml Fresh Lemon Juice
- 1 Large Green Bell Pepper (Cut Into Large Chunks And Seeds Removed)
- 180ml Plain Yogurt
- 60ml Vegetable Oil
- Teaspoons Tomato Paste
- Cloves Garlic (Minced)
- 229gram Freshly Chopped Flat Leaf Parsley
- 1 Teaspoon Dried Oregano
- 1 ½ Teaspoons Salt
- ¼ Teaspoon Ground All Spice
- ¼ Teaspoon Ground Black Pepper
- ¼ Teaspoon Ground Cardamom
- ¼ Teaspoon Ground Cinnamon

How it's made

1. In a bowl, whisk together the oil, lemon juice, garlic, yogurt, tomato paste, allspice, oregano, cardamom, cinnamon, pepper, oregano, and salt. Then add the chicken and toss it through the mixture to make sure that all pieces are well coated. Then transfer to a large plastic bag (resealable kind is best) and place it in the refrigerator for 4 hours.

2. Whilst you are threading the chicken, onions, and bell pepper on to skewers, start up the barbecue, so it has reached the required temperature to cook these chicken kebabs. It is important that you cook the chicken over medium to high heat for 5 minutes on each side. The

exterior of the meat should be golden in color, whilst when you make insertion into the meat, it should look white inside. Once they have been cooked through properly, remove kebabs from heat, then sprinkle over some of the flat-leaf parsley before serving.

Grilled butter chicken

This particular recipe originally comes from India and is best made using a whole, which you or your butcher then cut up into pieces. The spices really help to make this dish much more flavorsome.

Prep Time: 15 minutes Cook Time: 20 minutes Total Time: 35 minutes

Servings: 8

Nutritional value

386 calories

Total Fat 6.6 g

Total Carbohydrate 15.5 g

Protein 25.5 g

What to use

- 1.3 to 1.8 kg Whole Chicken (Cut Into Quarters And Skin Removed)
- 114gram of Pureed Onion
- 120ml Plain Yogurt
- 120ml Melted Butter or Clarified Butter (Ghee)
- 4 to 5 cloves of Garlic (Minced)
- 1 Serrano Chili (Seeds Removed And Minced)
- ½ Tablespoons Ground Ginger
- 1 Tablespoon Ground Coriander Seeds

- 1 Tablespoon Oil
- 1 ½ Teaspoons Salt

How it's made

1. Combine together the onion, yogurt, garlic, chili, ginger, coriander, oil, and salt in a bowl. When combined together thoroughly now pour of the chicken pieces that have been placed in a shallow glass bowl. Now cover the chicken and allow it to marinate in the sauce for between 8 and 12 hours.

2. Next, remove the chicken from the refrigerator and let it stand for 20 to 30 minutes. Whilst this is happening, take half of the butter and melt it in a saucepan and let it cook for 3 to 5 minutes.

3. Whilst the chicken is coming back up to room temperature, turn on the barbecue so that you are able to then grill the meat on it at a medium to high heat. Make sure that the grill on which you place the meat has been lightly oiled first, and then cook each piece of chicken for 25 to 30 minutes. You must make sure that you turn the chicken over regularly and baste it with the melted butter often; once the chicken has cooked through, remove from the grill. Now place on to a clean plate and pour over the rest of the butter.

Blackened chicken

This particular recipe packs quite a punch. You will find that there is not only enough sauce for basting the chicken as it cooks but also to use as a dipping sauce as well.

Prep: 10 mins Cook: 10 mins Total: 20 mins

Servings: 2

135 calories

protein 24.7g

carbohydrates 0.9g

at 3g

What to use

- 4 Boneless And Skinless Chicken Breasts Halved
- 1 Tablespoon Paprika
- 4 Teaspoons Sugar (Divided)
- 1 ½ Teaspoons Salt
- 1 Teaspoon Garlic Powder
- 1 Teaspoon Dried Thyme
- 1 Teaspoon Lemon Pepper Seasoning
- Teaspoon Cayenne Pepper
- 1½ Teaspoons Pepper (Divided)
- 320ml Mayonnaise
- 2 Tablespoons Water
- 2 Tablespoons Cider Vinegar

How it's made

1. In a small bowl, place the paprika, 1 teaspoon sugar, 1 teaspoon salt, the garlic powder, lemon pepper, thyme, cayenne pepper, and ½ to 1 teaspoon of pepper. Mix well together, then sprinkle over all sides of the chicken and set the meat to one side.

2. In another bowl, you place the mayonnaise, water, vinegar, and the rest of the sugar, salt, and pepper. Once all ingredients have been combined together, you put around 240ml of this to one side, which you place in the refrigerator to chill. The rest of the mixture is what you will be basting the chicken in.

3. To cook the chicken, place over indirect medium heat on the barbecue. Remember to oil the grill first to ensure that the chicken doesn't stick to it, then cook on each side for 4 to 6 minutes or until the juices that are released by the chicken as it cooks run clear. Don't forget, as you are cooking the chicken on the grill to baste it regularly with the sauce made using the mayonnaise. After cooking, serve with the sauce in the refrigerator.

Grilled herb chicken burgers

As well as these burgers being low in fat, they also taste extremely delicious. You will know if the burgers aren't cooked properly because they will be soft to the touch.

Total: 30 mins Prep: 15 mins Cook:15 mins

Servings:4 servings

Nutritional value:

Calories: 547kcal

Carbohydrates: 30g

Protein: 29g

Fat: 34g

What to use

- 450gram Ground Chicken Breast
- 1 Small Carrot (Grated)
- 2 Green Onions (Minced)
- Cloves Garlic (Minced)
- 1 Teaspoon Dried Parsley
- 1 Teaspoon Dried Basil
- ¼ Teaspoon Salt
- ¼ Teaspoon Freshly Ground Black Pepper

How it's made

1. Into a large mixing bowl, put the ground chicken meat, the carrot, onions, garlic, herbs, salt, and pepper. Mix thoroughly together. It is best if you use your hands to do this. Whilst you are mixing these ingredients together, then you should have the barbecue turned on, or you should have lit the charcoal. So by the time the burgers are made, you can then start cooking them.

2. After mixing the ingredients together, you should take between 4 and 6 burgers from it. Before you cook them, however, place them on a sheet of wax paper and let them rest in the refrigerator for a few minutes.

3. Once the barbecue has heated up; you must first lightly oil the grill before then placing the burgers on to it. To make sure that the chicken is cooked properly, they should remain on the grill for between 12 and 15 minutes. It is important that during this time, you turn them over at least once. You will know when they are cooked through, as the juices running out of them will run clear.

Grilled chicken wing with sweet red chili & peach glaze

The adding of the peaches into the marinade helps to counteract some of the heat from the chilies.

PREP TIME: 15m COOK TIME: 30m

YIELD: 2

Nutritional value

Calories 770

Fat 37g

Carbohydrate 65g

Protein 42g

What to use

- 1.13Kg Chicken Wings
- 350ml Jar Of Peach Jam
- 240ml Thai Sweet Red Chili Sauce
- 1 Teaspoon Fresh Lime Juice
- 1 Tablespoon Fresh Cilantro (Minced)

How it's made

1. In a bowl, mix together the peach jam, the chili sauce, the lime juice, and cilantro. Take half of this mixture and pour it into a bowl, as you will use this as a dipping sauce to serve with the cooked chicken wings.

2. After your barbecue has reached the right temperature, and you have sprayed the grill with oil to prevent the chicken wings from sticking, place them on it. Grill the wings for between 20 and 25 minutes, remembering to turn them over frequently to ensure that they are cooked through evenly.

3. Only when the juices are running clear from the chickens, can you then apply the remaining half of the sauce to glaze them. After applying the glaze, make sure that you cook them for a further 3 to 5 minutes. Again you need to turn them over once during this time to make sure that they are well coated with the glaze.

Grilled chicken koftas

You can either eat these by themselves, or you can use them as a filling for a sandwich or in pitta bread. If you are going to put them into pitta bread, then warm the bread through first by placing it on the edge of the barbecue away from the direct heat source for a minute, turning them over after 30 seconds.

Prep: 15 Minutes - Cook: 10 Minutes

Serves: 4

Nutritional value

Calories 273

Fat 9.3g

Protein 40.8g

Carbohydrate 4.7g

What to use

- 450gram Ground Chicken Breast
- 229gram Bread Crumbs
- 1 Egg (Lightly Beaten)
- 2 Cloves Garlic (Minced)
- 1 Tablespoon Cilantro (Finely Chopped)
- 1 Teaspoon Hot Sauce
- 1 Teaspoon Salt
- ¼ Teaspoon Freshly Ground Black Pepper

How it's made

1. In a large mixing bowl, combine together the ground chicken breast, bread crumbs, egg, garlic, cilantro, hot sauce, salt, and pepper. Then cover and allow to rest in the refrigerator as this will make it much easier to then form the Koftas (sausage shape patties), which you form around a metal skewer.

2. As soon as you have formed the Koftas around the skewer, they are now ready to cook. Place them about 3 inches above the barbecue and allow them to cook for around 10 minutes. During this time,

make sure that you turn them frequently to ensure that they don't burn and that the meat cooks evenly. As soon as they are cooked, you can then serve them.

Thai grilled chicken with a chili dipping sauce

You will find this recipe quite refreshing, and the dipping sauce really adds a new element to the whole dish.

Prep: 15 mins   **Cook:** 30 mins

Servings: 4

Nutritional value

332 calories

protein 24.4g

carbohydrates 16.1g

fat 19g

What to use

- 1.36Kg Chicken Breast (Cut Into Pieces)
- 120ml Coconut Milk
- Tablespoons Fish Sauce
- Tablespoons Garlic (Minced)
- Tablespoons Fresh Chopped Cilantro
- 1 Teaspoon Ground Turmeric
- 1 Teaspoon Curry Powder
- ½ Teaspoon White Pepper

Dipping Sauce

- 6 Tablespoons Rice Vinegar
- 4 Tablespoons Water
- 4 Tablespoons Sugar
- ½ Teaspoon Minced Birds Eye Chilli
- 1 Teaspoon Garlic (Minced)
- ¼ Teaspoon Salt

How it's made

1. In a shallow dish, mix the coconut milk, fish sauce, garlic, cilantro, turmeric, curry powder, and white pepper. Then when thoroughly combined, add the chicken pieces and turn them over in the sauce so that they are completely coated. Cover and place in the refrigerator for 4 hours or overnight to let the chicken pieces marinate in the sauce.

2. Whilst the chicken is marinating, you can now make the sauce. To do this, you place the vinegar, water, sugar, garlic, chili, and salt into a saucepan and bring this mixture to a boil. Now lower the heat and let the mixture simmer for about 5 minutes. It is important you stir the sauce from time to time to prevent it from sticking to the base of the saucepan and burning. Remove from heat and allow it to cool before placing it into a serving bowl.

3. When cooking the chicken on the barbecue, make sure that the grill has been lightly oiled first. Cook each piece of chicken for 10 minutes on each side or until the juices start to run out of them clearly. Brush them with a little of the sauce you made earlier before serving, whilst the rest remains in the serving dish and which people can then dip the chicken wings into if they wish.

Catalan chicken quarters

This is a Spanish-inspired recipe where not only does the smoke help to enhance the flavor of the chicken, so does the thick tomato sauce.

Prep Time:15 - 25 minutes Cook Time: 45 - 55 minutes

Servings: 4

Nutritional value

Calories 273

Fat 9.3g

Protein 40.8g

Carbohydrate 4.7g

What to use

- 4 Chicken Leg Quarters
- 1 Onion (Chopped)
- 172gram Chorizo (Spicy Sausage Chopped)
- 1 Can Whole Tomatoes (Drained And Chopped)
- 120ml Red Wine
- 114gram Olives (Pitted And Chopped)
- 5 Cloves Of Garlic (Minced)
- Tablespoons Olive Oil
- 1 Teaspoon Salt
- ½ Teaspoon Cumin
- ½ Teaspoon Cinnamon
- ¼ Teaspoon Cayenne Pepper
- ¼ Teaspoon Freshly Ground Black Pepper

How it's made

1. In a bowl, combine together the salt, cumin, black pepper, and cayenne pepper and rub over the surface of the chicken, making sure you get as much of this rub under the skin of the chicken as well.

2. Allow the chicken to rest in the refrigerator for a while (covered) whilst you start preparing the sauce to go with them. To make the sauce sauté the onions and garlic in the olive oil before adding the sausage, tomatoes, and red wine. Allow this to simmer on low heat whilst you are then cooking the chicken quarters on the barbecue. You should cook the chicken quarters until the juice runs clear from them, remembering to turn them over often to prevent the skin from burning.

3. Whilst the chicken is cooking, you should now add the olives to the sauce and continue simmering it for a further 20 minutes.

4. To serve, simply place one of the chicken quarters on to a plate and then pour over some of the sauce.

Thai chicken satay

Unfortunately, this is a recipe you shouldn't be trying if you or someone you know is allergic to peanuts.

PREP TIME: 15 MINUTES COOK TIME: 10 MINUTES TOTAL TIME: 25 MINUTES

SERVINGS: 4

Nutritional value

Calories 526

Fat 28g

Carbohydrates 25g

Protein 47g

What to use

- 907gram Chicken Breasts Without The Skin (Cut Into Strips)
- 2 Tablespoons Vegetable Oil
- 2 Tablespoons Soy Sauce
- 2 Teaspoons Tamarind Paste
- 2 Stalk Lemon Grass (Chopped)
- 1 Cloves Garlic (Crushed)
- 1 Teaspoon Ground Cumin
- 1 Teaspoon Ground Coriander
- 1 Tablespoon Fresh Lime Juice
- Teaspoon Muscovado Sugar
- ½ Teaspoon Chili Powder

Sauce

- 1 Tablespoon Peanut Butter (Crunchy)
- 2 Tablespoons Peanuts (Chopped)
- 1 Can Coconut Milk
- 1 Teaspoon Red Thai Curry Paste
- 1 Tablespoon Fish Sauce
- 1 Teaspoon Tomato Paste
- 1 Tablespoon Brown Sugar

How it's made

o You first need to make up the sauce in which the chicken pieces will be marinated. To do it, get a large bowl and into place the vegetable oil, soy sauce, tamarind paste, lemongrass, garlic, cumin, coriander, lime juice, sugar, and chili powder. Make sure that you combine these ingredients well before adding the chicken and stir around until you know all the chicken pieces have been coated in the marinade. Cover the bowl and place in the refrigerator for one hour.

o Whilst the chicken is marinating, and you can make the satay (peanut) sauce. To do this into a small saucepan, put the peanut butter, peanuts, coconut milk, red Thai curry paste, fish sauce, tomato paste, and sugar. Cook the ingredients on medium to low heat, making sure that you stir it frequently and until it looks smooth. It is important that you keep the sauce warm after it has been made, so turn the heat down as low as possible and cover.

o To cook the chicken pieces, you first need to thread them onto skewers, and when this is turn place them on to the lightly oiled barbecue grill and allow them to cook on each side for around 3 to 5 minutes. Once the chicken is thoroughly cooked, remove from the heat and either pour the satay sauce over them or provide it in a bowl in which guests can then dip their chicken kebabs if they wish.

Barbecue chicken breasts

You will find that this particular recipe becomes one that you will use time and time again. When cooked correctly, the exterior of the chicken becomes crispy whilst the interior remains moist.

PREP TIME: 5 MINUTES COOK TIME: 7 HOURS TOTAL TIME: 7 HOURS 5 MINUTES

SERVINGS: 4 -6

Nutritional value:

Calories 443.02

Fat 6.55g

Carbohydrates 43.73g

Protein 49.03g

What to use

- 4 x 250gram Skinless Chicken Breasts
- Zest Of 1 Orange
- 1 Dried Chili
- 1 ½ Teaspoon (Heaped) Smoked Paprika
- 1 ½ Teaspoons Dijon or English Mustard
- Tablespoons Honey
- Tablespoons Tomato Ketchup
- 1 Teaspoon Olive Oil
- 1/16 Teaspoon Sea Salt
- Freshly Ground Black Pepper To Taste

How it's made

1. Into a bowl, put the finely grated zest of the orange, along with the dried chili (crumbled), the paprika, mustard, honey, tomato ketchup, and the olive oil. Then, after combining all these ingredients together, add a pinch of salt along with some pepper then stir again.

2. Take out a couple of spoonful of the mixture made and put to one side. To the rest of the marinade in the bowl, you add the chicken breasts. Turn them over so that they are completed coated by the marinade made and cover with plastic wrap before leaving to one side for 5 to 10 minutes.

3. Once the barbecue has heated up correctly, you need to put the chicken on the grill, but before you do, make sure that you lightly oil it. When you place them on the grill, make sure that the heat underneath isn't too high. If you notice the outer part of the chicken is starting to char quickly, then move them over to a cooler part of the barbecue and reduce the heat if possible. You should be aiming to cook the chickens on each side for about 5 minutes, turning them every minute and basting them with some more of the marinade left in the bowl. You should only remove them from the heat when they have turned a golden brown and are cooked all the way through.

The best way of testing to see that they are cooked all the way through is to push a skewer in to. If the juices that flow out are clear, then you know the chicken is properly cooked. Remove from heat, then place on clean plates and spoon some of the sauce that you put aside earlier over them.

Spicy plum chicken thighs

The plum sauce that coats the chicken thighs creates a slightly sweeter tasting barbecue sauce. It is important that you don't cook the thighs over too high a heat;

otherwise, this could result in the sauce burning.

Prep: 10 mins **Cook:** 25 mins
 Total: 35 mins

Servings: 4

Nutritional value

calories 333

protein 19.6g

carbohydrates 30.3g

fat 15g

What to use

- 8 Chicken Thighs (Skin On And Bone-In)
- Salt and Freshly Ground Black Pepper

Plum Sauce

- 2 Tablespoons Peanut Oil
- 1 Small Coarsely Chopped Onion
- 4 Cloves Garlic (Coarsely Chopped)
- 1 Tablespoon Fresh Coarsely Chopped Ginger
- 2 Coarsely Chopped Thai Chili
- ¼ Teaspoon Ground Cinnamon
- ¼ Teaspoon Ground Cloves
- 680gram Red or Purple Plums (Pitted and Coarsely Chopped)
- 60ml Honey
- 60ml Soy Sauce
- 1Tablespoons Fresh Lime Juice
- 1 Tablespoon Granulated Sugar

How it's made

1. Before you do anything else, you need to make the plum sauce. To do this, in a medium-size saucepan, place the oil and heat it up. When it is hot enough, add the onions and garlic and cook until they are soft. Then add to these the ginger, cinnamon, Thai chili, and cloves and cook for 2 minutes. Now you need to add the rest of the ingredients listed above and cook until the plums have softened and the sauce has started to thicken. Then place the mixture into a food processor or blender and mix them until smooth. Pour into a bowl and allow to cool.

2. After making the sauce, you need to heat the barbecue up to medium-low indirect heat for cooking the chicken thighs. Just before you place the chicken thighs on to the grill, lightly oil it first and season the thighs with salt and pepper. Cook on either side until they turn a light golden brown between 1 and 5 minutes.

3. Now brush one side of the chicken with the plum sauce made earlier and turn the thighs over and continue cooking for 3 to 4 minutes. Once this time has elapsed, brush the sides of the thighs facing you with more sauce and again turn them over to cook for another 3 to 4 minutes. You should continue turning and basting the thighs with the plum sauce until they are cooked through. You will find that they will be cooked through properly after 15 to 20 minutes. However, if you are unsure, just insert a skewer into the thickest part of the thigh. If you notice the juices running out are clear, then the chicken is cooked.

4. Please don't forget to keep the thighs at a good height above the heat to prevent them and the sauce from burning.

Maple barbecued chicken

You will find that the sweet flavor of the maple helps to really make this dish stand out and may have guests at your barbecue asking for seconds. To obtain the best results possible, use a good quality syrup. Of course, if you want to give this recipe a little kick, then add some hot chili sauce as well.

PREP TIME: 5 MINUTES COOK TIME: 7 HOURS TOTAL TIME: 7 HOURS 5 MINUTES

SERVINGS: 4 -6

Nutritional value:

Calories 443.02

Fat 6.55g

Carbohydrates 43.73g

Protein 49.03g

What to use

- 4 Skinless Chicken Thighs
- 3 Tablespoons Maple Syrup
- 3 Tablespoons Hot Chili Sauce (Optional)
- 1 Tablespoon Cider Vinegar
- 1 Tablespoon Canola Oil
- 2 Teaspoon Dijon Mustard
- Salt
- Freshly Ground Pepper

How it's made

1. Whilst the barbecue is heating up in a saucepan, combine together the maple syrup, cider vinegar, and mustard. Plus, of course, the hot chili sauce if you are looking to give this recipe an extra kick. After mixing the ingredients together, place the saucepan on medium heat and let the mixture simmer for 5 minutes.

2. Next, you need to brush the chicken with the oil before then sprinkling on some salt and pepper to season. Then place them on to the grill and cook for between 10 and 15 minutes. As you cook them, turn them regularly and each time that you turn them, brush a generous amount of the sauce over them. Once cooked, place on a clean plate and serve immediately. Any sauce leftover can either be poured over the chicken thighs or placed in a bowl, which the thighs can then be dipped into.

Spatchcock barbecue chicken

It is best if you get your butcher to cut the chicken up for doing this recipe.

Prep:20 mins Cook:1 hr.

Serves: 2 – 4

Nutritional value

Kcal 650

Fat 45g

Carbs1g

Sugars 0g

Fiber 1g

Protein 59g

What to use

- 1.3kg Spatchcock Chicken
- 3 Tablespoon Olive Oil 1 Teaspoon Paprika
- 1 Garlic Clove Crushed
- Juice and Zest Of 1 Lemon
- A Little Water or Beer to Taste
- Salt
- Freshly Ground Pepper
- 2 Lemons Quartered

How it's made

1. Whilst the barbecue is heating up in a bowl, mix together the oil, garlic, paprika, lemon zest, salt, and pepper. Once all these ingredients have been mixed together, you brush it all over the skin of the chicken before then placing it covered in the fridge for 30 minutes to allow it to marinate.

2. When it comes to cooking the chicken on the barbecue, you should cook it initially for 5 minutes on each side in the middle of the barbecue. Then move over to the side so that the heat cooking is much gentler. It is important whilst the chicken is cooking that you turn it regularly and baste in between each turn with either beer or water. The best way of determining when the chicken is cooked through is to pierce between the thigh and breast bone with a sharp knife. When you do, the flesh should feel firm and should look white.

You should be cooking each side of the chicken for between 20 and 30 minutes. Plus, place something over the top, as the steam produced will help the chicken to cook through.

3. Once the chicken has cooked, you now need to remove it from the heat and leave it to rest. Make sure that you cover it with foil and leave it to rest for around 10 to 15 minutes. Once this time has passed, cut it up into pieces and drizzle some lemon juice, oil, salt, pepper, and paprika over them. Then serve on a fresh palate with the lemon quarters.

Chicken tikka skewers

As well as being a quick and easy dish to prepare for your barbecue this summer, this particular recipe is also low in calories.

Prep Time:10 mins Cook Time:15 mins
Total Time:25 mins.

Calories 437

Fat 9g

Carbohydrates 46g

Protein 44g

What to use

- 4 Skinless Boneless Chicken Breasts Cut Into Cubes
- 150gram Low Fat Natural Yogurt
- 2 Tablespoon Hot Curry Paste
- 250gram Cherry Tomatoes
- 4 Whole meal Chapattis
- ½ Cucumber Cut In Half Lengthways, Deseeded and then Sliced
- 1 Red Onion Thinly Sliced
- Handful Coriander Leaves Chopped
- Juice 1 Lemon
- 50gram Lamb's Lettuce or Pea Shoots

How it's made

1. Place the wooden skewers (8 in all) in some water in a bowl to soak. After doing this, you need to place the yogurt and curry paste in a bowl and mix together. Then to this, you add the cubes of chicken. Make sure that you stir the chicken into the mixture well to ensure all pieces are coated. Now cover the top of the bowl and place in the refrigerator to marinate for an hour or so.

2. Next, in another bowl, place the cucumber, red onion, coriander, and lemon and toss them all together. Again

place this bowl in the refrigerator (covered over) and leave there until you are ready to serve the chicken.

3. Whilst the barbecue is heated up now, you need to start preparing the skewers. You must make sure that you shake off any excess marinade before then threading the pieces of chicken on to the skewers. After threading on a piece of chicken, now thread on a cherry tomato and do this until all skewers have been used.

4. Once the Chicken Tikka skewers are ready and the barbecue has heated up, you are now ready to start cooking. You should keep the skewers on the barbecue for between 15 and 20 minutes, making sure that you turn them regularly so that they get cooked through and become a nice brown color.

5. When it comes to serving the skewers, place them to one side on a clean plate to rest for a few minutes whilst you prepare the salad. Into the salad before serving, mix the lettuce and pea shoots and divide this equally between four plates and on top of which you then place two of the skewers. Serve them with chapattis that have been warmed through on the barbecue. The best way to warm the chapattis on the barbecue is to wrap them in some aluminum foil.

Sweet & spicy wings with summer coleslaw

Just like many other recipes in this book, this is one that is very quick and easy to make and will certainly help to add a little spice to your barbecue this summer.

Prep: 15 mins   **Cook:** 45 mins.

Serves: 4

What to use

- 1kg Chicken Wings
- 4 Tablespoon Curry Paste (Tikka would be wonderful)
- 3 Tablespoon Mango Chutney
- 200g Sliced Radishes
- 1 Cucumber Halved Lengthways And Sliced
- 1 Small Bunch Roughly Chopped Mint
- Juice Of 1 Lemon

How it's made

1. Start getting the barbecue heated up. Now in into a large bowl, place the curry paste and 2 tablespoons of the mango chutney with a little salt and pepper to season, then stir well.

2. Place the chicken wings in the mixture and toss around so that they are all well coated, and then leave to marinate for a short while.

3. Now place on to the barbecue griddle making sure that the surface has been lightly oiled first to prevent the chicken from sticking to it. Now cook for between 40 and 45 minutes, occasionally turning until all sides are golden brown and the wings are cooked through. The quickest way to determine if the wings have been cooked through is to stick a skewer into the thickest part and, when removed, do the juices run clear.

4. Finally, just before you are about to serve the chicken wings in another bowl, place the radishes, cucumber, mint, the rest of the mango chutney, and the lemon juice and stir thoroughly. Now place the chicken wings on a clean plate, and then beside it place the freshly made coleslaw.

Sticky chicken drumsticks

This isn't only a recipe that kids will enjoy eating; so will many adults, especially those with somewhat of a sweet tooth.

Prep time5 mins Cook time:e40 mins Total time: 53 mins

Nutritional value

Calories: 263

Total fat: 9g

Saturated fat: 2g

Trans fat: 0g

Unsaturated fat: 5g

Protein: 23g

What to use

- 8 Chicken Drumsticks
- 2 Tablespoon Soy Sauce
- 1 Tablespoon Honey
- 1 Tablespoon Olive Oil
- 1 Tablespoon Tomato Puree
- 1 Tablespoon Dijon Mustard

How it's made

1. You need to make 3 slashes into each chicken drumstick as this will then help the meat to absorb quite a bit of the marinade you are about to make. Then place the drumsticks into a shallow dish.

2. To make the marinade, you need to place the soy sauce, honey, olive oil, mustard, and tomato puree into a bowl and whisk together thoroughly. Once all these ingredients have been combined, pour some over the drumsticks before turning them over and pouring the remainder of the marinade over them. Once this has been done, you must place

them in the refrigerator overnight (remembering to cover them).

3. Whilst the barbecue is heating up, ready for you to cook the drumsticks, remove them from the refrigerator and allow them to come up to room temperature. When the barbecue is heated up sufficiently, you can now place the drumsticks onto the grill. Although there is oil in the marinade, don't forget to brush some over the grill to prevent the chicken drumsticks from sticking to them.

4. It is important that you cook these for around 35 minutes or until the juice inside them starts to run clear. Also, it is important to remember to turn them over regularly to prevent the exterior from becoming burnt and also to ensure that they cook right through. Once they are cooked, now place them on a clean plate and serve to your waiting guests.

Jerk chicken kebabs and mango salsa

The inclusion of mango salsa with these kebabs helps to take some of the kick out of the spices used in making the Jerk Chicken.

Prep:20 mins Cook:20 mins.

Serves: 4

Nutritional value

Kcal 263

Fat 5g

Carbs19g

Fiber 4g

Protein 37g

Jerk Chicken

- 2 Teaspoon Jerk Seasoning
- 4 Skinless Chicken Breasts Cut Into Chunks
- 1 Large Yellow Pepper Cut Into 2cm Cubes
- Juice of 1 Lime
- 1 Tablespoon Olive Oil

Mango Salsa

- 1 Large Red Pepper Deseeded and Diced
- 320g Mango Diced
- 1 Red Chili Chopped (This Is Optional)
- Bunch Spring Onions Finely Chopped

How it's made

1. In a bowl place, the jerk seasoning, olive oil, and lime juice and then mix thoroughly together. A whisk would be best to do this. Then once all these ingredients have been thoroughly combined, toss the chunks of chicken in it and place it in the refrigerator for at least 20 minutes. However, if you really want the meat to absorb as much of the marinade as possible, then it is best to leave it in the refrigerator for at least 24 hours.

2. Once the meat has time to marinade; you are now ready to start cooking it. But whilst the barbecue is heating up, you can now start making the salsa. To do this, you simply place all the ingredients mentioned above in a bowl and stir together. Add a little salt and pepper to season, then place in the refrigerator until you are ready to serve it with the kebabs.

3. To make the kebabs, you need some wooden skewers, which have been left in some water for at least 30 minutes. Remember doing this will prevent them from burning. Now on to each skewer, you thread a piece of chicken followed by a piece of the yellow pepper. You should be aiming to put on each of the 8 skewers 3 pieces of meat and 3 pieces of pepper.

4. Once the kebabs have been made and the barbecue is hot enough, you can start cooking them. Each side of the kebab should be cooked for around 8 minutes. This will not only ensure that they are cooked through but also helps to create a little charring on them once they are cooked; place two kebabs on a plate and add some salsa.

Chapter 10: Carnivore Dinner

Roasted Leg of Lamb

This recipe requires 15 minutes of preparation time, 1 hour 45 minutes to cook, and will make 12 servings.

Net Carbs: 0.4 grams

Protein: 35.8 grams

Fats: 25.3 grams

Calories: 382

Sodium: 136 milligrams

What to use

- Leg of lamb (5 lbs.)
- Garlic (4 cloves, chopped)
- Fresh rosemary (2 tbsp.)
- Pinch of black pepper
- Pinch of salt

How it's made

1) Start by preheating the oven to 175 degrees C (350 degrees F).

2) Using a knife, cut a line at the top of the lamb's leg, not too deep but enough to push slices of garlic inside the meat. Continue this every three to four inches of all five lamb legs.

3) Stuff each slice with garlicup Sprinkle salt and pepper over the top of the lamb. Sprinkle some rosemary on both the bottom and top before placing the lamb on a roasting pan.

4) Roast the lamb in the preheated oven until it is cooked to your liking. It will take around 1.75 to two hours. Be careful not to overcook the lamb since the flavor is the best when the meat is still slightly pink.

5) Let it rest for at least ten minutes before serving.

6) If you want a medium-rare roasted lamb, read the instant-read thermometer located at the center of the oven, it should read at least 57 degrees C (135 degrees F). It will still prepare itself for a while after removing it from the oven.

7) Serve and enjoy!

Garlic Butter Baked Pork Chops

This recipe requires 5 minutes of preparation time, 18 minutes to cook, and will make 2 servings.

Net Carbs: 1 gram

Protein: 14 grams

Fats: 35 grams

Calories: 371

Sodium: 478 milligrams

What to use

- Breed pork chops (2 medium-sized)
- Garlic (2 cloves, minced)
- Grass-fed butter (4 tbsp.)
- Virgin olive oil (1 tbsp.)
- Pinch of salt and ground black pepper
- Fresh thyme (1 tbsp, chopped)

How it's made

1) Begin by preheating the oven to 190 degrees C (375 degrees F).

2) In a bowl, sprinkle a pinch of salt and pepper on the pork, mix together, and set aside.

3) In a separate bowl, mix together the thyme, garlic, and butter. Set aside.

4) Using a cast-iron skillet, heat the pan over medium heat before adding olive oil.

5) When the skillet is well heated, add the pork chops. Cook until golden, about two minutes on each side.

6) Place the pork chops into a foil baking pan and pour over some of the butter mixtures, leaving at least two to three tablespoons behind.

7) Place the foil pan into the oven and cook until the oven reaches an internal temperature of 62 degrees C (145 degrees F). Cook for about ten to twelve minutes; the time strictly depends on the thickness of the pork chops.

8) After it's done cooking, take it out from the oven and, using a spoon, pour some of the remaining butter sauce over the pork.

Crispy Tandoori Chicken Drumsticks

This recipe requires 20 minutes of preparation time, 1 hour to cook, and will make 4 servings, 12 drumsticks. (Note: refrigeration of some ingredients is required but not included in the meal preparation time, read direction for more information)

Net Carbs: 8 grams

Protein: 73 grams

Fats: 53 grams

Calories: 807

Sodium: 1184 milligrams

What to use

- Ground cumin (1 tbsp.)
- Ground turmeric (0.5 tsp.)
- Vegetable oil (0.25 cup)
- Cayenne pepper (0.5 tsp. or 0.25 tsp. for less heat)
- Salt (2-2.5 tsp.)
- Chicken drumstick (12 average sizes, 4 lbs..)
- Garam masala (1 tbsp.)
- Paprika (1 tbsp.)
- Ground coriander (1 tbsp.)
- Fresh ginger (3 tbsp. peeled and chopped)
- Garlic (7 cloves, peeled and chopped)
- Mango chutney for serving (1 jar, 9 ounces)
- Whole milk Greek yogurt (0.25 cup)
- Lime wedges for serving
- Zest from one lime (1 tsp.)
- Juice from one lime (2 tbsp.)
- Pinch of cilantro

How it's made

1) Using a small pan over low-medium heat, combine the garam masala, cayenne pepper, paprika, cumin, turmeric, and coriander.

Stir frequently while cooking for two minutes, until the spices start to get fragrant.

2) Throw in the spices with ginger, garlic, Greek yogurt, oil, salt, lime zest, and juice into a mini food processor or a blender. Process it until it's smooth.

3) With a sharp knife, make two to three slashes per each drumstick, but we warned for they are slippery. In a bowl, gently mix together the drumsticks and the marinade. Cover the top of the bowl and refrigerate for at least three hours or leave overnight.

4) Preheat oven to 233 degrees C (450 degrees F). Line a baking sheet with aluminum foil before setting an oven-proof rack over the top inside the oven. Grease the rack with vegetable oil or spray with nonstick cooking spray.

5) Spread the chicken on the rack, leave space in between each drumstick. Using a spoon, use any excess marinade left inside the bowl and spread it evenly over the drumsticks.

6) Roast for forty-five minutes, turning them midway through once until the chicken turns a golden-brown color.

7) Use the broiler and to broil the drumsticks about six inches from the heat for three to five minutes until they are crisp and lightly charred all over. Place some mango chutney on the side.

8) Serve and enjoy!

Marinated Grilled Flank Steak

This recipe needs 15 minutes of preparation time, 10 minutes to cook, and will make 6 servings. (Note: refrigeration of some ingredients is required but not included in the meal preparation time, read direction for more information)

Net Carbs: 3.4 grams

Protein: 14.8 grams

Fats: 22.5 grams

Calories: 275

Sodium: 935 milligrams

What to use

- Flank steak (1.5 lbs.)
- Vegetable oil (0.5 cups)
- Soy sauce (0.33 cups)
- Ground black pepper (0.5 tsp.)
- Red wine vinegar (0.25 cups)
- Garlic (2 cloves, minced)
- Fresh lemon juice (2 tbsp.)
- Dijon mustard (1 tbsp.)
- Worcestershire sauce (1.5 tbsp.)

How it's made

1) Using a medium bowl, mix soy sauce, lemon juice, ground black pepper, garlic, oil, vinegar, mustard, and Worcestershire sauce. Place the steak into a shallow glass dish or a bowl.

2) Pour the marinade over the meat; with a spatula or a spoon, turn over the steak to coat it thoroughly. Cover the bowl and refrigerate for six hours.

3) Preheat the grill for high-medium heat. Make sure to oil the grill gate

before placing the meat on the grill. Do not pour over the remaining marinade in the bowl.

4) Grill steak for five minutes for each side or until the desired doneness.

5) Serve and enjoy!

Baked Lemon Butter Tilapia

This recipe needs 10 minutes of preparation time, 10 minutes to cook, and will make 4 servings.

Net Carbs: 1.8 grams

Protein: 35.5 grams

Fats: 14.5 grams

Calories: 276.4

Sodium: 94.2 milligrams

What to use

- Garlic (3 cloves, minced)
- Fresh parsley leaves (2 tbsp. chopped)
- Unsalted butter (0.25 cups, melted)
- Zest of 1 lemon
- Tilapia fillets (4 average-sized, 6 ounces)
- Freshly squeezed lemon juice (2 tbsp.)
- Pinch of freshly ground pepper and kosher salt

How it's made

1) Start by preheating the oven to 218 degrees C (425 degrees F).

2) Using a 9 x 13 baking dish, coat lightly with oil or nonstick cooking spray.

3) Using a small bowl, whisk together lemon juice, lemon zest, butter, and garlic Set aside.

4) Sprinkle the tilapia with salt and pepper on all sides and place it into the oiled baking dish.

5) Drizzle the tilapia with the butter mixture before placing it into the oven. Bake unit the fish can easily break off with a fork, which is about ten to twelve minutes. When done, sprinkle with parsley for a richer flavor.

6) Serve and enjoy!

Roasted Bone Marrow

This recipe needs 5 minutes of preparation time, 20 minutes to cook, and will make 2 servings.

Net Carbs: 0 grams

Protein: 4 grams

Fats: 48 grams

Calories: 440

What to use

- Bone marrow (4 halves)
- Sprinkle of freshly ground black pepper
- Sprinkle of sea salt flakes

How it's made

1) Begin by preheating the oven to 175 degrees C (350 degrees F).

2) Using a deep baking pan, place the bone marrow facing up.

3) Cook in the oven for twenty to twenty-five minutes until it turns crispy and golden. Most of the excess fat will be rendered off.

4) Season the marrow with freshly ground black pepper and sea salt flakes.

5) Serve and enjoy!

Goat Stew

Prep Time: 20 mins. Cooking Time: 60 mins.

Number of Servings: 8

Nutritional Values (Per Serving)

Calories: 488 Fat: 19g

Saturated Fat: 7.7g

Trans Fat: 0.8g

Carbohydrates: 0g

Fiber: 0g

Sodium: 253mg

Protein: 47g

What to use

- 4 lbs. goat, with bone 4-5 tbsp tallow
- Salt Pepper
- 2 pints of chicken broth
- To serve:
- Parmesan cheese, grated
- You will also need a pressure cooker

How it's made

- Set the pressure cooker over high heat and add 2 tablespoons tallow.
- In a bowl, place the goat meat along with 2-3 tablespoons tallow and season with salt and pepper to taste. Coat evenly.

- Place in the pressure cooker and sauté on both sides until golden brown.
- Add the broth and close with the lid.
- Turn the valve to the proper indicator and let the meat boil over medium-low heat for about 50 minutes.
- Serve with plenty of broth and grated parmesan cheese over it.

Pork Pockets with Cheese and Bacon

Prep Time: 30 mins. Cooking Time: 20 mins.

Number of Servings: 4

Nutritional Values (Per Serving)

Calories: 1420

Fat: 75g

Saturated Fat: 25g

Trans Fat: 0g

Carbohydrates: 0g

Fiber: 0g

Sodium: 1762mg

Protein: 66g

What to use

- 4 thick pork steaks 7oz cheddar cheese 8 slices bacon
- 4 tablespoons lard
- 2 tablespoons beef stock

To serve:

- Parmesan, grated

How it's made

1. Preheat your oven to 390F on the fan setting.

2. Place a skillet over high heat.

3. Score the steak at several points on the fat over the bone.

4. Make a pocket on the fleshy part for the stuffing.

5. Cut the bacon and the cheddar into thin slices and divide between the steaks. Secure the pocket with a toothpick.

6. Brush the steaks with a bit of lard, then place vertically on the skillet, making sure the fat touches the pan. Cook until it's golden brown.

7. Cook on either side until they're golden brown, about 4 minutes.

8. Brush half the stock on one side, then transfer to a baking dish with a rack. Place the unbrushed side up.

9. Brush the rest of the stock on the other side of the steaks.

10. Bake for about 20 minutes.

11. Serve with grated parmesan

Spit-Roast Lamb

Prep Time: 55 mins. Cooking Time: 5 hours.

Number of Servings: 16

Nutritional Values (Per Serving):

Calories: 270

Fat: 30g

Saturated Fat: 10g

Trans Fat: 1g

Carbohydrates: 0g

Fiber: 0g

Sodium: 400mg

Protein: 21g

What to use

- 20lbs lamb (1 lamb) 5oz salt
- 1tbsp pepper
- 5oz kefalotyri cheese 7oz tallow, melted

How it's made

1. Place the lamb on a clean table and season inside and out with some salt and pepper.

2. Insert the skewer through the back of the lamb all across the spine until you reach the skull's base.

3. Rotate the head so you can pass the skewer under the eyes.

4. Use a pair of spit forks to prick the lamb's legs so it retains its balance on the spit.

5. Using a stainless steel wire, wrap the lamb along the hips, rack, and neck, then pass it through the lamb and tie it securely on the spit.

6. Follow up with tying the legs and neck on the skewer as well.

7. Place the kefalotyri cheese on the inside of the lamb, cut into pieces.

8. Using kitchen twine and a thick needle, sew the stomach of the lamb.

9. Brush tallow on the outside of the lamb and further season with salt and pepper

10. In a bowl, add the remaining tallow and keep warm so that it stays melted.

11. Place the spit in the highest position and roast for around 5 hours.

12. Lower the spit every hour.

13. Make sure to baste the lamb every 15 minutes with the melted tallow.

14. Ideally, the majority of the charcoal should be under the legs and back of the lamb.

15. Serve hot.

Butter Quail

Prep Time: 10 mins. Cooking Time: 30 mins.

Number of Servings: 4

Nutritional Values (Per Serving):

Calories: 470 Fat: 32g

Saturated Fat: 11g

Trans Fat: 1g

Carbohydrates: 0g

Fiber: 0g

Sodium: 197mg

Protein: 42.9g

What to use

- 2 tablespoons grass-fed butter (or other fat of your preference)
- 8 quails
- salt pepper
- 1 cup of water

How it's made

- Season the quails with salt and pepper to taste
- In a deep skillet or wok, heat the butter over medium heat.
- Sauté the quails for 3 minutes with the breast side down.
- Flip them over.
- Deglaze with water, then cover the skillet and let it simmer for about 10 minutes.
- Set the quails on a plate and keep them warm.

- Continue simmering the broth in the pan until it resembles a thick sauce.
- Serve with the broth over the quails.

Full Carnivore Turducken Masterpiece

Prep Time: 2 hours. Cooking Time: 5 hours.

Number of Servings: 20

Nutritional Values (Per Serving):

Calories: 1,422

Fat: 58.1g

Saturated Fat: 23g

Trans Fat: 4g

Carbohydrates: 0g

Fiber: 0g

Sodium: 822mg

Protein: 206g

What to use

- 1 whole turkey, boned, with wings and legs still intact ~ 25lbs
- 1 whole duck, boned ~6lbs
- 1 whole chicken, boned ~3lbs
- Kitchen twine and a large thick needle
- 1 lb. ground beef
- 2 cups beef broth Carn "bread" stuffing Shrimp stuffing

How it's made

- Ask your butcher to bone the birds unless you are experienced in doing it yourself. Make sure to ask for the turkey's wings and legs to be left intact.

- Ideally, you can prepare the stuffing's at an earlier time so that they're at room temperature when you need to stuff the birds.

- Begin by lightly cooking the ground beef in the 2 cups of broth until it absorbs the liquid and resembles stuffing

- Preheat your oven to 325F

To assemble:

- Each layer of stuffing should be about 1/2 inch thick.

- Place the turkey on your worktop with the skin-side-down. Season it with pepper and salt to taste.

- Spread the carn "bread" on the insides of the turkey, coating it well.

- Place the duck, skin side down, on top of the "bread" stuffing, then spread the ground beef on the inside of the duck, coating it well.

- Finally, place the chicken skin-side down on the beef and stuff it with the shrimp stuffing.

- You can save any leftover stuffing for later.

- When you are finished layering the birds, take the sides of the turkey and fold them together. Use stainless steel sealer clips or another person's help to hold the turkey closed, then begin to sew the bird closed. The stitches should be around 1-1 1/2 inch apart.

- When you're done stitching, tie the turkey's legs together above the hip bones.

- Place the bird in a large roasting tray, breast side up, and cook for about 4 1/2 to 5 hours.

- Make sure to check with a meat thermometer you will insert in the thickest part on the bundled birds. The birds are ready once the thermometer reaches 180F.

Ultimate Beef Burgers

Prep Time: 15 mins. Cooking Time: 20 mins.

Number of Servings: 14

Nutritional Values (Per Serving):

Calories: 195

Fat: 12.7g

Saturated Fat: 5.6g

Trans Fat: 0.2g

Carbohydrates: 0g

Fiber: 0g

Sodium: 65mg

Protein: 18.6g

What to use

- 3lbs beef chuck, ground

- 1lb beef brisket, ground

- 12oz beef short ribs, boneless and ground

- Sea salt

- Black pepper

- 1 tbsp ghee

How it's made

1.	In a bowl, add all three of the ground meats and mix well until evenly combined

2.	Form into burger patties, around 5oz each

3.	Season both sides with salt and pepper to taste

4.	Place a non-stick skillet over high heat and let it get very hot

5.	Add the ghee, waiting for it to melt if hardened, then cook the burgers for about 5 minutes per side until they are charred. Cook longer if you want them more well done.

6.	Serve immediately

Buttered Scallops

Prep Time: 20 mins. Cooking Time: 5 mins.

Number of Servings: 12

Nutritional Values (Per Serving):

Calories: 152

Fat: 9g

Saturated Fat: 4.7g

Trans Fat: 0g

Carbohydrates: 0g

Fiber: 0g

Sodium: 133mg

Protein: 16g

What to use

- 4 tablespoons butter
- 2lbs scallops cleaned Salt
- Pepper

How it's made

1.	In a skillet over medium heat, melt 4 tablespoons of the butter and heat.

2.	Add half of the scallops into the skillet and season them with salt and pepper to taste.

3.	Cook for 2 minutes or until they become golden, then flip and cook for another 2 minutes.

4.	Remove from heat and set aside, then cook the second batch of scallops. This might not be needed depending on the size of your skillet.

5.	Serve hot with extra pepper and salt.

Rabbit Roast

Prep Time: 10 mins. Cooking Time: 90 minutes

Number of Servings: 4

Nutritional Values (Per Serving):

Calories: 630

Fat: 33g

Saturated Fat: 8g

Trans Fat: 0.2g

Carbohydrates: 0g

Fiber: 0g

Sodium: 1684g

Protein: 64g

What to use

- 1 rabbit, cleaned and chopped into pieces around 3lbs
- 1 tablespoon black pepper
- 1 teaspoons salt
- 2 cups broth
- ¼ cup butter

How it's made

1.	Preheat your oven to 350F

2.   Season the rabbit with salt and pepper to taste.

3.   In a large pan over medium-high heat, melt the butter.

4.   Place the rabbit in the pan and cook until brown on all sides.

5.   Transfer to a deep baking dish, then pours the broth over the rabbit.

6.   Bake for 90 minutes until very tender, frequently basting with melted butter.

Pluck Kabobs

Prep Time: 20 mins. Cooking Time: 10 mins.

Number of Servings: 6

Nutritional Values (Per Serving):

Calories: 450

Fat: 23g

Saturated Fat: 10g

Trans Fat: 1g

Carbohydrates: 0g

Fiber: 0g

Sodium: 245mg

Protein: 62g

What to use

- 4lb veal pluck including sweetbreads,
- cleaned Sea salt
- Black pepper Skewers

How it's made

- Make sure the pluck is cleaned off any arteries and connective tissues. If you're not sure, ask your butcher
- Chop pluck into half-inch pieces

- Turn on your grill and bring it to medium-high heat
- Begin threading the pluck on the skewers making sure to include some variations on each skewer
- Season thoroughly with salt and pepper to ensure the livers won't stick to the grill
- Grill until they're charred on all sides

Barbecue bourbon steak

Although the flavor may be quite sweet, when teamed with a fresh crispy green salad, you will find that this type of barbecued steak tastes wonderful.

Prep Time: 10 minutes Cook Time: 25 minutes Passive Time:20 minutes

Servings: 4 people

Nutritional value

Carbs52 g

Dietary Fiber2 g

Sugar16 g

Fat21 g

Protein37 g

What to use

- 4 x 200g Rump, Fillet or Sirloin Steaks
- 200g Dark Brown Sugar

How it's made

1.   You need to lightly score the surface of each steak with the tip of a sharp knife on one side (diagonally). Then place into a shallow dish with the side you

have scored facing upwards. Now you must pour the bourbon over the steaks and then over the top sprinkle on the dark brown sugar before then rubbing it in.

2.   Once you have done the above, you must now cover the steak up and place it in the refrigerator and leave for 1 to 3 hours for the marinade to infuse into the meat. Around 15 minutes before you take the steaks out of the refrigerator, you should get your barbecue going. Once the barbecue is hot enough and you have placed the grill about 6 inches above the heat, you can place the steaks on to the grill sugar side down. Allow them to cook for around 4 to 5 minutes or until the sugar has caramelized.

3.   Whilst the steak is going, you should baste the side of the steak that is facing towards you with the remaining marinade before then turning it over. Just as with the previous side, you should cook it again for around 4 to 5 minutes or cook until it is done to how you or your guests like it. Once the steak is ready, serve immediately with a fresh green salad.

Tomato herb marinated flank steak

A very simple recipe that helps to make something that tastes truly amazing. If you can, it is a good idea to allow the meat to remain in the marinade for at least 12 hours, as this will help to make it much tender when it is cooked.

Prep time: 25 minutes Cook time: 30 minutes

SERVING SIZE: 3 1/2 ounces each

Nutrition per serving

Calories: 164

Sugar: 0 g

Sodium: 289 mg

Fat: 6 g

Carbohydrates: 1 g

Fiber: 0 g

Protein: 25

What to use

- 1 Medium Tomato
- 1 Shallot
- 60 ml Red Wine Vinegar
- Tablespoons Fresh Chopped Marjoram
- 1 Tablespoon Fresh Chopped Rosemary
- 1 Teaspoon Salt
- ½ Teaspoon Freshly Ground Pepper
- 680 Grams Of Flank Steak

How it's made

1.   In a blender, put the tomato, shallot (which have both been chopped), the marjoram, rosemary, salt, and pepper. Blend until they form a smooth paste and set aside covered in the refrigerator. If there is any of the puree remaining in the blender, scrape it out into a sealable plastic

bag into which you then put the steak. Make sure that you spend time moving the steak around in the bag so that it is all coated in the puree. Once all the steak has been coated, you now place it in the bag into the refrigerator and leave it to marinate for between 4 and 24 hours. The longer you leave the meat to marinate in the puree, the more flavor it will take on.

2. Once the allotted time has passed, you should now get the barbecue heated up and set the grill above the heat at a height that it cooks the meat on medium heat. Also, make sure that you oil the rack first. Once the barbecue is heated up enough, you should grill the steaks for between 4 to 5 minutes per side if you want your medium-rare or 6 to 7 minutes if you want yours to be medium. You should only turn the steaks one making sure that you brash the side that is already cooked with some of the sauce you reserved earlier.

3. As soon as the second side of the steak has been cooked, you should turn it over again and brush it with more of the puree and then remove from the heat and place it on a clean plate. Now allow it to rest for 5 minutes before then thinly cutting the steak crosswise. Before serving, you should spoon on the rest of the puree.

Grilled steak with a whiskey and dijon sauce

Although this particular recipe contains alcohol when you cook it off, you will find a lot of the whiskey taste has been removed; instead, a much sweeter oaky flavor is produced.

Preparation time: 35 minutes   total time: 35 minutes

Nutritional value

Calories247

Fat 9g

Carbohydrates 9g

Dietary fiber 0g

Protein 24g

Sodium 440 mg

Sugars 7g

What to use

- 120ml Reduced Sodium Beef or Chicken Broth
- Tablespoons Whiskey
- Tablespoons Dijon Mustard
- Tablespoons Light Brown Sugar
- 1 Large Shallot (Finely Chopped)
- 1 Teaspoon Worcestershire Sauce
- 1 Teaspoon Freshly Chopped Thyme
- 450 Gram Skirt Steak (Which has been trimmed and cut into 4 pieces)
- ½ Teaspoon Freshly Ground Pepper
- ¼ Teaspoon Salt

How it's made

1. Preheat your barbecue to medium-high heat. Whilst the barbecue is heating up, you can prepare the sauce. To do this, you need to combine in a saucepan the

whiskey, mustard, brown sugar, shallot, thyme, and Worcestershire sauce. Bring all these ingredients to the boil, then reduce the heat so that a lively simmer is maintained.

It is important that you stir this sauce frequently to prevent it from sticking to the sides of the saucepan and burning. Keep it simmering for around 6 to 10 minutes until it has been reduced down by about half. Then remove from the heat.

2.   Now you need to cook the steaks on the barbecue. But before you do, sprinkle both sides with salt and pepper. If you want yours to be medium, you should cook each steak for between 1.5 and 3 minutes on each side. However, you should cook them for less time if you want yours to be medium-rare. Once they have been cooked for the recommended about of time, remove them from the grill and let them rest for 5 minutes before serving with the sauce.

Grilled Thai style beef kebabs

The use of Middle Eastern seasoning in these kebabs makes them taste absolutely wonderful, as well as helping them to become much more tender when cooked.

Total:35 mins   Prep:20 mins   Cook: 15 mins

Servings:4 servings

Nutritional value

Calories 586

Fat 42g

Carbs 18g

Protein 36g

What to use

- 450-gram Beef Sirloin (cut into 1-inch pieces)
- 1 Bell Pepper (cut into 1-inch pieces)
- 1 Small Onion (cut into 1-inch pieces)

Marinade Ingredients

- 120ml Vegetable or Olive Oil
- 1 Tablespoon Rice Wine Vinegar
- Tablespoon Roasted Sesame Seeds
- 2-3 Teaspoons Curry Powder
- Teaspoons Soy Sauce
- 2 Teaspoons Sesame Oil
- 2 Gloves Minced Garlic
- 2 Teaspoons Dry Mustard
- 1 Teaspoon Hot Sauce
- 1 Teaspoon Cumin Powder
- 1 Teaspoon Sugar
- ½ Teaspoon Dried Ginger
- ½ Teaspoon Salt
- ½ Teaspoon Paprika
- ¼ Teaspoon Black Pepper

How it's made

1.   Place the meat into a large sealable plastic bag and put it to one side whilst you make the marinade. Best to place it in the refrigerator.

2.   To make the marinade, you combine all the ingredients above together in a bowl or jug. Once combined, remove the meat from the refrigerator and pour the

marinade directly into the bag and move the meat around to ensure that it is coated well. Replace the bag back in the refrigerator and leave it, therefore, for between 3 and 6 hours to allow the meat to become infused with the marinade.

3. When the allotted time has passed, now remove the meat from the bag discarding it and the marinade. On to skewers, you now place meat, onions, and bell pepper alternately. If you are using wooden skewers, then soak them in water for around 30 minutes, as this will prevent them from burning when placed on the barbecue.

4. To cook the kebabs, place them on a grill over medium to high heat and cook for 10 to 12 minutes, remembering to turn them occasionally once they are cooked, remove from heat and serve.

Grilled balsamic steak

If you are at all conscious about the number of carbs you are consuming, then you will find this recipe ideal.

Total:20 mins   Prep:10 mins   Cook:10 mins

Nutritional Guidelines (per serving)

Calories 655

Fat 26g

Carbs 76g

Protein 31g

Servings:4 servings

What to use

- 900gram Sirloin Steak (Should be about an inch thick)
- 240ml Water
- 120ml Soy Sauce
- 1 Small Onion (minced)
- Tablespoons Worcestershire Sauce
- 2 Tablespoons Balsamic Vinegar
- 2 Tablespoon Dijon Mustard
- Gloves Garlic (minced)
- ¼ Teaspoon Hot Sauce

How it's made

- Please the steak either into a glass dish or a bag that is sealable. Now combine the rest of the ingredients above in a bowl or a jug and whisk thoroughly.

- Once you have combined all the ingredients above together, you then pour off the steak and leave to marinate for between 1 and 12 hours. When you are ready to cook the steak, you should get your barbecue heated up and cook it over medium to high heat.

1. When the barbecue is at the right temperature, you should remove the steak from the marinade and place it on the grill cooking it on each side for between 5 and 7 minutes if you like it medium. Any leftover marinade should be discarded, and once the steak is cooked to the way you or your guests like it, you can now remove it from the heat and serve.

Grilled meatball kebabs

These meatball kebabs not only taste great when served on their own but also when you choose to put them into a sandwich.

Total:25 mins   Prep:15 mins
Cook:10 mins

Servings:4 to 6 servings

Nutritional Guidelines (per serving)

Calories 315

Fat 13g

Carbs 20g

Protein 29g

What to use

- 450gram Ground Beef
- 1 Large Onion (cut into 1-inch pieces)
- 1 Large Red Or Yellow Bell Pepper (cut into 1-inch pieces)
- 115gram Dried Bread Crumbs
- 60ml Milk
- 75gram Parmesan Cheese (grated)
- 2 Gloves Garlic (Minced)
- 2 Tablespoons Dried Parsley
- 1 Tablespoon Dried Basil
- ½ Teaspoon Salt
- ½ Teaspoon Black Pepper
- 2 Eggs

How it's made

- In a small bowl, mix the bread crumbs and mil and let stand for 5 minutes. After five minutes, squeeze the bread crumbs to help remove any excess milk and then combine this with the beef, cheese, herbs, garlic, salt, pepper, and eggs and blend them together well.

After combining all these ingredients together, you shape the meat into around 16 to 18 meatballs. They should measure around ½ inch.

- Once you have created the meatballs, you place them onto skewers one at a time, and in between each one, place a piece of onion and pepper.
- Now you need to place the kebabs on to your grill that is lightly oiled to prevent them from sticking and cook them on medium heat for around 10 minutes. Remember to rotate them every 2 to 3 minutes to ensure that they are cooked evenly. Once they have been cooked properly, you can remove them from the heat and serve.

Easy grilled veal chops

This is one of the simplest and easiest barbecue beef recipes you may want to try. It tastes absolutely delicious, especially if you serve it with some freshly grilled vegetables.

Total:23 mins   Prep:7 mins
Cook:16 mins

Servings:6 servings

Nutritional Guidelines (per serving)

Calories 544

Fat 31g

Carbs 0g

Protein 63g

What to use

- 6 Veal Chops (Should be about 1 ½ inches thick)

- 3 Tablespoons Extra Virgin Olive Oil
- 2 Teaspoons Freshly Chopped Thyme
- ½ Teaspoon Salt
- ½ Teaspoon Black Pepper

How it's made

1. Preheat heat the barbecue and cook the veal chops on medium to high heat. Whilst the barbecue is heating up, you can now prepare the chops.

2. The first thing you need to do is coat the veal chops in the olive oil before then sprinkling over them (both sides) the thyme, salt, and pepper. Once you have done this, you now place them on the barbecue grill and cook on each side for between 7 and 8 minutes. Once they have been cooked for the allotted time, remove from heat and serve.

Quickly grilled beef quesadillas

The great thing about this particular recipe is that it doesn't take that long to prepare, so makes the perfect food to have midweek or as a starter for when organizing a big barbecue that lots of friends and family are going to be attending.

Total:20 mins   Prep:4 mins
Cook:16 mins

Servings:8 servings

Nutritional value

Calories 600

Fat 35

Carbs 0g

Protein 63g

What to use

- 229gram Sliced Roast Beef
- 1 Can Black Beans (drained and rinsed)
- 689gram Monterey Jack Cheese
- 8-10 Flour Tortillas
- 172gram Salsa
- 57gram Freshly Chopped Cilantro
- 3 Tablespoons Lime Juice

How it's made

- Turn on the barbecue, so it is heated up to the right temperature for you to then cook these quesadillas properly.

- Whilst the barbecue is heating up in a bowl, combine the salsa, cilantro, and lime juice and then set to one side. However, before you do set it aside, mix a third of this mixture with the beans in a separate bowl.

- Now you are ready to start making the quesadillas. Onto one of the tortillas, places some of the sliced roast beef and cheese before then topping off with a spoonful of the beans and salsa mix. Fold the tortilla over and place on the barbecue grill and cook for between 4 and 5 minutes, turning them over once. Remove them from the heat as they turn golden brown and serve with the other salsa mix you made earlier.

Spicy lime marinated round eye steaks

Another barbecued beef recipe that doesn't require a lot of preparation but will still produce wonderful tasting food. Best served with grilled potatoes or a fresh green salad.

Total:20 mins   Prep:10 mins
Cook:10 mins   Marinate:30 mins

Servings:2 servings

Nutritional Guidelines (per serving)

Calories 421

Fat 15g

Carbs 6g

Protein 64g

What to use

- x 226gram Round Eye Steaks (measuring 1 inch thick)
- Juice from 1 Lime
- 1 Teaspoon Garlic Powder
- 1 Teaspoon Cumin Powder
- 1 Teaspoon Ground Coriander
- 1 Teaspoon Salt
- 1 Teaspoon Freshly Ground Pepper

How it's made

1. In a bowl, combine together the lime juice, garlic powder, cumin, coriander, salt, and pepper.

2. Next, trim off any fat that is visible from the steaks and place them in a plastic bag that can be resealed. But before closing the bag up, pour in the mix you made earlier, ensuring that the steaks have been coated well, and leave in the refrigerator for 30 minutes.

3. Whilst the steaks are marinating; you can start heating up the grill ready for cooking. Once the 30 minutes have passed, you can remove the steaks from the bag and place them on the grill. Cook each side of the steak for 4 to 5 minutes before serving them.

Grilled strip steak with garlic and oregano

Another barbecued steak recipe that doesn't need a lot of preparation and so can be prepared and served to your guests very quickly.

PREP TIME: 5 MINUTES   COOK TIME :20 MINUTES   TOTAL TIME :25 MINUTES

SERVINGS: 4 SERVINGS

Nutritional value

Calories469kcal

Carbohydrates17g

Protein26g

Fat34g

Saturated Fat17g

What to use

- 4 Strip Steaks (1 Inch Thick)
- Gloves Of Garlic Minced
- 1 ½ Tablespoon Olive Oil
- 1 Tablespoon Dried Crushed Oregano
- ¼ Teaspoon Salt
- ¼ Teaspoon Freshly Ground Pepper

How it's made

- In a small bowl, combine together the oil, garlic, oregano, salt, and pepper, then slather over the steak on both sides. Then place them in a dish that you cover and put in the refrigerator for 2 to 3 hours to allow the steak to become infused with the marinade.

- It is important that when cooking these steaks, you do so on the highest heat possible on the barbecue. Place them on the barbecue grill and cook each side for between 6 to 8 minutes; once both sides have been cooked, remove from heat and serve.

Grilled beef tenderloin with an herb, garlic & pepper coating

You may want to consider trying out this recipe first before you decide to serve your guests. This will then help to ensure that you cook the meat properly.

Prep time: 10 minutes   cook time: 25 minutes   total time: 35 minutes

Servings: 8 people

Nutritional value

Calories 862kcal

Carbohydrates2g

Protein42g

Fat76g

Fiber1g

Sugar1g

What to use

- 2.26Kg Whole Beef Tenderloin
- 6 Tablespoons Olive Oil
- 8 Large Garlic Cloves Minced
- 1 Tablespoon Freshly Minced Rosemary
- 1 Tablespoon Dried Thyme Leaves
- Tablespoons Coarsely Ground Black Pepper
- 1 Tablespoon Salt

How it's made

- You need to prepare the beef first. This means trimming off any excess fat with a sharp knife before folding over the thinnest part of the meat so that it is about the same thickness as the rest. Of course, if you want, you could ask your butcher to do this for you. They will then tie it with butchers' twine as well. It is also important that you snip the silver skin on the meat, as this will prevent it from bowing when it is cooking.

- Once the meat is prepared, now you need to mix the other ingredients together and then rub these all over the meat. Place the meat in the refrigerator whilst you prepare the barbecue to cook it on. If you are using a charcoal grill, then build a fire on just one half of it. However, if you are using a gas barbecue, turn the burners up high for 10 minutes.

- Before you place the meat onto the grill, make sure that you coat it well with oil using a cloth that is soaked in oil between a pair of tongs. Once the grill has been coated with oil, place the beef onto it and close the lid. After 5 minutes, you now need to turn the meat over and repeat the same process.

- After the meat has been seared (sealed) on both sides, you now need to place it on to the side of the charcoal grill, which is cooler, or if using a gas barbecue, turn off the heat directly underneath the meat. Cook for around 45 to 60 minutes, or when a thermometer is inserted, the internal temperature of the beef has reached 130 degrees Fahrenheit. Once it has cooked for the time stated, now remove it from the heat and let it stand for 15 minutes (cover it over) before carving.

Beef in hoisin and ginger sauce

Looking for something with a little kick, then look no further than this particular recipe. You can either serve this with some rice or noodles or some grilled Pak Choi.

PREP TIME: 5 MINUTES COOK TIME: 15 MINUTES TOTAL TIME: 20 MINUTES
SERVINGS: 4 PEOPLE

Nutritional value

Calories 407kcal

Carbohydrates 61g

Protein 20g

Fat 10g

Fiber 3g

Sugar 15g

What to use

- 900gram Flank Steak
- 240ml Hoisin Sauce
- Tablespoons Fresh Lime Juice
- 1 Tablespoon Honey
- 1 Glove Garlic Minced
- 1 Teaspoon Salt
- 1 Teaspoon Freshly Peeled And Grated Ginger Root
- 1 Teaspoon Sesame Oil (Optional)
- 1 Teaspoon Chilli Garlic Sauce
- ½ Teaspoon Crushed Red Pepper Flakes
- ¼ Teaspoon Freshly Ground Black Pepper

For Decoration

- 1 Tablespoon Toasted Sesame Seeds
- 2 Chopped Green Onions

How it's made

- At an angle, thinly slice the steak across the grain, so you are creating slices that measure around 1.25 inches thick.

- Next, in a bowl, whisk together the hoisin sauce, lime juice, honey, garlic, salt, sesame oil, chili garlic sauce, red pepper flakes, and pepper. Then pour into a plastic resealable bag and into this also put the steak and move it around, so it is well coated by the marinade. Then place in the refrigerator for between 2 to 12 hours to allow the meat to become infused with the marinade.

- When you want to cook the steak, you should preheat your barbecue to medium to high heat and thread the slices of meat onto skewers. If you are using wooden skewers, soak them in water for around 30 minutes, as this will prevent them from burning when you place them on the grill. Any leftover marinade should then be discarded.

- Cook the meat on the barbecue for between 2 and 3 minutes on each side depending on how you like your beef to be cooked. 2 minutes for rare to medium and 3 minutes for well done. Once the steak has been cooked, sprinkle them with the toasted sesame seeds and chopped green onions before serving.

Ranch burgers

This is a very quick and easy way to make burgers that taste not only wonderful but also look wonderful as well. Because very little preparation is involved, you may want to consider getting your kids to help you make them.

Prep time: 10 minutes cook time: 20 minutes   total time: 30 minutes

Servings: 4 servings

Nutritional value

Calories 490kcal

Carbohydrates 28g

Protein 36g

Fat 25g

Fiber 1g

Sugar 3g

What to use

- 900gram Lean Ground Beef
- 1 Pack of Ranch Dressing Mix

- 1 Egg (Lightly Beaten)
- 172gram Saltine Crackers (Crushed)
- 1 Onion (Chopped)

How it's made

1. In a bowl, place the ground beef, the dressing mix, the egg, crushed crackers, and onion. Combine well together before then, forming them into hamburger patties. You should be making the burgers as you allow the barbecue to heat up to a high temperature.

2. Once the burgers are ready, and the barbecue has reached the desired, you now place them on it. It is a good idea to coat the grill with some oil first to prevent the burgers stick to it. You should cook each side of the burger for 5 minutes, and when do you serve them in a sesame topped bun.

Three herb steak

A very simple and quick recipe to prepare, but the herbs used help to bring out even more of the flavor of the steak— ideal for serving to those who don't like their food a little hot.

Prep time:10 minutes   cook time: 20 minutes   total time: 30 minutes

Servings: 2 steaks

Nutritional value

Calories506kcal

Carbohydrates1g

Protein23g

Fat46g

Fiber1g

Sugar1g

What to use

- 2 Beef Top Loin Steaks (1 ½ Inch Thick)

- 2 Medium Red or Yellow Sweet Peppers (Seeds Removed And Cut Into ½ Inch Rings)

- 1 Tablespoon Olive Oil

- Salt And Pepper To Season

- Marinade

- 114gram Freshly Cut Parsley

- 60ml Olive Oil

- 57gram Freshly Cut Basil

- 1 Tablespoon Freshly Cut Oregano

- 1 to 2 Teaspoons Of Freshly Cracked Black Pepper

- ½ Teaspoon Salt

How it's made

- In a bowl, mix the olive oil, basil, parsley, oregano, cracked black pepper, and salt to create the marinade.

- Before rubbing the mixture made up over the steak (both sides), you need to trim off any fat. Once coated in the marinade, you need to place them on a clean plate (covered) and put in the refrigerator for one hour.

- Whilst the steak is in the refrigerator, slice up the pepper before then coating with olive oil, salt, and pepper. Put these to one side, ready for when you start cooking.

- As soon as you remove the steak from the refrigerator, start up the barbecue. This will allow time for the meat to come up to room temperature, making it much easier to cook. If you want your steaks to be a rare medium cook for between 15 and 19 minutes (turning once during this time). However, if you want your steaks to be medium, then cook for between 18 and 23 minutes. Put the peppers on to grill around 10 minutes before you take the meat off. You should turn them once during this time to sure that they are cooked well.

- After the time for cooking, the steaks have passed, remove from heat place on a clean plate sprinkle with the rest of the herb mixture before covering and leaving to stand for 10 minutes. To serve, you simply slice the steak across the grain and then top off with some of the pepper rings.

Peppered rib eye steak

Applying the dry rub mixture to the meat before cooking helps to make it taste more succulent. Plus, it also helps to reduce the number of calories and fat you are consuming.

Total Time: Prep: 10 min. + chilling Grill: 25 min

Makes 8 servings

Nutritional value

3 ounces cooked beef:

257 calories

18g fat (7g saturated fat)

67mg of cholesterol

453mg sodium

2g carbohydrate

21g protein.

What to use

- 4 x 285-340gram Rib Eye Steaks (Cut 1 Inch Thick)
- 1 Tablespoon Olive Oil
- 1 Tablespoon Paprika
- 1 Tablespoon Garlic Powder
- 2 Teaspoons Crushed Dried Thyme
- 2 Teaspoons Crushed Dried Oregano
- 1 ½ Teaspoon Lemon Pepper Seasoning
- 1 Teaspoon Salt
- ½ to 1 Teaspoon Freshly Ground Black Pepper
- ½ to 1 Teaspoon Cayenne Pepper

How it's made

- Trim any excess fat from the steak, then brush with the olive oil. Also, snip the edges of the steak before coating to prevent them from curling up when grilling on the barbecue.

- In a bowl, combine the other ingredients together before then sprinkling over the meat evenly before then rubbing it into the meat with your fingers. Place on a clean plate and cover the steaks once both sides have been coated in the dry mixture before then placing in a refrigerator for 1 hour.

- To cook the steaks, remove from the refrigerator whilst the barbecue is heating up, and when ready cook them directly over medium heat and cook until they are done to the way you and your guests like to eat them. For steaks that are medium-rare, cook for between 11 and 15 minutes, turning them once. Whilst if you want yours cooked to medium, then keep then on the grill for between 14 and 18 minutes. Again turning them over once during this time.

Grilled beef tenderloin with Mediterranean relish

The Mediterranean Relish that you make to go with this particular barbecued beef dish really helps to create a summery feel to the meal.

Prep: 25 mins   Grill: 35 mins   Stand: 15 mins

Servings: 10

Nutritional value

Calories 240

Total fat 12g

Carbohydrates 6g

Protein 27g

What to use

- 1.3to1.8Kg Center Cut Beef Tenderloin
- 2 Japanese Eggplants (Cut Lengthwise In Half)
- 2 Red Or Yellow Sweet Peppers (Seeded and Cut Lengthwise in Half)
- 1 Sweet Onion (Cut Into ½ Inch Slices)
- 2 Plum Tomatoes (Chopped)

- 2 Tablespoons Kalamata Olives (Pipped and Chopped)

- 2 Tablespoons Olive Oil

- 2 Teaspoons Crushed Dried Oregano

- 2 Teaspoons Cracked Black Pepper

- 1 ½ Teaspoon Freshly Shredded Lemon Peel

- 3 Cloves Garlic (Minced)

- 2 Tablespoons Freshly Snipped Basil

- 1 Tablespoon Balsamic Vinegar

- ¼ to ½ Teaspoon Salt

- 1/8 Teaspoon Ground Black Pepper

How it's made

- In a small bowl, combine together the cracked black pepper, lemon peel, oregano, and 2 of the minced garlic cloves. Once thoroughly combined together, rub this all over the meat.

- To cook the meat, you need to place a drip tray at the bottom of the barbecue, and around it place the hot charcoal; once the temperature has reached the right level, place the meat on the grill above the drip tray. As for the vegetables, these should be placed around the meat directly over the coals, brushing them with olive oil first. Close the lid on the grill and allow it to remain closed for 10 to 12 minutes. By this time, the vegetables should be tender and need to be removed from the grill.

- Once the vegetables have been removed and placed on a clean plate and covered, close the lid on the barbecue once more and allow the meat to continue cooking for between 25 and 30 minutes or until the internal temperature of the meat has reached 135 degrees Fahrenheit when a meat thermometer is inserted. If this temperature has been reached, remove meat from the barbecue, place it on a clean plate, and cover, leaving it to rest for 15 minutes before you slice it.

- Now the vegetables have had sufficient time to cool down; you can make the relish to go with the beef. Simply put all the vegetables into a bowl after coarsely chopping them and add to them the olives, basil, tomatoes, and garlic clove, vinegar, salt, and ground black pepper.

Jerk beef with plantain kebabs

You may think combining Plantain (a form of banana) with beef seems wrong, but the use of the Jamaican jerk seasoning helps to combat this.

Active: 25 mins   Total: 40 mins

Servings:4

Nutritional value

258 calories

protein 20g

carbs 34g

fat 9g

What to use

- 340gram Boneless Sirloin Steak (Cut To 1 Inch Thick)
- 2 Tablespoons Red Wine Vinegar
- 1 Tablespoon Cooking Oil (Vegetable Is Best)
- 1 Tablespoon Jamaican Jerk Seasoning
- 2 Ripe Plantains (Peeled Then Cut Into 1 Inch Chunks)
- 1 Medium Sized Red Onion (Cut Into Wedges)

How it's made

1. Trim any excess fat from the meat before then cutting into 1 inch thick pieces then place to one side whilst you make the marinade for it.

2. Into a bowl, place the vinegar, oil, and jerk seasoning. Use a whisk to make sure that all the ingredients have been combined well together. Now divide the mixture into two separate amounts and use one half of the mixture to coat the steak. Then leave the steak to marinate in this mixture whilst you prepare the plantain and onion to make the skewers.

3. To make the kebabs, you thread on to the meat, plantain, and onion. Make sure you leave a gap of about ¼ inch between each item placed on the skewer. Then brush the onions and plantain with the other half of the marinade mixture.

4. In order to cook the kebabs, you place them directly over the coals or turn the burners down to medium heat and grill for between

12 and 15 minutes. It is important that you turn the kebabs occasionally to ensure that they are cooked evenly.

Asian barbecued steak

You may find the thought of combining fish sauce with beef a little off-putting. However, when combined with the other ingredients in this recipe, it helps to make the meat much more flavorsome and tender.

Prep:5 min

Total: 3 HR 15 MIN

Servings: 4

Nutritional value

Calories 370

Total Fat 13g

Carbohydrate 5g

Protein 56g

What to use

- 907gram Flank Steak
- 60ml Chilli Sauce
- 60ml Fish Sauce
- ½ Tablespoons Dark Sesame Oil
- 1 Tablespoon Freshly Grated Ginger Root
- 2 Gloves Garlic (Peeled And Crushed)

How it's made

- In to a bowl, pour the chili sauce, fish sauce, sesame oil, grated ginger root, and garlic and mix well together. Now set aside a few tablespoons of this mixture, as you will use it to baste the meat whilst it is on the barbecue.

- Next, you must score the meat and then place it in a shallow dish before then pouring over the remainder of the marinade you made earlier. Turn the meat over to ensure that it is coated in the sauce completely. Then cover the meat and place in the refrigerator for no less than 3 hours.

- To cook the steak, you need to heat the barbecue up to a high temperature. Then just before placing the meat onto the barbecue, brush the grill lightly with oil to prevent the meat from sticking to it. Now grill the meat for around 5 minutes on each side to have meat that is medium-rare. Of course, if you want your meat to be cooked to medium or well-done levels, then cook on each side for a little cooker. Whilst cooking, brush over some more of the marinade you put to one side. When cooked, let stand for a few minutes before then serving.

Garlic Bacon Wrapped Chicken Bites

This recipe needs 10 minutes of preparation time, 30 minutes to cook, and will make 4 servings.

Net Carbs: 5 grams

Protein: 22 grams

Fats: 13 grams

Calories: 230

What to use

- Chicken breast (1 large, cut into 22-27 small pieces)
- Garlic powder (3 tbsp.)
- Bacon (8-9 thin slices, cut into thirds, raw)

How it's made

1) Begin by preheating the oven to 205 degrees C (400 degrees F). Line a baking tray with aluminum foil for easy cleanup.

2) Using a bowl, place the garlic powder inside and dip each chicken piece in it. Make sure the powder gets on all the sides of the chicken bite.

3) Wrap the short strand of the bacon around each chicken bite before placing it on the baking tray. Make sure to spread them out enough, so the pieces are not touching. Cook for 25 to 30 minutes until the bacon is nice and crispy.

4) Serve and enjoy!

Pinchos Puerto Rico Marinated Grilled Chicken Kebabs

This recipe needs 10 minutes of preparation time, 10 minutes to cook and will make 4 servings. (Note: refrigeration of some ingredients is required but not included in the meal preparation time, read direction for more information)

Net Carbs: 3 grams

Protein: 39 grams

Fats: 10 grams

Calories: 290

Sodium: 321 milligrams

What to use

- Chicken breast, no bones, no skin (1.5 lbs. or 680 grams)
- Minced garlic (1 tbsp.)
- Freshly squeezed lime juice (1 tbsp.)
- Himalayan salt (0.5 tsp.)
- Extra-virgin olive oil (1 tbsp.)
- Ground black pepper (0.5 tsp.)
- Fresh oregano, (2 tsp, minced) or dried oregano (1 tsp.)

How it's made

1) You will be using seven to nine skewers. If you use wooden or bamboo, soak them in water for about thirty minutes before grilling.

2) In a small bowl, mix the salt, pepper, oregano, oil, garlic, and

lime juice, stir until you form a paste.

3) Chop chicken breast to form 2.5 cm chicken chunks (1 inch). Place in a glass container, mix the marinade with the chicken, stir gently, and cover with a lid. Refrigerate for at least two hours or leave overnight.

4) Get the grill ready for direct cooking. Preheat at medium heat, 325 degrees to 375 degrees F (170 degrees to 190 degrees C). It should take around 15-20 minutes, depending on the grill type.

5) Take the chicken out. Using the skewers, thread through the chicken piece gently. Don't leave any space in between.

6) Once the grill is done preheating, make sure the cooking grates are clean to prevent sticking.

7) Close the lid as much as you can and grill over direct medium heat until the chicken is well done, golden in color, and not pink in the center. It should take 8-10 minutes. Turn once or twice while cooking to prevent it from burning and make sure to not overcook.

8) Once done, remove from the grill, serve and enjoy!

Chicken and Prosciutto Spiedini

This recipe needs 10 minutes of preparation time, 15 minutes to cook and will make 8 skewers.

Note: nutrition varies per skewer

Net Carbs: 0.75 grams

Protein: 20 grams

Fats: 10 grams

Calories: 174

What to use

- Skewers (8)
- Kosher salt (0.5 tsp.)
- Fresh basil leaves
- Ground black pepper (0.13 tsp.)
- Block provolone cheese (8 oz.)
- Garlic powder (0.25 tsp.)
- Prosciutto (8 slices)
- Chicken tenders (8 pieces, raw)

How it's made

1) In a small bowl, mix garlic powder, salt, and pepper.

2) Cut the chicken tenders off the tendon. Pound them into a half-inch thickness. Sprinkle the chicken with the garlic mixture, make sure to get it on all sides.

3) Cut the provolone into one inch by two inches long. Take and lay a slice of prosciutto on a cutting board.

4) Place a pounded chicken tender on top, and then one or two leaves of fresh basil on top of the chicken.

5) Top it with a piece of provolone cheese on top of the fresh basil, and then carefully roll the prosciutto, skewer it, so it doesn't fall apart, and place it on a plate. Repeat for the rest of the chicken tenders.

6) Preheat the grill at medium heat, 325 degrees to 375 degrees F (170 degrees to 190 degrees C).

7) Grill for three minutes per side, or until the thermometer reads 165

degrees C (325 degrees F). Make sure the skewers are cooked through.

8) Serve and enjoy!

Homemade Beef Jerky

This recipe needs 10 minutes of preparation time, 1 hour, and 30 minutes to cook and will make 6 servings.

Net Carbs: 0 grams

Protein: 35 grams

Fats: 20 grams

Calories: 320

What to use

- Beef (1 lb..)
- Pinch of pepper and salt to taste
- Extra virgin oil (depends on how many beef strips)
- Herbs and spices of your choice for flavor

How it's made

1) Start by cutting the beef into thin strips, preferably one to two cm wide.

2) Using a bowl, place the beef strips inside before coating it with a pinch of salt and pepper, the flavorings of your choice, and olive oil to coat the strips.

3) Mix together but make sure the beef is coated with the oil and spices or herbs from top to bottom.

4) Coat a baking tray either with nonstick cooking spray or a nonstick baking paper.

5) Bake at 80 degrees C (176 degrees F) for one hour. Turn each beef strip around before baking it or dehydrate it for another half an hour.

6) Turn them over again and turn off the oven but leave the beef strips inside while it's still hot.

7) They can last up to two weeks.

8) Serve and enjoy!

Feta Cheese Meatballs

This recipe needs 10 minutes of preparation time, 15 minutes to cook and will make 20 meatballs.

Net Carbs: 1 gram

Protein: 4 grams

Fats: 7 grams

Calories: 75

What to use

- Chilly paprika flakes (1 tsp.)
- Ground lamb (200 grams, 7 oz.)
- Black pepper (1 tsp.)
- Ground Pork (200 grams, 7 oz.)
- Goat butter or ghee or regular grass-fed butter (2 tbsp.)
- Grass-fed ground beef (200 grams, 7 oz.)
- Garlic infused water, recipe below (0.5 cups, 100 ml.)
- Eggs (2, medium-sized)
- Feta cheese goat (100 grams, 3.5 oz)

How it's made

1) First, make the garlic-infused water. Clean and cut the cloves of one full garlic into halves. In a container with 200 ml of water,

place the garlic inside before closing with a lid. Refrigerate for at least 24 hours. When done, remove the cloves and use the water.

2) Using your hands, mix all the three types of meat. Add garlic-infused water and eggs before mixing it again.

3) Break the feta cheese into small pieces and add them into the egg and meat mixture. Still using your hands, mix once more and make sure the cheese is equally distributed throughout the mixture.

4) Take some of the mixtures into your hands and form into a meatball. Repeat until the mixture is finished.

5) You can add any spices or herbs that you'd like, but it is optional.

6) In a skillet, melt the goat butter. You can always use goat ghee or regular grass-fed butter. Make sure to set the temperature high in the beginning. It will create the crust and be able to prevent the cheese from melting.

7) Place the meatballs in the pan and fry them. Gently roll them to prevent burning and cook from all sides. Stop when you reach a nice golden-brown color, evenly spread throughout the meatball. Reduce the heat and cook for another ten minutes. Keep turning the meatballs every three minutes.

Beef Broth

Prep Time: 20 mins. Cooking Time: 8-24 hours.

Number of Servings: 1 gallon of broth

Nutritional Values (Per Serving):

Calories: 17

Fat: 0.4g

Saturated Fat: 0.3g

Trans Fat: 0g

Carbohydrates: 0g

Fiber: 0g

Sodium: 893mg

Protein: 2.7g

What to use

- 8 pounds bones - preferably marrow, tails, feet, knuckles, ketchup Salt

H0w it's made

1. Preheat oven to 450°F.

2. Place the bones in a baking pan and roast for about 20 minutes until they turn golden brown.

3. Fill a large stockpot with 24 cups of water.

4. Put the roasted bones into the pot along with any fat and juices. If necessary, add more water so that the bones are covered.

5. Season with salt.

6. Bring the water to a gentle boil then cover the pot with the lid slightly off-center.

7. Bring the heat down to a very gentle simmer and maintain for at least 8 hours and up to 24. Do not leave unattended.

8. Scrape off any foam or film off the top.

9. If needed, add water to make sure the bones remain covered. It becomes better the longer you cook it.

10. Remove from the heat and allow the broth to cool.

11. Using a mesh or cheesecloth, strain the broth and store it in a container.

12. It can last for up to 5 days in the fridge and up to 6 months in the freezer.

Tallow and Cracklings

Prep Time: 25 mins, plus 2 hr. chilling time Cooking Time: 3-4 hours

Nutritional Values (Per Tablespoon):

Calories: 115

Fat: 12.8g

Saturated Fat: 6.4g

Trans Fat: 0.5g

Carbohydrates: 0g

Fiber: 0g

Sodium: 0mg

Protein: 0g

What to use

- 6lb Grass-fed Beef suet

How it's made

1. Chill your suet for a couple of hours so it will become easier to slice.

2. Start by cutting the suet into tiny pieces. The smaller the parts, the easier the fat will be extracted. If you wish, you may use a food processor to do it. Make sure to cut the larger pieces anyway, so it doesn't clog your machine.

3. Start pulsing the suet until it looks crumbled. If the processor clogs, remove some of the pieces and blend again. You may need to run multiple batches.

4. Add the ground suet to a stockpot over low heat. Do not add water.

5. Keep the heat very low so as to melt the fat but not burn it and keep checking the pot hourly, stirring so that it doesn't stick.

6. The process may take from 3-5 hours, depending on the size of the pieces, the pot you're using, and the intensity of your stove.

7. You can tell the tallow is done cooking when the suet begins to shrink into tiny and shriveled pieces.

8. Strain the liquid fat, let it slightly cool, then store in a clean and dry (preferably sterilized) jar. You may also use a silicone mold to make butter-like chunks of tallow.

9. You can eat the cracklings too after they cool!

Carnivore "Bread"

Prep Time: 15 mins. Cooking Time: 20 mins.

Number of Servings: Around 16 squares

Nutritional Values (Per Serving):

Calories: 229

Fat: 18.3g

Saturated Fat: 8.4g

Trans Fat: 2g

Carbohydrates: 0g

Fiber: 0g

Sodium: 643mg

Protein: 14.5g

What to use

9oz cream cheese

3 free-range eggs

12oz fatty bacon, cooked

6.5oz cheddar cheese, grated

1/3 cup parmesan cheese

How it's made

1. Chop the cooked bacon as small and possible. Use a food processor if you like.

2. In a blender, add the cream cheese and the eggs and blend.

3. Add the bacon in the mixture and blend some more.

4. Fold in the rest of the cheeses.

5. Line a baking sheet with parchment paper.

6. Using a spatula, spread the mixture on the baking sheet laying it as flat as possible.

7. Bake at 390F for around 20 minutes.

8. Eat as a side, cut into portions, or use it as a carnivore pizza base!

Livers in a Blanket

Prep Time: 10 mins. Cooking Time: 12 minutes

Number of Servings: 16 pieces

Nutritional Values (Per Serving):

Calories: 178

Fat: 9.9g

Saturated Fat: 3.4g

Trans Fat: 0.1g

Carbohydrates: 0g

Fiber: 0g

Sodium: 625mg

Protein: 18.5g

What to use

- 2lbs grass-fed venison liver

- 16 slices of fatty bacon

- Salt

How it's made

1. Preheat your oven to 390F

2. Cut the liver into 16 pieces, around 1 inch thick each.

3. Wrap the bacon around the liver and pin it with a toothpick to secure

4. Salt to taste

5. Bake until crispy, around 12 minutes

6. Don't forget to take out the toothpicks before serving!

Crispy Skin Chips

Prep Time: 10 mins. Cooking Time: 30 mins.

Number of Servings: 8

Nutritional Values (Per Serving):

Calories: 572

Fat: 51.2g

Saturated Fat: 14.4g

Trans Fat: 0.5g

Carbohydrates: 0g

Fiber: 0g

Sodium: 82mg

Protein: 25.7g

What to use

2 pounds of chicken skin Salt

How it's made

1. Prepare a sheet pan with wax paper.

2. Preheat your oven to 330F

3. Cut skins into strips or squares according to your preference.

4. Season with salt to taste

5. Arrange skins on the sheet. It's okay if the skins touch as they will shrink while roasting.

6. Take another wax paper and place it over the skins then cover it with a second baking sheet. This will make lovely and flat chips.

7. Bake for about 15 minutes.

8. Flip the skins over and bake for an additional 15 minutes.

9. Let the chips cool before you eat them.

Beef Pâté

Prep Time: 10 mins.

Cooking Time: 10 mins+ 4-5 hours to chill.

Number of Servings: 12

Nutritional Values (Per Serving):

Calories: 216

Fat: 18.3g

Saturated Fat: 9.2g

Trans Fat: 0.8g

Carbohydrates: 0g

Fiber: 0g

Sodium: 287mg

Protein: 10.2g

What to use

- 1lb beef liver
- 12 Tbsp tallow, divided
- 1 teaspoon salt
- 1 teaspoon ground black pepper

- 1/2 cup high-fat heavy cream (optional)

How it's made

1. In a skillet, melt 6 tablespoons of the tallow.

2. Slice the liver into thin strips and add to the skillet.

3. Sprinkle with salt and cook for a minute on each side of the strip.

4. Let the liver cool for around 5 minutes.

5. Add the liver in a blender and pulse until it's smooth.

6. Add the remaining tallow and the cream if you're using it.

7. Add salt to taste and blend until all ingredients are combined into a smooth paste.

8. Remove from the blender and place in an airtight glass container.

9. Let it chill for at least 4 hours to harden.

10. Enjoy!

Liver Chips

Prep Time: 10 mins. Cooking Time: 7-8 hours

Number of Servings: 32

Nutritional Values (Per Serving):

Calories: 34 Fat: 2g

Saturated Fat: 2g Trans Fat: 0g
Carbohydrates: 0g Fiber: 0g

Sodium: 26mg Protein: 6g

What to use

2lbs rudiment liver (Beef, lamb, ketchup), ground

How it's made

1. In your food processor or blender, blend the minced liver until it resembles a paste.

2. Line a baking sheet with wax paper and spread the liver paste on it evenly using a spatula. Try to make it as thin as possible. Do it in two batches if needed.

3. Set your oven at the lowest possible temperature. This is usually 120F.

4. Once the center is dry (around 3 hours depending on your oven), flip the liver around and leave it to keep cooking.

5. Keep checking on it after the 6th (out of 8) hour mark. It's ready when the edges begin to separate, and the liver has dried.

6. Break into pieces and store in an airtight container.

Salmon Skin Chips

Prep Time: 20 mins. Cooking Time: 15 mins.

Number of Servings: 4

Nutritional Values (Per Serving):

Calories: 408 Fat: 33.6g

Saturated Fat: 19.3g

Trans Fat: 1g Carbohydrates: 4g Fiber: 0g

Sodium: 842mg Protein: 21g

What to use

- Skin from 4 salmons or other fish of your choice
- 1/3 cup ghee
- Salt

How it's made

1. Preheat your oven to 395F

2. Prepare a sheet pan with wax paper.

3. Separate the skins from the fish using a sharp knife, or ask for the skin separated when you purchase it.

4. If there's any leftover fish flesh on the skin, separate it with a spoon to make sure the skins will be absolutely crispy.

5. Cut the skins into 2-inch pieces.

6. Arrange skins on the sheet, making sure they are skin face-down and that they don't touch

7. Using a kitchen brush, brush the skins with ghee.

8. Season with salt to taste.

9. Take another wax paper and place it over the skins then cover it with a second baking sheet. This will make lovely and flat chips and ensure that the fish skin won't bubble as much.

10. Bake for approximately 15 minutes.

11. Using a spatula, remove the fish skins from the tray and serve them on a plate

Wrapped Hearts

Prep Time: 15 mins. Cooking Time: 15 mins

Number of Servings: 24 pieces

Nutritional Values (Per Serving):

Calories: 309

Fat: 19.9g

Saturated Fat: 9.3g

Trans Fat: 1g

Carbohydrates: 0g

Fiber: 0g

Sodium: 646mg

Protein: 30.2g

What to use

- 3lbs grass-fed beef heart, cleaned with arteries removed
- 24 slices of fatty bacon
- 24 slices cheddar Salt

How it's made

1. Preheat your oven to 390F

2. Wash the heart and make sure any arteries are cut out.

3. Slice in half then cut into 24 pieces, around 1 inch thick each.

4. Wrap the bacon and cheddar around the heart pieces and pin it with a toothpick to secure

5. Salt to taste

6. Bake until crispy, around 15 minutes

7. Don't forget to take out the toothpicks before serving!

Shrimp Stuffing

Prep Time: 15 mins. Cooking Time: 60 mins.

Number of Servings: 6

Nutritional Values (Per Serving):

Calories: 428

Fat: 30.5g

Saturated Fat: 13.7g

Trans Fat: 1g

Carbohydrates: 0g

Fiber: 0g

Sodium: 1045mg

Protein: 33.1g

What to use

- 6 tbsp ghee
- 1/2 cup chicken livers, chopped
- 1 lb. shrimp, clean and deveined
- 1 tbsp parmesan flakes
- 1 1/2 cup carnivore "bread" crumbs
- 1 cup full-fat milk
- tbsp beef gelatin
- 3/4 cup grated cheddar cheese Sprinkles of red pepper
- salt to taste

How it's made

1. In a large pan, add 3 tablespoons of ghee over medium-high heat. Sauté the livers until they're tender

2. Add the shrimp and keep cooking until they turn nice and pink.

3. Add the parmesan cheese and remove from heat.

4. Add the crumbs and mix very well.

5. Take another pan and add the rest of the ghee and melt if hardened.

6. Reduce the heat then add the milk and gelatin, stirring until thickened.

7. Add the cheddar cheese and remove from the heat.

8. Whisk continuously until the cheese melts and combines

9. Pour this mixture over the shrimp mixture and stir so that they mix well.

10. Transfer to a baking dish and cover with tin foil.

11. Bake for about 35 minutes, then uncover and bake for another 10 minutes.

12. Make sure it is room temperature before you stuff your bird.

Carn "Bread" Stuffing

Prep Time: 15 mins. Cooking Time: 55 mins.

Number of Servings: 12

Nutritional Values (Per Serving):

Calories: 320

Fat: 22.3g

Saturated Fat: 12.4g

Trans Fat: 2g

Carbohydrates: 0g

Fiber: 0g

Sodium: 1643mg

Protein: 20.5g

What to use

2   tbsp tallow

4 cups carnivore "bread" crumbled

1/2lb chicken livers, chopped

1/2lb chicken gizzards, chopped Salt and pepper to taste

Chicken broth

How it's made

1. For stuffing, it's best to use dried "bread." If you don't have any at hand, you can dice fresh "bread" then put it in the for about 10 minutes at 300°F

2. You can make the stuffing ahead of time and store it in the fridge for up to 48 hours to use it when you need it. However, it should be at room temperature before you can use it.

3. Preheat your oven to 350°F.

4. In a large pan, melt your tallow over medium heat. Add the livers and gizzards and sauté until tender, about 15 minutes.

5. In a bowl, place your "bread" cubes. Season with salt and pepper

6. Pour broth on the "bread" until they're moistened but not soggy.

7. Transfer both "bread" and meats in a baking dish and cover with tin foil.

8. Bake for about 35 minutes, then uncover and bake for another 10 minutes.

9. Make sure it is room temperature before you stuff your bird.

Carni Protein Bar

Prep Time: 20 mins.

Cooking Time: 5 mins+time to set

Number of Servings: 24

Nutritional Values (Per Serving):

Calories: 404

Fat: 39.2g

Saturated Fat: 19.5g

Trans Fat: 2g

Carbohydrates: 0g

Fiber: 2g

Sodium: 1053mg

Protein: 11.7g

What to use

- pounds lamb mince, dried (you may also use other kinds of meat or tallow such as venison, elk, beef, ketchup)

- Salt

- pounds tallow

How it's made

1. Melt the tallow in a double-boiler or a microwave-safe bowl.

2. In a separate bowl, mix the meat and the salt.

3. Star pouring the tallow on the meat. Make sure it's not too hot.

4. Start stirring, so they combine well. The tallow should be enough to make the meat moist throughout but shouldn't pool.

5. If the mixture is too dry, you can add more tallow.

6. You can let the mix set in a baking dish or use muffin liners to separate portions. You can even form it into balls with your hands!

Everything deviled eggs

Servings: 12 | Prep: 15m | Cooks: 20m | Total: 35m

Nutrition facts

Calories: 40 | Carbohydrates: 0.4g | Fat: 2.7g | Protein: : 3.3g | Cholesterol: 93mg

What to use

- 6 large eggs
- 1 teaspoon white vinegar
- 2 tablespoons full-fat plain Greek
- 1/2 teaspoon Worcestershire sauce
- yogurt
- 1 teaspoon prepared yellow mustard
- 1/4 teaspoon white sugar
- 1/4 teaspoon everything bagel seasoning, or to taste
- 1 teaspoon sliced scallion greens

How it's made

1. Place eggs in a saucepan and cover with water. Bring to a boil, remove from heat, and let eggs stand in hot water for 15 minutes. Remove eggs from hot water, cool under cold running water, and peel.

2. Slice eggs in half lengthwise and set the whites aside. Place yolks in a mini blender or food processor; pulse several times until finely chopped. Add yogurt, mustard, vinegar, Worcestershire sauce, and sugar and blend until smooth.

3. Transfer yolk mixture to pastry bag fitted with a large star tip and pipe filling into the egg whites (or stuff filling into egg whites with a spoon).

Sprinkle with everything bagel seasoning and garnish with sliced scallions.

Chill in the refrigerator until ready serve.

Easy rumaki with pineapple

Servings: 24 | Prep: 20m | Cooks: 20m | Total: 40m | Servings: 24

Nutrition facts

Calories: 40 | Carbohydrates: 3.7g | Fat: 2g | Protein: 1.7g | Cholesterol: 5mg

What to use

- Cooking spray
- 24 toothpicks

- 24 (1 inch) cubes, fresh pineapple
- ½ cup low-fat sesame
- 24 water chestnut slices
- 1 tablespoon chopped green onion to taste
- 8 thick-cut bacon slices, cut crosswise into 3 pieces

How it's made

- Preheat oven to 375 degrees F (190 degrees C). Line the bottom section of a broiler pan with aluminum foil, top with the broiler rack, and spray rack with cooking spray.

- Place a water chestnut slice atop each pineapple cube; wrap each with 1 bacon slice, securing with a toothpick. Arrange wrapped pineapple on the prepared broiler rack.

- Bake in the preheated oven for 7 minutes; turn and continue baking until bacon is almost crisp, about 8 more minutes. Brush rumaki with sesameginger dressing and continue baking until bacon is crisp, about 5 more minutes. Garnish rumaki with green onion.

Fried mozzarella puffs

Servings: 6 | Prep: 20m | Cooks: 15m | Total: 1h40m

Nutrition facts

Calories: 289 | Carbohydrates: 12.1g | Fat: 23.7g | Protein: 7.4g | Cholesterol: 55mg

What to use

- 1/3 cup water

- 1 pinch freshly ground black pepper
- 2 tablespoons unsalted butter
- 1/2 teaspoon dried oregano
- 1 teaspoon kosher salt
- 1 cup marinara sauce, or to taste
- 1/3 cup all-purpose flour
- 1/2 teaspoon red pepper flakes
- 1 large egg
- 1 teaspoon balsamic vinegar
- 1 anchovy fillet

How it's made

- Combine water, butter, and salt in a saucepan over medium-high heat.

  Bring to a simmer; pour in flour all at once and reduce heat to medium.

  Stir with a wooden spoon or spatula until a dough starts coming together. Cook, scraping up and stirring the dough, for 2 to 3 minutes.

- Remove from heat; transfer dough to a mixing bowl. Let cool until no longer hot but still very warm, 5 to 10 minutes. Add egg and season with cayenne and freshly ground black pepper. Whisk vigorously until mixture combines into a very soft, sticky dough. Switch to a spatula and scrape dough into a ball.

- Seal dough and spatula with plastic wrap and refrigerate in the bowl until cool, about 1 hour.

- In the meantime, season marinara sauce with oregano, red pepper flakes, balsamic vinegar in a small pot over medium heat. Add anchovy fillet. Stir together and bring to a simmer. Let simmer for 10 minutes; turn off heat

and let sit until ready to use.

- Grate mozzarella cheese over the dough and stir to combine.

- Heat oil to 350 degrees F (175 degrees C) in a deep fryer or heavy-duty pan over medium heat. Preheat oven to 200 degrees F (93 degrees C) or any temperature for keeping warm.

- Scoop out about 2 tablespoons of dough per puff and form into a football shape using two spoons. Fry puffs, 5 or 6 at a time, in the hot oil until browned, 2 to 3 minutes. Drain on paper towels. Keep puffs warm in low oven while frying the rest. Serve with hot marinara sauce.

Strawberry bruschetta

Servings: 12 | Prep: 10m | Cooks: 5m | Total: 15m

NUTRITION FACTS

Calories: 120 | Carbohydrates: 23.1g | Fat: 1.6g | Protein: 3.7g | Cholesterol: 3mg

What to use

- 24 slices French baguette

- 2 cups chopped fresh strawberries

- 1 tablespoon butter, softened

- 1/4 cup white sugar, or as needed

How it's made

1. Preheat your oven's broiler. Spread a thin layer of butter on each slice

of bread. Arrange bread slices in a single layer on a large baking sheet.

2. Place bread under the broiler for 1 to 2 minutes, just until lightly toasted. Spoon some chopped strawberries onto each piece of toast, then sprinkle sugar over the strawberries.

3. Place under the broiler again until sugar is caramelized, 3 to 5 minutes.

Serve immediately.

Garlicky appetizer shrimp scampi

Servings: 6 | Prep: 15m | Cooks: 6m | Total: 21m

NUTRITION FACTS

Calories: 302 | Carbohydrates: 0.9g | Fat: 21.8g | Protein: 25g | Cholesterol: 261mg

What to use

- 6 tablespoons unsalted butter, softened

- 2 tablespoons minced fresh chives

- 1/4 cup olive oil

- salt and freshly ground black pepper taste

- 1 tablespoon minced garlic

- 1 tablespoon minced shallots

- 1/2 teaspoon paprika

- 2 pounds large shrimp - peeled and deveined

How it's made

- Preheat grill for high heat.

- In a large bowl, mix together softened butter, olive oil, garlic, shallots, chives, salt, pepper, and paprika; add the shrimp, and toss to coat.

- Lightly oil grill grate. Cook the shrimp as close to the flame as possible for 2 to 3 minutes per side, or until opaque.

Artichoke hearts gratin

Servings: 4 | Prep: 10m | Cooks: 10m | Total: 35m

NUTRITION FACTS

Calories: 89 | Carbohydrates: 6.3g | Fat: 6.2g | Protein: 3.3g | Cholesterol: 4mg

What to use

- 6 canned artichoke hearts, drained and halved

- 1/4 cup finely grated Parmigiano-Reggiano cheese

- 1 teaspoon vegetable oil

- 1 tablespoon olive oil

- salt and freshly ground black pepper to taste

- 1/2 lemon, cut into wedges

- 2 tablespoons dry bread crumbs

How it's made

- Place artichoke heart halves on a paper towel cut-side down to drain for about 15 minutes.

- Set oven rack about 6 inches from the heat source and preheat the oven's broiler. Line a baking sheet with aluminum foil and lightly coat with vegetable oil.

- Place artichoke heart halves on the prepared baking sheet, cut side up. Season with salt and pepper, sprinkle with breadcrumbs and ParmigianoReggiano cheese, and drizzle with olive oil.

- Broil artichoke hearts until browned on top, about 7 minutes. Serve with lemon wedges.

Buffalo chicken dip

Servings: 20 | Prep: 5m | Cooks: 40m | Total: 45m

NUTRITION FACTS

Calories: 284 | Carbohydrates: 8.6g | Fat: 22.6g | Protein: 11.1g | Cholesterol: 54mg

What to use

- 2 (10 ounce) cans chunk chicken, drained

- 1 1/2 cups shredded Cheddar cheese

- 2 (8 ounce) packages cream cheese, softened

- 1 bunch celery, cleaned and cut in

- 4 inch pieces

- 1 cup Ranch dressing

- 1 (8 ounce) box chicken-flavored crackers

- 3/4 cup pepper sauce

How it's made

1. Heat chicken and hot sauce in a skillet over medium heat, until heated through. Stir in cream cheese and ranch dressing. Cook, stirring until well blended and warm. Mix in half of the shredded

cheese, and transfer the mixture to a slow cooker. Sprinkle the remaining cheese over the top, cover, and cook on Low setting until hot and bubbly. Serve with celery sticks and crackers.

Mouth-watering stuffed mushrooms

Servings: 12 | Prep: 25m | Cooks: 20m | Total: 45m

NUTRITION FACTS

Calories: 88 | Carbohydrates: 1.5g | Fat: 8.2g | Protein: 2.7g | Cholesterol: 22mg

What to use

- 12 whole fresh mushrooms
- 1/4 cup grated Parmesan cheese
- 1 tablespoon vegetable oil
- 1/4 teaspoon ground black pepper
- 1 tablespoon minced garlic
- 1/4 teaspoon onion powder
- 1 (8 ounce) package cream
- 1/4 teaspoon ground cayenne pepper cheese, softened

How it's made

1. Preheat oven to 350 degrees F (175 degrees C). Spray a baking sheet with cooking spray. Clean mushrooms with a damp paper towel. Carefully break off stems. Chop stems extremely fine, discarding tough end of stems.

2. Heat oil in a large skillet over medium heat. Add garlic and chopped mushroom stems to the skillet. Fry until any moisture has disappeared, taking care not to burn garlic. Set aside to cool.

3. When garlic and mushroom mixture is no longer hot, stir in cream cheese, Parmesan cheese, black pepper, onion powder and cayenne pepper. Mixture should be very thick. Using a little spoon, fill each mushroom cap with a generous amount of stuffing. Arrange the mushroom caps on prepared cookie sheet.

4. Bake for 20 minutes in the preheated oven, or until the mushrooms are piping hot and liquid starts to form under caps.

Restaurant-style buffalo chicken wings

Servings: 5 | Prep: 15m | Cooks: 15m | Total: 2h | Additional:

1h30m

NUTRITION FACTS

Calories: 364 | Carbohydrates: 10.7g | Fat: 32.4g | Protein: 7.9g | Cholesterol:44mg

What to use

- 1/2 cup all-purpose flour oil for deep frying
- 1/4 teaspoon paprika1/4 cup butter
- 1/4 teaspoon cayenne pepper1/4 cup hot sauce
- 1/4 teaspoon salt1 dash ground black pepper
- 10 chicken wings1 dash garlic powder

How it's made

- In a small bowl mix together the flour, paprika, cayenne pepper and salt. Place chicken wings in a large nonporous glass dish or bowl and sprinkle flour mixture over them until they are evenly coated. Cover dish or bowl and refrigerate for 60 to 90 minutes.

- Heat oil in a deep fryer to 375 degrees F (190 degrees C). The oil should be just enough to cover wings entirely, an inch or so deep. Combine the butter, hot sauce, pepper and garlic powder in a small saucepan over low heat. Stir together and heat until butter is melted and mixture is well blended. Remove from heat and reserve for serving.

- Fry coated wings in hot oil for 10 to 15 minutes, or until parts of wings begin to turn brown. Remove from heat, place wings in serving bowl, add hot sauce mixture and stir together. Serve.

Double tomato bruschetta

Servings: 12 | Prep: 15m | Cooks: 7m | Total: 35m

NUTRITION FACTS

Calories: 215 | Carbohydrates: 24.8g | Fat: 8.9g | Protein: 9.6g | Cholesterol: 12mg

What to use

- 6 roman (plum) tomatoes, chopped

- 1/4 cup fresh basil, stems removed

- 1/2 cup sun-dried tomatoes, packed

- 1/4 teaspoon salt in oil

- 3 cloves minced garlic

- 1/4 teaspoon ground black pepper

- 1/4 cup olive oil

- 1 French baguette

- 2 tablespoons balsamic vinegar

- 2 cups shredded mozzarella cheese

How it's made

- Preheat the oven on broiler setting.

- In a large bowl, combine the roman tomatoes, sun-dried tomatoes, garlic, olive oil, vinegar, basil, salt, and pepper. Allow the mixture to sit for 10 minutes.

- Cut the baguette into 3/4-inch slices. On a baking sheet, arrange the baguette slices in a single layer. Broil for 1 to 2 minutes, until slightly brown.

- Divide the tomato mixture evenly over the baguette slices. Top the slices with mozzarella cheese.

- Broil for 5 minutes, or until the cheese is melted.

Asian lettuce wraps

Servings: 4 | Prep: 20m | Cooks: 15m | Total: 35m

NUTRITION FACTS

Calories: 388 | Carbohydrates: 24.3g | Fat: 22.3g | Protein: 23.4g | Cholesterol: 69mg

What to use

- 16 Boston Bibb or butter lettuce leaves

- 1 tablespoon rice wine vinegar

- 1 pound lean ground beef
- 2 teaspoons minced pickled ginge
- 1 tablespoon cooking oil
- 1 dash Asian chile pepper sauce, to taste (optional)
- 1 large onion, chopped
- 1 (8 ounce) can water chestnuts, drained and finely chopped
- 1/4 cup hoisin sauce
- 1 bunch green onions, chopped
- 2 cloves fresh garlic, minced
- 2 teaspoons Asian (dark) sesame
- 1 tablespoon soy sauce

How it's made

1. Rinse whole lettuce leaves and pat dry, being careful not tear them. Set aside.

2. Heat a large skillet over medium-high heat. Cook and stir beef and cooking oil in the hot skillet until browned and crumbly, 5 to 7 minutes. Drain and discard grease; transfer beef to a bowl. Cook and stir onion in the same skillet used for beef until slightly tender, 5 to 10 minutes. Stir hoisin sauce, garlic, soy sauce, vinegar, ginger, and chile pepper sauce into onions. Add water chestnuts, green onions, sesame oil, and cooked beef; cook and stir until the onions just begin to wilt, about 2 minutes.

3. Arrange lettuce leaves around the outer edge of a large serving platter and pile meat mixture in the center.

Brown sugar smokies

Servings: 12 | Prep: 10m | Cooks: 20m | Total: 30m

NUTRITION FACTS

Calories: 356 | Carbohydrates: 18.9g | Fat: 27.2g | Protein: 9g | Cholesterol: 49mg

What to use

- 1 pound bacon
- 1 cup brown sugar
- 1 package little smokie sausages

How it's made

- Preheat oven to 350 degrees F (175 degrees C).
- Cut bacon into thirds and wrap each strip around a little sausage. Place the wrapped sausages on wooden skewers, several to a skewer. Arrange the skewers on a baking sheet and sprinkle them liberally with brown sugar.
- Bake until bacon is crisp and the brown sugar melted.

Coconut shrimp

Servings: 6 | Prep: 10m | Cooks: 20m | Total: 1h

NUTRITION FACTS

Calories: 317 | Carbohydrates: 26.3g | Fat: 19.3g | Protein: 8.4g | Cholesterol: 67mg

What to use

- 1 egg
- 2 cups flaked coconut
- 1/2 cup all-purpose flour24 shrimp

- 2/3 cup beer3 cups oil for frying
- 1 1/2 teaspoons baking powder
- 1/4 cup all-purpose flour

How it's made

1. In medium bowl, combine egg, 1/2 cup flour, beer and baking powder. Place 1/4 cup flour and coconut in two separate bowls.

2. Hold shrimp by tail, and dredge in flour, shaking off excess flour. Dip in egg/beer batter; allow excess to drip off. Roll shrimp in coconut, and place on a baking sheet lined with wax paper. Refrigerate for 30 minutes. Meanwhile, heat oil to 350 degrees F (175 degrees C) in a deep-fryer.

3. Fry shrimp in batches: cook, turning once, for 2 to 3 minutes, or until golden brown. Using tongs, remove shrimp to paper towels to drain. Serve warm with your favorite dipping sauce.

Cocktail meatballs

Servings: 10 | Prep: 20m | Cooks: 1h25m | Total: 1h45m

NUTRITION FACTS

Calories: 193 | Carbohydrates: 15.2g | Fat: 10.2g | Protein: 9.8g | Cholesterol:53mg

What to use

- 1 pound lean ground beef
- 1 (8 ounce) can jellied cranberry sauce
- 1 egg
- 3/4 cup chili sauce

- 2 tablespoons water
- 1 tablespoon brown sugar
- 1/2 cup bread crumbs
- 1 1/2 teaspoons lemon juice
- 3 tablespoons minced onion

How it's made

1. Preheat oven to 350 degrees F (175 degrees C).

2. In a large bowl, mix together the ground beef, egg, water, bread crumbs, and minced onion. Roll into small meatballs.

3. Bake in preheated oven for 20 to 25 minutes, turning once.

4. In a slow cooker or large saucepan over low heat, blend the cranberry sauce, chili sauce, brown sugar, and lemon juice. Add meatballs, and simmer for 1 hour before serving.

Baked buffalo wings

Servings: 20 | Prep: 15m | Cooks: 45m | Total: 2h | Additional:1h

NUTRITION FACTS

Calories: 125 | Carbohydrates: 3.8g | Fat: 9.2g | Protein: 6.8g | Cholesterol: 32mg

What to use

- 3/4 cup all-purpose flour
- 1/2 teaspoon cayenne pepper
- 1/2 teaspoon garlic powder
- 1/2 teaspoon salt
- 20 chicken wings
- 1/2 cup melted butter
- 1/2 cup hot pepper sauce

How it's made

1. Line a baking sheet with aluminum foil, and lightly grease with cooking spray. Place the flour, cayenne pepper, garlic powder, and salt into a resealable plastic bag, and shake to mix. Add the chicken wings, seal, and toss until well coated with the flour mixture. Place the wings onto the prepared baking sheet, and place into the refrigerator. Refrigerate at least 1 hour.

2. Preheat oven to 400 degrees F (200 degrees C).

3. Whisk together the melted butter and hot sauce in a small bowl. Dip the wings into the butter mixture, and place back on the baking sheet. Bake in the preheated oven until the chicken is no longer pink in the center, and crispy on the outside, about 45 minutes. Turn the wings over halfway during cooking so they cook evenly

Conclusion

Thank you for making it through to the end of *Carnivore Diet: a new powerful diet for weight loss with a healthy meat-based meal plan that exceeds the use of plant-based products.* Let's hope it was informative and able to provide you with all the tools and information that you need to perfectly transition to the carnivore diet.

The next step is to finally put everything you learned into good use. Use the recipes in this book to discover what you like and what you don't like, experiment with different spices and herbs to make your meal taste better. Learn different methods to cook meat and remember to keep track of your journey in your food journal. Use the one-week meal plan provided for you to start your new journey, and know that if you are suffering from any illnesses or diseases, consult with a doctor before attempting a change in any diet on your own.

Thank you for reading and good luck on your journey!

Finally, if you find this book useful in any way, a review on Amazon is always appreciated!

CPSIA information can be obtained
at www.ICGtesting.com
Printed in the USA
BVHW011014080221
599628BV00005B/460